2020

ADVANCES IN
SMALL ANIMAL CARE

EDITOR-IN-CHIEF
Philip H. Kass

SECTION EDITORS
Chiara Mariti
Angela J. Marolf
Silke Salavati
Vanessa R. Barrs
Jonathan Stockman

ELSEVIER

Publishing Director, Medical Reference: Dolores Meloni
Editor: Stacy Eastman
Developmental Editor: Laura Fisher

Reprints: For copies of 100 or more of articles in this publication, please contact the Commercial Reprints Department, Elsevier Inc., 360 Park Avenue South, New York, NY 10010-1710. Tel: 212-633-3874; Fax: 212-633-3820; E-mail: reprints@elsevier.com.

Editorial Office:
Elsevier, Inc.
1600 John F. Kennedy Blvd,
Suite 1800
Philadelphia, PA 19103-2899

International Standard Serial Number: 2666-4518
International International Standard Book Number: 978-0-323-79210-3

ADVANCES IN SMALL ANIMAL CARE

EDITOR-IN-CHIEF

PHILIP H. KASS, BS, DVM, MPVM, MS, PhD
Diplomate, American College of Veterinary Preventive Medicine
(Specialty in Epidemiology)
Vice Provost for Academic Affairs
Professor of Analytic Epidemiology
Department of Population Health and Reproduction, School of Veterinary Medicine
Department of Public Health Sciences
School of Medicine, University of California, Davis
Davis, California, USA
phkass@ucdavis.edu

SECTION EDITORS

CHIARA MARITI, DVM, PhD, MSC, EBVS
European Veterinary Specialist in Animal Welfare Science
Ethics and Law gruppo ETOVET c/o Dip.to Scienze Veterinarie
Università di Pisa viale delle Piagge
Pisa, Italy
chiara.mariti@unipi.it

ANGELA J. MAROLF, DVM, DACVR
Professor, Environmental and Radiological Health Sciences
College of Veterinary Medicine and Biomedical Sciences
Colorado State University
Fort Collins, Colorado, USA
angela.marolf@colostate.edu

SILKE SALAVATI, DR.MED.VET., PhD, DIPL.ECVIM-CA, FHEA, MRCVS
Senior lecturer in Small Animal Internal Medicine
University of Edinburgh
Royal (Dick) School of Veterinary Studies and The Roslin Institute
Hospital for Small Animals
Easter Bush, Midlothian, UK
Silke.Salavati@ed.ac.uk

VANESSA R. BARRS, BVSC(HONS), PhD, MVETCLINSTUD, FANZCVS (FELINE MEDICINE)
Professor of Feline Medicine & Infectious Diseases
The University of Sydney
Faculty of Science, Sydney School of Veterinary Science and Marie Bashir Institute of Infectious Diseases & Biosecurity
The University of Sydney, Sydney, Australia
vanessa.barrs@cityu.edu.hk

JONATHAN STOCKMAN, DVM, DACVN
Assistant Professor, Department of Veterinary Clinical Sciences
College of Veterinary Medicine
Long Island University
Old Brookville, New York, USA
jonathan.stockman@liu.edu

[illegible]

PHILIP H. KASS, BS, DVM, MPVM, MS, PhD
Diplomate, American College of Veterinary
Preventive Medicine
(Specialty in Epidemiology)
Vice Provost for Academic Affairs
Professor of Analytic Epidemiology
Department of Population Health and
Reproduction, School of Veterinary Medicine
Department of Public Health Sciences
School of Medicine, University of California, Davis
Davis, California, USA
phkass@ucdavis.edu

SECTION EDITORS

VANESSA R. BARRS, BVSc(HONS), PhD,
MVetClinStud, FANZCVS (Feline Medicine)
Professor of Feline Medicine & Infectious Diseases
The University of Sydney
Faculty of Science, Sydney School of Veterinary
Science and Marie Bashir Institute of Infectious
Diseases & Biosecurity
The University of Sydney, Sydney, Australia
vanessa.barrs@cityu.edu.hk

JONATHAN STOCKMAN, DVM, DACVN
Assistant Professor, Department of Veterinary
Clinical Sciences
College of Veterinary Medicine
Long Island University
Old Brookville, New York, USA
jonathan.stockman@liu.edu

CHIARA MARITI, DVM, PhD, MSc, EBVS
European Veterinary Specialist in Animal Welfare
Science
Ethics and Law group, ECAWBM Dip in Scienze
Veterinarie
Università di Pisa, Viale delle Piagge
Pisa, Italy
chiara.mariti@unipi.it

ANGELA J. MAROLF, DVM, DACVR
Professor, Environmental and Radiological Health
Sciences
College of Veterinary Medicine and Biomedical
Sciences
Colorado State University
Fort Collins, Colorado, USA
angela.marolf@colostate.edu

SILKE SALAVATI, DR MED VET, PhD,
DipECVIM-CA, FHEA, MRCVS
Senior Lecturer in Small Animal Internal Medicine
University of Edinburgh
Royal (Dick) School of Veterinary Studies and
The Roslin Institute
Hospital for Small Animals
Easter Bush, Midlothian, UK
Silke.Salavati@ed.ac.uk

CONTRIBUTORS

SARAH K. ABOOD, DVM, PhD
Assistant Professor, Ontario Veterinary College, University of Guelph, Guelph, Ontario, Canada

KARIN ALLENSPACH, DVM, PhD, DECVIM
Professor of Small Animal Internal Medicine, Department of Veterinary Clinical Sciences, College of Veterinary Medicine, Iowa State University, Ames, Iowa, USA

MARTA AMAT, DVM, PhD, Dip ECAWBM
AWEC (Animal Welfare Education Centre), School of Veterinary Science, Autonomous University of Barcelona, Bellaterra (Barcelona), Spain

EMI N. BARKER, BSc(Hons), BVSc(Hons), PhD, DipECVIM-CA, MRCVS
Feline Centre, Langford Vets, Bristol Veterinary School, University of Bristol, Langford. United Kingdom

GIOVANNA BERTOLINI, DVM, PhD
Doctor Europaeus, San Marco Veterinary Clinic and Laboratory, Head, Diagnostic and Interventional Radiology Division, Veggiano, Padova, Italy

JONATHAN BOWEN, BVetMed, MRCVS, DipAS(CABC)
Queen Mother Hospital for Small Animals, Royal Veterinary College, Hertfordshire, United Kingdom

TOMÁS CAMPS, DVM, PhD, Dip ECAWBM
Etovets (Behavioural Medicine and Animal Welfare Service), Palma de Mallorca, Spain

FRANCESCO COLLIVIGNARELLI, DVM
PhD Student, Faculty of Veterinary Medicine, University of Teramo, Teramo, Italy

RONALD JAN CORBEE, DVM, PhD, Dipl ECVCN
Assistant Professor, Department of Clinical Sciences, Faculty of Veterinary Medicine, Utrecht University, Utrecht, The Netherlands

NICOLA DECARO, DVM, PhD, DipECVM
Professor of Infectious Diseases of Animals, Department of Veterinary Medicine, University of Bari, Bari, Italy

FRANCESCA DEL SIGNORE, DVM
PhD Student, Faculty of Veterinary Medicine, University of Teramo, Teramo, Italy

SEAN J. DELANEY, BS, DVM, MS, DACVN
Davis Veterinary Medical Consulting, Inc., Woodland, California, USA

ROSWITHA DORSCH, Priv-Doz, Dr med vet, Dr habil, Dipl ECVIM-CA
Clinic of Small Animal Medicine, LMU Munich, Munich, Germany

ILARIA FALERNO, DVM
PhD Student, Faculty of Veterinary Medicine, University of Teramo, Teramo, Italy

ANDREA J. FASCETTI, VMD, PhD, DACVIM (SA), DACVN
Department of Molecular Biosciences, School of Veterinary Medicine, University of California, Davis, Davis, California, USA

JAUME FATJÓ, DVM, PhD, Dipl.ECAWBM-BM
Chair, Affinity Foundation Animals and Health, Universitat Autònoma de Barcelona, Barcelona Biomedical Research Park, Barcelona, Spain

KATRIN HARTMANN, Prof Dr med vet, Dr habil, Dipl ECVIM-CA
Clinic of Small Animal Medicine, LMU Munich, Munich, Germany

ROMY M. HEILMANN, Dr med vet, Dipl ACVIM (SAIM), Dipl ECVIM-CA (SAIM), MANZCVS (Small Animal Medicine), PhD
Small Animal Internal Medicine, Department for Small Animals, Veterinary Teaching Hospital, College of Veterinary Medicine, Leipzig, Saxony, Germany

PHILIP H. KASS, BS, DVM, MPVM, MS, PhD
Diplomate, American College of Veterinary Preventive Medicine (Specialty in Epidemiology); Vice Provost for Academic Affairs, Professor of Analytic Epidemiology, Department of Population Health and Reproduction, School of Veterinary Medicine, Department of Public Health Sciences, School of Medicine, University of California, Davis, Davis, California, USA

JENNIFER A. LARSEN, DVM, MS, PhD, DACVN
Department of Molecular Biosciences, School of Veterinary Medicine, University of California, Davis, Davis, California, USA

SUSANA LE BRECH, DVM, PhD, Dip CLEVe
AWEC (Animal Welfare Education Centre), School of Veterinary Science, Autonomous University of Barcelona, Bellaterra (Barcelona), Spain

XAVIER MANTECA, DVM, PhD, Dip ECAWBM
AWEC (Animal Welfare Education Centre), School of Veterinary Science, Autonomous University of Barcelona, Bellaterra (Barcelona), Spain

JONATHAN P. MOCHEL, DVM, MS, PhD, DECVPT
Associate Professor of Pharmacology, Department of Biomedical Sciences, College of Veterinary Medicine, Iowa State University, Ames, Iowa, USA

YUKI OKADA, BA, DVM, PhD
ACVN Resident (Alternate Residency Program), Veterinary Nutrition Specialty Service, San Rafael, California, USA

MARIA GRAZIA PENNISI, Prof Dr med vet, Dr habil, Spec Applied Microbiology
Department of Veterinary Sciences, University of Messina, Messina, Italy

FABIO PROCOLI, DMV, MVetMed, DipACVIM, DipECVIM-CA, MRCVS
Unità Operativa di Medicina Interna, Ospedale Veterinario I Portoni Rossi, Bologna, Italy

ELISSA RANDALL, DVM, MS, DACVR
Associate Professor of Radiology, Veterinary Teaching Hospital, Colorado State University, Fort Collins, Colorado, USA

BARBARA SCHÖNING, Dr.med.vet, MSc, PhD
Specialist in Animal Behavior and Animal Welfare, Behavior Consultations, Hamburg, Germany

FRANCESCO SIMEONI, DVM
PhD Student, Faculty of Veterinary Medicine, University of Teramo, Teramo, Italy

JAN S. SUCHODOLSKI, MedVet, DrMedVet, PhD, AGAF, DACVM
Professor and Associate Director, Gastrointestinal Laboratory, Department of Small Animal Clinical Sciences, Texas A&M University, College Station, Texas, USA

ROBERTO TAMBURRO, DVM, PhD
Senior Researcher, Faculty of Veterinary Medicine, University of Teramo, Teramo, Italy

SÉVERINE TASKER, BSc, BVSc(Hons), PhD, DSAM, DipECVIM-CA, FHEA, FRCVS
Bristol Veterinary School, University of Bristol, Langford, United Kingdom; The Linnaeus Group, Shirley, Solihull, United Kingdom

MASSIMO VIGNOLI, DVM, PhD, Dipl. ECVDI
Associate Professor, Faculty of Veterinary Medicine, University of Teramo, Teramo, Italy

ALLISON M. WARA, DVM, DACVN
Veterinary Clinical Nutritionist, Royal Canin Canada, Morriston, Ontario, Canada; Adjunct Assistant Associate Professor, College of Veterinary Medicine, University of Missouri, Columbia, Missouri, USA

CONTENTS

VOLUME 1 • 2020

Infectious Disease

Advances in Small Animal Care 1 (2020) xiii–xiv
ADVANCES IN SMALL ANIMAL CARE

Preface

Aspirations for a Successful New Series

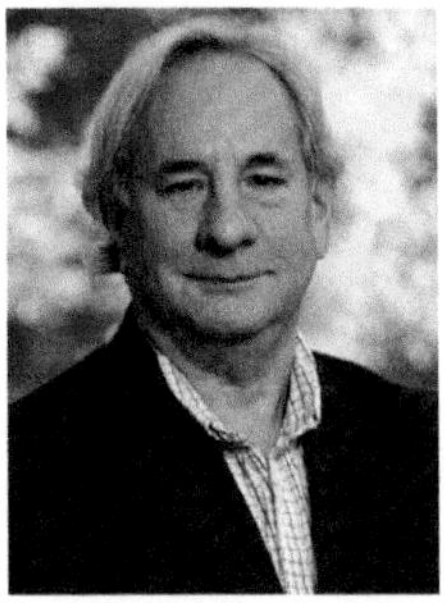

Philip H. Kass, BS,
DVM, MPVM, MS, PhD
Editor

This inaugural volume of *Advances in Small Animal Care* represents the culmination of almost 3 years of careful planning and execution in the establishment of a new series—one that could occupy a niche in the exploration of new knowledge through continuing education unfilled by other veterinary medical journals and textbooks. Within many of the broad areas of veterinary medical health, disease, and wellness, we designated topics that are both emerging and evolving, and sought authors who could extend knowledge to veterinarians in private, public, and academic occupations through incorporation of new, up-to-date research. Taking this approach allows synthesis and translation of research articles to a wider audience, without having to wait for them to ultimately be recapitulated in textbooks that can be years in the making. The virtue of making each volume of this series multidisciplinary is that the most important advances are prioritized for publication, narrowing the time it takes to disseminate and institutionalize new knowledge.

It is with great pride that we present an editorial board and author list for volume 1 that is diverse and international, with 8 countries represented. In future volumes, we will continue to seek out the finest researchers from all over the world to contribute their expertise.

For this first volume, we have selected new topics from the areas of behavior, imaging, gastroenterology, infectious disease, and nutrition. It is our hope these articles will become important references for researchers and practitioners alike, as they concern health challenges that are ubiquitous in canine and feline medicine. They include behavioral challenges like separation anxiety, aggression, and concurrent health problems; imaging breakthroughs in whole-body cancer staging, angiography, and lymph node evaluation; chronic inflammatory and viral gastroenteropathy in dogs; breaking new treatment of feline infectious

https://doi.org/10.1016/j.yasa.2020.08.001
2666-4518/20/

peritonitis; and nutritional challenges that include care of hospitalized patients, the ongoing enigma of taurine in canine cardiac health, the critical interaction between nutrition and physical rehabilitation, and how cat and dog health is impacted by vitamin D.

The success of this series ultimately depends on how well it serves our audience of readers. If you have particular topics that you believe are timely and worth visiting or are on the cusp of discovery, I invite you to reach out to me directly at phkass@ucdavis.edu. I hope you enjoy this volume, and look forward to the many others that are forthcoming.

Philip H. Kass, BS, DVM, MPVM, MS, PhD
Office of Academic Affairs
University of California, Davis
One Shields Avenue
Davis, CA 95616, USA

E-mail address: phkass@ucdavis.edu

Behavior

Advances in Small Animal Care 1 (2020) 1–8
ADVANCES IN SMALL ANIMAL CARE

Separation-Related Problems in Dogs

A Critical Review

Marta Amat, DVM, PhD, Dip ECAWBM[a,*], Susana Le Brech, DVM, PhD, Dip CLEVe[a], Tomás Camps, DVM, PhD, Dip ECAWBM[b], Xavier Manteca, DVM, PhD, Dip ECAWBM[a]
[a]AWEC (Animal Welfare Education Centre), School of Veterinary Science- Autonomous University of Barcelona, Bellaterra (Barcelona) 08193, Spain; [b]Etovets (Behavioural Medicine and Animal Welfare Service), Palma de Mallorca 07009, Spain

KEYWORDS
• Behavior • Dog • Anxiety • Separation • Fear • Inappropriate bond • Attachment • Frustration

KEY POINTS

- Separation-related problems (SRPs) are common in dogs and have negative effects on dog welfare and human-dog bond.
- The most reported signs of SRPs are inappropriate elimination, destructive behavior, and vocalization. Dogs can show other signs that may be overlooked by owners.
- SRPs can result from several factors, including hyperattachment, fear, an inappropriate human-dog bond, and frustration.
- Some of the treatment strategies for SRPs are at variance with the current understanding of stress and fear in animals and must be revisited.
- It is recommended to increase the predictability of owner departures and to include interventions designed to reduce frustration.

INTRODUCTION

The term separation-related problem (SRP) is used to refer to a set of problem behaviors shown by dogs when the owner or the attachment figure is absent [1–4]. Although this problem is also known as separation anxiety or separation distress, the term SRP is used in this article, because current evidence suggests that affective states other than anxiety or distress are involved (discussed later) [5–11].

The most commonly reported signs of SRP are excessive vocalization, inappropriate elimination, and destructiveness. Because these behaviors are annoying for owners, they are hardly missed [4,9,11–15]. However, dogs with SRP can also show many other symptoms that are more likely to be overlooked by owners, particularly because they happen when the owner is absent. Examples of such behaviors include panting, salivation, vomiting, restlessness, repetitive behaviors, trembling, immobility, and anorexia. In addition, some dogs with SRP show fear responses or aggression when the owner leaves [2,6,7,11,13,16–19].

It has been suggested that between 14% and 55% of all dogs show signs of SRP at some point in their lives [16,19–23]. However, prevalence estimates should be taken cautiously because they are likely to have several limitations. A first problem is that owners may fail to recognize SRP in dogs that show subtle signs [11]. According to a recent study, depressionlike symptoms while the owner is absent account for up to 52.9% of all cases of SRP [11] and it has been reported that most dog owners are not able to identify subtle signs of stress [24]. As a result, some studies are likely to underestimate the prevalence of SRP.

*Corresponding author, *E-mail address:* marta.amat@uab.es

https://doi.org/10.1016/j.yasa.2020.07.001
2666-4518/20/

A second problem with prevalence estimates is related to the information source: although some studies are based on owner surveys [4,7], others are based on the caseload of either general practitioners and/or behavior referral services [9,16,19,22,23].

In addition, the criteria used to include SRP cases vary across studies. As already mentioned, problem behaviors that occur when the owner is absent can result from an anxiety response but they can also have other causes. For example, destructive behavior can result from a lack of stimulation [8,11,25], excessive barking can be an alarm response when an unknown person approaches the dog's home, and inappropriate elimination in the owner's absence may develop because the dog learns how to avoid being punished by the owner. Dogs that show problem behaviors that do not result from anxiety or any other negative affective state are considered by some investigators (but not others) as having an SRP as long as the problem occurs only when the owner is absent.

Obviously, SRPs have negatives consequences on the welfare of both the dog and the owner. SRPs are annoying for the owners and, in some cases (eg, when the dog vocalizes), for the neighbors as well. Furthermore, these problems can cause an additional financial expense [26]. The frustration and anger experienced by the owner as a result of an SRP is likely to have a strong negative impact on the owner-dog bond [7,14,27], and, as a result, many dogs with SRP are euthanized or relinquished [28–32].

SRPs also have a severe negative impact on the welfare of the dog. Animal welfare includes both the physical health and the emotional state of the animals [33]. Dogs that have SRP as a result of an anxiety response obviously have poor welfare during the periods when the owner is absent, which may account for a significant part of the dog's life.

Moreover, dogs with SRP caused by anxiety are likely to have poor welfare even when the owner is not absent, mainly as a result of cognitive bias. Cognitive bias is widely used to assess the affective state of animals and can be defined as a change in a cognitive process (eg, judgment, attention, or memory) that results from a change in the affective state of the animal [34–36]. The type of cognitive bias most commonly used in studies of animal welfare is the so-called judgment bias: animals that are in a negative affective state tend to judge an ambiguous stimulus as being negative (ie, they show a "pessimistic" judgment), whereas animals in a positive emotional state tend to be more "optimistic" and interpret an ambiguous stimulus as being positive [34]. Judgment bias was studied in shelter dogs with and without SRP, and dogs with SRP had significantly more negative bias than dogs without SRP [37]. Furthermore, Karagiannis and colleagues [38] studied judgment bias in owned dogs with and without SRP and also found that dogs with SRP were more pessimistic than dogs without SRP. They also found that treatment of SRP significantly reduced pessimistic bias, thus showing a cause-effect relationship between SRP and cognitive bias [38].

SRP can also have other long-term negative effects on the welfare of dogs. There is an increasing body of evidence showing that chronic stress has deleterious effects on physical health, and it has been shown that dogs with SRP are more likely to develop skin problems than dogs without SRP. Moreover, dogs with SRP tend to have a shorter lifespan than control dogs [39].

Despite its prevalence and importance, there are many aspects of SRP in dogs that are still a matter of controversy and hence deserve further research. This article critically reviews such aspects. In particular, it addresses 3 issues: (1) the main risk factors for the development of SRP; (2) the causes of SRP and, in particular, what is the role of hyperattachment in the development of SRP; and (3) what is the best treatment strategy for dogs with SRP and, more precisely, how current treatment strategies can be reconciled with current understanding of stress and anxiety in animals.

WHAT IS KNOWN ABOUT SEPARATION-RELATED PROBLEM RISK FACTORS?

Many studies have been published on the risk factors for SRP, and this article focuses on 4 of them: gender, neutering status, origin, and breed.

Several studies have found that SRPs are more common in males than in females [4,14,18,30,40,41]. However, it is not clear whether this finding results from a difference between males and females in their likelihood to develop SRP or from owners of male dogs with SRP being more likely to seek help than owners of female dogs with SRP. It has been suggested that male dogs with SRP can be more annoying than females because they are larger and vocalize more loudly [42].

As for the neutering status, some investigators have found a lower frequency of SRP in neutered dogs compared with non-neutered ones [9,14], whereas other studies have concluded the opposite [41]. To the best of our knowledge, there is no information on the possible effects of sexual hormones on SRP. However, it is interesting that McGreevy and colleagues [43] found a higher risk of behavior problems (including fear-related problems) in neutered dogs. These investigators suggest that sexual hormones may play an important role in the control of fear, and hence early castration would increase the likelihood of fear and anxiety-related problems [9,43].

Some studies have concluded that dogs from pet shops are more likely to develop SRP and other behavioral problems than dogs from other origins [41,44,45]. This tendency could be explained by 2 mechanisms that are not mutually exclusive: first, the socialization process for puppies may not be adequate in dogs coming from pet shops [44,46] and, second, puppies from pet shops may have been exposed to a stressful environment and this may increase the risk of developing anxiety-related problems later in life [45].

In addition, other studies conclude that coming from a dog shelter increases the likelihood of having SRP [1,17,44]. Again, this could be explained by 2 hypotheses: shelter conditions could increase the likelihood of dogs developing SRP on adoption, and/or many dogs in shelters may have been relinquished because they showed SRPs [7,47,48].

Concerning the possible effect of breed on the development of SRP, Bradshaw and colleagues [4] did not find any differences between breeds, whereas other studies found a higher prevalence of SRP in crossbred dogs [49,50]. Nevertheless, other investigators have found that some breeds, such as the cocker spaniel and the dachshund were common in the population of dogs with SRP [9,11,14]. This finding could be explained by the breed being abundant in the general dog population, by owners of some breeds being more likely to seek help than others [51], and/or by genetic breed differences [9].

CAUSES OF SEPARATION-RELATED PROBLEMS: MORE THAN HYPERATTACHMENT

For many years, it has been suggested that SRPs were mainly caused by the dog showing hyperattachment to its owner [42,52]. Hyperattached dogs have been described as constantly looking for contact with the owner [6] and being more likely to follow their owners around and greet them effusively on their returning home [14,42].

Hyperattachment can result from several mechanism. Neoteny (ie, the retention of infantile characteristics into adulthood) is a consequence of the domestication process and may have increased the tendency of some dogs to develop a strong attachment to their owners [53,54]. Also, hyperattachment can be a consequence of the owner reinforcing the attention-seeking behavior shown by dogs [6]. In addition, it has been suggested that early weaning may prevent puppies from developing independent behavior [44].

The main problem with the hypothesis that SRPs result solely from hyperattachment is that dogs with and without SRP seek contact equally with their owners and many dogs without SRP are very dependent on their owners [55]. By comparing the behavior of dogs with and without SRP when left alone in an unfamiliar place and on being reunited with their owners, it has been found that dogs with SRP showed more stress-related behaviors during separation than dogs without SRP. However, there were no differences between both groups of dogs in their attempts to have physical contact with their owners on reunion, which fails to support the hypothesis that dogs with SRP show hyperattachment. Interestingly, dogs with SRP did not calm down as much as dogs without SRP once they were reunited with their owners. Therefore, it seems that hyperattachment is not enough to explain the development of SRP.

Partly as a result of this difficulty, it has been suggested that fear could be involved in some cases of SRP when dogs associate an aversive event (eg, a thunderstorm) with being alone. This hypothesis is supported by the fact that a high number of dogs with SRP also have noise phobias [7–9,13,14,41], although not all studies have found such comorbidity between SRP and phobias [17].

More recently, some researchers have suggested that an inappropriate dog-owner bond can play a key role in the development of SRP, and this hypothesis was initially based on studies on children with SRP [55]. Children whose parents are not sensitive to their needs, discourage their autonomy, and act in an unpredictable way tend to develop what is called an insecure or ambivalent attachment style, show a great deal of distress during separation, are not easily calmed when reunited with their parents, and do not see them as safety figures [56]. More importantly, these children are more prone to develop separation anxiety [57].

The hypothesis that a similar mechanism may be at work in dogs with SRP has been at least partially supported by several studies of different types of owner-dog bond and their effect on dogs' reactions to being left alone [58,59]. For example, dogs with a secure bond with their owners show a lesser increase in plasma cortisol concentration when left alone compared with dogs with an insecure bond (ie, dogs whose owners respond in an unpredictable way). In addition, dogs without SRP react to their owners as if they were safe attachment figures [60].

In addition, frustration is not usually included among the affective emotional states leading to SRP in dogs. However, a recent study by de Assis and colleagues [11] found that frustration-related signs such as destructiveness were very common in dogs with SRP. Interestingly, children with an inappropriate attachment style are more prone to show frustration [61]. Clearly, further research is needed in order to clarify the role of frustration in SRP.

In conclusion, it seems that the mechanisms leading to SRP in dogs are much more complex than initially thought and it is likely that several affective states (including anxiety, fear, and frustration) can be involved. Therefore, it is important to identify the relative contribution of each of these affective states in order to design the best treatment strategy for each case.

SHOULD TREATMENT STRATEGIES BE MODIFIED ACCORDING TO THE CURRENT UNDERSTANDING OF FEAR AND STRESS?

The standard treatment of separation anxiety includes changes in the environment, pharmacologic treatment, behavior-modification techniques, and changes in the behavior of the owners toward their dogs. The main objective of the environmental changes is to provide appropriate stimulation to the dog, such as physical activity or play. The pharmacologic treatment is intended to improve dog welfare by reducing fear and/or anxiety levels [62].

Traditionally, behavior modification, which is the main part of the treatment protocol, was based on 2 points: to set up unpredictable owner departures by giving false departure cues and to habituate the dog to being left alone by doing fake departures of increasing duration. In addition, it was also recommended that owners avoid any kind of punishment and ignore the dog some time before the departure, on returning home, and whenever the dog was aroused [2,6,7,42,63–65].

Taking into account the different factors that could influence the development of this problem and the emotions that could be involved, the authors suggest several changes in the standard treatment protocol, namely establishing predictable owner departures, creating a safe area, and modifying the advice given to the owners in relation to their behavior toward their dogs.

Predictability is one of the main psychological factors that modulate the stress response [66–68] because it has been shown that it reduces the anxiety associated with highly aversive stimuli. This outcome is caused by the fact that, when animals can predict the aversive event, they relax and feel safe when the aversive event will not occur [69–71]. This principle is likely to apply to dogs with separation anxiety, because they perceive the owner absence as a highly aversive situation [72]. The predictability of owner departures can be increased by adding a new cue (Fig. 1) just before the owner or the attachment figure departs; this cue will be removed when the owner returns [73]. In addition, in order to habituate the dog to being left alone, a different cue (called a safe cue; Fig. 2) is used before each fake departure. Using 2 different cues allows the dog to distinguish actual departures from fake ones done during the habituation sessions. Once the habituation session is over, the safe cue should also be removed [73]. When the dog tolerates being left alone for 60 minutes without showing signs of anxiety, the habituation sessions are

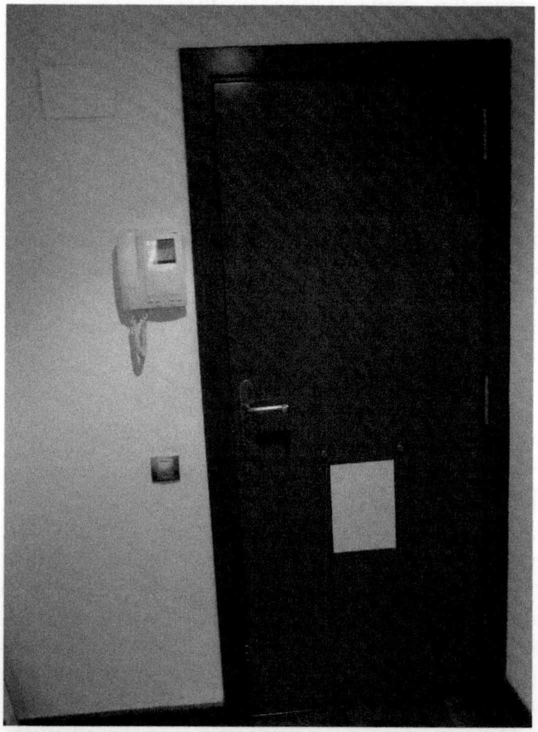

FIG. 1 A piece of white cardboard is put on the exit door just before leaving. This cue should be removed once the owners return. (*From* Amat M, Camps T, Le Brech S, Tejedor S. Tratamiento de la ansiedad por separación. In: Manual práctico de etologia clínica del perro, 2nd ed. Sant Cugat del Vallés: Multimédica Ediciones Veterinarias; 2018. p. 266; with permission.)

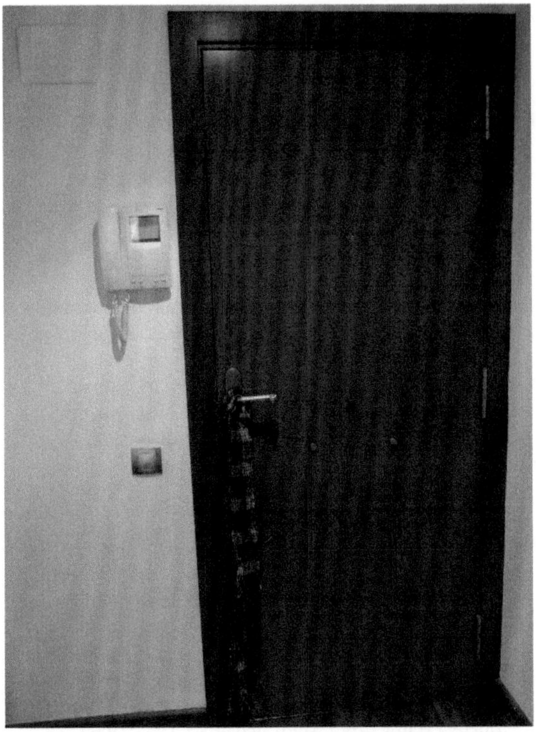

FIG. 2 A scarf is used as a signal for habituation sessions (fake departures). This safe signal should also be removed after the habituation session. (*From* Amat M, Camps T, Le Brech S, Tejedor S. Tratamiento de la ansiedad por separación. In: Manual práctico de etologia clínica del perro, 2nd ed. Sant Cugat del Vallés: Multimédica Ediciones Veterinarias; 2018. p. 267; with permission.)

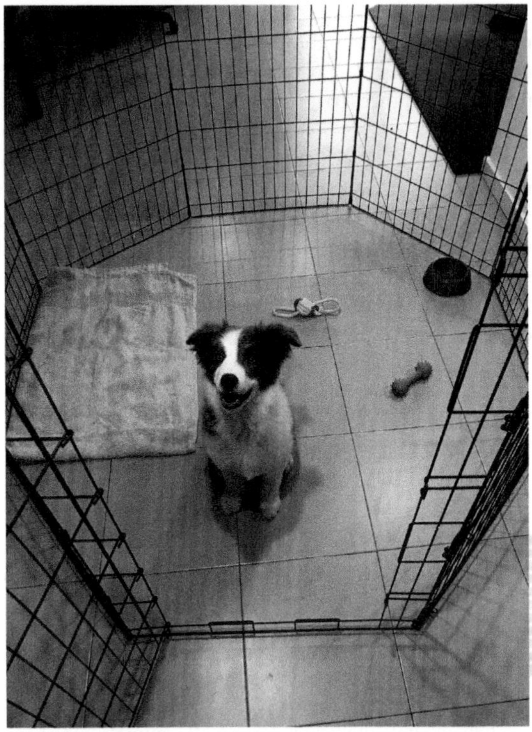

FIG. 3 Training sessions should be done in a safe area (ie, a place that the dog does not associate with actual departures). (*Courtesy of* C. González, Barcelona, Spain.)

discontinued, and the safe cue replaces the cue used to signal actual departures [73].

Often dogs with SRP are left alone in a restricted, well-defined area in order to reduce the nuisances caused by their behavior. In these cases, it is likely that dogs will show contextual fear when placed in such location. Contextual fear develops when an animal associates a specific location with a frightening stimulus and, as a result, shows fear of that location even when the stimulus is not present [74]. Contextual fear is particularly pronounced in anxiety problems, which are triggered by poorly defined stimuli [75]. In addition, in dogs with SRP, contextual fear may be more pronounced if they cannot predict the owner departure.

Ideally, and in order to avoid contextual fear during the habituation sessions, during these sessions the dog should be in a safe area. A safe area is a place that the dog does not associate with actual departures and should always be accessible to the dog, including the periods when owners are absent (Fig. 3) [73].

In addition, the behavior of the owner toward its dog is fundamentally important, because an inappropriate dog-owner bond is involved in the development of SRP. For example, it has been shown that petting the dog before departure reduces the stress signals during the owner absence [76].

Several studies have found that owners that fail to react to signs of distress given by their dogs can increase the risk of SRP [58,59,77,78]. Therefore, the authors suggest that ignoring the dog is not recommended and that owners should respond to the dog when it demands attention [78]. In order to avoid the reinforcement of nervous behaviors such as jumping during greeting, owners should promote an alternative and calmer behavior and reward it. Consistent handling is another important recommendation and all family members should come to an agreement about daily routines because otherwise lack of control and predictability could increase stress in the dog and cause frustration [79].

In addition, because frustration seems to play an important role in the development of SRP, the authors recommend that behavioral interventions designed to increase tolerance to frustration be included in the treatment.

In summary, the authors suggest that some of the most recommended treatment strategies for SRP are at variance with the current understanding of stress and fear in animals and therefore must be revisited, and we recommend increasing the predictability of owner departures and including interventions designed to reduce frustration.

DISCLOSURE

The authors have nothing to disclose.

REFERENCES

[1] Voith VL, Borchelt PL. Separation anxiety in dogs. Compend Contin Educ Vet 1985;7:42–52.

[2] Horwitz DF. Diagnosis and treatment of canine separation anxiety and the use of clomipramine hydrochloride (Clomicalm®). J Am Anim Hosp Assoc 2000;37:313–8.

[3] Overall KL. Fear, anxieties, and stereotypies. In: Clinical behavioural medicine for small animals. St Louis (MO): Mosby; 1997. p. 209–50.

[4] Bradshaw JWS, McPherson JA, Casey RA, et al. Aetiology of separation related behaviour in the domestic dog. Vet Rec 2002;151:43–6.

[5] Lund JD, Jørgensen MC. Behaviour patterns and time course of activity in dogs with separation problems. Appl Anim Behav Sci 1999;63:219–36.

[6] Appleby D, Pluijmakers J. Separation anxiety in dogs: the function of homeostasis in its development and treatment. Clin Tech Small Anim Pract 2004;19:205–15.

[7] Sherman B, Mills D. Canine anxieties and phobias: an update on separation anxiety and noise aversions. Vet Clin North Am Small Anim Pract 2008;38:1081–106.

[8] Horwitz DF. Separation-related problems in dogs and cats. In: Horwitz DF, Mills DS, editors. BSAVA manual of canine and feline behavioural medicine. Quedgeley (England): British Small Animal Veterinary Association; 2009. p. 146–58.

[9] Storengen LM, Kallestad Boge SC, Strøm SJ, et al. A descriptive study of 215 dogs diagnosed with separation anxiety. Appl Anim Behav Sci 2014;159:82–9.

[10] Ogata N. Separation anxiety in dogs: what progress has been made in our understanding of the most common behavioral problems in dogs? J Vet Behav 2016;16: 28–35.

[11] de Assis LS, Matos R, Pike TW, et al. Developing diagnostic frameworks in veterinary behavioral medicine: disambiguating separation related problems in dogs. Front Vet Sci 2020;6:1–20.

[12] Pageat P. General psycho-psychology and nosography of behaviour disorders of dogs. Pathologic du comportament du chien. 2nd edition. Paris: Editions du Point Vetérinaire; 1998.

[13] Overall KL, Dunham AE, Frank D. Frequency of nonspecific clinical signs in dogs with separation anxiety, thunderstorm phobia, and noise phobia, alone or in combination. J Am Vet Med Assoc 2001;219:467–73.

[14] Flannigan G, Dodman NH. Risk factors and behaviors associated with separation anxiety in dogs. J Am Vet Med Assoc 2001;219:460–6.

[15] Palestrini C, Minero M, Cannas S, et al. Video analysis of dogs with separation-related behaviors. Appl Anim Behav Sci 2010;124:61–7.

[16] Borchelt PL, Voith VL. Diagnosis and treatment of separation-related behaviour problems in dogs. Vet Clin North Am Small Anim Pract 1982;12:625–35.

[17] Mc Crave EA. Diagnostic criteria for separation anxiety in the dog. Vet Clin North Am Small Anim Pract 1991;21: 247–55.

[18] Beaver BV. Canine social behaviour. In: Canine behavior: a guide for veterinarians. Philadelphia: WB Saunders; 1999. p. 137–81.

[19] Simpson BS. Canine separation anxiety. Compend Contin Educ Vet 2000;22:328–39.

[20] Wright JC, Nesselrote MS. Classification of behavior problems in dogs: distributions of age, breed, sex and reproductive status. Appl Anim Behav Sci 1987;19:69–78.

[21] Mills DS, Mills CB. A survey of the behaviour of UK household dogs. Paper presented at: 4th International Veterinary Behaviour Meeting; August 18–20, 2003, Caloundra, Australia.

[22] Denenberg S, Landsberg G, Horwitz D, et al. A comparison of cases referred to behaviorists in three different countries. In: Mills D, Levine E, Landsberg G, et al, editors. Current issues and research in veterinary behavioral medicine: papers presented at: the fifth veterinary behavior meeting. West Lafayette (IN): Purdue University Press; 2005. p. 56–62.

[23] Bamberger M, Houpt KA. Signalment factors, comorbidity, and trends in behavior diagnoses in dogs: 1,644 cases (1991-2001). J Am Vet Med Assoc 2006; 229:1591–601.

[24] Mariti C, Gazzano A, Lansdown Moore J, et al. Perception of dogs' stress by their owners. J Vet Behav 2012;7: 213–9.

[25] Heath S. Separation-related behaviour problems in pet dogs. Vet Times 2001;31:11–2.

[26] Lindell EM. Diagnosis and treatment of destructive behavior in dogs. Vet Clin North Am Small Anim Pract 1997;27:533–48.

[27] Houpt KA, Honig SU, Reisner IR. Breaking the human-companion animal bond. J Am Anim Hosp Assoc 1996;208:1653–9.

[28] Patronek GJ, Glickman LT, Back AM, et al. Risk factors for relinquishment of dogs to an animal shelter. J Am Vet Med Assoc 1996;209:738–42.

[29] Salman MD, Hutchison J, Ruch-Gallie R, et al. Behavioral reasons for relinquishment of dogs and cats to 12 shelters. J Appl Anim Welf Sci 2000;3:93–106.
[30] Takeuchi Y, Ogata N, Houpt KA, et al. Differences in background and outcome of three behavior problems of dogs. Appl Anim Behav Sci 2000;70:297–308.
[31] Mondelli F, Prato Previde E, Verga M, et al. The bond that never developed: adoption and relinquishment of dogs in a rescue shelter. J Appl Anim Welf Sci 2004;7:253–66.
[32] Gonzalez Martinez A, Santamarina Pernas G, Dieguez Casalta FJ, et al. Risk factors associated with behavioral problems in dogs. J Vet Behav 2011;6:225–31.
[33] Fraser D, Weary DM, Pajor EA, et al. A scientific conception of animal welfare that reflects ethical concerns. Anim Welf 1997;6:187–205.
[34] Harding EJ, Paul ES, Mendl M. Animal behaviour - cognitive bias and affective state. Nature 2004;427:312.
[35] Paul ES, Harding EJ, Mendl M. Measuring emotional processes in animals: the utility of a cognitive approach. Neurosci Biobehav Rev 2005;29:469–91.
[36] Mendl M, Burman OHP, Parker RMA, et al. Cognitive bias as an indicator of animal emotion and welfare: emerging evidence and underlying mechanisms. Appl Anim Behav Sci 2009;118:161–81.
[37] Mendl M, Brooks J, Basse C, et al. Dogs showing separation-related behaviour exhibit a "pessimistic" cognitive bias. Curr Biol 2010;20:R839–40.
[38] Karagiannis CI, Burman OHP, Mills DS. Dogs with separation-related problems show a "less pessimistic" cognitive bias during treatment with fluoxetine (Reconcile TM®) and a behaviour modification plan. BMC Vet Res 2015;11:1–10.
[39] Dreschel NA. The effects of fear and anxiety on health and lifespan in pet dogs. Appl Anim Behav Sci 2010; 125:157–62.
[40] Podberscek AL, Hsu Y, Serpell JA. Evaluation of clomipramine as an adjunct to behavioural therapy in the treatment of separation-related problems in dogs. Vet Rec 1999;145:365–9.
[41] McGreevy PD, Masters AM. Risk factors for separation-related distress and feed-related aggression in dogs: additional findings from a survey of Australian dog owners. Appl Anim Behav Sci 2008;109:320–8.
[42] Takeuchi Y, Houpt KA, Scarlett JM. Evaluation of treatments for separation anxiety in dogs. J Am Vet Med Assoc 2000;217:342–5.
[43] McGreevy PD, Wilson B, Starling MJ, et al. Behavioural risks in male dogs with minimal lifetime exposure to gonadal hormones may complicate population-control benefits of desexing. PLoS One 2018;13:1–14.
[44] Serpell J, Jagoe A. Early experience and the development of behaviour. In: Serpell J, editor. The domestic dog: its evolution, behaviour and interactions with people. Cambridge (UK): Cambridge University Press; 1995. p. 79–102.
[45] McMillan FD, Serpell JA, Duffy DL, et al. Differences in behavioral characteristics between dogs obtained as puppies from pet stores and those obtained from noncommercial breeders. J Am Vet Med Assoc 2013;242: 1359–63.
[46] Bennett PC, Rohlf VI. Owner-companion dog interactions: relationships between demographic variables, potentially problematic behaviors, training engagement and shared activities. Appl Anim Behav Sci 2007;102: 65–84.
[47] Miller DD, Staats SR, Partlo C, et al. Factors associated with the decision to surrender a pet to an animal shelter. J Am Vet Med Assoc 1996;209:738–42.
[48] Herron ME, Lord LK, Husseini SE. Effects of preadoption counselling on the prevention of separation anxiety in newly adopted shelter dogs. J Vet Behav 2014;9: 13–21.
[49] Mugford RA. Canine behavioural therapy. In: Serpell J, editor. The domestic dog: its evolution, behaviour, and interactions with people. Cambridge (UK): Cambridge University Press; 1995. p. 139–52.
[50] Guthrie A. Dogs behaving badly-canine separation disorder research. Vet Pract 1999;31:12–3.
[51] Amat M, Manteca X, Mariotti V, et al. Aggressive behavior in the English Cocker Spaniel. J Vet Behav 2009;4:111–7.
[52] Sherman BL. Separation anxiety in dogs. Compend Contin Educ Vet 2008;30:27–42.
[53] Fox M. Vocalizations in wild canids and possible effects of domestication and stages and periods in development: environmental influences and domestication. In: The dog: its domestication and behaviour. New York: S & PM Press; 1978. p. 69–89.
[54] Topál J, Gácsi M, Miklósi A, et al. Attachment to human beings: a comparative study of hand-reared wolves and differently socialized dog puppies. Anim Behav 2005; 70:1367–75.
[55] Parthasarathy V, Crowell-Davis SL. Relationship between attachment to owners and separation anxiety in pet dogs (Canis lupus familiaris). J Vet Behav 2006;1:109–20.
[56] Ainsworth MDS, Blehar MC, Waters E, et al. Patterns of attachment: a psychological study of the strange situation. Hillsdale (NJ): Lawrence Erlbaum Associates, Publishers; 1978.
[57] Warren SL, Huston L, Egeland B, et al. Child and adolescent anxiety disorders and early attachment. J Am Acad Child Adolesc Psychiatry 1997;36:637–44.
[58] Solomon J, Beetz A, Schoeberl I, et al. Attachment Classification in pet dogs: Application of Ainsworth's Strange Situation and classification procedures to dogs and their human caregivers. Paper presented at: International Society of Antrozoology Annual Meeting; July 17–21, 2014, Vienna, Austria.
[59] Schöberl I, Beetz A, Solomon J, et al. Social factors influencing cortisol modulation in dogs during a strange situation procedure. J Vet Behav 2016;11:77–85.
[60] Mariti C, Ricci E, Zilocchi M, et al. Owners as a secure base for their dogs. Behaviour 2013;150:1275–94.
[61] Ainsworth MDS. Infant-mother attachment. Am Psychol 1979;34:932.

[62] King JN, Simpson BS, Overall KL, et al. Treatment of separation anxiety in dogs with clomipramine: results from a prospective, randomised, double-blind, placebo-controlled, parallel-group, multicentre clinical trial. Appl Anim Behav Sci 2000;67:255–75.
[63] Bowen J, Heath S. Canine fear, anxiety and phobia-related disorders. In: Bowen J, Heath S, editors. Behaviour problems in small animals. Practical advice for the veterinary team. Philadelphia: Elsevier Saunders; 2005. p. 73–95.
[64] Blackwell E, Casey RA, Bradshaw JWS. Controlled trial of behavioural therapy for separation-related disorders in dogs. Vet Rec 2006;158:551–4.
[65] Overall KL. Abnormal canine behaviors. In: Manual of clinical behavioral medicine for dogs and cats. St Louis (MO): Mosby; 2013. p. 231–309.
[66] Weinberg J, Levine S. Psychobiology of coping in animals: the effects of predictability. In: Levine S, Ursin H, editors. Coping and health. New York: Plenum Press; 1980. p. 39–59.
[67] Sapolsky RM. Why zebras don't get ulcers: a guide to stress, stress related diseases, and coping. 3rd edition. New York: Holt Paperbacks; 2004.
[68] Lovallo WR. Stress & health: biological and psychological interactions. 2nd edition. Newbury Park, California: Sage Publications; 2005.
[69] Seligman MEP, Binik YM. The safety signal hypothesis. In: Davis H, Hurwiwtz HMB, editors. Operant-Pavlovian interactions. Hoboken, New Jersey: John Wiley & Sons Inc; 1977. p. 165–88.
[70] Grillon C, Baas JP, Lissek S, et al. Anxious responses to predictable and unpredictable aversive events. Behav Neurosci 2004;118:916–24.
[71] Shankman SA, Robison-Andrew EJ, Nelson BD, et al. Effects of predictability of shock timing and intensity on aversive responses. Int J Psychophysiol 2011;80:112–8.
[72] Mineka S, Zinbarg R. A contemporary learning theory perspective on the etiology of anxiety disorders. Am Psychol 2006;61:10–26.
[73] Amat M, Camps T, Le Brech S, et al. Separation anxiety in dogs: The implications of predictability and contextual fear for behavioural treatment. Anim Welf 2014;23: 263–6.
[74] Blanchard DC, Blanchard RJ. Innate and conditioned reactions to threat in rats with amygdaloid lesions. J Comp Physiol Psychol 1972;81:281–90.
[75] Davis M. Are different parts of the extended amygdala involved in fear versus anxiety? Biol Psychiatry 1998;4: 1239–47.
[76] Mariti C, Carlonea B, Protti M, et al. Effects of petting before a brief separation from the owner on dog behavior and physiology: A pilot study. J Vet Behav 2018;27:41–6.
[77] Schöberl I, Wedl M, Bauer B, et al. Effects of caregiver-dog relationship and caregiver personality on cortisol modulation in human-dog dyads. Anthrozoös 2012;25: 199–214.
[78] Solomon J, Beetz A, Schöberl I, et al. Attachment security in companion dogs: adaptation of Ainsworth's strange situation and classification procedures to dogs and their human caregivers. Attach Hum Dev 2019;21:389–417.
[79] Beerda B, Schilder MBH, van Hooff JARAM, et al. Manifestations of chronic and acute stress in dogs. Appl Anim Behav Sci 1997;52:307–19.

Advances in Small Animal Care 1 (2020) 9–23
ADVANCES IN SMALL ANIMAL CARE

Aggressive Behavior in Dogs

An Overview of Diagnosis and Treatment

Barbara Schöning, Dr.med.vet, MSc, PhD
Specialist in Animal Behavior and Animal Welfare, Behavior Consultations, Hohensasel 16, Hamburg 22395, Germany

KEYWORDS
• Dog • Aggression problem • Aggressive behavior • Behavior analysis • Diagnosis • Management • Training • Positive training

KEY POINTS

- Aggression problems have a causation, triggers for showing behavior in a specific situation, and a system of reinforcers that helped to develop the problem and keep the behavior alive.
- For development of a sufficient prognosis and treatment plan, a thorough analysis of these causations and triggers is important.
- Treatment must focus on management to avoid critical situations, curing any underlying health problems when possible; studying the social interaction between dog and owner; using psychoactive drugs when necessary; and administering special training, including desensitization, teaching alternative behavior, and aiming at changing the emotional state of the dog.
- Training must focus on positive techniques. Aversive methods are to be avoided.

INTRODUCTION

Aggressive behavior in dogs causes a major risk to public safety; damages the relationship between dogs and their owners; and is one of the major reasons for harsh treatment, relinquishment to shelters, or euthanasia [1]. Thus aggressive behavior in dogs, besides being a public health concern, also leads to a welfare issue [2,3]. The number of dog bites per year is unknown because many bite incidents go unreported. According to the World Health Organization (WHO) [4], dog bites to humans account for tens of millions of injuries annually, with children at the highest risk for bites and fatalities. Valid data for biting incidents between dogs, or dogs and other animals, are even more scarce, as are the data on, for example, euthanasia as a result of aggressive behavior. Thus it is not known what proportion of the dog population does not fulfill their owners' expectations by showing aggressive behavior, but it can be estimated that many owners are in the position of requiring help.

Aggressive behavior of dogs can be directed toward familiar people, strangers, or toward other dogs (also against other animals) and is manifested in behaviors ranging from subtle threats to massive biting. Aggressive behavior as a problem is a highly emotional issue and people often forget that aggressive behavior is part of the domestic dog's social behavior and belongs to its normal behavioral repertoire [5]. There is no such thing as an unaggressive dog. The statement made by Rooney [6] about play behavior of dogs can still equally be applied to their aggressive behavior: "Literature is vast but suffers from a deficiency of empirical hypothesis testing and an abundance of unsubstantial claims which have, in some cases, been raised to theorem." For example, for a long time, catchword-phrases such as dominance-aggression or fear-aggression have been

E-mail address: bs@ethologin.de

https://doi.org/10.1016/j.yasa.2020.07.002
2666-4518/20/

used for diagnosis. Such simple classification systems subsequently led to certain treatment recommendations, which were often issued like cooking recipes. This approach is counterproductive for solving the problem and helping dog and owner.

To solve a problem properly, every problem dog and its behavior has to be assessed individually, and an individual treatment plan has to be designed. Fatjo and Bowen [7] recently emphasized that a multiaxis model for the collection and organization of information about companion animal behavior problem cases would be useful. It allows some of the limitations of simple classification systems to be avoided and would be aligned with the current research approach in human psychiatry. Such a model would also better assists clinicians in making a complete and thorough assessment of cases, allow a thorough prognosis, and help in developing an individual treatment plan.

This article gives an overview of a differentiated approach for diagnosis and treatment possibilities. Every behavior problem, not only aggression problems, has a causation, triggers for showing the problem behavior in specific situations, and a system of reinforcers that keep the behavior alive and may have helped to develop and intensify it from the beginning to the moment the dog is presented in a consultation. Even when a problem behavior can be diagnosed as abnormal/pathologic, there is a causation somewhere, and this is one of the first relevant pieces of information an owner needs to get: aggressive behavior belongs to the normal behavioral repertoire of any dog. It has a biological function and, as long as the dog shows it effectively to fulfill its needs (fulfillment of demands and prevention of harm), it is not pathologic or abnormal in a clinical sense. Abnormal or pathologic aggressive behavior is behavior that is not species typical, or that, despite being species typical, does not fulfill the needs of the dog or does not enable the dog to adapt effectively to its environment in the long run. There is a difference between what is biologically normal and what is regarded as wanted or not wanted in human society. Humans might tend to label behavior they do not like or want as abnormal, so it is important for compliance of owners that they understand species-typical behavior, causations, triggers, and open or hidden rewards for behavior shown.

This article starts by studying causations and triggers that may contribute to both the development and the continuation of an aggression problem, and that may be responsible for a dog showing aggressive behavior in any individual situation. For some causal factors (eg, health, or owner influence), it is, or at least can be, possible to reduce their impact via treatment and training. For other factors (eg, genetic predisposition) this might not be the case. However, knowledge about such factors is also important for the prognosis. Assessing the dog practically, together with gaining as much information as possible (eg, on problem behavior, health status, owner influence, general environment and living conditions) is described next, followed by general methods and approaches in treatment.

This article focuses on aggressive behavior as a problem. It does not give specific details on dealing, for example, with individual/specific dog-dog aggression or dog-human aggression. Instead it gives an overview on which methods can principally be used. Each individual case demands an individual evaluation and application of methods and measures.

CAUSATIONS AND TRIGGERS: FACTORS INFLUENCING THE DEVELOPMENT OF AN AGGRESSION PROBLEM, AND ELICITING INDIVIDUAL AGGRESSIVE ACTIONS

Before further procedures for anamnesis, diagnosis and possible treatments are described, some causal factors are discussed, that may contribute both to the development and the continuation of an aggression problem. These factors have to be considered for the prognosis and treatment plan: health, genetics, possible morphologic deficits and deficits in socialization and habituation, and learning processes throughout the dog's life. In anamnesis and in practically evaluating the dog, these factors must be considered to get a complete picture of the problem and for as accurate a prognosis as possible. Table 1 gives an overview of these factors. Development in general and deprivation in the socialization phase are dealt with separately, although they influence each other. For example, a problem dog that has prenatal deficits will have a poorer prognosis. Focusing only on the postnatal socialization period of such a dog (which might have been optimal) would lead to important information being missed. Therefore, information on the background with respect to living conditions of the mother, development of siblings (eg, any dead born), and so forth is important.

Besides looking for factors involved in the development of the problem, it is necessary to look for individual triggers: what makes a dog show aggressive behavior toward an individual human or dog, in an individual context, at an exact individual time and location? Besides acute pain and shock, most such triggers are learned. Table 1 also gives some examples.

TABLE 1
Factors Contributing to the Development and Continuation of an Aggression Problem

Factor	Examples
Health	Health conditions influence how an animal perceives its environment and reacts to it. Reduced well-being can decrease the stress tolerance, lower thresholds for anxiety or fear, and altogether can make the dog more prone to react with aggressive behavior toward individual stimuli. This factor applies, for example, for acute or chronic painful situations, brain-specific pathogens, or systemic pathogens (eg, causing inflammation and fever) [41–44]. Conditions such as hypothyroidism or Cushing disease can also decrease the stress tolerance and lower the threshold for anxiety or fear, with subsequent behavior problems [7,45–49]. Listed are just a few examples of how health conditions can influence behavior. Every dog with an aggression problem should undergo a thorough veterinary examination, which should include, besides a general examination, blood and hormone status, orthopedic examination, and a neurologic examination (when possible with regard to fear, stress, and maybe defensive behavior of the dog). Computed tomography or MRT may be useful for further verifying a diagnosis
Genetics	Thresholds for experiencing fear/anxiety and becoming stressed, frustrated, or excited have a genetic background. There is vast literature on personality traits in dogs, such as anxiousness, impulsiveness, excitability, sociability, boldness, or assertiveness. Although they have a genetic background, these traits develop through an interplay between genes and environment [50]. Rooy et al [51] summarized the problems scientists encounter when studying behavioral genetics: probably most traits are polygenetic, it is difficult to differentiate between nature and nurture when studying an individual at a specific time in its life, and it is unknown how traits influence each other. As a last big problem for identifying the genetic background for certain problem behaviors, heterogeneous terminology and diagnostic criteria are used in the literature on behavioral medicine Despite an incomplete picture of the genetic basis for traits and thresholds, there are certain gene defects that are associated with low tolerance levels for becoming anxious and stressed (eg, MDR-1 gene defect). Genetics and health, and the next factor (development), are interwoven and overlap, and it is sometimes not clear which factor had the main influence in the development of a problem behavior. In individual aggression cases, it should be evaluated and (when possible) tested whether certain gene deficits are prevalent and might influence the emotional state and behavior of the dog
Brain development	When the brain shows morphologic, anatomic, or physiologic deficits/faults, these affects emotional and behavioral reactions. There can be obvious conditions such as hydrocephalus, but small, well-defined brain areas can also be affected that are not detected with standard diagnostic tools such as MRT. The prenatal phase plays an important role in the development of a functional brain. Stressed mothers (eg, by illness) have a greater chance of their puppies showing low stress tolerance and social incompetence later in life, conditions that create a higher chance of developing aggression problems. These emotional and behavioral conditions can remain in the puppy, even when it lives in optimal conditions after birth [52–54]. It is therefore important not only to look at the problem dog but also to try to get information on its background, parents, and siblings
Socialization	Dogs from puppy mills and pet shops often experience deprivation and develop a higher chance of behavioral problems (eg, fear and aggression problems) later in life [55,56]. This deprivation is not only caused by a general lack of contact (eg, with humans and other dogs) that leaves the puppy socially incompetent and reduced in its communicative abilities, it can also be caused by a lack of habituation in general. Pirrone et al [57] found that dogs from pet shops showed a higher risk of developing owner-directed aggressive behavior later in life, even when the puppies were well kept and had social contacts after being purchased. It is supposed that, because of prenatal and postnatal deficits, certain areas in the brain do not develop sufficiently, especially in the dopaminergic system, and deficits emerge in the prefrontal area Deprivation of social contact and poor habituation later in puppyhood, and also too early separation from mother/siblings, also lead to deficits in development and promote problems in impulse control, heightened anxiety, and low tolerance for frustration and stress [58,59]. Deprived dogs might have a broader prey spectrum; thus, they might have a higher chance of showing hunting behavior (including grabbing and biting) toward nonprey individuals (eg, small dogs)

(*continued on next page*)

TABLE 1
(*continued*)

Factor	Examples
Trauma	Traumatic experiences can facilitate fast and massive long-term memory. Triggers eliciting aggressive behavior in individual situations can be learned through trauma. Triggers can be individual acoustic, olfactory, tactile, or optic stimuli, but can also be made up from a whole context, comprising a range of such individual stimuli. Trauma can lead to the development of a posttraumatic stress disorder with subsequent chronic stress and impaired learning abilities [60–62], which can also facilitate aggressive behavior in individual contexts
Learning	Dogs react to and learn from their environments throughout their lives. The environment consists of unanimated (optic, tactile, acoustic, and olfactory stimuli) and animated elements, and, for most, the social environment. The most important individuals here are mother and siblings, breeder or keeper in puppyhood, and the owner later on. In general, memory building occurs when the dog subjectively experiences a positive consequence following its behavior (see also Table 4). A positive outcome of aggressive behavior could be the opponent fleeing, and a resource been won or kept. When a dog experiences through a range of threatening situations that, for example, means for deescalation are not successful (success = decrease of threat and fear), the dog will show other behaviors to reach its goal of optimizing its own situation; eg, it might react more and more with aggressive behavior, and might even generalize the context for showing aggression. A dog will also learn which stimuli or contexts predict danger, and will learn about fear-eliciting stimuli, and how best to cope with this situation. Triggers for aggression can be manifold: daytime, location, absence or presence of certain other individuals, behavior of the other party, certain sounds or commands or actions (eg, grabbing the leash) by the owner, and so forth. The consequence the dog experiences from its behavior determines the reaction next time; ie, it keeps the problem behavior alive or makes it even more intense

Abbreviation: MRT, magnetic resonance tomography.

ANAMNESIS, HISTORY TAKING, PRACTICAL EVALUATION, AND DIAGNOSIS

For finding a diagnosis, and for the development of an individual and effective treatment plan, the information listed in Table 2 is necessary. It helps to focus on the problem in a scientifically based way, and not get easily caught in anthropomorphisms or catchword diagnoses. Also it gives information about the causations, triggers, and rewards mentioned earlier, and helps in avoiding them or reducing their impact. The table does not give a chronological order of what has to be done/asked first, but it lists the areas in which information has to be obtained. Each consultation is different according to individual owners, dogs, and problems, and requires individual approaches for negotiation and action. There is only 1 prerequisite that must always be kept in mind with aggression problems: safety for anybody involved in the consultation.

In-home consultations have advantages and disadvantages, as have consultations in a special room in a practice. The big disadvantage of in-home visits lies in safety management. On their own premises, clinicians can set rules and take precautions, which allows them to control a situation more easily. Adequate muzzles, leashes, and collars can be kept in stock. Personal experience shows that owners often come with inadequate collars, have no muzzle at hand, and use flexible leashes. Rules of where and how the dog shall be allowed to roam throughout the consultation can be set and looked up more easily at the clinician's premises. In their own homes, owners are used to letting the dog roam freely and, even when the clinician sets the rules, there is a greater chance that these will be disobeyed. Of course, there are certain (problem) behaviors the dog might only show on its own territory, in the presence of specific resources, or in the area where it is regularly walked. The author's research showed no significant difference between behavior at home and at a special testing site when evaluating 256 dogs for aggressive behavior and dangerousness [8]. Thiesen-Moussa and colleagues [9] emphasized that an in-home visit as well as testing for special triggers can increase the validity of tests for dangerousness. Thus it has to be an individual decision, depending on the results of history taking, where to let a consultation take place.

TABLE 2
Anamnesis and History Taking: the Necessary Information

Focus on	Questions	Practical Evaluation
The dog	General information • Age, sex, reproductive status, breeds • When purchased and from where • Former living conditions	—
	Environment • Living conditions and daily routines (including food and feeding, walks, play sessions, dog's bed) • Training: how, how often, and for what purpose	• Let the owners show how they work with their dogs, and which commands are used • How does the dog react to the commands and to the owner? • How does owner control dog, and how well can owner control dog? Note: this knowledge is also important for own safety
	Health • Vaccinations, deworming • General examination • Any known health problems and medications	Advice for special examinations when necessary
	Behavior • Owner describes and interprets behavior shown in consultation • Owner describes general character and traits of the dog • Owner describes behavior when playing with the dog • When necessary, ask owner especially on hunting behavior • When necessary, give examples of distinct situations for which owner shall describe behavior	Own observations: • Social competence and communication abilities of the dog • Tolerance levels for becoming stressed and frustrated • Thresholds for anxiety and becoming excited; how long does such a state last? • Which behavior is shown when thresholds/ tolerance levels are reached/exceeded? • When necessary: special evaluation of hunting behavior • Special evaluation of bite inhibition (when possible, without endangering own safety) • Timeline: does behavior change during consultation? • How does owner description relate to own observations during consultation? Note: own safety and safety of all people present, and safety of stooge-dogs, has priority When testing the dog, welfare must not be compromised
The problem	Owner describes problem in own words: • W questions (what, who, where, with whom, when, how long) • Chronology of problem development • The first and the last incident should be described in detail, including how owner reacted to dog	Own observations: • Reaction to special test situations and how these reactions compare with described behavior for incidents • How does owner description relate to own observations during consultation? • If it applies, how does dog react to muzzle or any other safety measure?

(continued on next page)

TABLE 2
(*continued*)

Focus on	Questions	Practical Evaluation
	• The behavior the dog showed, in detail, during the last incident • What solutions/training did the owner already try and for how long? How successful were these? • What safety measures/management have the owner implicated already?	• If applicable for safety, welfare, and ethical reasons, carefully apply trigger situations for the problem behavior Note: own safety and safety of all people present, and safety of stooge-dogs, has priority. When testing the dog, welfare must not be compromised
The owner	General information • Age and sex (of all owners and any person the dog meets on a regular basis) • Children (age, sex), interest in the dog, behavior of dog toward children • Illness and/or disabilities of respective persons • Owner describes bonding between dog and individual family members • Owner's knowledge on dog behavior and training in general	Own observations: • With special regard to bonding: how does owner description relate to own observations during consultation? • How is owner handling the dog and looking for safety? • How are the owner's practical actions and theoretic knowledge related?
The bitten person or dog	Although dealt with when studying the problem, a person/dog who has been bitten should be especially looked at, if possible • Behavior of bitten person/dog before, during, and after the incident • Special type of behavior/situation functioning as trigger • Wounds: type, location, severity, multiple biting, hospital yes or no, surgery needed • When person/dog and problem dog still live together, how intense is the person/dog's fear? • Is it possible at all to apply useful management? • Welfare conditions have to be regarded for dogs and humans	• Let person/dog tell in own words/behavior, when present in consultation • Pictures or videos, when available • How does what is seen relate to what is told? Note: when person/dog is present during consultation, special safety measures are necessary to avoid stress, fear, or even trauma

Questionnaires are not only helpful in getting relevant information from the owner in general but give preliminary information about the dog and problem, which helps for planning the live consultation with respect to safety, welfare considerations, and the decision on the location. There is a wide range of questionnaires available in the literature. For example, Overall [10] gives templates on general questionnaires and questionnaires focusing on special problem areas. The Canine Behavioral Assessment and Research Questionnaire (C-BARQ) is a widely used questionnaire for gaining information on the general character and temperament of a dog [11]. There are special questionnaires together with practical tests for measuring deficits in, for example, impulse control or cognitive abilities, or for predicting aggression [12–18].

Owner-report questionnaires are potentially vulnerable to psychological biases and perception errors, but they do account for the dog's behavior in a wide range of situations, and over long timescales [7]. There might be cultural and individual differences in how prone owners are to filling in questionnaires. Therefore, a questionnaire cannot be the only source of information. An face-to-face interview with the owner plus the clinician's own practical evaluation of the dog needs to be done in all cases. When questioning the owner and evaluating the dog, everyone who regularly has close social contact with the dog should be present. This rule applies to owners, families, children, and dog walkers or trainers. When children and/or targets of the dog's aggressive behavior are present in a consultation, safety precautions have to be taken very seriously.

Diagnoses should be descriptive, following the approach of Fatjo and Bowen [7], who noted that, when a diagnosis is too focused on syndromes and categories, sight may be lost of the individuality of the problem, with the subsequent risk of inadequate treatment protocols. A descriptive diagnosis gives information on the problem (eg, aggressive behavior toward a particular target) and allows a focus on underlying emotions (eg, fear or frustration) and motivations (eg, fulfillment of certain needs). The descriptive diagnosis provides information on whether it is normal behavior (shown, according to human interpretation, in the wrong place or time, toward the wrong individual, and so forth), or whether the behavior is abnormal/pathologic in a clinical sense.

After history taking and diagnosis, a prognosis should be given together with a treatment plan. The prognosis can vary from very good to very poor, according to what picture is given by the information gathered. Even euthanasia might be necessary in individual cases, although, in most cases, aggression problems are not "1-way streets" [19,20]. The prognosis is influenced not only by factors regarding the dog but also by owner personality and abilities. The owners have to act as cotrainers or cotherapists. They have to administer medication and, usually, have to set up management and perform the training. The owner needs to get from the clinician all of the information that is necessary for understanding the why and how of treatment, and thus for developing the necessary compliance.

TREATMENT

Treatment plans have to be developed individually according to the individual problem and diagnosis, but there are some general points that always apply. Treatment consists of different approaches: medical intervention, management, studying the social interaction between dog and owners, special training, and psychopharmacologic intervention, when necessary. Medical intervention is not discussed further here, because it depends on the individual health problem.

Management

Management is very important, at least at the beginning of any treatment. Management focuses on having the dog not showing the aggressive behavior any longer, or at least showing it controlled and in a much reduced quality and quantity. In aggression problems, the goal of effective management is first to avoid further harmed individuals (including the dog itself). However, there is another goal that is as important. Every time the dog shows the aggressive behavior, it undergoes some training in the behavior and learns something about triggers or special situations that will be counterproductive to effective training against the problem. Also, the owner might resume undesirable behavior such as, for example, punishing the dog [21], making effective management important for the dog's welfare in general. Table 3 gives an overview of management elements and measures, and what has to be considered when applying them. Each element has to be assessed individually for its appropriateness regarding the individual problem.

Because management can never be perfect, owners should be trained in how to react in a situation in which the dog shows aggressive behavior (ie, an emergency situation). They need to learn that, in such a situation, it is not possible to teach the dog something, but rather the focus must be on reducing danger. This approach can include the owners just holding the leash tightly and trying to leave the situation as quickly as possible with the dog, or the owner shutting a door between the dog and a possible target. Management is of utmost importance until the special training begins to pay off. The best owner reaction in an emergency situation always depends on the owner's abilities, the dog, the situation, and the problem behavior. It is beyond the scope of this article to go into more detail here.

Social Interaction Between Dogs and Owners

The borders between management, social interaction, and special training are not fixed. It is important to assess what is going on between dog and owner as a field of its own in treatment. Does a certain behavior of the owner act as a trigger for aggressive behavior? What role does the owner play in consciously and/or unconsciously rewarding the aggressive behavior, thus facilitating further learning? What role does the owner play as a social partner (bonding in general) and as a secure base for the dog? Are there certain owner behaviors that elicit fear and stress in the dog? Does the dog appear to expect certain behavior from the owner in individual situations (eg, anticipation of punishment)? When, and triggered by what, does the dog show attention-seeking behavior, and what happens when the owner reacts or does not react to this behavior? Is there a difference in the dog's reaction toward different

TABLE 3
Management Measures and Issues

Management Type	What	Remarks, Safety Precautions
Directly controlling the dog	Well-fitting collar or harness	Welfare must not be compromised by using the device. Dog might need training before the device can be used
	Fixed short or long leash	No flexible leash. Owner might need special training to work with a long leash; dog might need training to get used to it
	Head halter	Dog and owner might need special training before it is used. Welfare must not be compromised
	Muzzle	The muzzle must fit (neither too loose nor too tight, not leading to abrasions) and must allow the dog to pant and drink. Dogs need to be trained to wear it relaxed. Muzzles that still allow treats to be given are preferred. Note: a muzzle is no excuse to not train the dog. A dog wearing a muzzle must be under constant control. Even a muzzled dog can cause pain, wounds, and trauma in others, and the dog itself can be harmed
	Obedience	Good obedience makes controlling problem situations easier, and stops the owner needing to use harsh manipulation or punishment. In parallel, it increases the subjective feeling of security for the owner and thus avoids stress. Useful obedience elements are, at minimum, the recall, having the dog walk properly on loose leash, and 1 signal to bring the dog to a stationary position. A useful command at home is a signal to have the dog go to its bed or into a kennel and stay there relaxed until a new command is given
Controlling environment at home	Critical resources need to be controlled	Critical resources can be food items, toys, chewing objects, or social partners. Certain resources might play a role in eliciting and/or reinforcing aggressive behavior. The dog should not be able to use them freely, but only in controlled situations. Control by the owner also allows these resources to be more effectively used as primary rewards in controlled training situations, if applicable
	Decide on more appropriate type of, and places for, the dog's bed (when necessary)	Some resources cannot easily be controlled by the owner; eg, the dog's bed. When the aggression problem occurs at home, it can be necessary to think about the best place for the dog's bed. The bed should be a place of retreat that guarantees well-being for the dog (the dog should never be sent to bed as a punishment). For some dogs, it is important that the bed is somewhere hidden; others need it more open to have a good view. For some dogs, a box or kennel might be the best option Note: the owner should be advised that a box or kennel is not something a dog should be stored in whenever it is bothersome; and a dog needs to be trained to use a box relaxed [63]
	Structure of the day. Avoiding or managing individual critical situations	Think beforehand and plan: at what time might certain resources be more important, might certain triggers occur, or might be fear and stress of the dog be at such a high level that there is a greater chance of aggressive behavior being shown? Such situations should be mitigated beforehand (eg, taking the dog to a different room before a visitor rings the bell) Structure and routine help to increase the subjective feeling of security for the dog. Focus must be especially on those situations in which the dog has shown aggressive behavior before. This point is especially important when dog and possible target individuals live in the same household

(continued on next page)

TABLE 3
(continued)

Management Type	What	Remarks, Safety Precautions
	Tools	Tools, such as in-house leash or muzzle, should be put on well before a critical situation occurs. Obstacles to divide a room and limiting access of the dog can also be useful tools (eg, using a fence designed to prevent children from falling down stairs)
Controlling outside environment	Structure of the day. Avoiding or managing individual critical situations	At what time and location might certain resources be more important, might certain triggers occur, or might be fear and stress of the dog be at such a high level that there is a greater chance of aggressive behavior being shown? Such situations should be avoided wherever possible (eg, do not take the respective resources with you on walks; avoid walking the dog at special times or in special locations) Focus must be especially on those situations in which the dog has shown aggressive behavior before
	Tools	Tools such as leash or muzzle should be put on well before a critical situation occurs
Owner	Apply management measures	Owner needs to be instructed and reminded on a regular basis to use the respective tools and be thorough with applying the management measures listed earlier. Owners might need encouragement in behaviors such as changing to the other side of the street instead of directly passing another dog on the pavement
	Get rid of old habits (especially punishment)	Owner needs to be instructed and reminded on a regular basis to refrain from punishment and other measures/actions that might lead to escalation. Aversive measures can easily compromise welfare, and are generally not effective in decreasing the quality and quantity of the problem behavior

owners? For example, when a dog is more relaxed with one owner but not with the other, the owner eliciting less stress should start with the special training. While assessing these matters, the time should also be used to teach owners the necessary information on dog behavior, social behavior, and communication, and to teach them what to look for in their individual dogs (eg, discreet signals that are revealing about fear and stress, and discreet threats).

There is a remarkable similarity in the attachment bond that dogs establish toward their owners and that human children establish toward their caregivers. In the dog-owner bond, both a secure base and a safe haven effect have been found [22]. Gacsi and colleagues [23] highlighted the importance of a human analog safe haven effect of the owner in a potentially dangerous situation. Owners can provide a buffer against stress in dogs, which can even reduce the effect of an encounter with a threatening stimulus. The quality of an owner as secure base and safe haven is reduced if the owner acts, in the eyes of the dog, in ways that are unreliable and unfriendly. Such an effect can be easily provoked through punishment, for example. Therefore it is important to not only advise owners to refrain from punishment but also to give ideas on how the social bond between owner and dog can be improved. Predictable, friendly, and nonconfrontational handling of the dog is important, but there are some special training measures that can also be applied. Monteny and Moons [21] list some ideas about the forms such training can take, such as the predictability game. Teaching the dog safety cues that allow environmental and situational control reduces stress, as do special relaxation exercises together with teaching the dog a special signal for relaxation.

Almost all owners have a fixed set of expectations as to how the dog should behave in public, at home, in contact with other dogs, and so forth. When the dog conforms to this expectation, owners often do nothing, but, when the dog's behavior does not meet the owner's expectation, owners usually become active. They react toward the misbehaving dog, not only for control of the situation but also often either with punishment or trying to reassure the dog. Although reassuring a fearful dog is reasonable and effective when it is done correctly and is adequate for the situation [24], punishment has serious side effects [25–29]. Rather than focusing of what they do not want, owners should focus on wanted behavior and reward this as often as possible. Here management and social interaction affect each other, because the frequency of wanted behavior being shown spontaneously can be increased by well-planned management.

A good behavior that is always worth rewarding, especially at home, is relaxed, patient behavior by the dog, so instead of always reacting to the dog when it is active, and perhaps interacting with the owner (seeking attention), owners should focus on, and reward, the relaxed, quiet moments. It is important to teach owners about possible risks when doing so. Being ignored for behavior the owner had always reacted to before can frustrate the dog, elicit stress, and consequently elicit aggressive behavior. Owners therefore need advice about when exactly and for how long they should focus on such measures. With some dogs, especially when the aggressive behavior occurs at home and/or the dog has a very reactive, easily aroused character, such measures can only be applied for a short time, perhaps in times of the day when the dog is known to be already relaxed and silent. From here on, time spans can be increased slowly.

Special Training

Besides general training for obedience, special training is necessary to address individual key aspects of the problem. A dog that is easily aroused might need special training in becoming more patient. A dog that acts very impulsively and actively might need the same, but additionally needs training for inhibition and a special signal for becoming relaxed. A dog that acts aggressively toward other dogs or humans out of fear might need desensitization, focusing on changing the dog's emotional state when it is approached by another dog or human.

Special training approaches to solve an aggression problem are manifold and have to be chosen individually, with regard to the different causations and triggers. Table 4 provides an overview of the general methods and approaches. Irrespective of which method is chosen, there is some key information every owner needs:

- Do not aim at negative goals but instead focus on positive goals for training. A negative goal is something like saying, "My dog will not bite granny any longer." A positive goal could be, "When granny comes to visit, my dog will spontaneously go to its bed and stay there relaxed until granny leaves." This advice might seem pointless, but lay owners tend to think of what they do not want the dog to do, rather than thinking about useful behavior in a critical situation.
- Emergency situations and training situations must be clearly differentiated. Again, this is difficult for owners, because most owners want to tell the dog what it is doing wrong, and want the dog to learn to behave, at the exact moment when the dog is showing the problem behavior. In an emergency situation, such as when the dog is lunging at another dog, the dog is stressed and thus cannot easily show, or learn, alternative behavior or be open to a desensitization process. The stressed brain focuses on behaviors that were helpful (subjectively for the relevant individual) in past times. Often this is the problem behavior. Only in clearly designed training sessions can stressors be controlled so that learning can take place. Therefore, good management is important for avoiding emergency situations as much as possible.
- Owners need advice not to overdo training. They have to focus on short but frequent training sessions. Attention span, ability to concentrate, and tolerance level of the dog need to be considered and should not be exceeded in training. This point also applies for thresholds for becoming fearful. Stressors need to be introduced gradually and always up to the dog's competences and thresholds.
- Following from the last point, owners need the advice not to create a flooding situation while training. Flooding can easily lead to escalation in aggression, and/or the dog's welfare can be compromised. There is even a high chance that learned helplessness can develop, which is a sign for a dramatically negative mental state [30].
- Owners need advice to refrain from using punishment and any aversive means. Graeber [31] said that using violence in training means influencing behavior in a way that needs no understanding of the individual that is being worked with. Reward-based training demands much more knowledge and technical skill, and is the most powerful tool for changing behavior. It is the clinician's duty to teach the owner the necessary information [32].

Special training aims at controlling the dog in a critical situation more than is possible with simple obedience. In the long run, special training aims at the dog spontaneously showing so-called alternative behavior

TABLE 4
Training Methods and Techniques

Method/ Technique	Description	Remarks/Practical Application
Classical conditioning	Association between 2 stimuli: the US and a former neutral stimulus, which becomes a CS after the conditioning process. US elicits an unconditioned reaction. After conditioning, CS will elicit the same reaction, then named a conditioned reaction [64]	Conditioning of a reward signal follows this principle. A neutral stimulus (eg, a click) is paired with a treat (US), thus becoming a CS and obtaining a quality as reinforcer [65]
Operant conditioning	A behavior is associated with a stimulus and comes under control of that stimulus (stimulus acts as cue). Strength of association is modified by the consequences of the behavior (ie, reinforcement or punishment) [64]	Dogs can involuntarily be trained by their owners to show unwanted behavior, when owners unconsciously reward this behavior (eg, through attention or punishment; ie, attention with aversive quality). This point also applies for learned triggers for aggressive behavior
Classical counterconditioning	In classical counterconditioning a desirable stimulus (eg, food) is paired with a fear/stress-eliciting stimulus (eg, a stranger), thus reducing fear and stress in the dog by replacing the former negative association with a positive one [66]	Classical counterconditioning can be a powerful training tool, but it is also demanding for lay owners. Sessions have to be thoroughly planned, and timing in delivering the CS is essential. When perpetrator and target live together, it is difficult to be applied effectively. To be effective, it is necessary that the dog is only presented with the fear/stress-eliciting stimulus in planned training sessions, which is difficult, or might not be possible, when dog and stimulus are sharing the same habitat
Reconditioning or operant counterconditioning	The dog is trained to show an alternative behavior in critical situations, which preferentially is incompatible with the problem behavior	Eg, the dog can be trained to focus on the owner on cue. The cue is then given when another dog is present (in controlled training situations) and eventually other dogs become the cue for looking at the owner
Habituation and sensitization	Habituation leads to a stimulus becoming less important (eg, a former fear/stress-eliciting stimulus might become neutral). Sensitization means the opposite: a stimulus becomes more important and can, for example, elicit a fear response even when presented at low intensity. Also generalization (similar or related stimuli also elicit fear) can happen easily	When stimuli eliciting fear, stress, or arousal are detected in anamnesis and history taking, it is sensible to habituate the dog to such triggers. The more the dog is already sensitized against such stimuli, the more difficult it is to undo the sensitization process. Thorough management is necessary for having the dog not exposed too often and uncontrolled to these stimuli

(continued on next page)

TABLE 4
(continued)

Method/ Technique	Description	Remarks/Practical Application
Systematic desensitization	Systematic desensitization aims at removal of a fear and stress response to a stimulus. In human psychology, it is usually done via counterconditioning in addition to relaxation techniques. In behavior therapy in animals, the term is used for any training procedure that aims at changing the dog's emotional and behavioral reactions toward a fear/stress-eliciting stimulus	For a dog-dog aggression problem, this can include teaching the dog an alternative behavior and having the dog show this behavior on cue while gradually being exposed more intensely to other dogs; ie, aiming at habituation. In addition, a safety cue, cue-induced relaxation, and activities such as the predictability game can be used to speed up the process [21]. Overall [10] lists a range of desensitization protocols
Reinforcer, reward, reinforcement	A future behavior will be strengthened by a specific consequence (ie, the reinforcer) whenever it is preceded by a specific antecedent stimulus Positive reinforcement means that a reward is given (eg, a treat). Negative reinforcement means that something unpleasant is taken away whenever the wanted behavior is shown. A reward (ie, rewarding stimulus) can be anything a dog is wanting and liking in that special moment of training [67]	A negative reinforcer could be that the stooge dog (which was eliciting fear) is moving away at the moment the problem dog shows the wanted alternative behavior. A positive reinforcer in this situation would be the owner giving a treat as a reward at exactly that moment Timing and thorough planning of training sessions is essential to not involuntarily reward unwanted and/or unnecessary behavior in training

Abbreviations: CS, conditioned stimulus; US, unconditioned stimulus.

when a trigger occurs: certain behaviors incompatible with, for example, lunging and biting. Therefore, it is important that these alternative behaviors and general training methods are chosen carefully and are adequate for the relevant problem and dog. An alternative behavior, such as looking away from the opponent and focusing on the owner in a dog-dog-situation, does not only help the problem dog (as discussed later). From the opponent dog's point of view, such behavior looks like avoidance behavior, which could further help in deescalating the conflict. However, this special alternative behavior is not the best choice in every dog-dog problem. When the problem dog is a motoric, very active individual, it can be helpful to teach the dog active behaviors that mimic replacement activities, such as digging or showing a play bow. Another interesting approach is the engage-disengage game [33], where the dog learns to relaxed focus on former stressors/triggers; also helpful is the do-as-I-do concept [34,35], where the dog learns to imitate the actions of a human trainer. This concept can speed up learning of alternative behaviors, and in general makes the dog more prone to concentrate on the owner. Teaching owners how to use this method can additionally help in building up the social bond between owner and dog.

Once the alternative behavior is ritualized and is shown spontaneously in former critical situations, it helps the dog control its emotions and, in the long run, can change emotions. There is evidence from human psychology that alternative behavior that is trained in a way that makes the patients feel in control of the situation by being able to vary and modify their behavioral reactions on their own authority during training eventually leads to a decrease in fear, stress, and arousal. Former stress-eliciting and fear-eliciting situations are interpreted as being less dramatic and dangerous afterward [36,37], eventually allowing, for example, prosocial behavior toward other dogs or humans. Training dogs positively and considering state-of-the-art theoretic and practical knowledge on animal training can allow such changes in dogs. This process includes, for example, designing shaping processes toward the wanted behavior carefully and such in a way that the dog is most motivated to show exactly the behavior the trainer wants, without needing to push or drag the dog into that behavior.

Teaching the dog alternative behavior is an important part of special training but has to be done together with other training elements. Different training approaches have to be put in a chronologic order. For example, using an alternative behavior for desensitization against encounters with strange humans or dogs might only be possible after the dog has learned a cue for relaxation and/or has successfully completed training for general stress reduction [21]. As mentioned earlier, there are many possible causations and triggers for a dog showing aggressive behavior. This article cannot display all possible diagnoses together with the respective and differentiated treatment strategies in detail, but it gives an overview of what has to assessed and what general treatment possibilities exist. There is only 1 problem area that is mentioned individually here: when a dog has bitten another individual while clearly showing hunting behavior. Here the focus in training is different than for dogs having bitten in a social context (eg, in a conflict about a resource or out of fear when being subjectively threatened). Behaviors for deescalation and appeasement only work in a social context; that is, when the dog has noticed that the other individual is a conspecific or possible social partner, but not prey. Hunting behavior has a narrower genetic predisposition than social behavior and requires more intense and strict training, which should first focus on general control via obedience. Desensitization against the optic, olfactory, and acoustic stimuli that elicit hunting behavior is important, but takes a long time because of a genetically fixed motivation for action focusing on the prey.

Psychoactive Medication

Certain psychoactive substances can support training and allow fast and stable emotional changes. With highly deprived and/or fearful dogs, and very impulsive or reactive dogs, psychoactive substances may be indispensable for reaching an emotional condition where training can be administered effectively and safely.

There is a vast range of substances to choose from, with different target locations in the brain and different effects. The substances range from nutraceuticals (eg, tryptophan, L-theanine, or alpha-casozepine), to benzodiazepines, alpha-adrenoceptor agonists, tricyclic antidepressants, monoamine oxidase B inhibitors, and selective serotonin reuptake inhibitors. Some of the substances are labeled for use in dogs, and some have to be used off label. Dealing in detail with different substances and their indication and contraindications is beyond the scope of this overview. Readers are referred to the relevant literature [10,38–40]. This point also applies to supporting substances/elements such as pheromones and body wraps.

SUMMARY

Aggressive behavior in dogs is of multicausal origin, be it directed against humans or other dogs. A thorough anamnesis and history taking is important for a valid diagnosis and prognosis, and for the decision of an individual treatment plan. This article provides an overview on the principal methods that can be used in treatment, including advice on management, a focus on the social bonding between dog and owner, and individual application of methods and measures. The focus is on positive training; punishment must be avoided because aversive methods are counterproductive with regard to the final goal, and can compromise welfare.

DISCLOSURE

The author has nothing to disclose.

REFERENCES

[1] Greenebaum J. Training dogs and training humans: symbolic interaction and dog training. Anthrozoös 2010;23: 129–41.
[2] De Keuster T, Lamoureux J, Kahn A. Epidemiology of dog bites: A Belgian experience of canine behavior and public health concerns. Vet J 2006;172:482–7.
[3] Caffrey N, Rock M, Schmidtz O, et al. Insights about the epidemiology of dog bites in a canadian city using a dog aggression scale and administrative data. Animals 2019; 9:324.
[4] WHO. https://www.who.int/en/news-room/fact-sheets/detail/animal-bites. Accessed May 12, 2020.
[5] Bradshaw J, Nott H. Social and communication behaviour of companion dogs. In: Serpell J, editor. The domestic dog. Its evolution, behaviour and interactions with people. Cambridge, UK: Cambridge University Press; 1995. p. 115–30.
[6] Rooney N. Play behaviour of the domestic dog, Canis familiaris, and its effect upon the dog-human relationship. PhD-thesis. Southampton, UK: University of Southampton; 1999.
[7] Fatjo J, Bowen J. Making the case for multi-axis assessment of behavioural problems. Animals 2020;10:383.
[8] Schöning B. Evaluation and prediction of agonistic behavior in the domestic dog. PhD-thesis. Bristol, UK: University of Bristol; 2006.

[9] Thiesen-Moussa D, Hettwer A, Hackbart A. Der Niedersächsische Wesenstest: Ergebnisse des Testens der Gefährlichkeit von Hunden. Berl Münch Tierärztl Wochenschr 2018. https://doi.org/10.2376/0005-9366-18042.
[10] Overall K. Manual of clinical behavioral medicine for dogs and cats. St Louis (MO): Elsevier Mosby; 2013.
[11] Hsu Y, Serpell J. Development and validation of a questionnaire for measuring behavior and temperament traits in pet dogs. J Am Vet Med Assoc 2003;223:1293–300.
[12] Vas J, Topál J, Péch E, et al. Measuring attention deficit and activity in dogs: A new application and validation of a human ADHD questionnaire. Appl Anim Behav Sci 2007;103:105–17.
[13] Sheppard G, Mills D. The Development of a Psychometric Scale for the Evaluation of the Emotional Predispositions of Pet Dogs. Int J Comp Psychol 2002;15:201–22.
[14] Salvin HE, McGreevy PD, Sachdev SS, et al. The canine cognitive dysfunction rating scale (CCDR): a data-driven and ecologically relevant assessment tool. Vet J 2011;188:331–6.
[15] Wright H, Mills D, Pollux P. Behavioral and physiological correlates of impulsivity in the domestic dog (Canis familiaris). Physiol Behav 2012;105:676–82.
[16] Kubinyi E, Vas J, Hejjas K, et al. Polymorphism in the tyrosine hydrolase (TH) gene is associated with activity-impulsivity in German shepherd dogs. PLoS One 2012; 7:e30271.
[17] Wiener P, Haskell M. Use of questionnaire-based data to assess dog personality. J Vet Behav 2016;16:81–5.
[18] Bennett S, Litster A, Weng H, et al. Investigating behavior assessment instruments to predict aggression in dogs. Appl Anim Behav Sci 2012;141:139–48.
[19] David S, Woytalewicz K. Case study of methods for the rehabilitation of dogs that have bitten: Shelter dogs. In: Mills D, Westgarth C, editors. Dog bites – a multidisciplinary approach. Sheffield (England): 5m publishing; 2017. p. 368–78.
[20] Schöning B. Risk assessment principles and procedures in use. In: Mills D, Westgarth C, editors. Dog bites – a multidisciplinary approach. Sheffield (England): 5m publishing; 2017. p. 359–67.
[21] Monteny J, Moons C. A treatment plan for dogs (*Canis familiaris*) that show impaired social functioning towards their Owners. Animals 2020;10:161.
[22] Mariti C, Ricci E, Zilocchi M, et al. Owners as a secure base for their dogs. Behaviour 2013;150:1275–94.
[23] Gacsi M, Maros K, Sernkvist S, et al. Human analogue safe haven effect of the owner: Behavioral and heart rate response to stressful social stimuli in dogs. PLoS One 2013;8:e58475.
[24] Horn L, Huber L, Range F. The importance of the secure base effect for domestic dogs – evidence from a manipulative problem-solving task. PLoS One 2013;8: e65296.
[25] Hiby EF, Rooney NJ, Bradshaw JWS. Dog training methods: their use, effectiveness and interaction with behavior and welfare. Anim Welf 2004;13:63–9.
[26] Balint A, Rieger G, Miklosi A, et al. Assessment of owner-directed aggressive behavioral tendencies of dogs in situations of possession and manipulation. R Soc Open Sci 2017;4. https://doi.org/10.1098/rsos.171040.
[27] Ziv G. The effects of using aversive training methods in dogs – a review. J Vet Behav 2017;9:50–60.
[28] Fernandes J, Olsson I, de Castro A. Do aversive-based training methods actually compromise dog welfare?: A literature review. Appl Anim Behav Sci 2017;196: 1–12.
[29] Vieira de Castro A, Barrett J, de Sousa L, et al. Carrots versus sticks: The relationship between training methods and dog-owner attachment. Appl Anim Behav Sci 2019; 219. https://doi.org/10.1016/j.applanim.2019.104831.
[30] Maier S, Seligman M. Learned helplessness: theory and evidence. J Exp Psychol Gen 176;1976:105:3.
[31] Graeber D. Beyond power/knowledge: an exploration of the relation of power, ignorance and stupidity (Malinowski Memorial Lecture). London, UK: London School of Economics and Political Science; 2006. Available at: http://libcom.org.libcom.org/files/20060525-Graeber.pdf.
[32] Williams E, Blackwell E. Managing the risk of aggressive dog behavior: investigating the influence of owner threat and efficacy perceptions. Risk Anal 2019;39. https://doi.org/10.1111/risa.13336.
[33] Tong A. Available at: https://www.choosepositivedogtraining.com/single-post/2014/07/01/The-Practice-of-SelfInterruption-The-EngageDisengage-Game. Accessed August 20, 2020.
[34] Fugazza C, Pogany A, Miklosi A. Do as I … did! Long-term memory of imitative actions in dogs/Canis familiaris. Anim Cogn 2015. https://doi.org/10.1007/s10071-015-0931-8.
[35] Figazza C, Miklosi A. Social learning in dog training: The effectiveness of Do as I do method compared to shaping/clicker training. Appl Anim Behav Sci 2015; 171:146–51.
[36] Jiongjiong Y, Xiaohong X, Xiaoxa D, et al. Effects of unconscious processing on implicit memory for fearful faces. PLoS One 2011;6:e14641.
[37] Bebko G, Franconeri S, Ochsner K, et al. Attentional deployment is not necessary for successful emotion regulation via cognitive reappraisal or expressive suppression. Emotion 2014;14:504–12.
[38] Landsberg G, Hunthausen W, Ackerman L. Behaviour problems of the dog and cat. Toronto, Canada: Elsevier publishers; 2013.
[39] Riemer S. Effectiveness of treatments for firework fears in dogs. J Vet Behav 2020;37:61–70.
[40] Piotti P, Ucchedu S, Alliani M, et al. Management of specific fears and anxiety in the behavioral medicine of companion animals: punctual use of psychoactive medications. Dog Behav 2019;23–30. https://doi.org/10.4454/db.v5i2.109.
[41] Holton L, Reid J, Scott E, et al. Development of a behavior-based scale to measure acute pain in dogs. Vet Rec 2001;148:525–31.

[42] Wiseman-Orr M, Nolan A, Reid J, et al. Development of a questionnaire to measure the effects of chronic pain on health-related quality of life in dogs. Am J Vet Res 2004;65:1077–84.

[43] Fatjó J, Bowen J. Medical and metabolic influences on behavioral disorders. In: Horwitz D, Mills D, editors. BSAVA manual of canine and feline behavioral medicine. 2nd edition. Gloucester (UK): BSAVA; 2009. p. 1–9.

[44] Fagundes A, Hewison L, McPeake K. Noise sensitivities in dogs: an exploration of signs in dogs with and without musculoskeletal pain using qualitative content analysis. Front Vet Sci 2018;5:17.

[45] Radosta L, Shofer F, Reisner I. Comparison of thyroid analytes in dogs aggressive to familiar people and in non-aggressive dogs. Vet J 2012;192:472–5.

[46] Dodman N, Aronson L, Cottam N, et al. The effect of thyroid replacement in dogs with suboptimal thyroid function on owner-directed aggression: A randomized, double-blind, placebo- controlled clinical trial. J Vet Behav 2013;8:225–30.

[47] Hrovat A, De Keuster T, Kooistra H, et al. Behavior in dogs with spontaneous hypothyroidism during treatment with levothyroxine. J Vet Intern Med 2019;33:64–71.

[48] Notari L, Burman O, Mills D. Behavioral changes in dogs treated with corticosteroids. Physiol Behav 2015;1: 609–16.

[49] Notari L, Burman O, Mills D. Is there a link between treatments with exogenous corticosteroids and dog behavior problems? Vet Rec 2016;179:462.

[50] Shiner R, DeYoung C. The structure of temperament and personality traits: a developmental perspective. In: Zelazo PD, editor. The Oxford handbook of developmental psychology;. Oxford (UK): Oxford University Press; 2011. p. 113–41.

[51] Rooy D, Arnott E, Early J, et al. Holding back the genes: limitations of research into canine behavioural genetics. Canine Genet Epidemiol 2014;1:7–18.

[52] Adrover E, Pallares MW, Baier C, et al. Glutamate neurotransmission is affected in prenatally stressed offspring. Neurochem Int 2015;88:73–87.

[53] Casolini P, Zuena AR, Cinque C, et al. Sub-neurotoxic neonatal anoxia induces subtle behavioural changes and specific abnormalities in brain group-I metabotropic glutamate receptors in rats. J Neurochem 2005;95:137–45.

[54] Raper J, Stephens SBZ, Sanchez M, et al. Neonatal amygdala lesions alter mother-infant interactions in rhesus monkeys living in a species-typical social environment. Dev Psychobiol 2015;56:1711–22.

[55] McMillan F. Behavioral and psychological outcomes for dogs sold as puppies through pet stores and/or born in commercial breeding establishments: Current knowledge and putative causes. J Vet Behav 2017;19:14–26.

[56] Wauthier L. Scottish Society for the Prevention of Cruelty to Animals (Scottish SPCA), Williams J. Using the mini C-BARQ to investigate the effects of puppy farming on dog behavior. Appl Anim Behav Sci 2018; 206:75–86.

[57] Pirrone F, Pierantoni L, Pastorino GQ, et al. Owner-reported aggressive behavior towards familiar people may be a more prominent occurrence in pet shop-traded dogs. J Vet Behav 2016;11:13–7.

[58] Tiira K, Hakosalo O, Kareinen L, et al. Environmental effects on compulsive tail chasing in dogs. PLoS One 2012; 7:e41684.

[59] Zehle S, Bock J, Jezierski G, et al. Methylphenidate treatment recovers stress-induced elevated dendritic spine densities in the rodent dorsal anterior cingulate cortex. Dev Neurobiol 2007;67:1891–900.

[60] Van Boxelaere M, Clements J, Callaerts P, et al. Unpredictable chronic mild stress differentially impairs social and contextual discrimination learning in two inbred mouse strains. PLoS One 2017. https://doi.org/10.1371/journal.pone.0188537.

[61] Schoener J, Heinz A, Endres M, et al. Post-traumatic stress disorder and beyond: an overview of rodent stress models. J Cell Mol Med 2017;21:2248–56.

[62] Danek M, Danek J, Araszkiewic A. Large animals as potential models of human mental and behavioral disorders. Psychiatr Pol 2017;51:1009–27.

[63] Binder R, Arhant C, Affenzeller N, et al. Unterbringung von Hunden in Boxen und ähnlichen Unterkünften – Möglichkeiten und Grenzen der kurzfristigen Unterschreitung von tierschutzrechtlichen Mindestanforderungen. Wien Tierärztl Monatsschr 2020;107:8–68.

[64] Mazur J. Learning and behavior. Munich, Germany: Taylor & Francis publishers; 2016.

[65] Dorey N, Cox D. Function matters: a review of terminological differences in applied and basic clicker training research. Peer J 2018;6:e5621.

[66] McMillan F. Mental health and well-being in animals. 2nd edition. Oxford, UK: CABI; 2019.

[67] Hunter M, Rosales-Ruiz J. The power of one reinforcer: The effect of a single reinforcer in the context of shaping. J Exp Anal Behav 2019;111(3):449–64.

Advances in Small Animal Care 1 (2020) 25–33

ADVANCES IN SMALL ANIMAL CARE

Behavior and Medical Problems in Pet Animals

Jaume Fatjó, DVM, PhD, Dipl.ECAWBM-BM[a,*,1], Jonathan Bowen, BVetMed, MRCVS, DipAS(CABC)[b,1]

[a]Affinity Foundation Animals and Health, Universitat Autònoma de Barcelona, Barcelona Biomedical Research Park, C/ Drive Aiguader 88, Barcelona 08003, Spain; [b]Queen Mother Hospital for Small Animals, Royal Veterinary College, Hawkshead Lane, North Mymms, Hertfordshire AL9 7TA, UK

KEYWORDS

• Companion animal • Behavior problems • Physical health

KEY POINTS

- Physical and mental health are inseparable and combine to determine quality of life.
- The effect of physical health problems on behavior must always be integral to a behavioral assessment.
- Assessment should start with a full physical examination and a standard panel of hematology and biochemistry.
- Common conditions that affect behavior include pain, sickness behavior, epilepsy, and endocrine disease.
- Temperament and the physical and social environment strongly influence how a medical condition contributes to a behavior problem.

INTRODUCTION

Behavioral and physical health should not be considered as separate entities. Behavior is shaped and constrained by internal and external factors: temperament and health, and the physical and social environment [1]. Any change in these internal and external factors results in a change in behavior, sometimes with problematic results.

When considering the interaction between behavioral and medical factors, traditionally clinicians start from the perspective of the problem behavior, with a focus on ruling out the influence of concomitant medical factors. Until recently, veterinarians have considered behavior problems almost as diagnoses of exclusion. In reality, behavior is an output of the brain and body, and clinicians cannot totally rule out health influences, only take account of them; the management and treatment of physical health problems should be integral parts of behavioral therapy.

Likewise, rather than wait until behavior becomes problematic, it is better to consider the behavioral effects of any illness or treatment at the time of diagnosis, and to make recommendations as part of the normal management and treatment of that disease. For example, in the case of a polyphagic dog with diabetes mellitus, it should be normal to give advice to minimize risk of aggression around food; feeding the affected dog in a quiet location away from other pets and children reduces stress for the animal, and thereby reduces the hyperglycemic effects of cortisol, as well as preventing aggression.

This article considers behavioral and physical health as components of an integrated system that should be managed and treated holistically.

[1] These authors contributed equally to the article.

*Corresponding author, *E-mail address:* jaume.fatjo@uab.cat

https://doi.org/10.1016/j.yasa.2020.07.003
2666-4518/20/

MAKING AN INITIAL EVALUATION OF HEALTH IN BEHAVIOR CASES

The starting point before any behavioral assessment should be:

- A full physical examination
- A routine panel of hematology and biochemistry, including an evaluation by an experienced clinical pathologist
- A thorough review of the animal's medical history, including current and past health conditions, current and past drug treatments, supplements, nutraceuticals, and diets

Apart from this, clinicians should record a clinical impression of overall health. This impression takes into account the findings from the physical examination, blood tests, and medical history, as well as nonspecific health indicators such as body condition score, exercise tolerance, and demeanor. Health exists along a continuum between excellent and poor health, and the aim is to identify where on that continuum the individual is located; animals can be awarded a subjective score from 0 to 10, where 10 indicates that the animal has excellent physical health. This score should take into account past and recurrent episodes of illness, such as ear infections, diarrhea, or skin disease; a pet may currently be in good health, but a history of regular minor health problems bars it from having excellent health.

Unless the animal has excellent health, the clinician is then faced with some questions:

- The animal has existing health problems, but are they relevant to its current problem behavior?
- The animal is receiving medication, supplements, nutraceuticals, or a specialist diet, but are the effects, or adverse effects, of those biologic therapies relevant to its current problem behavior?
- The animal has no known health problems, but it does not have excellent health. What level of suspicion is there that the current problem behavior may be related to 1 or more undetected health problems?
- The animal has no known health problems, but it does not have excellent health. Is that a contributory factor to the current behavior, or an indication of other lifestyle factors that could be important?

Apart from the positive and negative effects of biologic therapies, there is increasing evidence about the influence of gut microbiome on behavior. A recent study linked the composition of the gut flora to interspecific aggression in shelter dogs [2]. Dietary evaluation should therefore form part of the assessment.

In addition, behavioral therapy can be challenging and stressful for an animal, so clinicians must decide whether lack of excellent health is a constraint on the planned treatment.

If it cannot be said that a pet has excellent health, for whatever reason, then this should raise the suspicion that health is at least a factor that contributes to the animal's behavior.

One of the main challenges is to decide the level of clinical investigation that is required in each case, to avoid performing costly and invasive tests for no reason. A useful set of indicators that suggest further analysis, or screening, for undiagnosed medical conditions could include [3]:

- In cases where it is difficult to establish a link between situational and environmental stimuli and the behavior of the animal.
- When the first signs of problem behavior are seen in an adulthood.
- If the patient is middle aged or older, it is more likely to have a physical condition.
- If a period of suboptimal health precedes the behavioral signs.
- If there are neurologic signs.
- If there are unexplained signs of weight loss.
- If there are heritable disorders in the animal's family, line, or breed.
- If there have been signs of changing level of consciousness or awareness, or other signs of mental impairment.
- If there are some physical signs that indicate serious physical disease (fever, abdominal swelling, edema, jaundice, and pain).
- If behavioral signs do not resolve, despite appropriate treatment.
- If there is evidence of generally worsening physical health (eg, exercise intolerance).

Once a basic medical examination and assessment have been conducted, this information could help the clinician to decide what additional medical tests could be helpful (Fig. 1).

THE INTERACTION BETWEEN MEDICAL AND BEHAVIORAL PROBLEMS

Behavior is simply 1 of the methods by which the individual seeks to establish an equilibrium between internals factors, such as health, and the environment. It is a single system, not 2 systems; physiology supports behavior, and behavior is a way to maintain physiologic homeostasis.

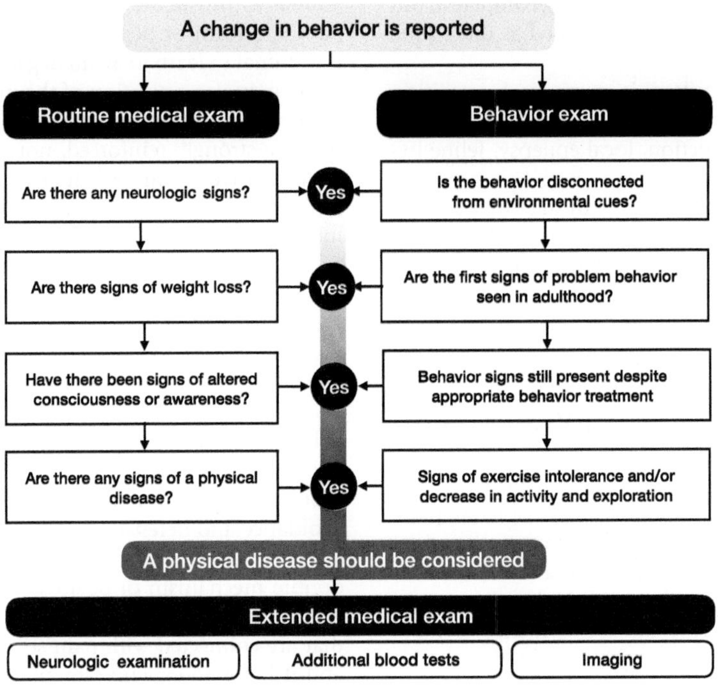

FIG. 1 During an initial physical and behavioral examination, certain features indicate a need for a more extended examination, imaging, or additional tests.

Disease-related behavior change can be seen as a sort of nonspecific collateral damage resulting from a system whose integrity has been affected (eg, a brain tumor), or an organized and purposeful way to improve the animal's response to a disorder (eg, social withdrawal and reduced activity during sickness, or defensiveness during pain). Most of the behavioral change that is seen in unwell animals is adaptive; it helps them to continue to function, or it helps them to recover. Lameness is a way to reduce load on a damaged limb to help it heal, and pain facilitates this adaptation.

Health problems can have deficit and productive effects on behavior [4]:

- Deficit effects are characterized by a decrease in certain behaviors, such as activity, alertness, social interaction, feeding, and play.
- Productive effects are characterized by an increase in the expression of behaviors that were previously expressed at a lower level, and the appearance of new behaviors that were previously absent. For example, aggression, elimination problems, and self-mutilation.

Health problems can alter the animal's response to its environment, including in the following ways:

- Altering motivation (eg, sickness behavior, painful conditions, altered hunger or thirst).
- Producing acute sensations that can alter behavior (eg, painful conditions, epilepsy).
- Causing functional impairment to sensory systems (eg, touch, vision, or hearing).
- Causing functional impairment to the central nervous system, leading to perceptual, emotional, or cognitive impairment (eg, brain tumor, cognitive dysfunction, epilepsy, hypothyroidism, or diabetes mellitus).

Of these, functional impairments and sensations that result from central nervous system disturbance (eg, seizures) can only be interpreted as damaging, and they have no benefit to the animal. However, motivational changes, such as those resulting from pain and sickness, can have a survival value even if they also lead to problem behavior. They represent normal, adaptive responses to change in priorities for the animal; for example, favoring self-defense rather than sociability.

In the clinical setting, there are 3 main ways in which behavioral problems and medical conditions are associated:

- A behavior problem is the presenting complaint, but a medical condition is later identified as one of the contributory factors.
- The presenting problem is a medical condition whose presenting signs are primarily behavioral (eg, cognitive dysfunction, focal epilepsy, feline hyperesthesia syndrome).
- The presenting problem is a medical condition that is linked to stress and certain behavioral risk factors. For example, in feline idiopathic cystitis, environmental stress and individual vulnerability are factors [5].

EXAMPLES OF MEDICAL PROBLEMS THAT INFLUENCE BEHAVIOR

The commonest health problems associated with behavioral alterations in animals and people are pain, sickness behavior, epilepsy, and endocrine dysfunction. For some of these, such as pain, the association with problem behavior is well established, whereas for others, such as endocrine disease, evidence is more mixed.

Pain

Pain can alter motivation and emotional estates, which results in a wide range of potential changes in behavior. It is a multidimensional phenomenon that includes perceptual, emotional, and learning-related components. For example, the afferent pathways of peripheral pain reach structures within the brain, such as the amygdala, that are deeply involved in the regulation of motivation and emotional states. In general, pain favors defensive and avoidance-related strategies to reduce loss and injury.

Common examples of adaptive changes in behavior to avoid or to reduce pain include:

- Altered gait to continue locomotion while experiencing reduced discomfort
- Aggression toward people and other animals to avoid petting-related pain
- In cases of tenesmus in cats, shifting the preferred location for defecation away from locations where the animal has previously experienced pain

Although these are all adaptive mechanisms from a biological point of view, they often result in behaviors that are perceived by the owner as problematic or inconvenient.

Avoidance-related behaviors are maintained and reinforced, and they help the individual to escape from negative experiences that are perceived by the animal as threatening. In these situations, relief from pain is a form of negative reinforcement that enables the animal to learn to avoid negative emotions. However, there is also activation of the mesolimbic dopamine pathways of reward; behaviors that help to reduce pain become strongly reinforced, not only as a way to prevent negative emotions but also because they help the individual to feel emotionally better (positive reinforcement) [6].

In positive reinforcement, the expression of a behavior consistently and repeatedly puts the animal in touch with the eliciting stimuli. If at some point the reward is no longer obtained, the behavior eventually disappears, through a process of extinction. However, in negative reinforcement, the expression of the behavior aims to prevent any future contact with the eliciting stimulus. Therefore, even after the external conditions have changed, the animal continues to perform avoidance and defensive behaviors because it lacks the stimulus contact that would permit extinction. This double mechanism of positive and negative reinforcement is what makes avoidance and defensive strategies that are connected with pain so resistant to extinction, and it helps to explain why pain-avoidance behaviors persist so long after the original pain has subsided.

Both chronic and acute pain have been studied as part of the development of pain assessment tools [7,8]. Pain is recognized as a factor in defensive behavior; for example, in a study of health-related quality of life of dogs with chronic pain [8], owners of dogs with chronic pain reported changes in multiple aspects of their dogs' behavior, including sociability, demeanor, attention seeking, aggression, anxiety/fearfulness, ability to rest, and compulsive behavior. More recently, an association between noise fear and orthopedic pain has been found [9].

Sickness Behavior

Sickness behavior can be defined as an organized and purposeful set of behaviors that have evolved to enable animals to conserve bodily resources while they recover from a pathologic state and to prevent disease transmission. Although the main characteristic of sickness behavior is an overall decrease in activity, it is not the result of a debilitated state. It is a phenomenon of motivational reorganization, as it is shown by the fact that it can be interrupted by salient and relevant stimuli.

From a physiologic perspective, sickness behavior is a cytokine-mediated motivational state linked to infection and inflammation that results in a reduction in activity, sociability, play, and exploratory behavior, and an increase in avoidance, social withdrawal, and sleep

[4]. Cytokines and sickness behavior have been associated with depression [10], and antiinflammatory drugs have been found to have beneficial effects on signs of depression when combined with antidepressant medication [11].

The impact of sickness behavior on adaptation and the human-animal bond could depend on the behavioral profile that existed before the illness. For instance, dogs showing high levels of excitability or aggressiveness might experience a paradoxic and transient amelioration, which often resumes after recovery.

Epilepsy

Psychiatric comorbidities, including mood, anxiety, and psychotic disorders, are common in people with epilepsy, and these comorbid conditions occur at rates that are 2-fold to 3-fold or higher than in the general population [12]. Focal seizures are the type that is most commonly associated with psychiatric problems. There is some evidence to support some of the same associations in veterinary patients. In a small study of abnormal behavior in bull terriers, Dodman and colleagues [13] found that tail chasing, irrational fear, and unprovoked aggression were associated with abnormal electroencephalogram results. A short case series identified paroxysmal episodes of acute fear and autonomic signs associated with focal seizures in Boerboel dogs [14], and in a survey of Groenendael and Tervueren dogs, 77.6% of those with epilepsy had focal seizures. In another study, owners reported that their dogs showed signs of depression up to several days before a seizure, and common behavioral signs associated with focal seizures included disorientation, attention seeking, and fearfulness [15]. In a retrospective study of behavioral changes associated with epilepsy, Shihab and colleagues [16] found that in drug-naive dogs' defensive aggression, fear and anxiety and abnormal perception were all increased after epilepsy. There was also a significant correlation between seizure frequency and score for defensive aggression.

Antiepileptic drugs can produce general changes in behavior, such as polyphagia and sedation. In the study by Shihab and colleagues [16], additional behavioral changes were found in treated dogs, including abnormal perception, abnormal reactivity, attachment disorder, demented behavior, and apathetic behavior. The difference in behavioral changes between treated and untreated dogs may reflect a difference in the severity of epilepsy, or a combination of epilepsy and iatrogenic, drug-related effects.

Endocrine Disease

In humans, there is a well-known association between endocrine disease and mental health problems [17], and the psychiatric manifestations of hypothyroidism were recognized as long ago as 1888. It is associated with depression, delusions and hallucinations, and cognitive impairment. A list of other psychiatric signs associated with endocrine disease in people is presented in Table 1.

Some of these are endocrine disorders that are common in both people and companion animals, but others, such as pheochromocytoma, are rare. Although the psychiatric comorbidity of these illnesses is well understood in human medicine, the same evidence is lacking in veterinary medicine.

Thyroid disease is common in companion animals and has been the focus of investigations into its effects on behavior. In 2002, Fatjó and colleagues [18] published a short case series of 4 dogs with aggression

TABLE 1
Psychiatric Signs Associated with Endocrine Disease in Human Patients

Endocrine Condition	Psychiatric Symptoms (Human)
Hyperadrenocorticism	Anxiety, panic disorders, irritability, mania, distress, mood disorders, depression
Type 1 diabetes	Depression, psychomotor agitation, insomnia, eating disorders
Type 2 diabetes	Depression, eating disorders
Hyperthyroidism	Anxiety, irritability, mania, psychosis, insomnia, attention and overactivity problems, depression, restlessness, fatigue, and delirium
Hypothyroidism	Delusions, hallucinations, attention deficits, and cognitive disturbances
Pheochromocytoma	Anxiety, panic disorders, tremulousness
Hypoparathyroidism	Depression
Androgens	Increased aggression, anger, acting out, dominant behavior, antisocial behavior

and hypothyroidism. In all 4 cases, aggressive signs reduced with thyroid supplementation. However, in a cross-sectional study, Radosta and colleagues [19] (2012) found no systematic relationship between aggression and thyroid hormones, and, in a randomized, double-blinded, placebo-controlled study of the effect of thyroid replacement therapy on aggressive dogs (owner directed) with suboptimal thyroid function, Dodman and colleagues [20] (2013) also did not find an effect. Hrovat and colleagues [21] (2019) tracked behavioral changes during levothyroxine therapy over 6 months in clinically hypothyroid dogs using the Canine Behavioral Assessment and Research Questionnaire (C-BARQ) questionnaire, and they found no change other than an increase in the score for the activity subscale. Taken as a whole, this suggests that, although clinical hypothyroidism is associated with behavioral disorder in individual cases, thyroid function does not have a predictably generalizable effect on aggression. Caution should be exercised with animals presented as having subclinical hypothyroidism (low-range but normal blood values plus nonspecific behavioral changes). Being one of the main hormones of metabolic regulation, thyroid hormone has effects on all cell types, including neurons in the central nervous system. Supplementation with thyroid hormones is therefore likely to affect behavior in all individuals, and this effect can therefore not be used as confirmation that an individual had a deficiency.

Hyperadrenocorticism is associated with a wide range of psychiatric signs in people, including emotional disorders and depression. Although this has not been studied in dogs, behavioral change is commonly identified as an early indicator of the disease. Synthetic antiinflammatory steroid preparations, such as prednisolone and dexamethasone, are widely prescribed in veterinary medicine. The iatrogenic effects of these preparations has been reported, and include reduced playfulness, increased fearfulness and restlessness, and aggression around food [22,23].

Other factors that influence the behavioral response to disease

Many dogs that are in pain never develop problems of aggression. Dogs with aggression problems often improve when their underlying pain is effectively treated, only for some to relapse when treatment fails, or is discontinued by the owner, or when the dog develops a new painful condition. The same can be said of many other health problems that influence behavior.

So, although increased defensiveness is a commonly identified characteristic of pain, there must be other factors that determine whether a particular individual shows problem behavior. These factors include traits, experience, and the physical and social environment.

THE INFLUENCE OF TRAITS

A trait can be defined as "a particular characteristic that can produce a particular type of behaviour" (Cambridge English dictionary). This definition is broad and includes temperamental traits, personality traits, coping styles, and other similar characteristics that have a pervasive, persistent influence on the typical responses of an individual.

Traits reflect relatively stable individual differences in cognitive, emotional, and regulatory aspects of behavior. They influence behavior by introducing a bias toward a particular kind of response to a situation. The nature and strength of that bias determine the effect that it has. An individual's behavioral traits can increase the likelihood of a particular problem, or they can reduce it.

Temperamental traits, such as anxiousness, impulsiveness, excitability, sociability, boldness, or assertiveness, are narrow in focus and probably closely related to neurobiological systems. They reflect underlying relatively stable individual differences in biological systems, which could be the target of biologic therapies, including drugs, synthetic pheromones, and dietary modification or supplementation. An example of this is the use of fluoxetine to treat problems of impulsive aggression in dogs; the dog's inability to withhold the aggressive response is the primary target of the drug [24].

Impulsive dogs experience the same emotional states and motivations as other dogs, but they have deficiencies in aspects of behavioral regulation (self-control) in their responses. Impulsiveness is a trait that can be measured through behavioral tests and scales, and it can be imagined that a very impulsive dog could respond differently to pain compared with a much less impulsive one. Part of the management of such a dog might include medication to reduce impulsiveness.

In both humans and dogs, high levels of arousal seem to impair top-down cognitive inhibition, which in turn has been linked to anxiety and impulse control. For example, in a study of the effects of arousal on inhibitory control, dogs scored worse for inhibitory control failure in a barrier detour task when they were excessively excited [25]. Therefore, excitability could be an underlying factor in a wide range of behavior problems through its impact on attention, cognition, and emotional intensity. Excitability has also recently been found to be associated with joint hypermobility in dogs, indicating that this trait may have a biological basis [26]. This behavioral trait therefore is linked to a physical condition, hip dysplasia, that is also likely to lead to pain.

Although there are fewer available tools for measuring behavioral traits, temperament, and personality in veterinary behavioral medicine than in human psychiatry, this is an area of active development. Examples include a scale developed to assess emotional predispositions in dogs (Positive and Negative Affect Schedule [PANAS]), a scale to assess attention and activity in dogs, and the wide range of battery tests designed to identify temperament traits related to aggression [27–29]. Although the C-BARQ is regarded by its creators as a data collection tool, it does include subscales that, individually or in combination, provide information about traits such as excitability, anxiety, and aggressiveness, and it has been used as the basis for several studies that have explored the biological basis of its subscales [26,30]. There are also battery tests, which are based on the dog's reaction to a limited series of single test events or situations [31,32], but these may be more indicative of state than trait.

THE INFLUENCE OF THE ENVIRONMENT (PHYSICAL AND SOCIAL)

Take the example of 2 small dogs, both with an anxious, impulsive, assertive, and defensive nature, and both with chronic back pain. They share the same temperamental and health characteristics to be high risk for owner-directed aggression when being handled. However, only 1 presents with an aggression problem; the dog that has always been allowed to get on the sofa, and has recently been repeatedly punished for growling when the owner goes to pick it up to get it off the sofa.

The same might be said for feline hyperesthesia (FHS) and interstitial cystitis (FIC), two recurrent episodic conditions with genetic risk factors, but that vary in severity and frequency of episodes according to physical and social environmental stressors. FIC is mostly connected with problems of inappropriate elimination, but it can be connected with other problems if the owner is confrontational or punitive. FHS can lead to owner-directed aggression and intercat aggression.

Apart from the amount of resources, such as food and resting places, that are available, there is also the matter of control over how those resources are accessed; for example, whether the animal is meal fed, fed on demand, or given ad libitum access to food. Meal frequency in cats may be around 12 times per day [33], so ad libitum access to food would be preferable to twice-daily meal feeding because it provides the cat with greater control. Control over access to places to hide from or avoid sources of fear, such as unfamiliar people or loud noises, may be particularly important.

Predictability of the environment is also important. In a laboratory study of the effects of unexpected environmental events (UEEs), including failure of light timers and temperature regulation, changes in caretaking personnel, intermittent loud noises, and movement of cats between rooms and cages, Stella and colleagues [34] (2011) found that cats that were exposed to UEEs (compared with control cats with a normal environmental schedule) were 9.3 times more likely not to eat or eliminate in a 24-hour period, 9.8 times more likely to defecate outside the litter box, and 1.6 times more likely to urinate outside the litter box. There were no differences in the level of environmental enrichment between the group with UEE and the group with a normal environmental schedule. In a similar controlled study by Carlstead and colleagues [35] (1993), cats that were exposed to a 21-day period of irregular feeding and cleaning times, absence of talking and petting by humans, and daily unpredictable manipulations showed significantly increased urinary cortisol levels, increased hiding and vigilance, and reduced exploratory behavior. This research suggests that, at least in cats, an unpredictable environment can, irrespective of the quality of the environment, lead to stress and problem behavior.

The owner is part of the animal's social environment as a source of security, a means of access to resources, and a source of stimulation. However, owners can also become a significant source of distress, as a consequence of how they interact with their pets. For instance, the use of punishment has been associated with a higher prevalence of behavior problems in dogs [36,37].

An owner's personality factors may influence the way the owner interacts with the dog [38]; for instance, extraverted owners tend to praise their dogs more. Owner personality and psychological factors seem to influence the expression of behavior problems in their pets. Personality traits such as neuroticism or emotional instability, as well as psychiatric conditions such as posttraumatic stress disorder, have been considered risk factors for dog behavior problems, including aggression and separation anxiety [37].

SUMMARY

This article discusses the many ways in which medical conditions can influence behavior and behavior problems. It also mentions the impact that adaptation and stress can have on physical health. This bidirectional relationship between physical health and behavior indicates that medical conditions can be seen as one of the fundamental dimensions of quality of life and well-being.

Quality of life is understood to be the product of the overall balance between positive and negative emotional states [39,40]. When the balance between positive and negative emotions is positive, quality of life can be said to be good. Quality of life is an essential objective in the treatment of both the physical and mental health of patients because it builds resilience against future physical and mental health problems.

Impaired physical health is considered to be a major contributing factor to a negative emotional balance, comparable with bad environmental conditions or improper handling. Therefore, veterinary care and preventive medicine should be seen as one of the cornerstones for a good quality of life. Veterinary intervention is particularly important in the management of chronic conditions, especially those with symptoms that could either go unnoticed or be ignored by the owner.

In general terms, the aim in behavioral therapy should be to produce a plan that takes into account environmental factors, temperamental factors, and health factors, so that there is an improvement in problem behavior along with an improvement in quality of life and well-being for the owner and for the animal. For animals with chronic, recurrent, or progressive health problems, this means that regular review and modification of the health management plan should be an integral part of behavioral therapy.

DISCLOSURE

The authors have nothing to disclose.

REFERENCES

[1] Fatjó J, Bowen J. Making the Case for Multi-Axis Assessment of Behavioural Problems. Animals (Basel) 2020; 10(3):383.
[2] Kirchoff NS, Udell M, Sharpton TJ. The gut microbiome correlates with conspecific aggression in a small population of rescued dogs (Canis familiaris). PeerJ 2019;7: e6103.
[3] Morrison J. When psychological problems mask medical disorders. New York: Guilford Press; 2015. p. 40.
[4] Fatjó J, Bowen JE. Medical and metabolic influences on behavioural disorders. In: Horwitz DF, Mills DS, editors. BSAVA manual of canine and feline behavioural medicine. 2nd edition. Gloucester (United Kingdom): BSAVA; 2009. p. 1–9.
[5] Lund HS, Saevik BK, Oystein WF, et al. Risk factors for idiopathic cystitis in Norwegian cats: a matched case-control study. J Feline Med Surg 2019;18(6): 483–91.
[6] Navratilova E, Xie JY, Okun A, et al. Pain relief produces negative reinforcement through activation of mesolimbic reward-valuation circuitry. PNAS 2012;109(50): 20709–13.
[7] Holton L, Reid J, Scott EM, et al. Development of a behaviour-based scale to measure acute pain in dogs. Vet Rec 2001;148(17):525–31.
[8] Wiseman-Orr ML, Nolan AM, Reid J, et al. Development of a questionnaire to measure the effects of chronic pain on health-related quality of life in dogs. Am J Vet Res 2004;65(8):1077–84.
[9] Fagundes ALL, Hewison L, McPeake KJ, et al. Noise Sensitivities in Dogs: An Exploration of Signs in Dogs with and without Musculoskeletal Pain Using Qualitative Content Analysis. Front Vet Sci 2018;5:17.
[10] Danzer R. Cytokines, sickness behavior, and depression. Immunol Allergy Clin North Am 2009;29(2):247–64.
[11] Müller N, Schwarz MJ, Dehning S, et al. The cyclooxygenase-2 inhibitor celecoxib has therapeutic effects in major depression: results of a double-blind, randomized, placebo controlled, add-on pilot study to reboxetine. Nat Mol Psychiatry 2006;11:680–4.
[12] Josephson CB, Jetté N. Psychiatric comorbidities in epilepsy. Int Rev Psychiatry 2017;29(5):409–24.
[13] Dodman NH, Knowles KE, Shuster L, et al. Behavioral changes associated with suspected complex partial seizures in bull terriers. J Am Vet Med Assoc 1996;208(5): 688-091.
[14] Stassen QEM, Grinwis GCM, van Rhijn NC, et al. Focal epilepsy with fear-related behavior as primary presentation in Boerboel dogs. J Vet Intern Med 2019;33: 694–700.
[15] Berendt M, Gulløv CH, Christensen SLK, et al. Prevalence and characteristics of epilepsy in the Belgian shepherd variants Groenendael and Tervueren born in Denmark 1995–2004. Acta Vet Scand 2008;22:50–1.
[16] Shihab N, Bowen J, Volk HA. Behavioral changes in dogs associated with the development of idiopathic epilepsy. Epilepsy Behav 2011;21:160–7.
[17] Conner SH, Solomon SS. Psychiatric Manifestations of Endocrine Disorders. J Hum Endocrinol 2017;1:007.
[18] Fatjó J, Stub C, Manteca X. Four cases of aggression and hypothyroidism in dogs. Vet Rec 2002;151:547–8.
[19] Radosta LA, Shofer FS, Reisner IR. Comparison of thyroid analytes in dogs aggressive to familiar people and in non-aggressive dogs. Vet J 2012;192(3):472–5.
[20] Dodman NH, Aronson L, Cottam N, et al. The effect of thyroid replacement in dogs with suboptimal thyroid function on owner-directed aggression: A randomized, double-blind, placebo-controlled clinical trial. J Vet Behav 2013;8:225–30.

[21] Hrovat A, De Keuster T, Kooistra HS, et al. Behavior in dogs with spontaneous hypothyroidism during treatment with levothyroxine. J Vet Intern Med 2019;(33): 64–71.

[22] Notari L, Burman O, Mills D. Behavioural changes in dogs treated with corticosteroids. Physiol Behav 2015; 1(151):609–16.

[23] Notari L, Burman O, Mills D. Is there a link between treatments with exogenous corticosteroids and dog behaviour problems? Vet Rec 2016;179(18):462.

[24] Rosado B, García-Belenguer S, León M, et al. Effect of fluoxetine on blood concentrations of serotonin, cortisol and dehydroepiandrosterone in canine aggression. J Vet Pharmacol Ther 2011;34(3):430–6.

[25] Bray EE, MacLean EL, Hare BA. Increasing arousal enhances inhibitory control in calm but not excitable dogs. Anim Cogn 2015. https://doi.org/10.1007/s10071-015-0901-1.

[26] Bowen J, Fatjó J, Serpell JA, et al. First evidence for an association between joint hypermobility and excitability in a non-human species, the domestic dog. Sci Rep 2019;9: 8629.

[27] Vas J, Topál J, Péch E, et al. Measuring attention deficit and activity in dogs: A new application and validation of a human ADHD questionnaire. Appl Anim Behav Sci 2007;103(1–2):105–17.

[28] Sheppard G, Mills DS. The development of a psychometric scale for the evaluation of the emotional predispositions of pet dogs. Int J Comp Psychol 2002;15: 201–22.

[29] Patronek GJ, Bradley J. No Better Than Flipping a Coin: Reconsidering Canine Behavior Evaluations in Animal Shelters. J Vet Behav 2016;15:66–77.

[30] Liinamo A, van den Berg L, Leegwater PAJ, et al. Genetic variation in aggression-related traits in Golden Retriever dogs. Appl Anim Behav Sci 2006;104:95–106.

[31] Miklosi A. The organisation of individual behaviour. In: Dog behaviour, evolution, and cognition. Oxford (United Kingdom): Oxford University Press; 2015. p. 324–45.

[32] Wiener P, Haskell MJ. Use of questionnaire-based data to assess dog personality. J Vet Behav 2016;16:81–5.

[33] Houpt KA. Domestic animal behavior. Ames (IO): Iowa State University Press; 2018. p. 307.

[34] Stella JL, Lord LK, Buffington CA. Sickness behaviours in response to unusual external events in healthy cats and cats with FIC. J Am Vet Med Assoc 2011;238(1):67–73.

[35] Carlstead K, Brown J, Strawn W. Behavioural & physical correlates of stress in laboratory cats. Appl Anim Behav Sci 1993;38(2):143–58.

[36] Hiby EF, Rooney NJ, Bradshaw JWS. Dog training methods: Their use, effectiveness and interaction with behaviour and welfare. Anim Welf 2004;13:63–9.

[37] Dodman NH, Brown DC, Serpell JA. Associations between owner personality and psychological status and the prevalence of canine behavior problems. PLoS One 2018;13(2):e0192846.

[38] Kis A, Turcsán B, Miklósi A, et al. The effect of the owner's personality on the behaviour of owner-dog dyads. Interact Stud 2012;13(3). https://doi.org/10.1075/is.13.3.03kis.

[39] McMillan FD. Quality of life in animals. J Am Vet Med Assoc 2000;216(12):1904–10.

[40] Mellor DJ. Updating Animal Welfare Thinking: Moving beyond the "Five Freedoms" towards "A Life Worth Living". Animals (Basel) 2016;6(3):21.

Diagnostic Imaging

Advances in Small Animal Care 1 (2020) 35–47
ADVANCES IN SMALL ANIMAL CARE

Whole-Body Computed Tomography Imaging in Cancer Staging

Francesco Collivignarelli, DVM, Francesca Del Signore, DVM, Francesco Simeoni, DVM*, Roberto Tamburro, DVM, PhD, Ilaria Falerno, DVM, Massimo Vignoli, DVM, PhD, Dipl. ECVDI
Faculty of Veterinary Medicine, University of Teramo, SP 18, Teramo 64100, Italy

KEYWORDS
• Computed tomography • Whole body • Cancer • Staging • Dog • Cat

KEY POINTS

- Whole-body computed tomography (WBCT) is a diagnostic tool that rapidly provides detailed information of the body.
- This technique is applied in veterinary medicine to fully characterize lesions in dogs and cats with polytrauma.
- In oncology, WBCT is of paramount importance to assess for the presence of metastasis, in particular in pulmonary and muscular locations.
- WBCT is recommended for the staging of oncology patients, especially for primary tumors characterized by high metastatic rate.

INTRODUCTION

Whole-body computed tomography (WBCT) is an imaging examination that provides a detailed view of the entire body and, for that reason, it is mainly applied to assess trauma or oncologic conditions in human and veterinary medicine. Particularly in human medicine, mortality and disability-adjusted life-years attributable to blunt multiple traumas have increased in the past decades, increasing the need for prompt diagnosis and management in industrialized countries [1]. WBCT is particularly useful for patients with polytrauma because it allows quick and early diagnosis of injury and improves survival rates [2–5]. However, WBCT diagnosis as standard of care is still under debate, because of the risk of developing cancer after long-term radiation exposure, expense, and limited access to unstable patients [6–10]. Recent studies have shown that radiation reduction with low-dose protocols does not lead to underestimating lesions in traumatized patients [11–15].

At present, WBCT is considered a useful tool in veterinary medicine to assess traumatic injuries in small animal patients. This technique provides the prompt detection of pneumothorax, and pleural and peritoneal fluid, thus permitting a complete evaluation of trauma-based injuries.

Alongside the use of WBCT for assessment of trauma, this technique is useful in oncology, in particular if applied to cancer staging.

Accurate and detailed tumor staging is essential in cancer management, to provide optimal therapeutic options and a more accurate prognosis in both human and veterinary medicine. The development of advanced diagnostic tools capable of scanning the whole body, such as WBCT, has proved to be an important tool to diagnose, stage, and manage malignancies [16]. In veterinary medicine, 3-view thoracic radiography and abdominal ultrasonography are conventionally performed to detect pulmonary and visceral metastasis [17–19], but, with the improvement of more advanced

*Corresponding author, *E-mail address:* fsimeoni@unite.it

https://doi.org/10.1016/j.yasa.2020.07.004
2666-4518/20/

tools, such as WBCT, a thorough staging of patients with cancer can now be performed to obtain more detailed information to characterize neoplastic conditions.

With computed tomography (CT) scanners, images are acquired in slices, and the superimposition of structures is eliminated [20]. Although CT has decreased spatial resolution compared with radiographs, the reduced anatomic superimposition and superior contrast resolution result in CT being more sensitive to detect lesions throughout the body [20,21]. To perform an optimal WBCT examination, slice thickness should be between 1.25 and 2.5 mm depending on the patient's size. Thin-slice imaging is more challenging on older scanners, because the heat load on the x-ray tube can slow the scanning time. Newer-generation CT scanners, particularly multislice helical scanners, have largely overcome this limitation by allowing faster examination for larger areas, also reducing slice thickness. This aspect deserves particular consideration, because it affects both image noise and partial volume averaging artifacts.

Partial volume averaging can result in indistinct margins, false attenuation measurements, and the appearance of pseudolesions. Thin-slice images have increased noise, which can be offset by increasing the milliampere setting. This increase improves image quality but also increases the radiation dose to the patient. The scan field of view (SFOV) is the area from which the image can be reconstructed. Because the reconstruction matrix size is constant, keeping the SFOV sized to the anatomy to be imaged improves spatial resolution. Multiplanar reformatting (MPR) or three-dimensional reformatting of images can provide more complete assessment [20].

Dogs and cats are usually under general anesthesia during the WBCT examination. With the increasing availability of faster multislice scanners, more CT examinations are being performed with sedation alone.

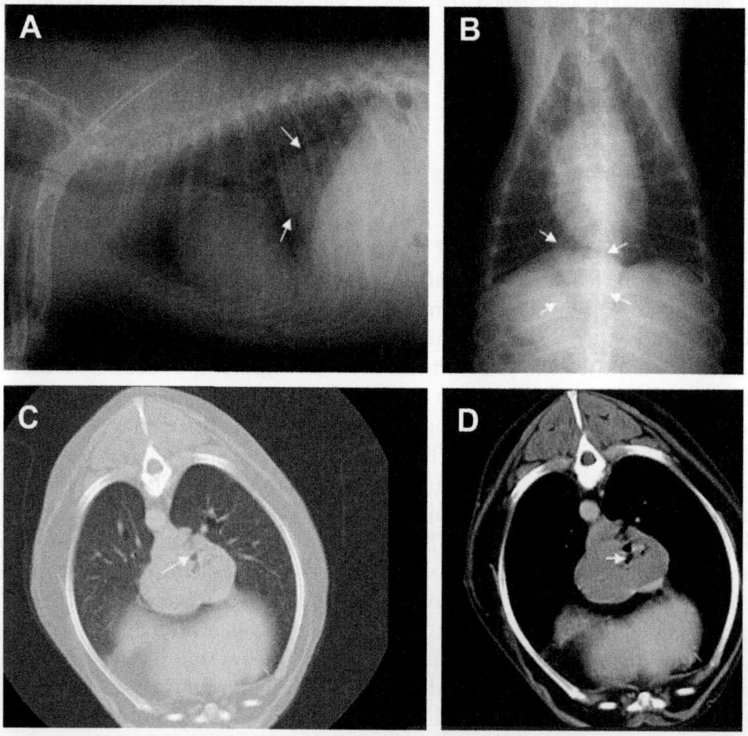

FIG. 1 **(A, B)** Thoracic radiographs of a 9-year-old spayed female mixed-breed dog. A soft tissue opaque mass is visible in the area of the caudal mediastinum along midline (*arrows*). Masses in this location can be difficult to localize in the lung or the mediastinum. **(C, D)** Transverse CT images of the same dog, in respective lung and postcontrast soft tissue windows, detail algorithm, showed internal air bronchograms (*arrows*), indicating the mass is pulmonary in origin and located in the accessory lung lobe (**C, D**). This mass was subsequently diagnosed as a carcinoma.

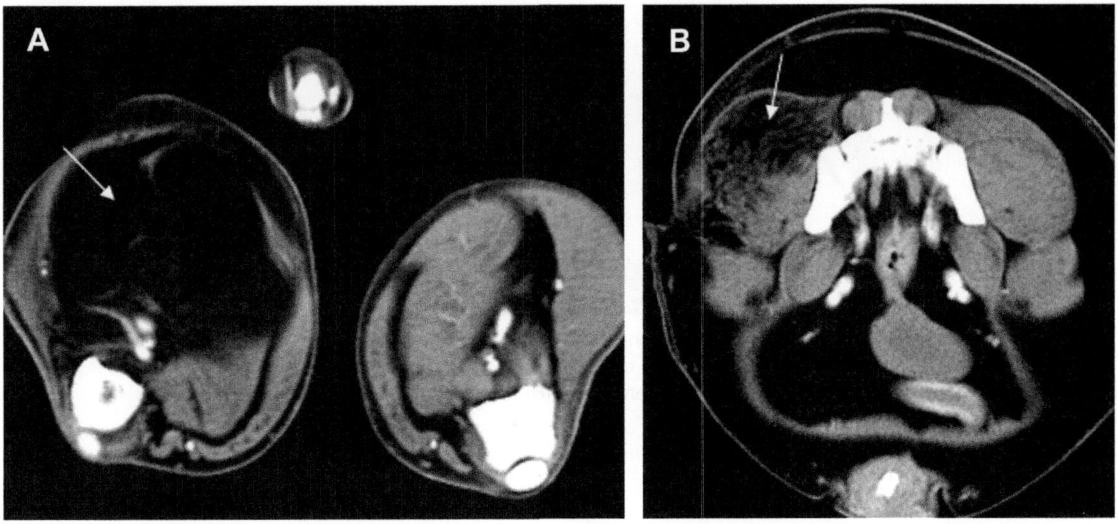

FIG. 2 Transverse CT images of the pelvic limbs postcontrast soft tissue window and algorithm. (**A**) Fat tissue attenuation mass is present in the caudal aspect of the right pelvic limb (*arrow*). Normal musculature in the left limb. (**B**) Scanning more cranially, fat tissue infiltrating the gluteal muscles is visible (*arrow*). Final diagnosis was an infiltrative lipoma.

However, it is the authors' opinion that this tool can be useful in emergency cases rather than in oncology.

WBCT imaging is discussed here, with a specific focus on the application of WBCT in small animal oncology. The current literature is discussed, this technique is described, and conditions are highlighted for which WBCT improves diagnosis and staging of neoplastic disorders in companion animals.

WHOLE-BODY COMPUTED TOMOGRAPHY TECHNIQUE

- After the patient has been anesthetized, placement in sternal recumbency is preferred, possibly with the aid of special foam cradles for optimal placement. To avoid imaging respiratory motion artifacts, patients may be manually hyperventilated just before slice acquisition to optimize lung visualization by

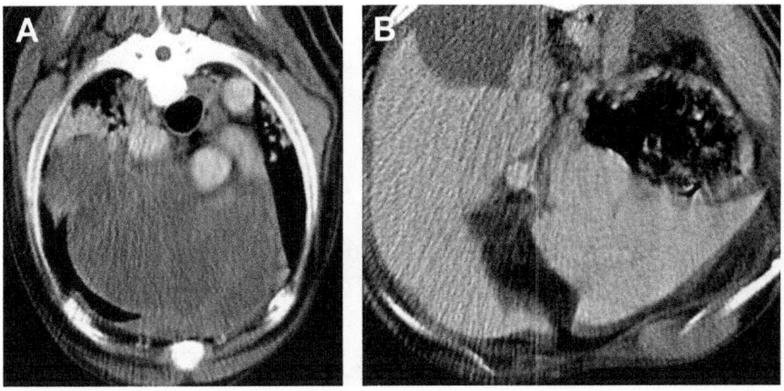

FIG. 3 An 8-year-old male Labrador retriever who underwent a CT scan for a mediastinal mass. Transverse CT image postcontrast with soft tissue window and algorithm (**A**) shows a large mediastinal soft tissue attenuation mass, with secondary dorsal displacement of the trachea, esophagus, vessels, and partial lung collapse. More caudally there was a second, smaller mass in the ventral left thoracic wall, involving a rib (**B**). The mediastinal mass was diagnosed as a thymoma, whereas the thoracic wall mass was a mastocytoma.

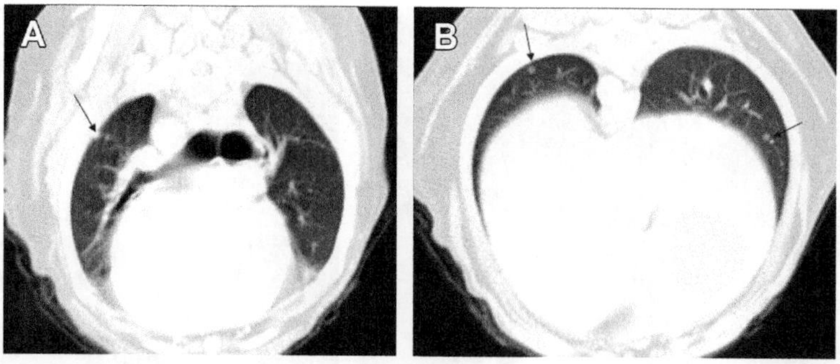

FIG. 4 A 12-year-old male Pomeranian dog underwent WBCT after a pancreatic mass was diagnosed via ultrasonography. Transverse CT images of the caudal thorax with lung window and medium algorithm highlighted several subpleural (*A*) and intraparenchymal (*B*) millimetric lung nodules (*arrows*).

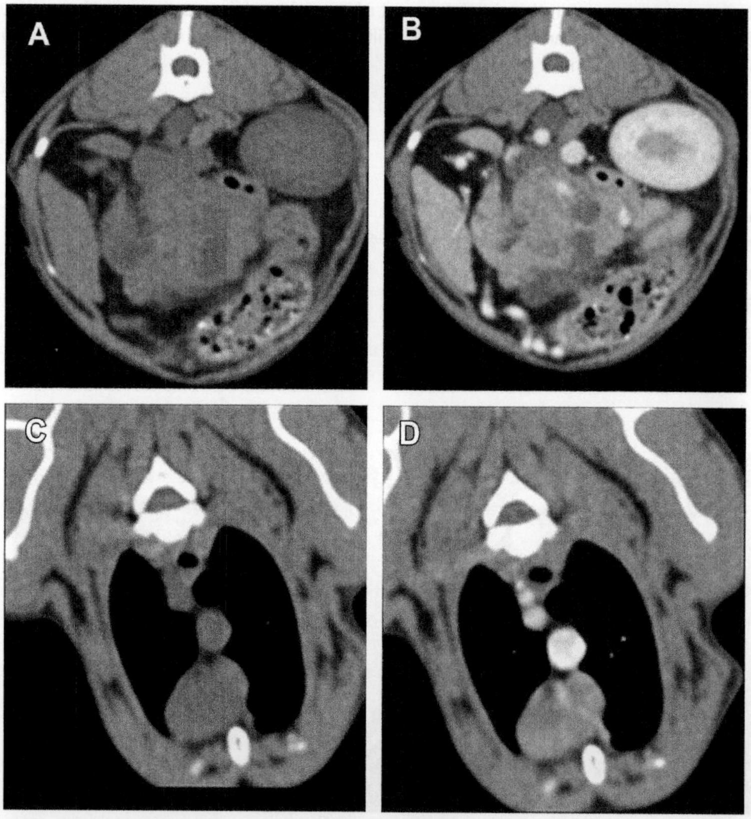

FIG. 5 A 12-year-old male castrated domestic shorthair cat with a pancreatic mass, cytologically diagnosed as pancreatic carcinoma. Transverse precontrast and postcontrast CT images with soft tissue window and algorithm reveal the pancreatic multicystic and heterogeneously contrast-enhancing mass (**A, B**), and sternal lymphadenomegaly. An enlarged heterogeneously contrast-enhancing sternal lymph node is present (**C, D**), cytologically confirmed as metastatic after ultrasonography-guided aspiration.

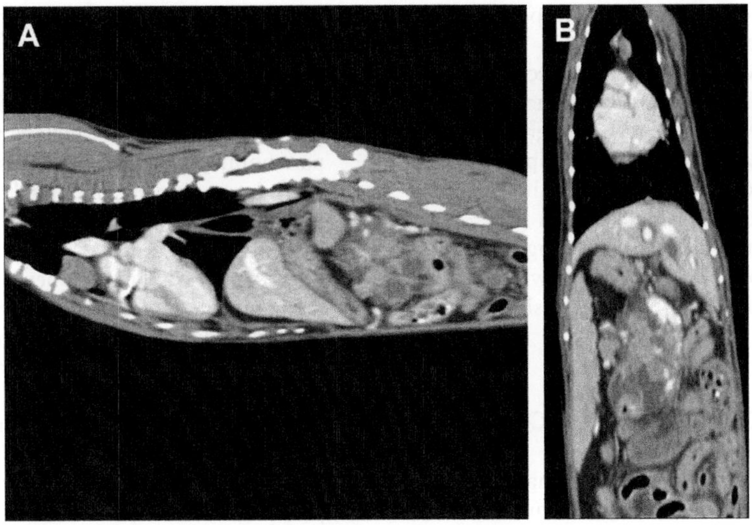

FIG. 6 Same cat as in Fig. 5. The postcontrast MPR images in sagittal (**A**) and dorsal (**B**) planes show the pancreatic mass and a sternal enlarged lymph node.

reducing any areas of atelectasis caused by anesthesia [21].

- Routinely, precontrast and postcontrast medium images are acquired. Nonionic water-soluble iodinated positive contrast medium administered at a dose of 2 mL/kg (600 mg of iodine per kilogram), injected into a peripheral vein, is routinely used to assess contrast enhancement of tissues.
- Contrast administration is crucial in WBCT for oncological staging to assess tumor vascularity, perfusion, and invasion into adjacent tissues. It is possible to perform a specific vascular assessment of arterial and early and delayed venous phase in masses and organs through triple-phase CT angiography (CTA): a single bolus injection facilitates imaging during the phase of preferential arterial enhancement (ie,

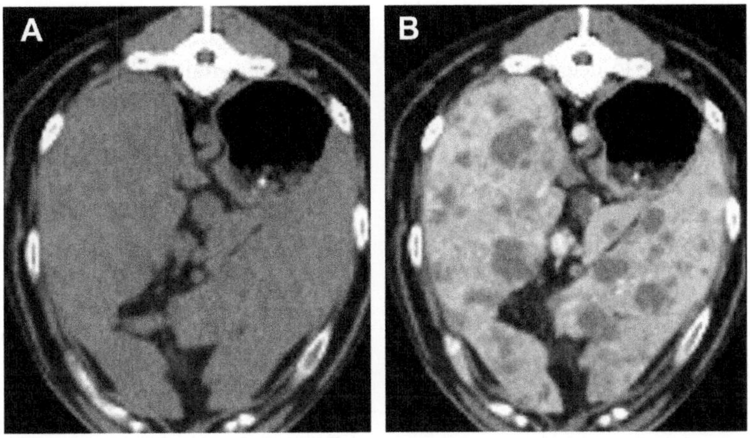

FIG. 7 A 6-year-old spayed female Czechoslovakian wolf with liver metastases from splenic hemangiosarcoma. Transverse CT images at the level of the liver precontrast and postcontrast with soft tissue window and algorithm. (**A**) Precontrast study showed mild heterogeneous liver parenchyma. (**B**) Postcontrast study highlighted multiple hypoattenuating nodules not previously visible.

the arterial phase), followed by the portal venous phase and delayed phase [22].

- Triple-phase CTA can improve the detection of small tumors, such as insulinoma and cardiac masses, and may help differentiate between benign and malignant lesions [23,24]. MPR can be helpful to better define lesions and may assist in predicting the malignancy of hepatic and splenic masses [24,25]. CT-guided biopsy is useful for the sampling of intracavitary lesions or pulmonary nodules, which are not readily identified or accessible with ultrasonography.

WHOLE-BODY COMPUTED TOMOGRAPHY ONCOLOGIC STAGING

- WBCT is an efficient and thorough imaging modality for the evaluation of multiple organs and structures. In oncology, WBCT is of paramount importance to assess (1) the correct localization of the tumor (Fig. 1), (2) its extension with or noninvolvement of the surrounding tissues/organs (Fig. 2), (3) concomitant diseases (Fig. 3), (4) metastatic lesions, and (5) follow-up after treatment. Specific structures evaluated on WBCT are discussed in more detail later.

THORAX EVALUATION

- CT imaging provides superior sensitivity in the identification of primary lung, mediastinal, heart base, and pleural tumors, and in assessment of pulmonary metastasis [26–30]. Because lesion identification with CT depends on the difference in Hounsfield units between lesions and their surroundings, with this technique it is possible to detect metastases as small as 1 mm in diameter (Fig. 4).
- CT allows detection of more lesions compared with conventional radiographs, so this technique is more sensitive in detecting pulmonary nodules [31].

LYMPH NODE EVALUATION

- Another important assessment is the cancer staging of lymph nodes for the evaluation of metastasis [32]. A study described lymph node findings using WBCT in cancer staging and found that lymphadenomegaly was commonly detected, thus alerting the clinicians to potential tumor spread [16].
- Enlarged lymph nodes may appear as oval to round soft tissue structures of homogeneous or heterogeneous attenuation and contrast enhancement. The pattern of tumor spread to regional or distant lymph nodes depends on the tumor type.
- Tracheobronchial lymph node enlargement is considered a prognostic factor for dogs with a primary lung tumor, thus making this information of paramount importance for clinicians to stage and formulate treatment planning [27].
- Sternal lymph node chain evaluation is important in cancer staging, because these nodes may drain either the thorax or cranial abdomen, including mammary tissue and dermal structures [16]. In particular, in human medicine, sternal and parasternal lymph nodes are staged in breast carcinoma, and, if enlarged, they represent metastasis to the internal mammary lymphatic chain, thus conferring poor prognosis for survival [33] Thorough evaluation of these nodes is of paramount importance with CT examinations [34] (Figs. 5 and 6).
- A recent retrospective study reported the usefulness of WBCT in the staging of gastric tumors in dogs [35,36]. The morphologic and contrast uptake parameters of primary gastric neoplasia and regional or peripheral lymph node involvement using dual-phase contrast WBCT in 16 dogs were evaluated. The dogs included were affected by adenocarcinoma, lymphoma, inflammatory polyps, and leiomyomas. Lymphadenopathy was regional in dogs affected by gastric adenocarcinoma, widespread in lymphomas, and not detected in leiomyomas. Also, lymph nodes measurements were reported to be larger in dogs with lymphomas than in dogs with adenocarcinomas [35].
- Definitive diagnosis of lymph node disorders is routinely performed with cytologic or histopathologic samples [32,37], but lymphatic draining patterns of certain type of tumors (eg, oral malignant melanoma or mast cell tumor) can diverge from the expected regional lymph node [38–40].
- In human medicine, the technique of sentinel lymph node mapping has been proved to be useful in cancer staging, considering the sentinel lymph node as the one receiving direct drainage from the tumor site [41,42]; in veterinary medicine, this technique is presently being investigated, with encouraging results and more detailed knowledge about the exact tumor lymphatic drainage [43,44].

LIVER EVALUATION

- Liver evaluation is crucial, not only for primary malignancies but also for potential metastatic spread from other primary tumors (Fig. 7). CT evaluation of the canine liver in both primary and metastatic hepatic neoplasm is reported in several studies describing the CT characteristics of liver masses [22,45,46]. Triple-phase CTA technique was used to evaluate the arterial, venous, and delayed phases to assess tumor type [22,45].

- Studies have compared hepatocellular carcinomas and nodular hyperplasia enhancement patterns and found that carcinomas had heterogeneous, marginal, or central arterial contrast enhancement and hypoattenuation in the later phases, whereas nodular hyperplasia had a diffuse enhancement pattern in the arterial phase and was isoattenuating in the delayed phase.
- Liver metastatic lesions were reported to be hypoattenuating in both arterial and delayed phases [22].

SPLEEN EVALUATION

- Another finding that can be detected with WBCT is splenomegaly, possibly caused by neoplasia, such as hemangiosarcoma, lymphoma, and mast cell tumor [16,47]. Standard precontrast and postcontrast CT findings are less specific in solid splenic masses, such as hematoma, nodular hyperplasia, hemangiosarcoma, and undifferentiated sarcoma in dogs.
- Three-phase CTA of splenic masses found nodular hyperplasia to have homogeneous normal enhancement pattern in all phases; hemangiosarcoma was characterized by 2 contrast enhancement patterns (a heterogeneous remarkable enhancement pattern in the arterial and portal venous phases and a homogeneous poor enhancement pattern in all phases) and, in addition, a heterogeneous normal enhancement pattern was detected

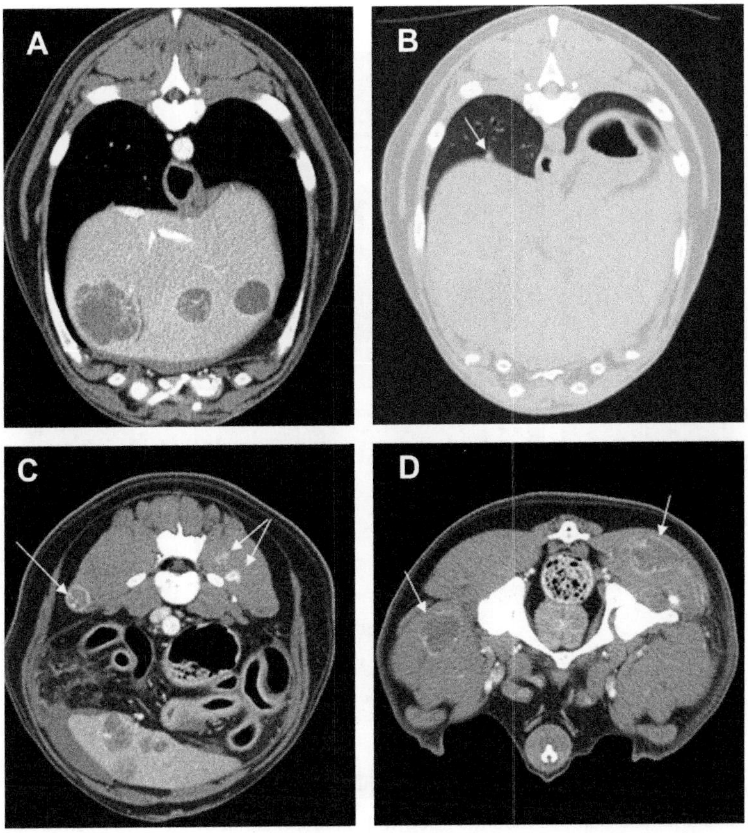

FIG. 8 A 7-year-old male boxer with a ruptured splenic hemangiosarcoma. Transverse CT images in multiple areas of the body. (**A**) Three hypoattenuating lesions are visible in the liver in the postcontrast study with soft tissue window and algorithm. (**B**) Lung window shows a small pulmonary nodule visible in the right caudal lung lobe (*arrow*). (**C, D**) several ring-enhancing (*arrows*) muscular nodules are visible in the epaxial, gluteal, and pelvic limb muscles. In (**C**), splenic nodules and free abdominal fluid are present.

in cases of hematoma and undifferentiated sarcoma [25] (Fig. 8D).

- When CT is used to stage multicentric lymphoma in dogs, in particular, the spleen and liver may appear normal or, when present, abnormalities are not pathognomonic for lymphoma. Fine-needle aspiration of the spleen and liver is recommended when using CT to stage dogs with multicentric lymphoma [48].
- Anesthetic drugs, in particular propofol, can also cause splenomegaly [49]. It has been suggested to minimize splenomegaly by using protocols that avoid drugs that could cause such effects and to combine spleen fine-needle aspiration or biopsy when the use of propofol cannot be avoided and splenomegaly is observed with CT scans [16].

MUSCULAR AND CARDIAC EVALUATION

- WBCT is also useful in cancer staging to detect muscular and cardiac metastasis, especially in primary tumors characterized by a high metastatic rate. Skeletal and cardiac musculature has been described in the literature as a rare metastatic target and this metastasis behavior is not completely understood. Inhibition of tumor cell proliferation by lactic acid, proteinase, and low pH in muscles are considered to be the most plausible reasons [50–53].
- In human medicine, cancers characterized by muscle metastasis are typically breast cancer, gastrointestinal adenocarcinoma, pulmonary adenocarcinoma, squamous cell carcinoma, and renal carcinoma [50,54–59]. In veterinary medicine, previous reports described muscle metastasis in pulmonary, mammary, and prostatic carcinoma, lymphoma, and

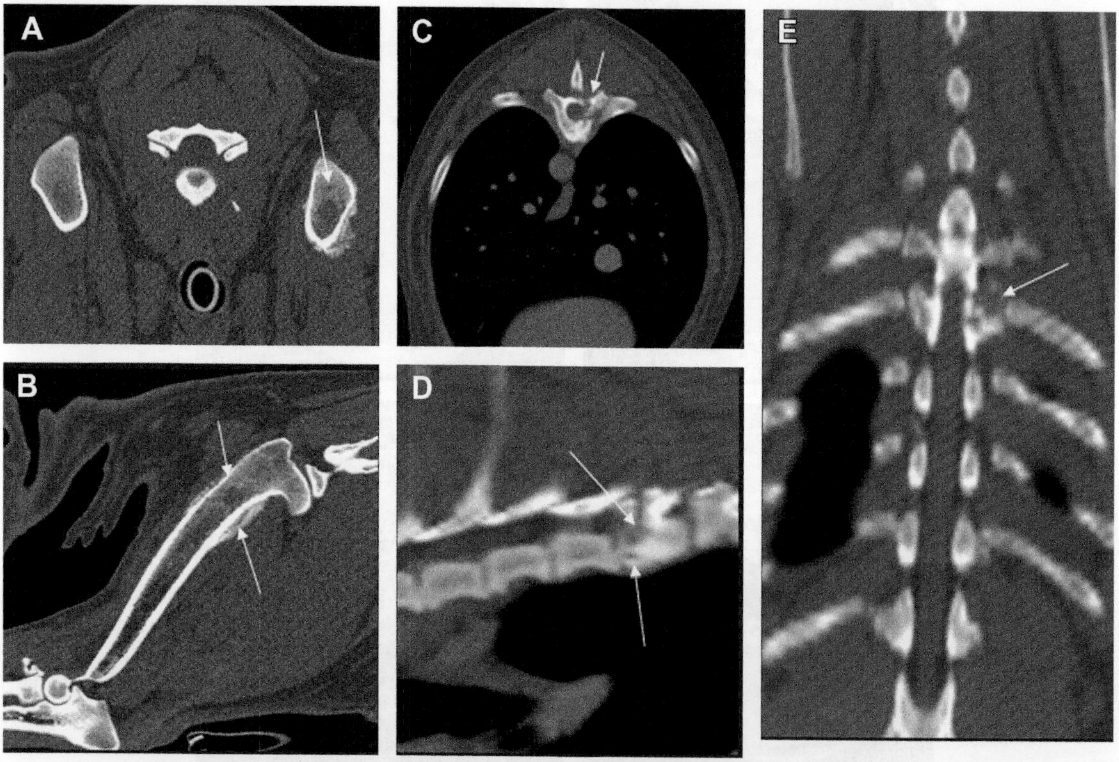

FIG. 9 A 4-year-old female Bernese mountain dog with osteosarcoma of the left proximal humerus. Bone window (**A–E**), bone algorithm (**A, B**), and soft tissue algorithm (**C–E**). (**A, B**) The transverse and sagittal MPR images, respectively, of the humeral lesion, with a mixed pattern of moth-eaten bone lysis and adjacent periosteal reaction (*arrows*). (**C**) Transverse view at the level of the eighth thoracic vertebra, where a lytic lesion of the left pedicle and lamina, and mixed bone lysis and sclerosis in the body, are visible (*arrow*). The vertebral lesion in sagittal (**D**) and dorsal (**E**) MPR reconstructions (*arrows*).

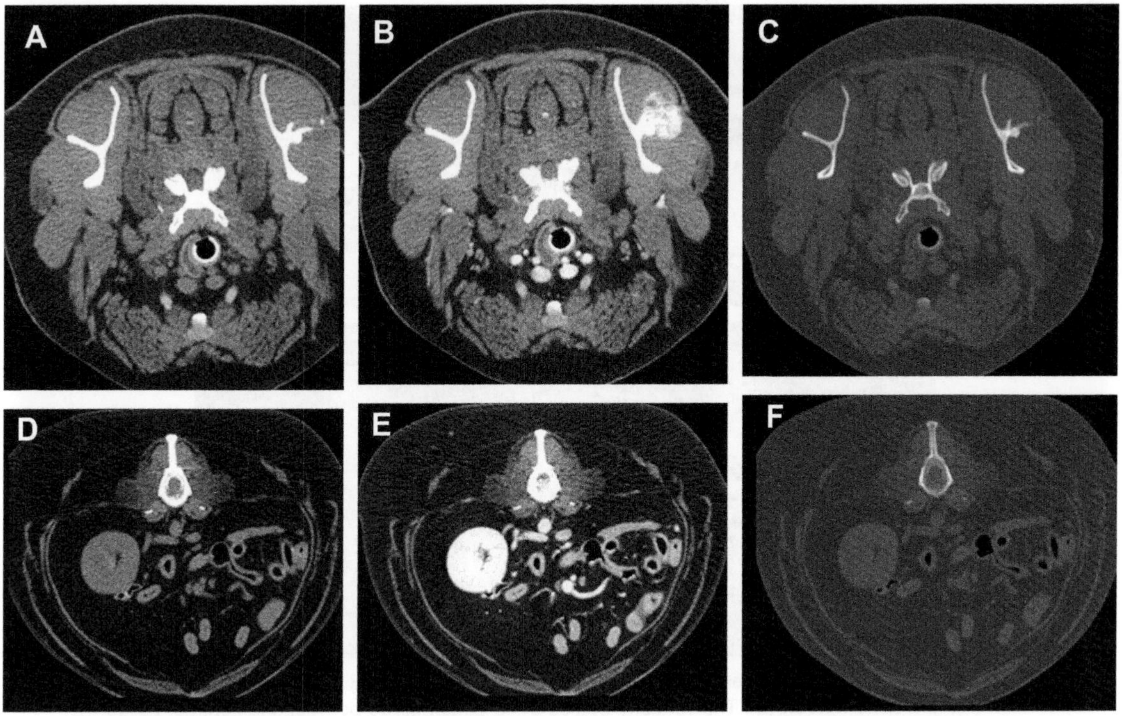

FIG. 10 An 8-year-old female spayed Rottweiler, 6 months after splenectomy for hemangiosarcoma. Transverse CT images, soft tissue algorithm, with precontrast (**A, D**) and postcontrast (**B, E**) soft tissue window. (**C, F**) Bone windows. The WBCT study showed multiple bone lysis, especially in the left scapula, with marked surrounding soft tissue enhancement (**A–C**), and lysis in several lumbar vertebrae, with vertebral canal invasion visible as contrast-enhanced tissue (**D–F**).

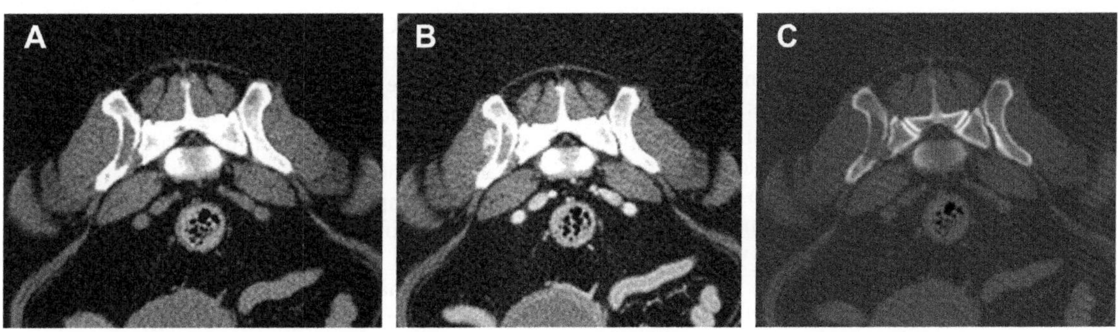

FIG. 11 Same dog as in Fig. 10. Transverse CT images, soft tissue algorithm, precontrast (**A**) and postcontrast (**B**) soft tissue window and bone window (**C**) of the pelvis. The lysis of the right ileum and sacrum is visible as well as the surrounding soft tissue contrast enhancement.

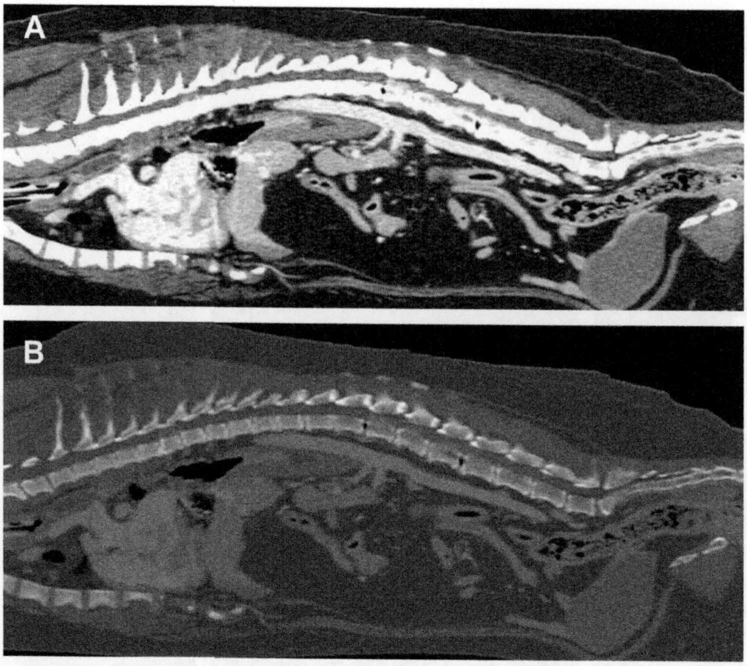

FIG. 12 Same dog as in Figs. 10 and 11. Soft tissue algorithm, sagittal MPR of the postcontrast soft tissue window (**A**), and bone window (**B**). The vertebral bodies L1 to L3 appear to be lytic, and contrast tissue enhancement is present in the vertebral canal. At the level of the intervertebral discs T13 to L1 and L3 to L4, gas is visible, representing a vacuum phenomenon secondary to disc degeneration.

mast cell tumors, with cardiac muscle metastasis described as originating from carcinoma, lymphoma, and hemangiosarcoma [60–63].

- Until CT was used to detect muscle metastasis, these metastases were detected either with necropsy or with biopsy [60–62] Studies have highlighted the importance of WBCT to visualize muscle metastasis in different kinds of neoplasia (mainly hemangiosarcoma and adenocarcinoma in dogs and adenocarcinoma in cats) to guide biopsy or cytology sample collection.
- CT patterns of the metastasis were also described, with the most frequent pattern being ring enhancement with hypoattenuating centers (Fig. 8), histologically characterized as necrotic areas [64]. Interestingly, most of the patients did not show clinical signs specifically attributable to their metastatic disease, underscoring the importance of WBCT to fully characterize and stage tumors with high metastatic rate [64].
- A recent study investigated the use of WBCT to detect muscle metastasis in canine hemangiosarcoma, with the prevalence of this kind of lesion higher compared with previous studies in both human and veterinary oncology. The investigators recommended WBCT as a routine staging procedure in canine hemangiosarcoma to detect lesions missed by clinical examination and traditional diagnostic imaging modalities [65].

SKELETAL EVALUATION

- With WBCT, bone metastasis (Figs. 9–12) can be properly assessed. A recent report described the role of WBCT in detecting urinary transitional cell carcinoma (TCC) metastasis and evaluated survival rate of the patients as well. The investigators observed that urethral TCC had higher metastasis rates and shorter survival time than dogs with urinary TCC [66].
- Sternal lymphadenomegaly and bone metastasis were identified as significant findings associated with WBCT screening at diagnosis because bone metastasis has been observed to be a poor predictor [67]. Furthermore, with WBCT it is possible to detect concurrent malignancies in patients, thus having more complete diagnosis by detecting lesions otherwise missed [19,68].

PRESENT RELEVANCE AND FUTURE CONSIDERATIONS

- WBCT in cancer staging of small animals is an extremely useful technique able to detect various sites for metastasis and further characterize the primary tumor.
- Further studies are needed to investigate the role of WBCT in feline oncology.
- In human medicine, careful attention is paid to the radiation dose per patient [12,69]. Similar studies may be useful in veterinary medicine.
- In addition, along with more advanced imaging such as PET/CT in oncology, the role of total-body MRI in cancer staging is now under investigation. The most recent reports described this technique as effective in detecting metastases, with reduced time, costs, and increased safety because of the lack of ionizing radiation [70–72].

SUMMARY

WBCT is considered useful in cases of malignant neoplasia characterized by a high metastatic rate, to thoroughly detect metastases affecting common and atypical tissues throughout the body. A complete and thorough characterization of the tumor is of paramount importance to properly manage the patient and plan effective treatment, and WBCT is an effective tool to be applied in routine oncologic practice.

DISCLOSURE

The authors have nothing to disclose.

REFERENCES

[1] Haagsma JA, Graetz N, Bolliger I, et al. The global burden of injury: incidence, mortality, disability-adjusted life years and time trends from the Global Burden of Disease study 2013. Inj Prev 2016;22(1):3–18.

[2] Ahmadinia K, Smucker JB, Nash CL, et al. Radiation exposure has increased in trauma patients over time. J Trauma Acute Care Surg 2012;72(2):410–5.

[3] Huber-Wagner S, Mand C, Ruchholtz S, et al. Effect of the localisation of the CT scanner during trauma resuscitation on survival – a retrospective, multicentre study. Injury 2014;45(Suppl 3):S76–82.

[4] Çorbacıoğlu ŞK, Aksel G. Whole body computed tomography in multi trauma patients: Review of the current literature. Turk J Emerg Med 2018;18(4):142–7.

[5] Huber-Wagner S, Biberthaler P, Häberle S, et al. Whole-Body CT in Haemodynamically Unstable Severely Injured Patients – A Retrospective, Multicentre Study. PLoS One 2013;8(7). https://doi.org/10.1371/journal.pone.0068880.

[6] Mathews JD, Forsythe AV, Brady Z, et al. Cancer risk in 680,000 people exposed to computed tomography scans in childhood or adolescence: data linkage study of 11 million Australians. BMJ 2013;346:f2360.

[7] Miglioretti DL, Johnson E, Williams A, et al. The Use of Computed Tomography in Pediatrics and the Associated Radiation Exposure and Estimated Cancer Risk. JAMA Pediatr 2013;167(8):700–7.

[8] Berrington de Gonzalez A, Salotti JA, McHugh K, et al. Relationship between paediatric CT scans and subsequent risk of leukaemia and brain tumours: assessment of the impact of underlying conditions. Br J Cancer 2016;114(4):388–94.

[9] Sierink JC, Saltzherr TP, Beenen LF, et al. A multicenter, randomized controlled trial of immediate total-body CT scanning in trauma patients (REACT-2). BMC Emerg Med 2012;12:4.

[10] Yeguiayan J-M, Yap A, Freysz M, et al. Impact of whole-body computed tomography on mortality and surgical management of severe blunt trauma. Crit Care 2012;16(3):R101.

[11] Elmokadem AH, Ibrahim EA, Gouda WA, et al. Whole-Body Computed Tomography Using Low-Dose Biphasic Injection Protocol With Adaptive Statistical Iterative Reconstruction V: Assessment of Dose Reduction and Image Quality in Trauma Patients. J Comput Assist Tomogr 2019;43(6):870–6.

[12] Stengel D, Mutze S, Güthoff C, et al. Association of Low-Dose Whole-Body Computed Tomography With Missed Injury Diagnoses and Radiation Exposure in Patients With Blunt Multiple Trauma. JAMA Surg 2020. https://doi.org/10.1001/jamasurg.2019.5468.

[13] Oliveira CR, Mitchell MA, O'Brien RT. Thoracic computed tomography in feline patients without use of chemical restraint. Vet Radiol Ultrasound 2011;52(4):368–76.

[14] Shanaman MM, Schwarz T, Gal A, et al. Comparison between survey radiography, B-mode ultrasonography, contrast-enhanced ultrasonography and contrast-enhanced multi-detector computed tomography findings in dogs with acute abdominal signs. Vet Radiol Ultrasound 2013;54(6):591–604.

[15] Dozeman ET, Prittie JE, Fischetti AJ. Utilization of whole body computed tomography in polytrauma patients. J Vet Emerg Crit Care 2020;30(1):28–33.

[16] Bonaparte A, Dhaliwal RS, Murtaugh RJ. Whole Body Computed Tomography for Tumor Staging in Dogs: Review of 16 Cases. J Vet Sci Technol 2016;7(4). https://doi.org/10.4172/2157-7579.1000344.

[17] Armbrust LJ, Biller DS, Hoskinson JJ. Case examples demonstrating the clinical utility of obtaining both right and left lateral abdominal radiographs in small animals. J Am Anim Hosp Assoc 2000;36(6):531–6.

[18] Mattoon JS, Bryan JN. The future of imaging in veterinary oncology: learning from human medicine. Vet J 2013; 197(3):541–52.

[19] Oblak ML, Boston SE, Woods JP, et al. Comparison of concurrent imaging modalities for staging of dogs with appendicular primary bone tumours. Vet Comp Oncol 2015;13(1):28–39.

20 Randall EK. PET-Computed Tomography in Veterinary Medicine. Vet Clin North Am Small Anim Pract 2016; 46(3):515–33, vi.

[21] Forrest LJ. Computed Tomography Imaging in Oncology. Vet Clin North Am Small Anim Pract 2016;46(3): 499–513, vi.

[22] Kutara K, Seki M, Ishikawa C, et al. Triple-phase helical computed tomography in dogs with hepatic masses. Vet Radiol Ultrasound 2014;55(1):7–15.

[23] Buishand FO, Vilaplana Grosso FR, Kirpensteijn J, et al. Utility of contrast-enhanced computed tomography in the evaluation of canine insulinoma location. Vet Q 2018;38(1):53–62.

[24] Leela-Arporn R, Ohta H, Shimbo G, et al. Computed tomographic features for differentiating benign from malignant liver lesions in dogs. J Vet Med Sci 2019;81(12): 1697–704.

[25] Kutara K, Seki M, Ishigaki K, et al. Triple-phase helical computed tomography in dogs with solid splenic masses. J Vet Med Sci 2017;79(11):1870–7.

[26] Prather AB, Berry CR, Thrall DE. Use of radiography in combination with computed tomography for the assessment of noncardiac thoracic disease in the dog and cat. Vet Radiol Ultrasound 2005;46(2):114–21.

[27] Paoloni MC, Adams WM, Dubielzig RR, et al. Comparison of results of computed tomography and radiography with histopathologic findings in tracheobronchial lymph nodes in dogs with primary lung tumors: 14 cases (1999-2002). J Am Vet Med Assoc 2006;228(11):1718–22.

[28] Ballegeer EA, Adams WM, Dubielzig RR, et al. Computed tomography characteristics of canine tracheobronchial lymph node metastasis. Vet Radiol Ultrasound 2010; 51(4):397–403.

[29] Marolf AJ, Gibbons DS, Podell BK, et al. Computed tomographic appearance of primary lung tumors in dogs. Vet Radiol Ultrasound 2011;52(2):168–72.

[30] Reetz JA, Buza EL, Krick EL. CT features of pleural masses and nodules. Vet Radiol Ultrasound 2012;53(2):121–7.

[31] Nemanic S, London CA, Wisner ER. Comparison of thoracic radiographs and single breath-hold helical CT for detection of pulmonary nodules in dogs with metastatic neoplasia. J Vet Intern Med 2006;20(3):508–15.

[32] Erhart EJ, Kamstock DA. The Pathology of Neoplasia. In: Withrow V, editor. Withrow and MacEwen's small animal clinical oncology. St. Louis (MO): Elsevier Saunders; 2013. p. 51–67.

[33] Maalej M, Hentati D, Afrit M, et al. Sternal or parasternal involvement from breast cancer: a misleading clinical sign. Tunis Med 2013;91(1):54–8.

[34] Smith K, O'Brien R. Radiographic characterization of enlarged sternal lymph nodes in 71 dogs and 13 cats. J Am Anim Hosp Assoc 2012;48(3):176–81.

[35] Tanaka T, Akiyoshi H, Mie K, et al. Contrast-enhanced computed tomography may be helpful for characterizing and staging canine gastric tumors. Vet Radiol Ultrasound 2019;60(1):7–18.

[36] Terragni R, Vignoli M, Rossi F, et al. Stomach wall evaluation using helical hydro-computed tomography. Vet Radiol Ultrasound 2012;53(4):402–5.

[37] Langenbach A, McManus PM, Hendrick MJ, et al. Sensitivity and specificity of methods of assessing the regional lymph nodes for evidence of metastasis in dogs and cats with solid tumors. J Am Vet Med Assoc 2001;218(9): 1424–8.

[38] Worley DR. Incorporation of sentinel lymph node mapping in dogs with mast cell tumours: 20 consecutive procedures. Vet Comp Oncol 2014;12(3):215–26.

[39] Skinner OT, Boston SE, Souza CHM. Patterns of lymph node metastasis identified following bilateral mandibular and medial retropharyngeal lymphadenectomy in 31 dogs with malignancies of the head. Vet Comp Oncol 2017;15(3):881–9.

[40] Williams LE, Packer RA. Association between lymph node size and metastasis in dogs with oral malignant melanoma: 100 cases (1987-2001). J Am Vet Med Assoc 2003;222(9):1234–6.

[41] Uren RF, Howman-Giles R, Chung D, et al. Imaging sentinel lymph nodes. Cancer J 2015;21(1):25–32.

[42] Nakagawa M, Morimoto M, Takechi H, et al. Preoperative diagnosis of sentinel lymph node (SLN) metastasis using 3D CT lymphography (CTLG). Breast Cancer 2016;23(3):519–24.

[43] Soultani C, Patsikas MN, Karayannopoulou M, et al. Assessment of sentinel lymph node metastasis in canine mammary gland tumors using computed tomographic indirect lymphography. Vet Radiol Ultrasound 2017; 58(2):186–96.

[44] Suga K, Ogasawara N, Yuan Y, et al. Visualization of breast lymphatic pathways with an indirect computed tomography lymphography using a nonionic monometric contrast medium iopamidol: preliminary results. Invest Radiol 2003;38(2):73–84.

[45] Fukushima K, Kanemoto H, Ohno K, et al. CT characteristics of primary hepatic mass lesions in dogs. Vet Radiol Ultrasound 2012;53(3):252–7.

[46] Taniura T, Marukawa K, Yamada K, et al. Differential diagnosis of hepatic tumor-like lesions in dog by using dynamic CT scanning. Hiroshima J Med Sci 2009; 58(1):17–24.

[47] Johnson KA, Powers BE, Withrow SJ, et al. Splenomegaly in dogs. Predictors of neoplasia and survival after splenectomy. J Vet Intern Med 1989;3(3):160–6.

[48] Jones ID, Daniels AD, Lara-Garcia A, et al. Computed tomographic findings in 12 cases of canine multicentric lymphoma with splenic and hepatic involvement. J Small Anim Pract 2017;58(11):622–8.

[49] Baldo CF, Garcia-Pereira FL, Nelson NC, et al. Effects of anesthetic drugs on canine splenic volume determined via computed tomography. Am J Vet Res 2012;73(11): 1715–9.

[50] LaBan MM, Nagarajan R, Riutta JC. Paucity of muscle metastasis in otherwise widely disseminated cancer: a conundrum. Am J Phys Med Rehabil 2010;89(11): 931–5.

[51] Al-Alao BS, Westrup J, Shuhaibar MN. Non-small-cell lung cancer: unusual presentation in the gluteal muscle. Gen Thorac Cardiovasc Surg 2011;59(5):382–4.

[52] Paget S. The distribution of secondary growths in cancer of the breast. 1889. Cancer Metastasis Rev 1989;8(2): 98–101.

[53] Seely S. Possible reasons for the high resistance of muscle to cancer. Med Hypotheses 1980;6(2):133–7.

[54] Pop D, Nadeemy AS, Venissac N, et al. Skeletal muscle metastasis from non-small cell lung cancer. J Thorac Oncol 2009;4(10):1236–41.

[55] Tuoheti Y, Okada K, Osanai T, et al. Skeletal muscle metastases of carcinoma: a clinicopathological study of 12 cases. Jpn J Clin Oncol 2004;34(4):210–4.

[56] Muzamil J, Bashir S, Guru FR, et al. Squamous Cell Carcinoma Lung with Skeletal Muscle Involvement: A 8-year Study of a Tertiary Care Hospital in Kashmir. Indian J Med Paediatr Oncol 2017;38(4):456–60.

[57] Ong N, George M, Dutta R, et al. CT imaging features of skeletal muscle metastasis. Clin Radiol 2019;74(5): 374–7.

[58] Marioni G, Blandamura S, Calgaro N, et al. Distant muscular (gluteus maximus muscle) metastasis from laryngeal squamous cell carcinoma. Acta Otolaryngol (Stockh) 2005;125(6):678–82.

[59] Lennartz S, Große Hokamp N, Abdullayev N, et al. Diagnostic value of spectral reconstructions in detecting incidental skeletal muscle metastases in CT staging examinations. Cancer Imaging 2019;19. https://doi.org/10.1186/s40644-019-0235-3.

[60] Meyer A, Hauser B. Lung tumor with unusual metastasis in a cat–a case report. Schweiz Arch Tierheilkd 1995; 137(2):54–7 [in German].

[61] Krecic MR, Black SS. Epitheliotropic T-cell gastrointestinal tract lymphosarcoma with metastases to lung and skeletal muscle in a cat. J Am Vet Med Assoc 2000; 216(4):524–9, 517.

[62] Langlais LM, Gibson J, Taylor JA, et al. Pulmonary adenocarcinoma with metastasis to skeletal muscle in a cat. Can Vet J 2006;47(11):1122–3.

[63] Aupperle H, März I, Ellenberger C, et al. Primary and secondary heart tumours in dogs and cats. J Comp Pathol 2007;136(1):18–26.

[64] Vignoli M, Terragni R, Rossi F, et al. Whole body computed tomographic characteristics of skeletal and cardiac muscular metastatic neoplasia in dogs and cats. Vet Radiol Ultrasound 2013;54(3):223–30.

[65] Carloni A, Terragni R, Morselli-Labate AM, et al. Prevalence, distribution, and clinical characteristics of hemangiosarcoma-associated skeletal muscle metastases in 61 dogs: A whole body computed tomographic study. J Vet Intern Med 2019;33(2):812–9.

[66] Charney VA, Miller MA, Heng HG, et al. Skeletal Metastasis of Canine Urothelial Carcinoma: Pathologic and Computed Tomographic Features. Vet Pathol 2017; 54(3):380–6.

[67] Iwasaki R, Shimosato Y, Yoshikawa R, et al. Survival analysis in dogs with urinary transitional cell carcinoma that underwent whole-body computed tomography at diagnosis. Vet Comp Oncol 2019;17(3):385–93.

[68] Talbott JL, Boston SE, Milner RJ, et al. Retrospective Evaluation of Whole Body Computed Tomography for Tumor Staging in Dogs with Primary Appendicular Osteosarcoma. Vet Surg 2017;46(1):75–80.

[69] Karpitschka M, Augart D, Becker H-C, et al. Dose reduction in oncological staging multidetector CT: effect of iterative reconstruction. Br J Radiol 2013;86(1021): 20120224.

[70] Lee DH, Lee JM. Whole-body PET/MRI for colorectal cancer staging: Is it the way forward? J Magn Reson Imaging 2017;45(1):21–35.

[71] Machado Medeiros T, Altmayer S, Watte G, et al. 18F-FDG PET/CT and whole-body MRI diagnostic performance in M staging for non-small cell lung cancer: a systematic review and meta-analysis. Eur Radiol 2020. https://doi.org/10.1007/s00330-020-06703-1.

[72] Taylor SA, Mallett S, Miles A, et al. Whole-body MRI compared with standard pathways for staging metastatic disease in lung and colorectal cancer: the Streamline diagnostic accuracy studies. Health Technol Assess 2019;23(66):1–270.

Advances in Small Animal Care 1 (2020) 49–74
ADVANCES IN SMALL ANIMAL CARE

CT Angiography and Vascular Anomalies

Giovanna Bertolini, DVM, PhD
San Marco Veterinary Clinic and Laboratory, Diagnostic and Interventional Radiology Division, Via dell'Industria 3, Veggiano, Padova 35030, Italy

KEYWORDS
• Computed tomography • CTA • Vascular anomaly • Portosystemic shunt

KEY POINTS

- Multidetector (MD) computed tomography (CT) technology has seen more rapid technological improvements than other radiological techniques.
- Vascular anatomic variants and anomalies frequently are encountered in dogs and cats.
- MDCT angiography now is the reference standard method for vascular abdominal vascular assessment in small animals.
- More advanced CT technologies offer new perspective in vascular imaging, combining morphologic and functional vascular assessment.

INTRODUCTION

In humans, computed tomography angiography (CTA) first became possible in the early 1990s with spiral or helical computed tomography (CT), which combined simultaneous continuous gantry rotation and table movement, succeeding the axial or step-and-shoot acquisition mode of conventional CT scanners [1]. The continuous movement of the tube-detector system around the patient moving through the gantry permitted the capture of the first pass of an intravenous contrast agent bolus as it transited a particular vascular territory. Until the advent of the MDCT technology, CTA was a special examination, performed for limited clinical indications at select institutions [2].

Similarly, in veterinary field, although proof-of-concept investigations of liver CT angiography [3] and CTA applications to discrete vascular territories were published using helical CT [4,5], the introduction of 16-row MDCT brought volumetric CT angiography to clinical practice [6]. MDCTA first was used for dogs and cats in the early 2000s and described for 3-dimensional (3-D) portosystemic shunt (PSS) assessment [7]. Over the years, the widespread availability of 16-row and more advanced MDCT technology has greatly advanced the role of CT angiography in veterinary clinical practice. The introduction of MDCT scanners that integrated multiple detector elements (from 16 detector rows onwards) transformed the imaging capability of CT from 2-dimensional (2-D) cross-sectional slices to rapid isotropic acquisitions and the generation of 3-D volumetric images.

MDCTA is a robust, easy-to-perform noninvasive technique highly standardizable technique that can provide simultaneous detailed information of the vascular lumen, wall, and surrounding structures. If performed in an optimal or appropriate manner, each contrast-enhanced CT examination now potentially can serve as a CTA [2]. Therefore, CTA can be incorporated into mainstream radiology practice and performed daily for a wide range of clinical indications.

E-mail address: bertolini@sanmarcovet.it

https://doi.org/10.1016/j.yasa.2020.07.005
2666-4518/20/

TECHNOLOGICAL AND TECHNICAL OVERVIEW

Computed Tomography Technological Evolution

- Prior to the introduction of scan pitch values greater than 1, using single helical CT, a scan with 3-mm nominal section thickness provided a maximum of 9-cm table travel in 30 seconds and thus limited initial applications. Early MDCT scanners introduced in 1998 had 4 detector rows and were capable of 0.5 s gantry rotations, effectively multiplying volume coverage per unit time per 8 at the same section thickness [8]. From that moment, MDCT has seen more rapid technological improvements than other radiological techniques, and continuous advances in CT technology yielded to systems with 8, 10, 16, 32, 40, 64, 128, and 320 detector rows with a rotation time down to 0.27 s, allowing submillimeter isotropic resolution to be acquired over very large volumes in, at most, a few seconds.
- Compared with 4-MDCT scanners, the performance (coverage × seconds/slice thickness) of 64-MDCT scanners has increased more than 20 times, due to the increase in the number of detector rows and rotation (Fig. 1) [9]. These technological advances, together with improvements in image reconstruction software, increased the temporal and spatial resolution as well as the processing workflow, which enabled widespread use of CT angiography and the advent of multiphasic imaging.
- The most recent dual-source CT (DSCT) scanner, which features 2 tube-detector arrays, can achieve a rotation time of up to 0.25 s and a volume coverage speed of up to 737 mm/s [10]. The implementation of dual-energy CT (DECT) with novel applications presents opportunities to assess vascular disease from a new perspective, expanding the role of CT angiography in vascular imaging from a traditional anatomic-morphologic tool to a functional and quantitative tool [11].

How to Review Computed Tomography Angiography Data

- An essential prerequisite for successful postprocessing is the acquisition of high-quality imaging data. With these data, there are an almost unlimited number of ways to reconstruct and view MDCT angiographic data sets. The review of transverse images is time-consuming and less accurate than 2-D multiplanar (MPR) and 3-D visualization, especially for

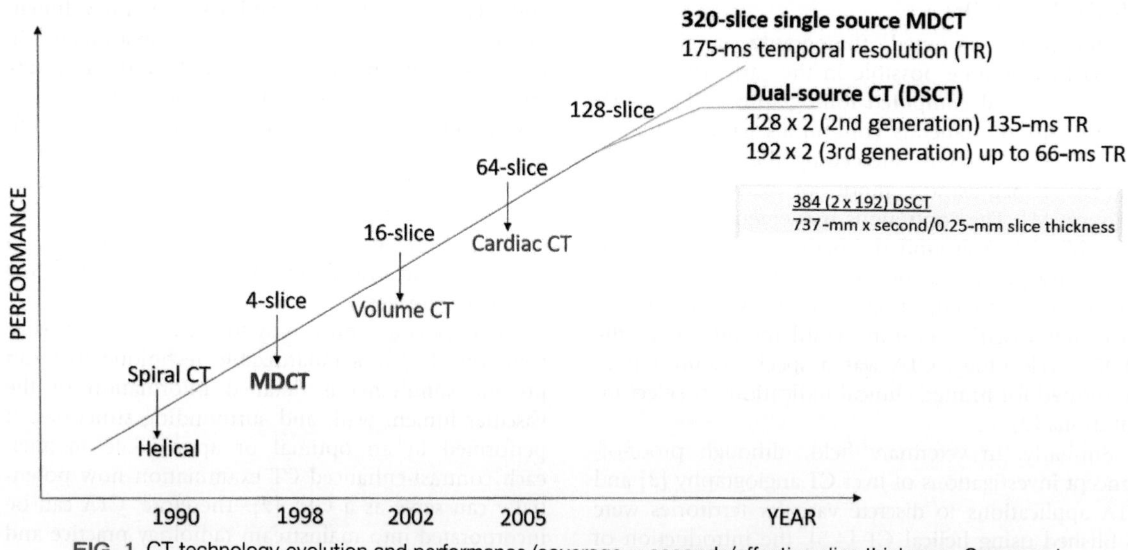

FIG. 1 CT technology evolution and performance (coverage × seconds/effective slice thickness. Compared with 4-MDCT, the performance of 64-MDCT scanner has increased more than 20 times, due to the increase in the number of detector rows and rotation speed. The most recent DSCT scanner, which features 2 tube-detector arrays, can achieve a rotation time of up to 0.25 s and a volume coverage speed of up to 737 mm/s. The higher spatial and temporal resolution, combined with the simultaneous assessment with 2 different level of energy, transformed the vascular imaging from a traditional anatomic-morphologic tool to a functional and quantitative tool TR, temporal resolution.

vascular structures. The analysis of CT angiographic data sets has evolved to the point where review of the transverse reconstructions is a secondary analysis to tailored visualization and quantitation tasks using application-specific postprocessing solutions [12]. Most 3-D reconstructions now are interactive in real time, and the most complex processing techniques, such as automatic bone removal, are immediate or take just seconds to complete.

- Visualization with interactive MPR, sliding thin-slab maximum intensity projection (MIP), or standardized volume rendering (VR) presets in combination with clip planes is used more frequently to review the data. If the CT angiographic data meet the requirements of isotropy (planes x = y = z), the quality of a reconstructed image in any plane is virtually identical to the original transverse images, and MPR creates views in arbitrary planes without loss of information. The key advantage of MPR is the simplicity and efficiency of the technique. Instead of individually viewing thousands of transverse slices, MPRs enable a radiologist to interact with the data as a volume [13].
- MIP algorithm, the highest-attenuation voxels along lines projected through the volume data set are selected [14]. The subset of these high-attenuation voxels from the volume then is incorporated into a 2-D image. In clinical practice, a slab-Maximum Intensity Projection of 10-mm to 20-mm thickness is excellent for the depiction of contrast material–filled structures. A limitation of the technique is that the presence of other high-attenuation voxels may obscure evaluation of the vasculature. Therefore, when other high-density structures, such as bone or calcifications, are present within the volume and superprojected over blood vessels, vessels may be obscured thus hampering their evaluation. Again, because the maximum CT number is displayed by MIP, visual cues that allow perception of depth relationships are lacking and the 3-D relationships among the structures in the display are not visible.
- VR currently is the most flexible 3-D visualization tool. In contrast to MIP, where only the voxel with the highest CT number is used, in VR each voxel in the original data is used to calculate the final image [15]. The resulting images, therefore, contain more information and potentially are more useful. VR not only allows display of the vascular anatomy but also provides definition of soft tissue, muscle, and bone, which may contribute to a more comprehensive understanding of pathologic processes.
- VR combines the use of opacity values and lighting effects to determine spatial relationships between structures. Color can be applied to enhance the discrimination between the tissues by selecting image presets or by changing parameters interactively until

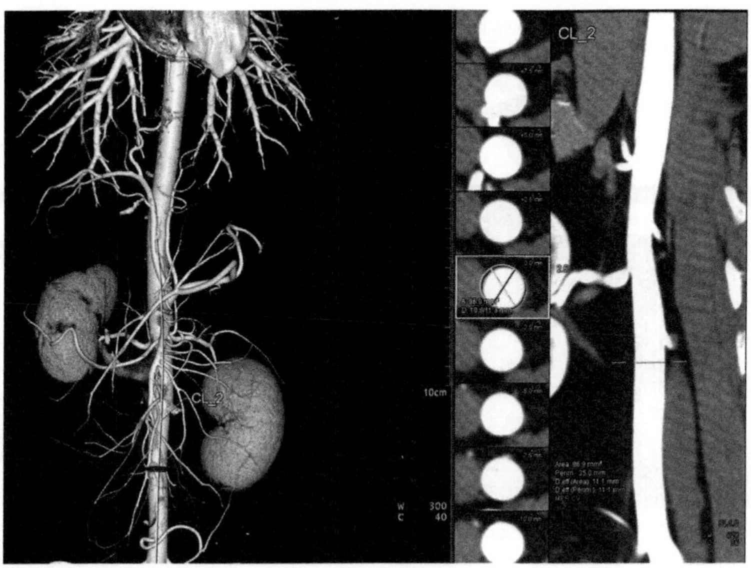

FIG. 2 Example of software designed for the evaluation and quantification of angiography images. (*Left panel*) Volume Rendering of the descending aorta. (*Right panel*) point by point diameter and section areas of the selected vessel. The centerline was selected manually point by point. The software then calculates automatically diameters and areas at any point of the target vessel.

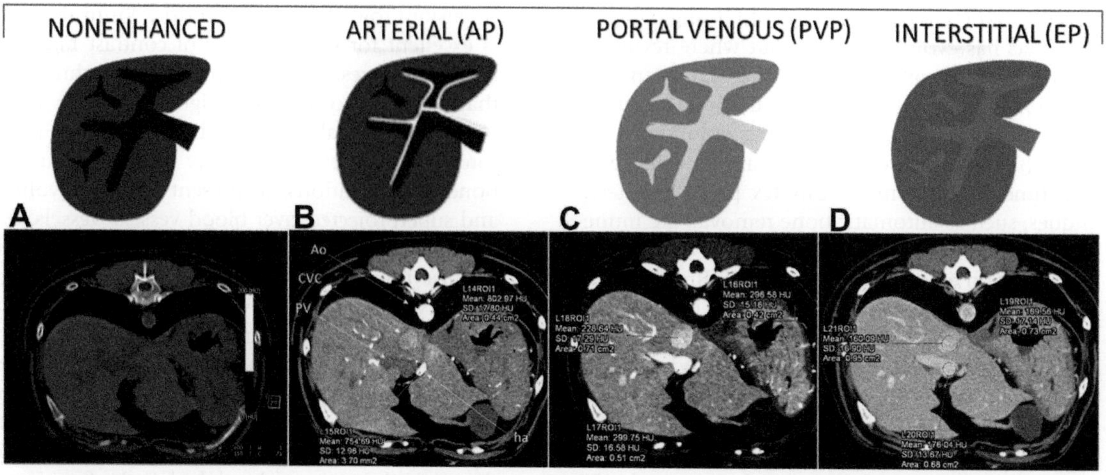

FIG. 3 Multiphase CT: (*A*) Nonenehanced; (*B*), Arterial phase; (*C*) Portal venous phase; (*D*), Interstitial or Equilibrium phase. The hepatic arterial phase (AP) is the postcontrast time range in which the hepatic artery and its branches are fully enhanced and the hepatic veins not yet enhanced by antegrade flow. In the portal venous phase (PVP) is the portal system is fully enhanced and the liver parenchyma is at peak of enhancement. In the interstitial or equilibrium phase (EP), both portal and hepatic veins are enhanced as well as the liver parenchyma but less than in the portal venous phase.

the desired effect is achieved. If used interactively, VR is operator dependent, and user comfort with this technique determines the optimization of rendering parameters. Unskilled users inadvertently can introduce significant errors into the VR image [14].

- Vascular lumen analysis is fundamental to managing complex vascular conditions. In an effort to automate vessel segmentation, several commercial vessel analysis software tools have been introduced by CT manufacturers. There are many computer software

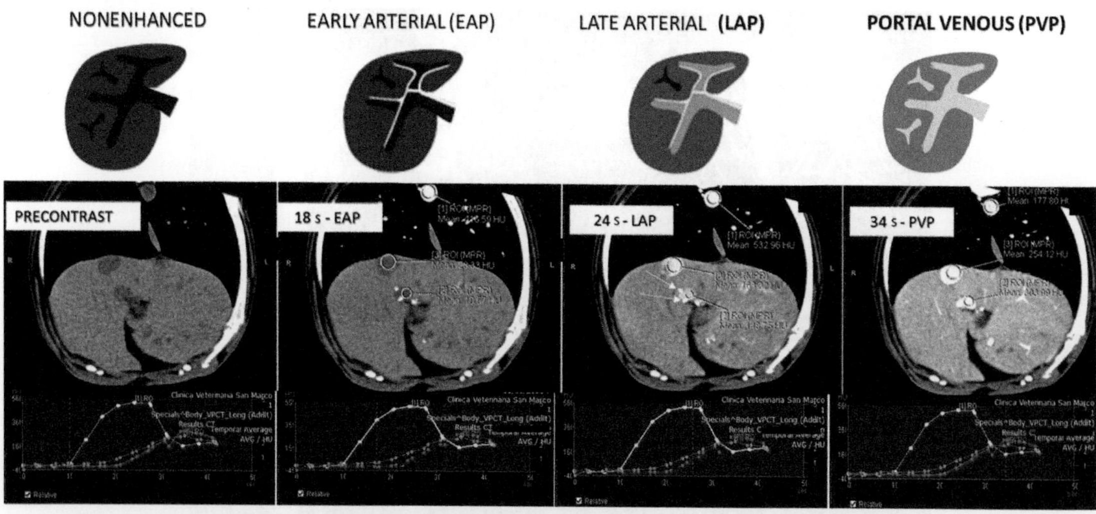

FIG. 4 Dynamic CE-CT. Changes in vascular density through a series of dynamically acquired CT images after the intravenous contrast injection. In the early arterial phase (EAP), the portal vein is not yet enhanced. In the late arterial phase (LAP), there is an initial enhancement of the portal vein (so called portal inflow phase). The portal venous (PVP) showed the portal vein, portal tributaries, and hepatic branches fully enhanced and the liver parenchyma is at peak of enhancement.

packages available. It is necessary to perform post-processing steps to produce the vessel path with MPR images or using automatic vessel segmentation.

- The software usually provides maximum, minimum, and mean intraluminal diameter measurements and cross-sectional areas of true orthogonal sections of the vessel at selected anatomic points (Fig. 2). High accuracy in the determination of the vessel centerlines is a prerequisite for precise cross-sectional rendering and measurements. An inaccurate vessel centerline may result in cross-sectional sections that are tilted against the true vessel path direction and thus in artificially enlarged cross-sectional areas and vessel diameters [16].
- Endoluminal imaging (virtual angioscopy) is a perspective VR technique that allows users to visualize the lumen of cavitary structures [15]. It requires substantial differences in CT numbers between the lumen and its surroundings. Therefore, it is most successful for displaying air-containing structures (virtual endoscopy) but also can be applied to high-density structures, such as contrast-enhanced blood vessels.

ABDOMINAL COMPUTED TOMOGRAPHY ANGIOGRAPHY

Multiphase Computed Tomography Angiography Technique and Factors

- Multiphase CT of the abdomen is the reference standard for abdominal vascular assessment in small animals [17]. With the multitude of different CT scanners, no single injection protocol strategy currently can be applied universally for CTA. Although CT technology continues to evolve, the physiologic and pharmacokinetic principles of vascular enhancement will remain unchanged in the foreseeable future. With the introduction of multidetector row (MD) CT from 16 slices onwards, virtually all limits on longitudinal anatomic coverage disappeared, paving the way for CT angiography to be applied to the whole body.
- Unless otherwise specified, the vascular phases of multiphase CT refer to the hepatic phases. The dual vascular supply of liver (80% portal venous and 20% hepatic arterial) results in sequential opacification of hepatic arteries, portal veins, and hepatic veins after injection of intravenous contrast. In

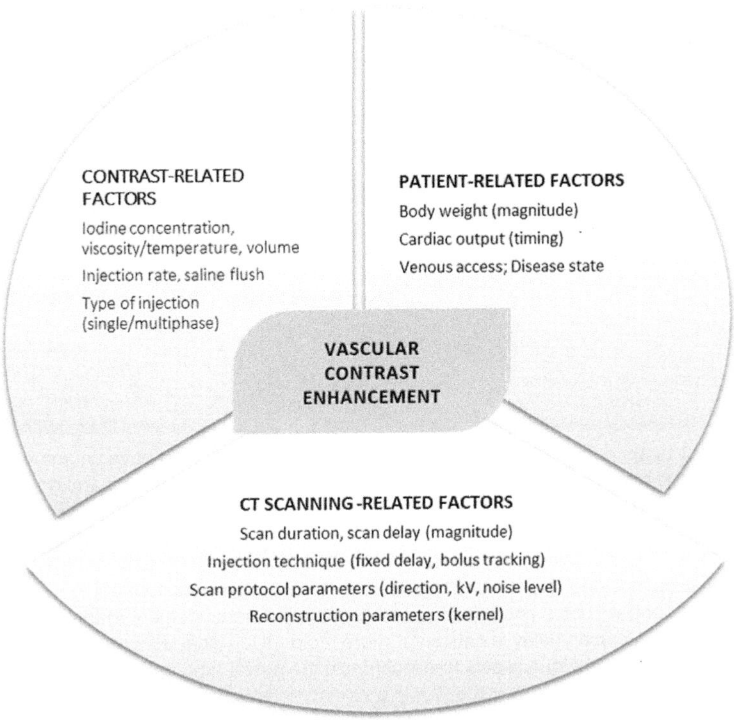

FIG. 5 Factors influencing the contrast medium distribution in the body.

multiphase CT angiographic technique scans are made at defined circulatory phases (static angiography). It includes at least 2 vascular phases, arterial and portal venous phases, and, ideally a third delayed interstitial or equilibrium phase (Figs. 3 and 4).

Timing

- Contrast enhancement timing for CT examinations is affected by numerous interacting factors. For optimal multiphase CT approach, the contrast agent concentration and injection protocol should be adapted to the patient characteristics, the vascular territory of interest, and the capabilities of the MDCT scanner used. Manual contrast injection according to empirically developed protocols for spiral CT is not applicable when more rapid MDCT scanners are used for CTA.
- A fixed-duration injection protocol may be a good compromise between an ideal vascular enhancement during the portal phase and an easily reproducible protocol on scanners with low and high numbers of detector rows CT scanners [18,19]. With faster CT scanners, however, individual timing of contrast material injection (bolus tracking or test bolus injection) is mandatory to predict how the contrast agent will behave in a given patient and to take advantage of phase-resolved image acquisition.
- The goal of CT angiography is to achieve an adequate opacification (magnitude of contrast enhancement) in the vascular territory of interest, within a certain time (timing of contrast), and to maintain a constant level of enhancement throughout scanning (shaping of contrast) [18,20]. An intravascular attenuation of at least 400 Hounsfield units (HU) along the full longitudinal extent of the target vasculature and throughout the duration of acquisition is considered a prerequisite for high-quality CT angiography.
- The magnitude of arterial enhancement in CTA increases proportionally with the rate of iodine delivery (grams of iodine per second), which corresponds to the product of the contrast medium concentration (milligrams of iodine per milliliter) and the injection rate (milliliters per second). Vascular contrast enhancement is influenced by various factors: patient-related, contrast agent-related, and CT scanner–related factors (Fig. 5).

Patient-Related Factors

- Principal patient-related factors that affect the contrast agent distribution in the vascular system and then the vascular enhancement are the cardiac output and the body weight. Both are extremely variable in veterinary patients [21,22]. In particular, the magnitude of contrast enhancement in vascular studies is inversely related to the body weight of the patient. The timing of vascular contrast enhancement is inversely related to the cardiac output of the patient. In patients with normal cardiac output, the

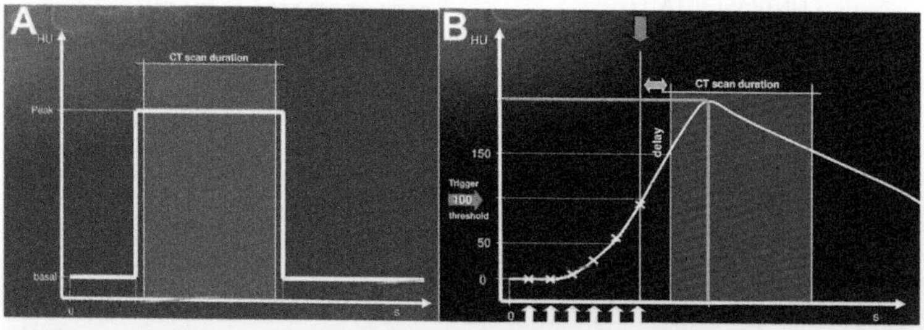

FIG. 6 The contrast bolus geometry. (*A*) The optimal bolus geometry should have an immediate rise and a plateau overlapping the scan duration. In truth, CTA is performed during an upslope and downslope contrast enhancement curve. The peak of the enhancement should be inside the scan range. For slow scanners (ranging from single-slice CT to 4-MDCT devices), the arrival time always is used directly as the scanning delay for subsequent CTA. (*B*) Using more advanced MDCT scanners with shorter contrast injection times, additional time must be included to obtain a diagnostic delay (taking into account also the scan length), to avoid outrunning the contrast bolus and assuring optimal contrast enhancement in the target vessel. Selection of the appropriate scan delay is critical for more rapid MDCT scanners (64-MDCT and above). The bolus tracking or triggering technique allows to synchronize the arrival time and the scanning time. With this option, multiple images are obtained over the ROI in a nonincremental manner (*arrows at bottom*) during the contrast agent injection and the scan is initiated automatically when the density within the vessel exceeds a predetermined HU value (eg, 50–100 HU, depending on the scanning speed).

peak arterial contrast enhancement is achieved shortly after injection. In those with decreased cardiac output, the contrast agent distributes and clears slowly, leading to delayed and persistent peak arterial enhancement. In those patients with higher cardiac output, the distribution of the contrast agent is unpredictable.

- All modern MDCT systems feature the bolus tracking technique. With this option, multiple images are obtained over the region of interest (ROI) in a nonincremental manner during the contrast agent injection, and the scan is initiated automatically when the density within the vessel exceeds a predetermined HU value (eg, 50–100 HU, depending on the scanning speed) (Fig. 6).

Power Injector

- A mechanical power injector is essential for MDCT angiography. This device allows preprogramming of the contrast agent volume and flow rate and the setting of an injection pressure limit, which synchronizes the scan for optimally timed intravenous contrast injection.
- Injection protocol parameters that may influence the opacification of target vascular territory are injection duration (volume: rate), rate of injection, and volume of contrast agent injected (duration × rate). A saline bolus (bolus chaser) injected immediately after the contrast injection (same volume and same rate) has several advantages: less contrast may be used for CTA, the peak of maximum enhancement is higher and longer, and the vascular enhancement more uniform [18].
- Finally, some scanner-dependent factors (temporal and spatial resolutions) play a critical role by enabling the acquisition of data at a specific enhancement time point and providing high-quality volume data.

Dynamic Contrast-Enhanced Computed Tomography

- Dynamic contrast-enhanced (DCE)-CT measures temporal changes in tissue density through a series of dynamically acquired CT images after the intravenous injection of the contrast agent. Rapid repetitive sampling of a specific tissue volume is performed

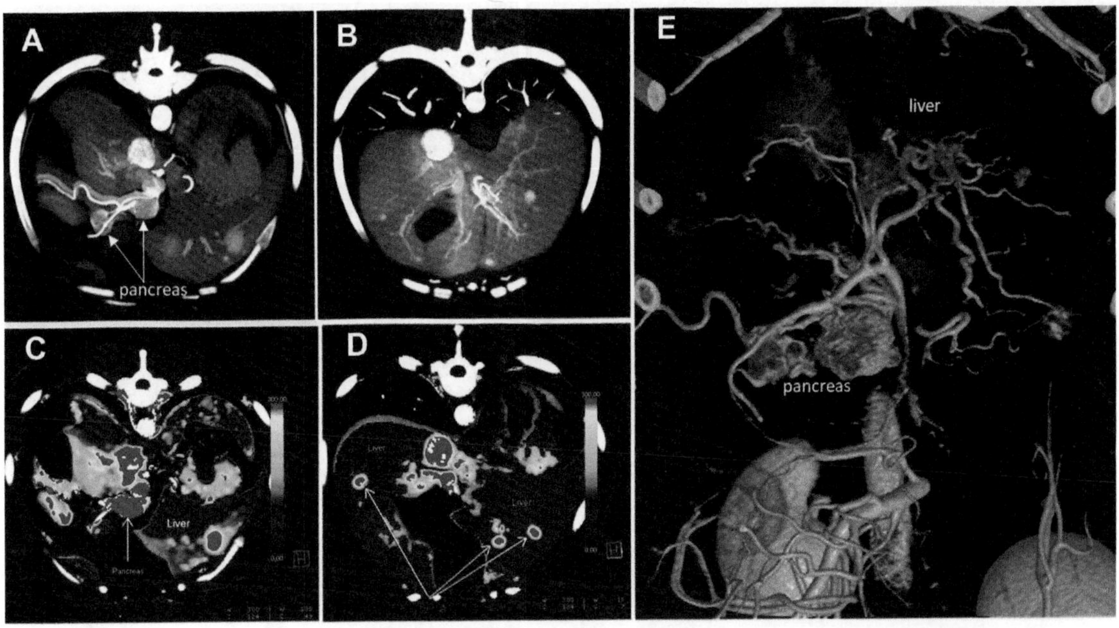

FIG. 7 DCE-CT in a dog with metastatic pancreatic insulinoma. Volume data were obtained using a third-generation DSCT scanner (192 rows × 2) during the bolus injection. (*A* and *B*) are transverse images of the liver during the pancreatic phase (between the late arterial and portal venous phases). (*A*). Transverse section through the pancreatic body. Arrows indicate pancreatic nodules. (*B*). Multiple hypervascular hepatic nodules are visible in the liver parenchyma. (*C* and *D*) are Color-coded maps of iodine distribution (*perfusion*). (*C*). transverse image at the level of the pancreatic body (*arrow*). (*D*). *Arrows* indicate the hypervascular nodules within the liver. (*E*) The same volume data set can provide excellent vascular 3-D maps.

while injecting a small volume of contrast agent at a high injection speed. DCE-CT provides iodine maps, which often are regarded as perfusion images. It allows the analysis of liver function through the calculation of a series of tissue perfusion parameters can be conceived to reflect physiologic markers related to angiogenesis (blood volume, flow, mean transit time, hepatic perfusion index, and so forth) Dynamic CT studies have been described for liver and pancreas perfusion assessment in healthy dogs and in dogs with vascular anomalies or tumors [4,23–25].

- The limited volume coverage of older CT systems restricted the clinical use of DCE-CT predominantly to areas of the abdomen. The advent of high-frequency spiral CT techniques and very wide detector coverage facilitated DCE-CT in whole-organ imaging [26]. The use of DCE-CT for perfusion evaluation is beyond the scope of this dicussion. It is interesting, however, to know that with state-of-the-art CT technologies, DCE-CT easily can be integrated into routine CT imaging protocols within the same imaging session and offers excellent spatial and temporal resolution for assessment of vascular anatomy, anomalies and vascular lesions (Fig. 7). This allows a simultaneous comprehensive morphologic and functional assessment of patients with vascular diseases.

Dual-Source Computed Tomography

- Conventional MDCT scanners use a single x-ray source mounted opposite to a detector array. The x-ray tube/detector array system rotates around the patient to generate tomographic images. To reconstruct a transverse CT image, the gantry requires a rotation of approximately 180°. DSCT uses 2 x-ray tubes with opposing detector arrays mounted 90° from each other. They can work using the same level of energy or 2 energy levels to acquire images that can be processed to generate additional data sets (Figs. 8 and 9). The main advantage of a DSCT system using same energy is that the temporal resolution is effectively halved because each x-ray tube/detector array system needs to rotate only half of the angle that otherwise would be required by a single-source system. As a result, for instance, the

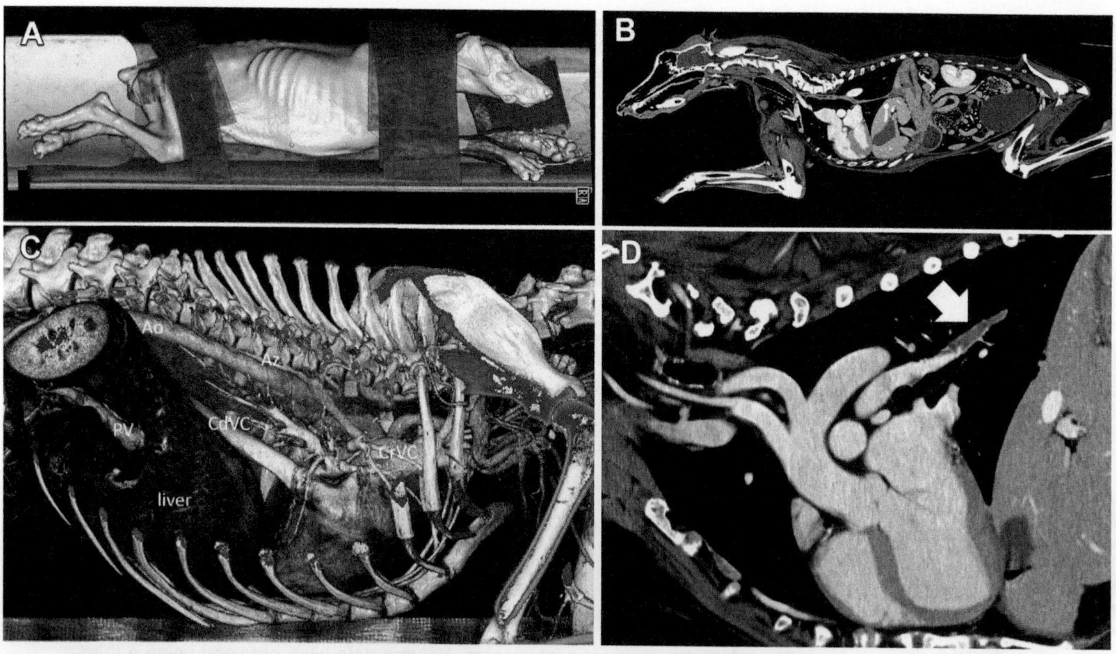

FIG. 8 DSCT angiography in an awake Doberman pinscher dog. Collimation 192-mm × 0.6-mm slices were acquired; reconstruction interval 0.4 mm; gantry rotation time 0.28 second/rotation, pitch 3.4, tube voltage 120 kV (both tubes). (*A*) VR image of the awake patient on the CT table. (*B*) Whole-body contrast-enhanced sagittal view. (*C*) Segmented VR image from right side, showing excellent depiction of vascular structures. Ao, aorta; Az, azygos vein; PV, portal vein; CdVC, caudal vena cava. (*D*) Left parasagittal view showing a filling defect in a pulmonary vessel (*arrow*), consistent with pulmonary embolism.

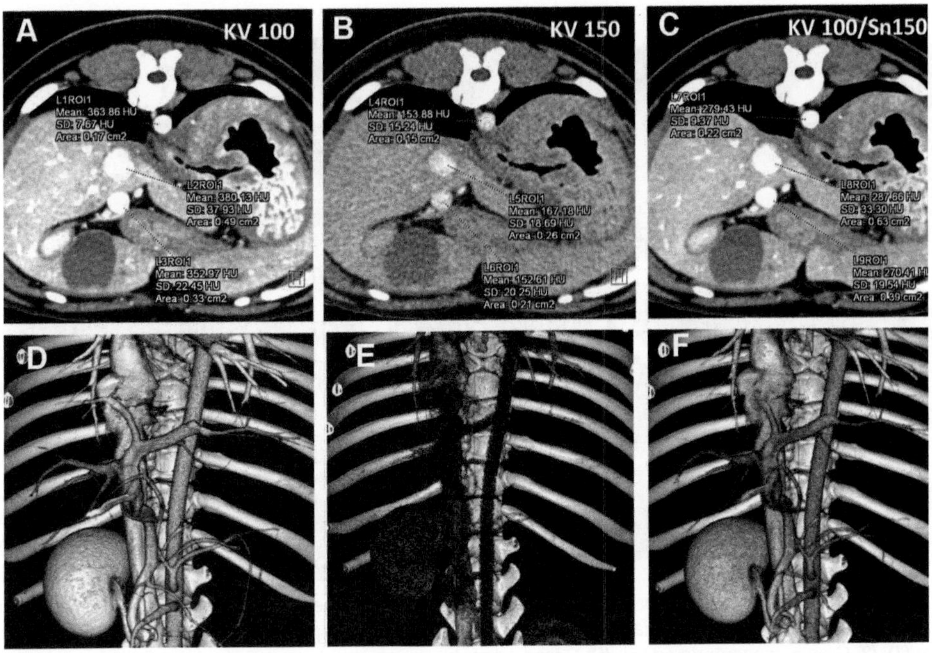

FIG. 9 Example of dual energy volume data sets obtained using a third-generation DSCT scanner (same kernel and same window settings). Please note the different soft tissue contrast and vascular attenuation of the same volume acquired simultaneously at different levels of energy. (*A*) Low-energy data set (100 kV). (*B*) High-energy data set (Sn140). (*C*) Mixed data set automatically generated by the software as a combination of the low and high energy volumes, containing then all the information (the final result is similar to that obtained with the traditional 120 kV). (*D-F*) VR images of the previous volume data sets using same postprocessing tool.

third-generation DSCT scanner, featured with 192 rows × 2 (384), can cover a volume up to 737 mm per second with 0.25 mm slice thickness. This high speed allows excellent, motion-free cardiac and vascular morphologic imaging even in awake or minimally sedated patients [17].

- When using different levels of energy (80/100 kV and 140 kV), DECT can play an important role in vascular imaging by improving image quality with less contrast and lower radiation dose compared with conventional CTA and useful postprocessing applications for vessels assessment. At lower x-ray energy levels, attenuation of iodine contrast increases as the energy level approaches the K-edge of iodine (33.2 keV). Several studies in people have described iodine dose reductions of up to 56% using 70 kV peak (p) to 80 kV(p) acquisition while maintaining image quality compared with routine CTA [27].

ABDOMINAL VASCULAR DISEASES

Congenital Arterial Anomalies

- Congenital arterial anomalies reported in small animals include variable patterns of renal arteries, aortic aneurysm, anomalies of the celiac-mesenteric axis, and arteriovenous fistulas. Hepatic arteriovenous malformations (HAVMs) also have been reported and are here included in portal venous anomalies (included in this article).
- Anatomic variations of the celiac trunk and cranial mesenteric artery recently were described in a multicentric study using CTA [28]. CTA of 267 patients (dogs and cats) underwent CT for various reasons were reviewed and abnormal anatomy of the celiac artery were found in 11.9% patients, including 3.4% anomalous origin or branching of the celiac artery and a common celiacomesenteric trunk in 2.9% (Fig. 10). In 8.6% of dogs with celiac artery anomaly was demonstrated a compression of the celiac artery

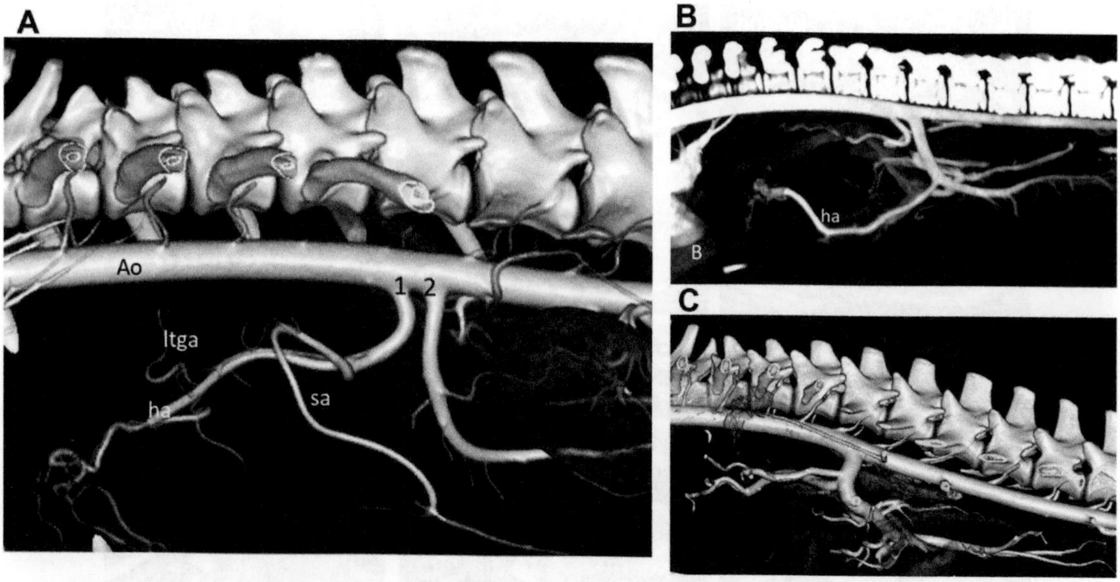

FIG. 10 Celiac-mesenteric vascular variants. (*A*) Normal anatomy of the visceral branches of the descending aorta (Ao). The left gastric artery (ltga), the hepatic artery (ha), and the splenic artery (sa) arise from the celiac artery (1). (2) Cranial mesenteric artery. (*B*) Celiac artery hypoplasia and abnormal origin of the hepatic artery from the mesenteric artery. (*C*) Both the celiac and mesenteric arteries originate from a common trunk (common celiacomesenteric trunk).

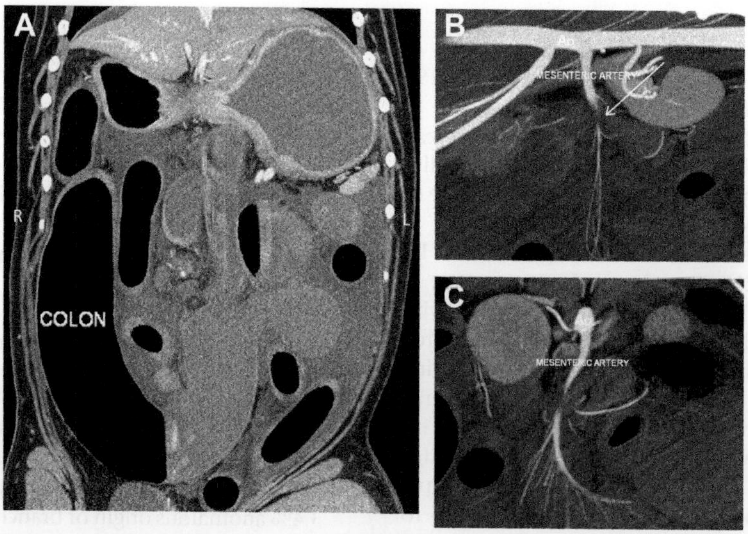

FIG. 11 High-pitch CTA (dual-source, flash mode) in an awake 40-kg dog with mesenteric torsion. (*A*) Dorsal MPR showing abundant free fluid in the abdominal cavity and distended and malpositioned bowel loops. (*B*, *C*) Midsagittal and transverse thin MIP images showing the torsed and obstructed mesenteric artery. Ao, aorta.

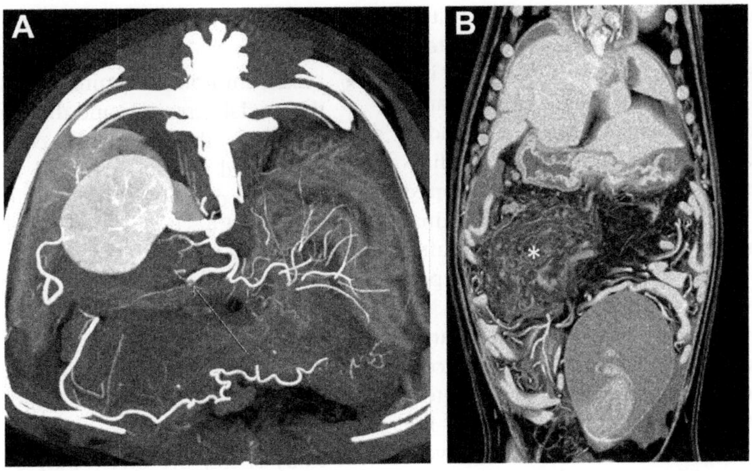

FIG. 12 Multiphase CTA in a dog with mesenteric ischemia and infarction. (*A*) Thin MIP; transverse view shows the arterial intraluminal defect (*arrow*). (*B*) Dorsal MIP; asterisk indicates the omental cake sign due to the omental infarction.

similar to that described in the median arcuate ligament syndrome in people.

Acquired Arterial Conditions

- Among acquired arterial conditions, local intraluminal thrombosis in the distal aorta with occlusion of the iliac and/or femoral artery is the most common indication for MDCTA in dogs and cats. Recently, 16-row CTA has been described as a safe and informative diagnostic imaging modality in awake (or lightly sedated) cats with severe cardiac disease and congestive heart failure using adapted microdose contrast injection protocol that allowed the identification of cardiac thrombi and other important cardiac and extracardiac information [29].
- Arterial aneurysm is focal dilatation involving all layers of the vessel (intima, media, and adventitia); in false pseudoaneurysm, blood leaks through the wall but is contained by the adventitia or surrounding perivascular soft tissue.
- Arterial pseudoaneurysm has been reported as segmental abrupt dilation of the vessel's lumen, with irregular asymmetric thickening of the vascular wall and perivascular increased attenuation and retroperitoneal fat stranding [30].
- Aortic wall inflammation (infectious or noninfectious vasculitis) results in circumferential vascular wall thickening [31]. Chronic stage may present arterial wall mineralization and retroperitoneal fibrotic changes.

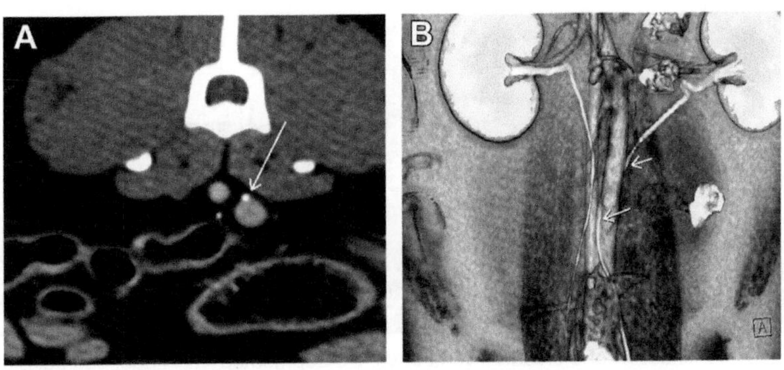

FIG. 13 Left-sided caudal vena cava, in its prerenal segment. (*A*) Transverse image from excretory phase showing the preureteral position of the cava resulting in retrocaval ureter (*arrow*). (*B*) VR image of the same dog showing the left ureter course dorsal to the left-sided vena cava (*arrows*).

- In humans, MDCT is considered the most sensitive and specific diagnostic tool for acute mesenteric ischemia and it is recommended as the first-line imaging modality in symptomatic patients because other causes of acute abdomen also can be excluded [32]. Imaging plays an important role in the diagnosis of mesenteric ischemia that has been reported in small animals in cases of mesenteric or intestinal volvulus or parasitic mesenteric thrombosis, after abdominal trauma, or associated with feline hypertrophic cardiomyopathy (Figs. 11 and 12) [33–36]. A 3-phase, 16-row CT scan protocol for mesenteric vasculature assessment was proposed in a recent study. The scan delay was set based on time-to-attenuation curves, drawn by placing the ROIs over the aorta, intestinal wall, and cranial mesenteric vein [37].

Congenital Anomalies of the Caudal Vena Cava

- Most common abdominal vascular diseases involve the caudal vena cava and the portal system. In adult mammals, the caudal vena cava typically is a single right-sided vessel developed in 5 segments: from caudal to cranial, the prerenal, renal, prehepatic, hepatic, and posthepatic segments. Each segment can be affected by a wide range of congenital variants, anomalies, and pathologic conditions alone or in combination with other vascular anomalies [38,39]. Preureteral vena cava, also known as "circumcaval ureter" or "retrocaval ureter," occurs when a persistent right cardinal vein traps part of the ipsilateral ureter dorsal to it. Although often clinically silent, the ureter may be significantly compressed, resulting in hydroureter and

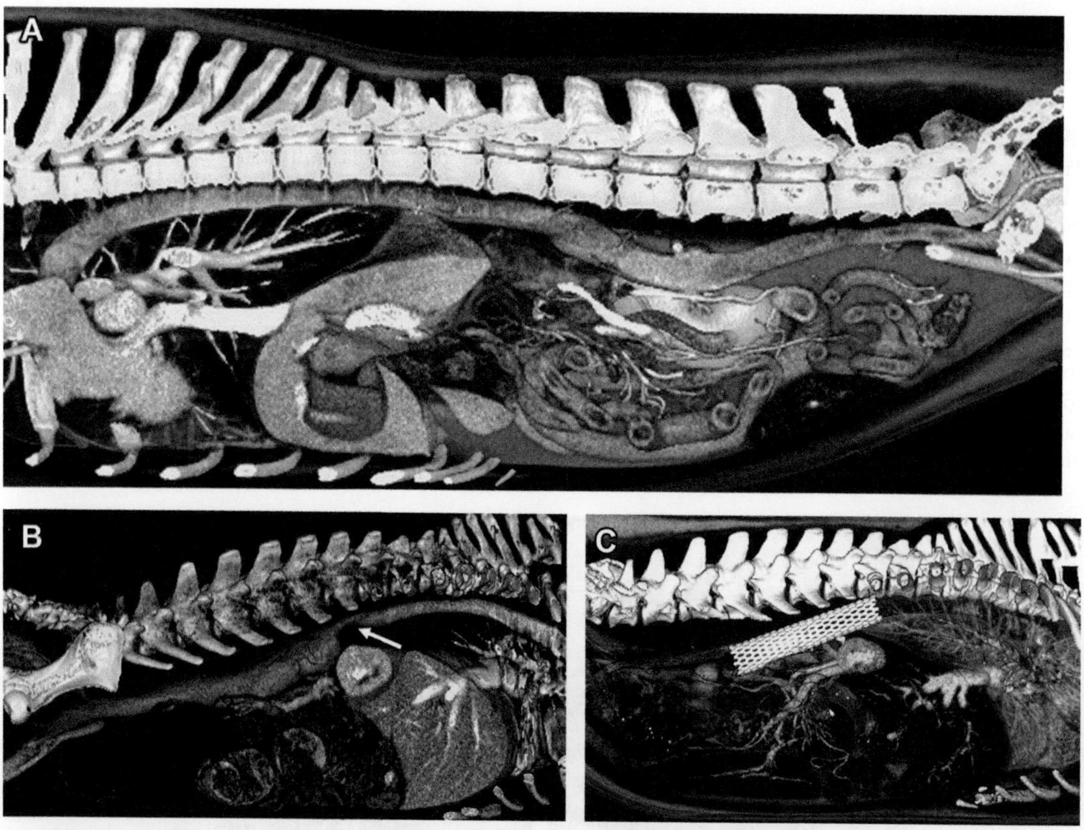

FIG. 14 Azygous continuation of the caudal vena cava. (*A*) Segmented VR image, sagittal plane. The vascular anomaly was discovered incidentally in patient with unrelated clinical signs. (*B*) and (*C*) are VR segmented images from patient's right side. The dog had chronic renal insufficiency and collapse. Note the stenosis at the diaphragmatic passage (*arrow*) treated with cava stenting (*C*).

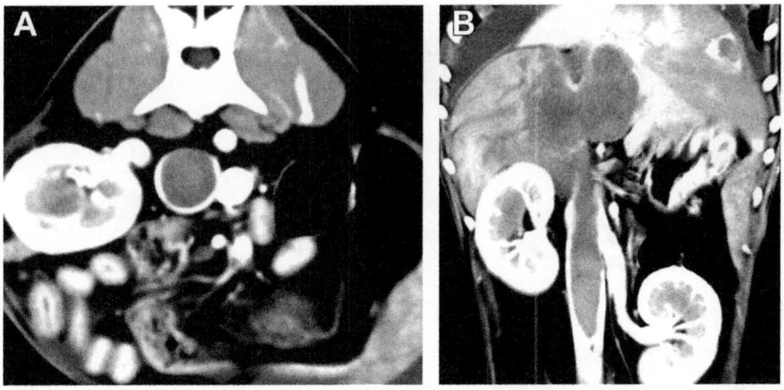

FIG. 15 Thrombosis of the caudal vena cava in a dog with hepatic hemangiosarcoma. (*A*) Transverse section at the level of the right kidney showing the large filling defect of the caudal vena cava. (*B*) Dorsal MPR showing the liver tumor invading the caudal vena cava and the extension of the venous thrombosis.

hydronephrosis. In cats, the preureteral vena cava is observed in approximately one-third of cats (from 22% to 35% prevalence) [40,41].

- In an in vivo study, cats with preureteral vena cava identified at CTA resulted in an increased risk for concurrent urinary signs, as reported in humans [41]. Failure of regression of the left embryonic supracardinal vein, with anomalous regression of the right one, results in the left-sided vena cava (may be associated with preureteral position) (Fig. 13).
- The persistence of both supracardinal veins and the intersubcardinal anastomosis and disturbances of the subsupracardinal anastomosis are embryonic mechanisms possibly involved in partial and complete duplication of the caudal vena cava, involving the prerenal segment alone or the prerenal and renal segments [38]. The interruption of the caudal vena cava with azygous continuation occurs when the right subcardinal–hepatic anastomosis fails to form, resulting in right subcardinal vein atrophy. In this anomaly, the hepatic segment of the caudal

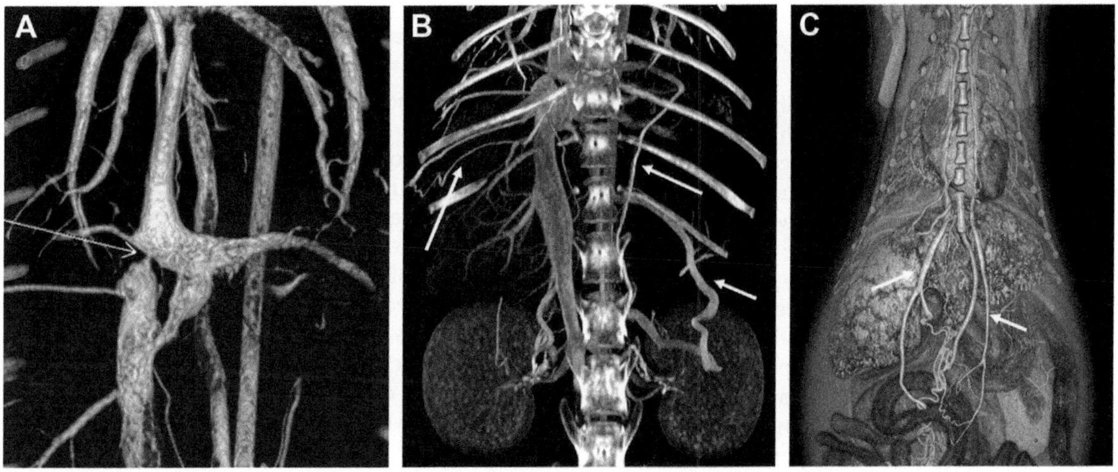

FIG. 16 Cava collaterals pathways in a kitten with hepatic venous outflow obstruction due to hepatic caudal vena cava weblike stenosis. (*A*) VR image showing the caval stenosis (*arrow*). (*B*) Dorsal MIP showing deep collaterals of the vertebral-hemiazygos pathway (*arrows*). (*C*) VR showing the superficial, mammary pathways, including the superficial thoracobdominal vein collaterals (*arrows*).

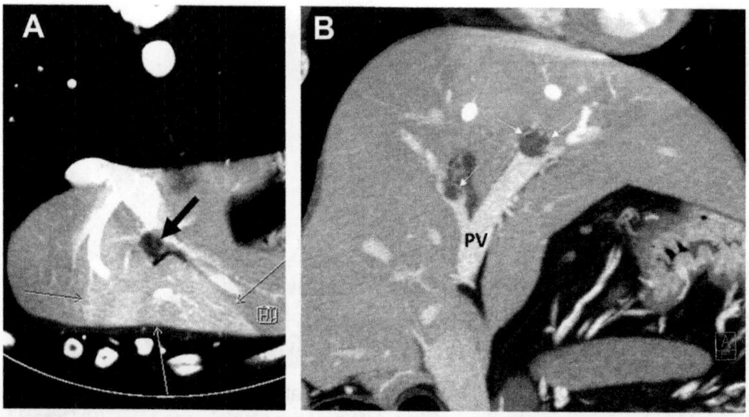

FIG. 17 (*A*) Transverse view of the liver in the arterial phase from multiphase CTA. The black arrow indicates the obstructed portal branch. Thin white arrows indicate a triangular area of early parenchymal enhancement (hepatic perfusion disorder, due to increased microscopic arterioportal communications). Note the early retrograde enhancement of the lobar hepatic veins. (*B*) Dorsal MPR of the same dog. Note the filling defects in both portal branches within the liver. Arrows indicate small, peripheral vessels attempting to recanalize the thrombus (vasa vasorum). PV, portal vein.

vena cava is absent. The caudal vena cava receives the renal veins in its renal segment and then runs dorsally past the diaphragmatic crura to join the right azygous vein in the thorax. In dogs, azygous continuation of the caudal vena cava has been described in association with portal vein aplasia and portocaval shunting, with or without situs inversus abdominalis, and associated with aneurysms of the renal veins and renal-prerenal caudal vena cava (Fig. 14) [42].

Acquired Vascular Conditions of the Caudal Vena

- Acquired vascular conditions of the caudal vena cava include benign and malignant thrombosis (Fig. 15) and collateral formation. Independent of the cause of obstruction, in chronic obstruction of the caudal vena cava, cava collateral pathways may form to maintain venous drainage to the right heart [43].
- Four main collateral pathways are possible that develop depending on the level obstruction: the vertebral-hemiazygos pathway (deep pathway); the internal and external mammary pathways, including the superficial thoracoabdominal veins (superficial pathway); the left renal-hemiazygos pathway, including the gonadal and periureteric veins (intermediate pathway); and a fourth cavoportal pathway is possible, through branches of the mesenteric veins (Fig. 16). These pathways should not be confused with acquired portosystemic connections. These may occur concomitantly with venous collateral pathways when the obstruction involves the hepatic/posthepatic caudal vena cava, causing the postsinusoidal portal hypertension.
- In a multiphase CTA evaluation, it may be possible to note that the opacity of the contrast agent in the collateral vessels matches that of the venous system from which the blood flows: the cava, in cases of cavoportal collateral vessels, and the portal system, in cases of acquired portosystemic collaterals [44].

Congenital and Acquired Portal Venous System Anomalies

- MDCT angiography currently is considered the best method of diagnosing and monitoring of portal vascular anomalies in veterinary patients. In normal adult mammals, no apparent vascular connection between the portal system and the systemic venous circulation exists.
- Portal venous system anomalies include congenital and acquired conditions of the portal vein alone or connections between the portal vein system with the systemic circulation. All these conditions may be isolated or combined in complex vascular patterns and can have serious clinical consequences [45].

Congenital Portal Venous System Anomalies

- Congenital absence of the portal vein (CAPV), due to excessive involution of the periduodenal vitelline veins or failure of the vitelline veins to establish anastomosis with hepatic sinusoids, always is described in association with the portal insertion into the caudal vena cava and total diversion of portal blood into the systemic circulation (end-to-side PSS). CAPV is a rare condition described in dogs in association with other developmental anomalies, including situs inversus, congenital heart diseases, vena cava anomalies, and polysplenia [42,46].

- Portal vein hypoplasia (PVH) refers to a disorder in which microscopic portal veins within the liver are underdeveloped. The primary, morphologic PVH is characterized by abnormally small extrahepatic or intrahepatic portal veins, which result in diminished hepatic perfusion and the potential for portal hypertension. A functional, secondary PVH always is found in liver biopsies of dogs with macroscopic PSSs [47].
- Because of the histologic similarities between primary and secondary PVH and similar nonvascular conditions, such as congenital hepatic fibrosis or other ductal plate anomalies [48], CT is necessary to exclude the presence of a congenital PSS (CPSS) or any other condition that may reduce the portal blood flow to the liver (eg, arteriovenous fistula or portal vein thrombosis [PVT]) as well as to reveal direct and indirect signs of portal hypertension or biliary disorders [49,50].
- Portal vein aneurysm (PVA) described using CTA has a reported prevalence of 0.49% in dogs and can be congenital or acquired [51]. On MDCT images, PVA appears as saccular or fusiform dilatation of the portal vein or its branches within the liver. Extrahepatic PVAs generally are located at the insertion of the gastroduodenal vein into the portal vein. Intrahepatic PVAs occur at bifurcations. Many PVAs are discovered incidentally on routine imaging studies. Potential complications of PVAs include portal system thrombosis, portal hypertension, and aneurysm rupture.

Portal Vein Thrombosis

- Thrombosis can affect any of the different venous segment of the portal venous system alone or combined: portal vein, splenic vein, gastroduodenal, and mesenteric veins. MDCT angiography is an excellent tool for the diagnosis of malignant and nonmalignant PVT to confirm and define the causative conditions of PVT and its complications [45].
- In cases of acute PVT, unenhanced scans may show slight hyperattenuation of material within the vascular lumen, which does not enhance in the portal venous phase. In cases of acute obstruction of the portal vein, dependent areas of the liver parenchyma may show increased arterial enhancement and decreased enhancement during the portal venous phase.
- Partial and complete PVT may show peripheral enhancement, and these conditions should be distinguished. In cases of partial occlusion, some contrast passes around the thrombus. In cases of complete obstruction, enhancement of the peripheral rim of the thrombus likely is due to dilatation of the vasa vasorum in the attempt to recanalize the vessel.
- As a consequence of portal vein obstruction, compensatory mechanisms are immediately activated to reestablish the portal flow to the liver. A first compensatory mechanism in cases of portal vein obstruction is the distention of the hepatic artery and its branches within the liver parenchyma, so-called arterialization. Small arterial-portal

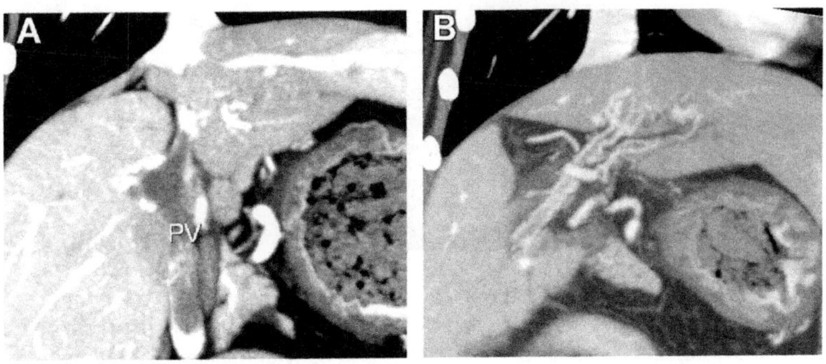

FIG. 18 Porto-portal collateral pathways in a case of obstructed portal vein. (*A*) Dorsal MPR showing the extensive filling defect in the portal vein and portal branches. (*B*) Long porto-portal collaterals reestablish the portal flow to the liver (thin MIP from interstitial phase).

connections may form within the liver and manifest as hepatic perfusion disorders in multiphase CTA.

- A second mechanism is the formation of portal venous collaterals [52]. Cavernous transformation of the portal vein refers to the radiological appearance of porto-portal collaterals around a thrombosed portal vein (Figs. 17 and 18). Two main types of porto-portal collateral may be found when reviewing MDCT data in chronic PVT in dogs and cats: short tortuous collaterals developing around/inside the thrombus and long collaterals.
- Isolated splenic vein thrombosis or obstruction has been described in dogs using CTA [31]. Depending on the level of obstruction, regardless of the cause (thrombosis, splenic pedicle torsion, or splenic vein tumor invasion), the splenic collateral circulation may be provided by the left gastric, left gastroepiploic, and/or splenogonadal veins.

High-Flow Versus Low-Flow Portal Anomalous Connections

Connections between the portal venous system and systemic circulation can be classified as high-flow (or fast-flow) and low-flow (or slow-flow) portal connections. Both include congenital and acquired conditions.

Hepatic Arteriovenous Malformations

- High-flow anomalous portal connections are rare structural or functional communications between a high-pressure hepatic arterial branch and a low-

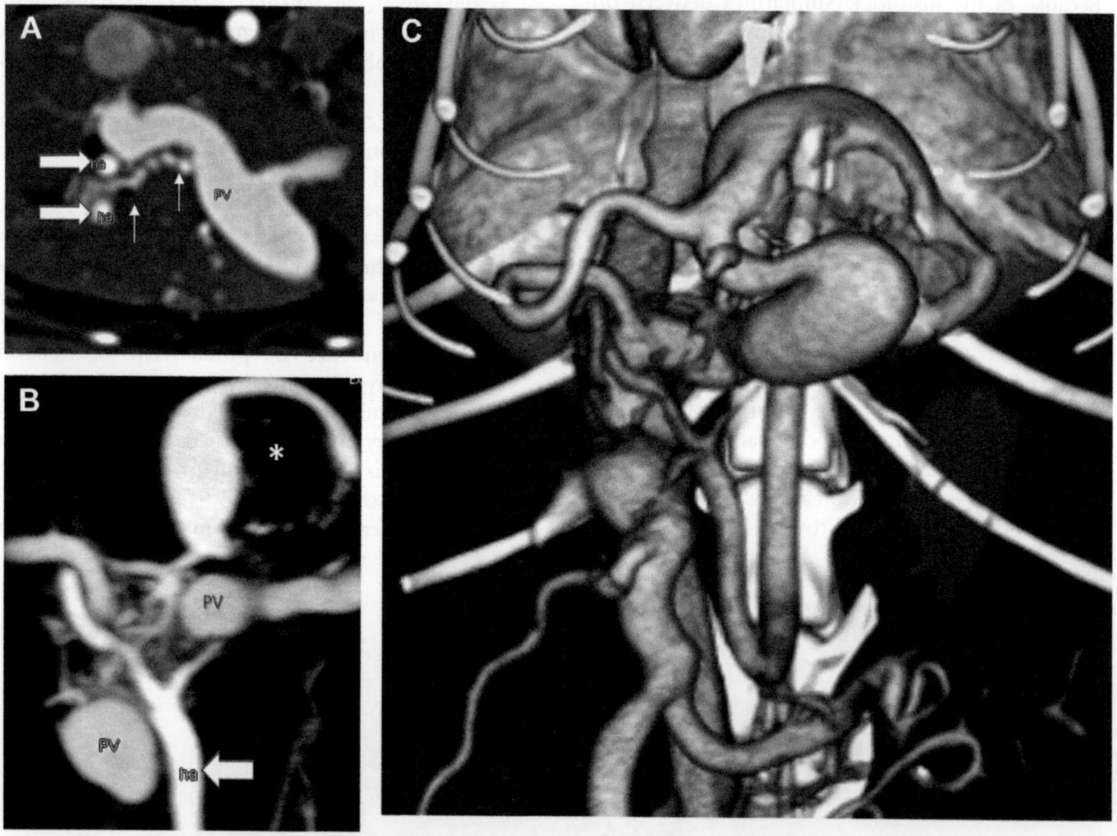

FIG. 19 HAVM in a kitten (intrahepatic left divisional and medial arterioportal malformation). (*A*) Transverse view of the liver in the arterial phase. Arterialization of the portal vein: many small branches of the hepatic artery (*large and thin arrows*) are visible around a dilatated and early enhanced branch of the portal vein (PV). (*B*) Dorsal thin MIP of same CTA. Note the multiple small vessels around the portal branch representing the nidus. The asterisk indicates a large thrombotic aneurysm. (*C*) VR showing the complex HAVM. ha, hepatic artery.

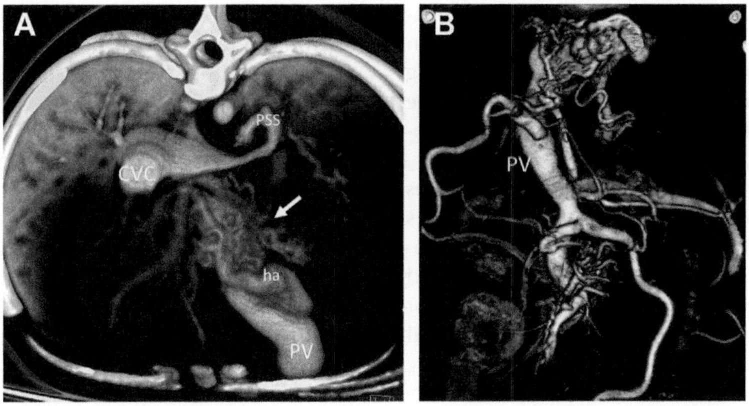

FIG. 20 HAVM in a dog. Note the enlarged hepatic artery (ha) and the nidus (*arrow*) and the aneurysmal branch of the portal vein (PV). In addition, note a splenophrenic PSS. (*B*) VR image showing the engorged portal venous system. PV, portal vein.

pressure portal branch, which may lead to presinusoidal portal hypertension. Recently, HAVMs have been subclassified using CTA as left medial and left lateral, depending on the site of the efferent portal vein drainage [53]. CTA of these patients may show direct and indirect signs, such as ascites and secondary acquired portosystemic collaterals (Figs. 19 and 20).

- Penetrating abdominal trauma, including liver biopsy and neoplasia, is a possible etiology of acquired arterioportal fistulas. CTA signs of acquired arterioportal fistula include earlier enhancement of the portal vein or its branches in the early arterial phase of a multiphasic examination.

Congenital and Acquired Portosystemic Shunts

- Low-flow anomalous portal connections include congenital and acquired PSSs (APSSs) and portoportal and cavoportal collaterals. CPSS refers to the presence of abnormal vascular connections due to

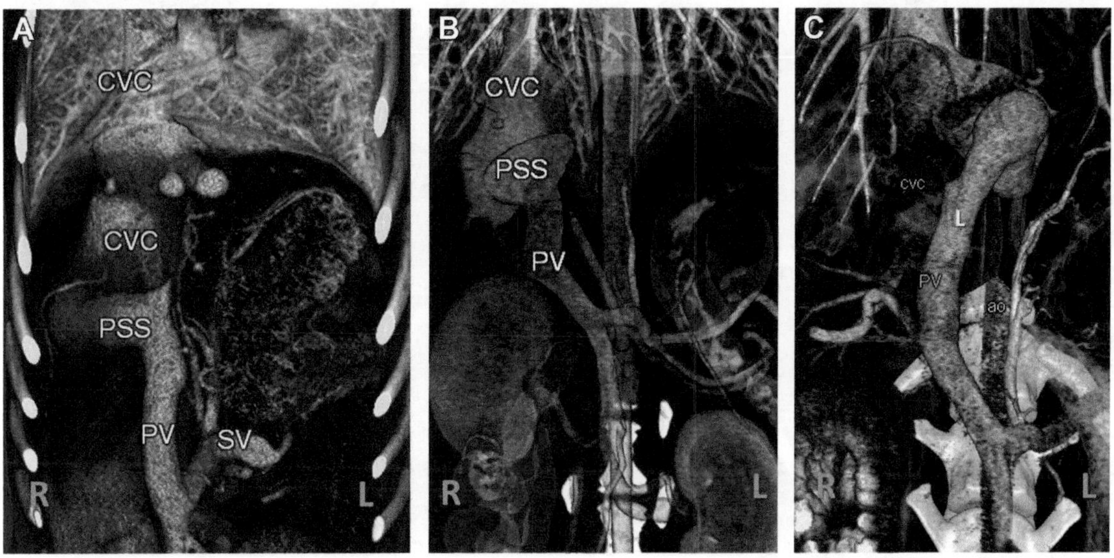

FIG. 21 Different patterns of single IHPSS in dogs. VR, from ventral point of view. (*A*) Right divisional. (*B*) Central divisional. (*C*) Left divisional. CVC, caudal vena cava; PSS, portosystemic shunt; PV, portal vein; SV, splenic vein. L, left portal branch. Ao, aorta.

embryonic errors or fetal vascular persistence; it connects the portal system directly to a systemic vein (caudal vena cava or azygous system), bypassing the liver. Based on anatomic location, they can be divided into intrahepatic PSSs (IHPSSs) and extrahepatic PSSs (EHPSSs).

- IHPSSs customarily were divided into 3 subtypes [54]. With the widespread use of MDCT in patients with suspected CPSS, new IHPSS patterns are identified and traditional classifications may be refined describing different phenotypes (Fig. 21). Single or multiple peripheral connections between portal branches and hepatic veins, affecting 1 or more liver lobes, and portosystemic intrahepatic connections through portal aneurysmal dilatations within the liver are possible presentations (Fig. 22) [45,55,56].
- EHPSSs are developmental anomalies resulting from anomalous connections between the vitelline veins, which form the portal system, and the cardinal veins, forming the systemic veins. The shunt can be between the portal vein directly or 1 of its tributaries (left gastric vein, splenic vein, or right gastric vein) and a systemic vein (caudal vena cava or right azygous vein). Various repetitive patterns of EHPSS have been described using MDCT angiography, which has completely changed the diagnostic work-up for CPSS in small animals [7,57].
- The morphologic classification defined the PSS on the basis of the starting vessel and the end. The left or right gastric veins more commonly emanate the shunting vessel that join a systemic vein, the caudal vena cava or azygos vein (thus referred to as left/right gastric-caval shunt or left/right-gastric azygos shunt) (Figs. 23 and 24) [58,59]. Mesenteric-reno-caval shunt has been reported in dogs and left colic vein or cranial rectal vein to pelvic systemic vein communication (directly to the caudal vena cava or through common iliac vein or internal iliac vein) has been reported in both dogs and cats [60,61].
- APSSs are characterized by hepatofugal pathways that can be caused by portal hypertension (increased resistance in the portal system) or increased resistance in the cranial vena cava (CrVC) system. Several patterns of APSS have been described in dogs and cats using MDCT angiography [62]. They can be divided grossly into large shunts (eg, left splenogonadal or splenophrenic shunt) and small shunts or varices (Figs. 25 and 26).
- Varices may be subdivided further according to their anatomic location and pathways into left gastric vein, gastrophrenic, omental, gallbladder,

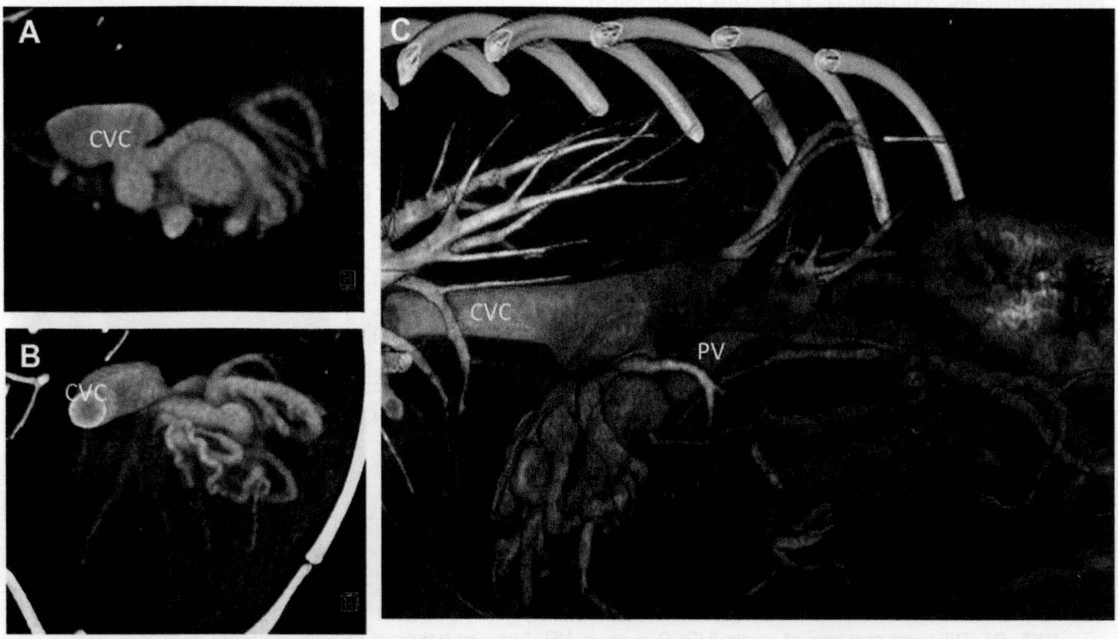

FIG. 22 Complex IHPSS in a puppy. There are multiple low-flow connections between portal branches and hepatic veins in the left liver lobes. All images are different 3-D VR segmentations. (*A*, *B*), from frontal point of view. (*C*) From left side point of view. CVC, caudal vena cava; PV, portal vein.

abdominal wall, duodenal, and colic varices. MDCT plays an important role in the diagnostic work-up for patients with acquired portal collaterals in cases of portal hypertension. Most prehepatic, hepatic, and posthepatic causes of portal hypertension can be identified easily by whole-body MDCT examination.

THORACIC COMPUTED TOMOGRAPHY ANGIOGRAPHY

- The thoracic vascularization includes systemic vasculature and pulmonary vessels. Factors that contribute to high-quality thoracic MDCTA depend on the CT scanner technology and techniques, including the access vein (site and size), the scan method, and contrast injection protocol. The delay between the contrast injection and the start of scanning should be tailored based on the patient's characteristics using the bolus test or the bolus tracking technique, as described for abdominal CTA.
- The ROI may be placed on different vascular structures, the ascending aorta, or the main pulmonary artery, depending on the purpose of the study. Pulsatile artifacts are critical for the accurate diagnosis of aortic arch anomalies, especially in small veterinary patients [63]. With slower 8 to 16 rows MDCT scanners, acquisition of near-isotropic data set with spiral acquisition mode and a half-scan interpolation reconstruction (50% overlap) algorithm may help to obtain diagnostic images.
- Scanners with 64 or more rows and DSCT scanners can routinely image the thoracic aorta using electrocardiogram gating or can acquired the thoracic volume in subsecond spiral mode, resulting in the freezing of cardiovascular and respiratory motions.

THORACIC VASCULAR DISEASES

CTA of the systemic thoracic vasculature has been described in a wide range of congenital and acquired vascular conditions, including anomalies of the aortic arch and its branches, bronchial and bronchoesophageal arterial anomalies, and systemic thoracic veins diseases [64,65].

Aortic Arch Anomalies

- In cases of aortic arch anomalies, CTA allows fast and high-quality assessment of the complex vascular anomalies and of tracheal or esophageal compression in the same study. Congenital anomalies of the aortic arch include diverse subgroups of malformations that may be clinically silent or may present with severe respiratory or esophageal signs, especially when associated with complete vascular rings (vascular ring anomalies) [64].
- Vascular ring anomalies in dogs and cats and assessed using CTA are described as follow: persistent right aortic arch with a left ligamentum arteriosus alone or with an aberrant normal or hypoplastic left subclavian artery, which may take a retroesophageal position resulting in an incomplete vascular ring, contributing to esophageal compression; a left aberrant subclavian artery can be found alone, with normal-sided aortic arch; a right aberrant subclavian artery, arising from the

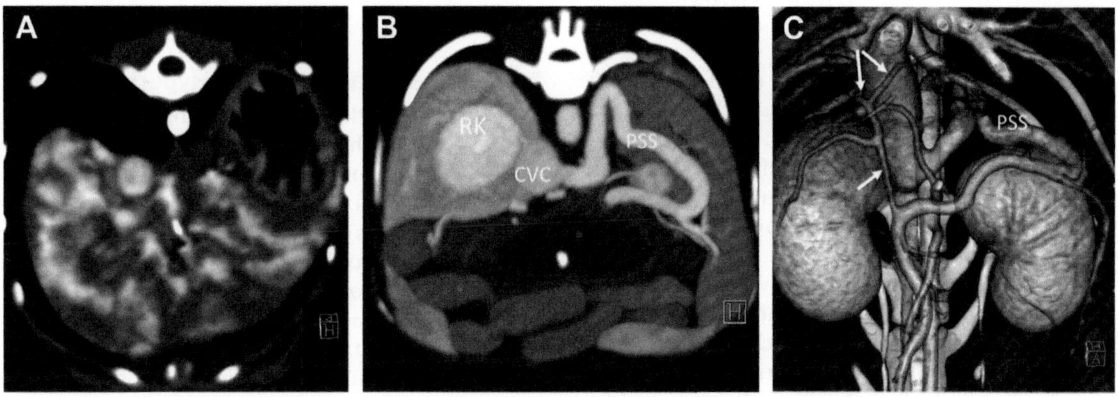

FIG. 23 Congenital EHPSS in a puppy (left gastric to prehepatic cava shunt). (*A*) Severe hepatic perfusion disorders (arterial phase) due to microscopic functional arterioportal shunts secondary to the PVH (functional PVH). (*B*) Transverse thin MIP showing the site of PSS insertion in the caudal vena cava (CVC). (*C*) VR image showing the course of PSS and thin, portal vein and portal branches (*arrows*). RK, right kidney.

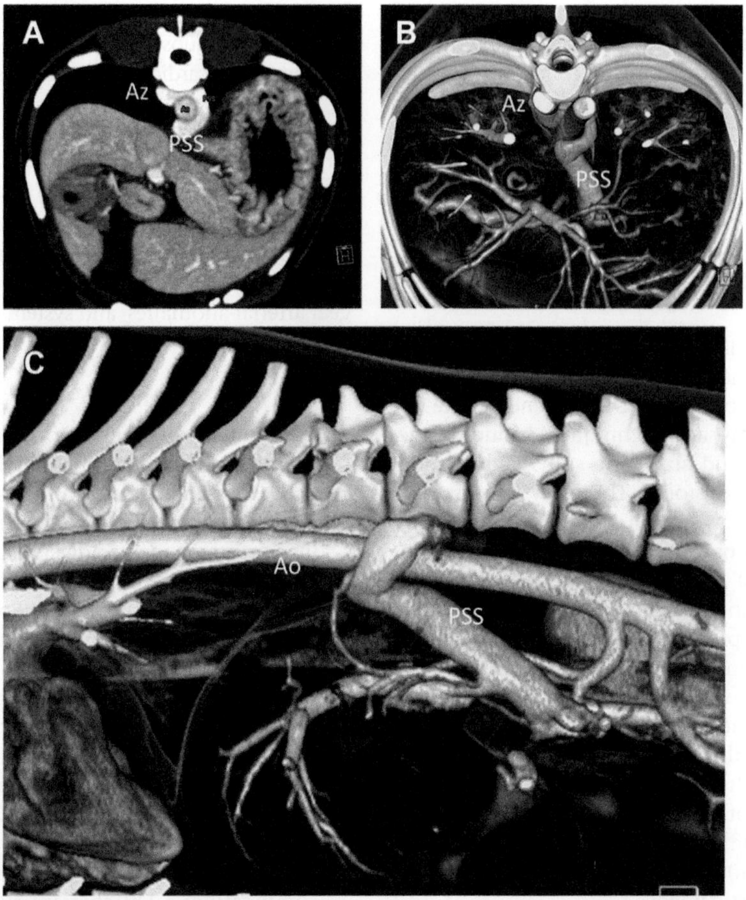

FIG. 24 Congenital EHPSS in a puppy (left gastric to right azygos shunt). (*A*) Transverse view (portal venous phase). Note the shunting vessel (PSS) encircling the descending aorta (Ao) to join the right azygous vein (Az). (*B*) Segmented VR from cranial point of view. (*C*) VR from left side, showing the starting point (from left gastric vein) and course of the anomalous vessel.

normally left-sided aortic arch, distal to the left subclavian artery, or from a bisubclavian trunk, generally is reported incidentally; a persistent right ligamentum arteriosum with a left aortic arch; and a double aortic arch for persistence of the fourth aortic arches, which encircle and constrict the esophagus and trachea (Fig. 27).

- Coarctation of the aorta (a narrowing of the aortic lumen) can occur in the segment of the aorta between the origin of the left subclavian artery and the insertion of the ductus arteriosus; in dogs, it has been described as the aortic hypoplasia (the interruption of the aorta), which may be associated with coarctation and other congenital defects, such as persistent ductus arteriosus.

Bronchoesophageal Artery Hypertrophy

- Enlarged bronchial branches of bronchoesophageal artery, bronchoesophageal artery hypertrophy (BEAH), and other nonbronchial thoracic arteries (eg, intercostal, internal mammary, and inferior phrenic arteries) frequently are observed in patients with chronic pulmonary embolism [65]. These vessels respond to chronic pulmonary ischemia and decreased pulmonary blood flow with hypertrophy or enlargement, trying to maintain blood flow to the affected lung and participate in gas exchange through the peripheral systemic-pulmonary arterial anastomoses.
- Thoracic CTA shows prominent bronchial branches at the bronchial bifurcation, continuing their course

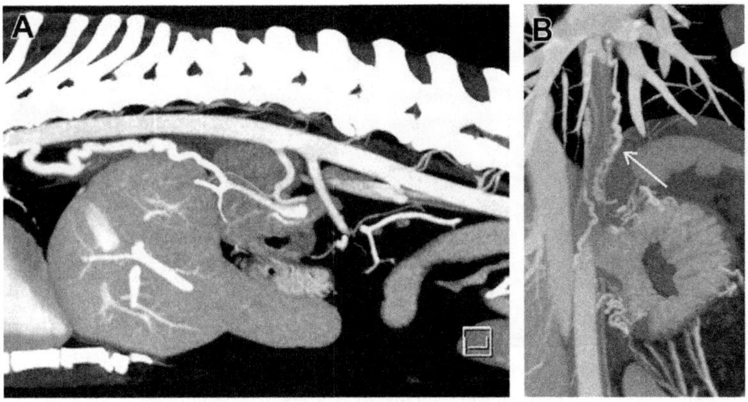

FIG. 25 (*A*) Acquired portosystemic connection in a dog with portal hypertension (left gastric vein varix, from left gastric vein to right azygos vein). Thin MIP, sagittal view of portal venous phase. (*B*) Thin MIP dorsal view from interstitial phase. Multiple gastroesophageal varices in another dog with portal hypertension (the arrow indicates uphill varices, between gastric veins and azygous vein system through esophageal venous drainage).

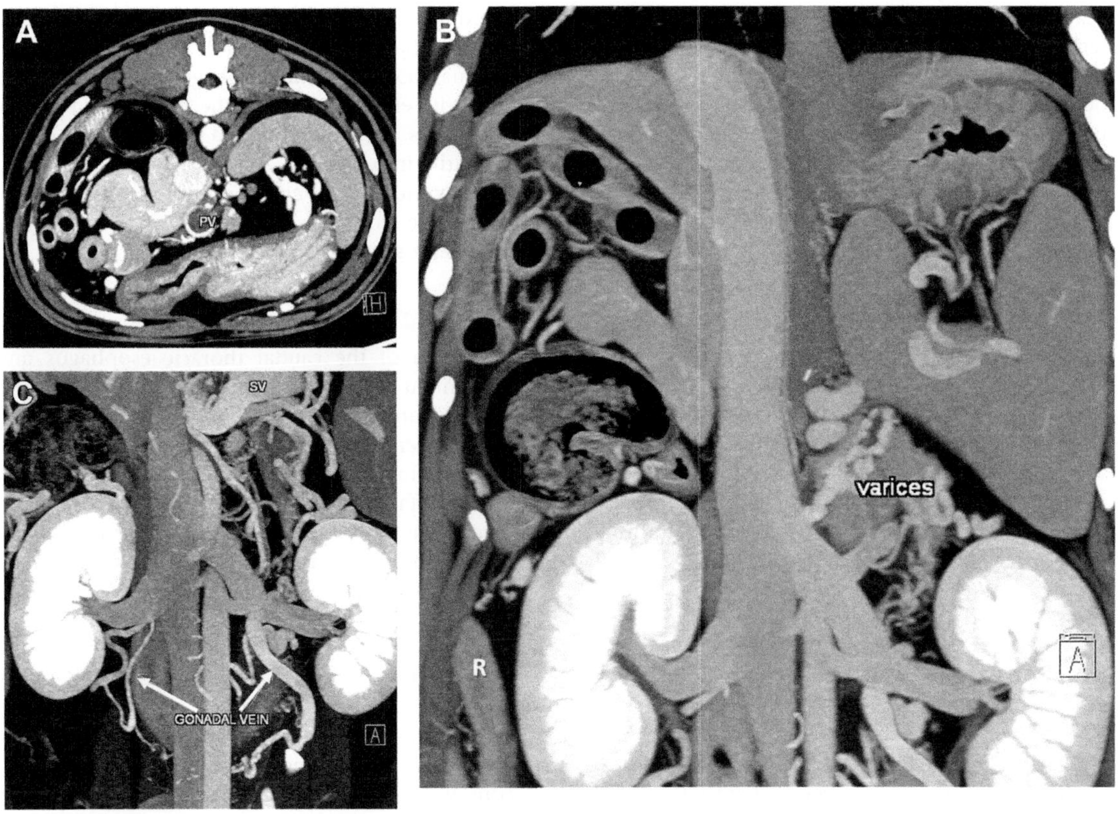

FIG. 26 Acquired portal collaterals in a dog with portal hypertension. (*A*) Transverse view from 16-MDCT angiography showing a large filling defect in the portal vein (portal thrombosis). (*B*) Dorsal, thin MIP showing distention of the left gonadal vein as compared with the contralateral (*arrows*) (splenogondal shunt; here is not visible the connection between splenic and gonadal vein). (*C*) Retroperitoneal varices (between gastrosplenic branches and phrenicoaddominal veins). PV, portal vein; SV, splenic vein.

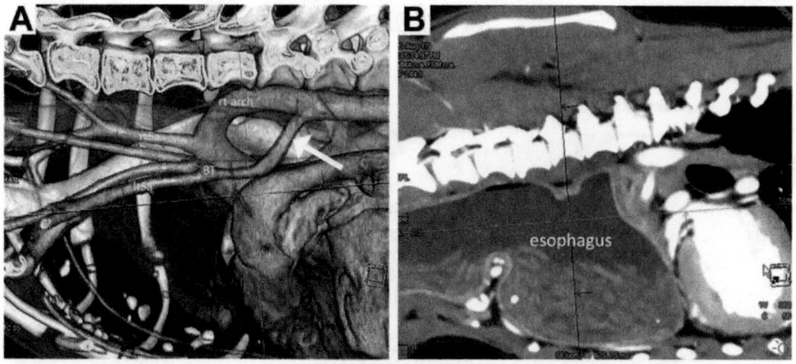

FIG. 27 Vascular ring anomalies in a dog. (*A*) VR image of double aortic arch for persistence of the fourth aortic arch (*arrow*) and abnormal origin of the subclavian arteries. (*B*) Sagittal MPR showing a large esophageal diverticulum containing fluid and food material inside. BT, brachycephalic trunk; ltSa, left subclavian artery; rt arch, right-sided aortic arch; rtSa, right subclavian artery.

along the bronchi, describing a tortuous path, and ultimately anastomose with the subsegmental pulmonary arteries (Fig. 28). Congenital pattern of BEAH is described in dogs in association with systemic-to-pulmonary fistula (with left or right main pulmonary artery). This pattern might result from persistent embryonic pulmonary-systemic connection, as hypothesized for patent ductus arteriosus. In these cases, a large vessel (5–8 mm diameter) is seen in middle mediastinum, emptying into the proximal part of the left or right pulmonary artery through a small orifice.

Persistent Left Cranial Vena Cava

- The CrVC and azygos vein system (azygos and hemiazygos veins) provide the venous drainage to the thorax. The left and right common cardinal veins empty into the transversely positioned sinus venosus, which subsequently develops into the right atrium. Most of the left cardinal system atrophies; only the left common cardinal vein persists, forming the coronary sinus. Incomplete atrophy of the left cranial cardinal vein leads to persistence of the left cranial cava.
- Two types of persistent left CrVC have been described in dogs and cats: a complete type, in which the nonatrophied left cranial cardinal vein retains its embryologic connection with the coronary sinus; and an incomplete type, in which the distal portion of the persistent vein atrophies, whereas the proximal portion persists and receives the hemiazygos vein [66].
- Persistent left CrVC alone often is an incidental CT finding, but it has been reported to cause esophageal stenosis and secondary megaesophagus. Moreover, subjects with left persistent CrVC may have other severe cardiovascular defects and should be assessed thoroughly.
- The esophageal (submucosal) and periesophageal venous plexi drain the esophagus and are situated along its entire length. In the cranial part of the esophagus, the periesophageal venous plexus drains primarily into the CrVC via the bronchoesophageal and thyroid veins. Venous drainage of the middle part of the esophagus is largely into the azygos and hemiazygos veins and thereby into the CrVC.

Esophageal Varices

- The veins of the caudal thoracic esophagus and abdominal esophagus drain into the azygos vein and accompany the esophageal branch of the left gastric artery, reaching the portal circulation by the splenic vein or directly by the portal vein (a tributary of the portal system). The latter is a possible hepatofugal pathway in cases of portal hypertension.
- Both types of esophageal varices have been described and classified in small animals using MDCTA [62,65,67]. Uphill varices have been described alone or in association with large abdominal APSSs in patients with portal hypertension. Downhill varices have been described in cases of BEAH, chronic CrVC compression, and tumoral invasion.
- The azygos system (right azygos vein and hemizygous vein) is an important intermediary between the caudal and CrVCs via the internal vertebral venous system, which drains into the cranial vein. In this setting, the azygos veins are systemic and involved in congenital and APSSs. In patients with

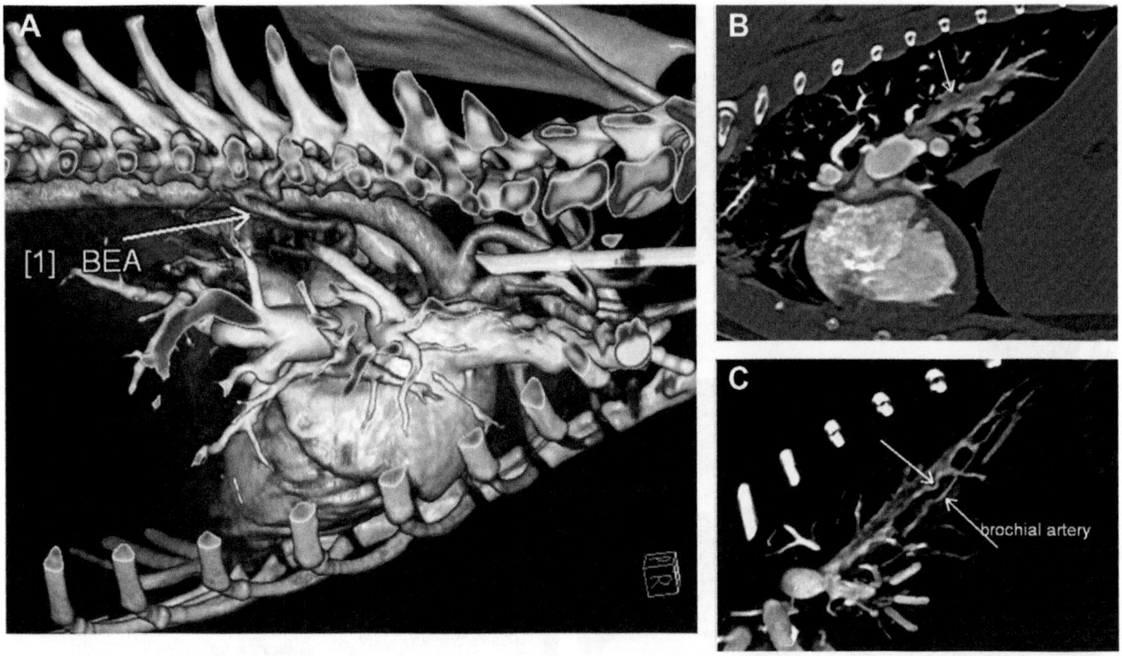

FIG. 28 BEAH in a dog with chronic pulmonary embolism. (*A*) Segmented VR image, from right side, showing the enlarged bronchoesophageal artery (BEA). (*B*) 2-D MPR parasagittal image showing the extensive pulmonary thrombosis (*arrow*). (*C*) Thin MIP at the same level, showing the prominent bronchial artery branches (*arrows*).

portoazygos connections, the right azygos vein is enlarged and tortuous.

PULMONARY VASCULAR DISEASES

Pulmonary Thromboembolism

- Pulmonary CTA is used for the assessment of the pulmonary vascular anomalies and is the preferred imaging method for intraluminal pathologic conditions of the pulmonary vessels, such as pulmonary thromboembolism [68]. Pulmonary CTA enables the visualization of pulmonary embolism in a majority of cases (Fig. 29). Small peripheral emboli, however, may remain unnoticed, or their impacts on lung perfusion may remain unclear.
- Whereas pulmonary CTA provides only morphologic information and does not allow direct assessment of the effects of thromboembolic clots on lung perfusion, dual-energy CTA simultaneously provides functional and morphologic information that might be clinically useful for patient management [68]. Both in people and in animals, dual-energy CTA perfusion imaging showed good agreement with scintigraphy findings [69].
- The density of iodine CM is stronger at lower voltage than at higher voltage, whereas this effect is negligible for the other elements (air and soft tissue). Therefore, this peculiar x-ray absorption characteristic makes selective iodine mapping (corresponding to lung perfusion) possible. Most recent generations of single-source (single x-ray tube) MDCT scanners can be used to acquire dual-energy data by ultrafast switching between 140 kVp and 80 kVp. Most recent (second-generation and third-generation) DSCT scanners have double tube detector systems (Dual Energy-DSCT) that enable the simultaneous acquisition of high-quality data at different energy levels (generally 140 kVp and 100 kVp).
- Dedicated software can be used to obtain virtual noncontrast images, color-coded MPRs, and specific measurements from original data sets. Local triangular perfusion defects are signs of pulmonary embolism. In a recent preliminary study in dogs, dual-energy DSCT lung perfusion imaging in addition to CT pulmonary angiography helped the detection of segmental and subsegmental pulmonary embolism [70].

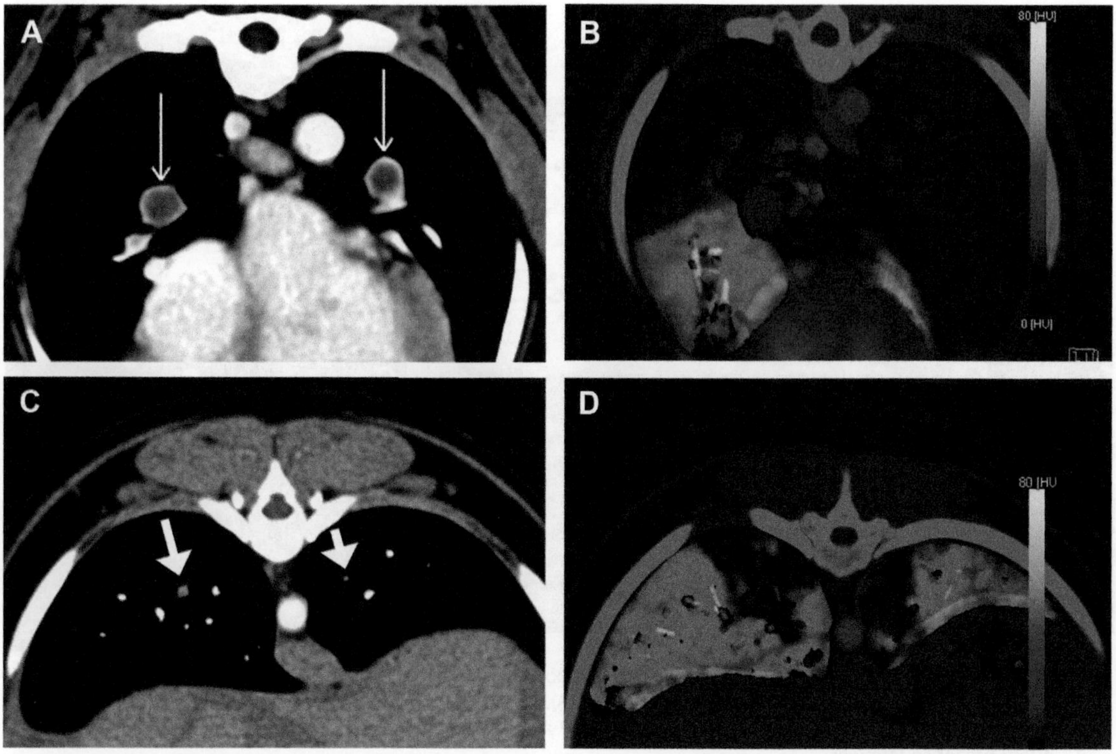

FIG. 29 Dual-source, dual-energy pulmonary angiography. (*A*) Transverse image of a pulmonary CTA in a dog with intraluminal filling defects in the pulmonary vessels of the caudal lobes (*arrows*). (*B*) Color-coded map showing the iodine distribution pattern. The dark areas are hypoperfused lung parenchyma. Yellow indicates more iodine concentration and better perfusion. (*C*) Note small nonenhanced subsegmental pulmonary vessels (*arrows*) that may pass unnoticed on rapid evaluation of the lung volume. (*D*) Lung perfusion imaging. Color coded map representing the iodine distribution map. Note the red triangular areas corresponding to the ischemic lung dependent areas.

DISCLOSURE

The author has nothing to disclose.

REFERENCES

[1] Napel S, Marks MP, Rubin GD, et al. CT angiography with spiral CT and maximum intensity projection. Radiology 1992;185(2):607–10.

[2] Prokop M. Principles of computed tomography angiography. In: Rubin DG, Rofsky NM, editors. CT and MR angiography. Philadelphia, PA: Lippincott Williams & Wilkins (LWW); 2008. p. 3–51.

[3] Zwingenberger AL, Schwarz T. Dual-phase CT Angiography of the Normal Canine Portal and Hepatic Vasculature. Vet Radiol Ultrasound 2004;45:117–24.

[4] Zwingenberger AL, Shofer FS. Dynamic computed tomographic quantitation of hepatic perfusion in dogs with and without portal vascular anomalies. Am J Vet Res 2007;68(9):970–4.

[5] Cáceres AV, Zwingenberger AL, Hardam E, et al. Helical computed tomographic angiography of the normal canine pancreas. Vet Radiol Ultrasound 2006;47:270–8.

[6] Bertolini G, Prokop M. Multidetector-row computed tomography: Technical basics and preliminary clinical applications in small animals. Vet J 2011;189:15–26.

[7] Bertolini G, Rolla EC, Zotti A, et al. Three-dimensional multislice helical computed tomography techniques for canine extra-hepatic portosystemic shunt assessment. Vet Radiol Ultrasound 2006;47:439–43.

[8] Rubin GD, Shiau MC, Schmidt AJ, et al. Computed tomographic angiography: historical perspective and new state-of-the-art using multi detector-row helical computed tomography. J Comput Assist Tomogr 1999; 23(Suppl 1):S83–90.

[9] Rogalla P, Kloeters C, Hein PA. CT technology overview: 64-slice and beyond. Radiol Clin North Am 2009;47(1):1–11.

[10] Petersilka M, Bruder H, Krauss B, et al. Technical principles of dual source CT. Eur J Radiol 2008;68(3):362-368.

[11] Fuentes-Orrego JM, Pinho D, Kulkarni NM, et al. New and evolving concepts in CT for abdominal vascular imaging. Radiographics 2014;34(5):1363–84.

[12] Rubin GD, Leipsic J, Joseph Schoepf U, et al. CT angiography after 20 years: a transformation in cardiovascular disease characterization continues to advance. Radiology 2014;271(3):633–52.

[13] Fishman EK, Ney DR, Heath DG, et al. Volume rendering versus maximum intensity projection in CT angiography: what works best, when, and why. Radiographics 2006; 26:905–22.

[14] Dalrymple NC, Prasad SR, Freckleton MW, et al. Introduction to the language of three-dimensional imaging with multidetector CT. Radiographics 2005;25:1409–28.

[15] Lipson SA. 3D Workstations: basic principles and pitfalls. In: MDCT and 3D Workstations—a practical guide and teaching file. New York: Springer; 2006. p. 41–63.

[16] Boskamp T, Rinck D, Link F, et al. New vessel analysis tool for morphometric quantification and visualization of vessels in CT and MR imaging data sets. Radiographics 2004;24(1):287–97.

[17] Bertolini G. Basic principles of MDCT Angiography. In: Body MDCT in small animals. Cham, Switzerland: Springer International Publishing AG; 2017. https://doi.org/10.1007/978-3-319-46904-1.

[18] Bae KT. Intravenous Contrast Medium Administration and Scan Timing at CT: Considerations and Approaches. Radiology 2010;256:1, 32-61.

[19] Thierry F, Chau J, Makara M, et al. Vascular conspicuity differs among injection protocols and scanner types for canine multiphasic abdominal computed tomographic angiography. Vet Radiol Ultrasound 2018;59:677–86.

[20] Fleischmann D, Kamaya A. Optimal vascular and parenchymal contrast enhancement: the current state of the art. Radiol Clin North Am 2009;47(1):13–26.

[21] Cassel N, Carstens A, Becker P. The comparison of bolus tracking and test bolus techniques for computed tomography thoracic angiography in healthy beagles. J S Afr Vet Assoc 2013;84(1):E1–9.

[22] Mai W, Suran JN, Cáceres AV, et al. Comparison between bolus tracking and timing-bolus techniques for renal computed tomographic angiography in normal cats. Vet Radiol Ultrasound 2013;54(4):343–50.

[23] Iseri T, Yamada K, Chijiwa K, et al. Dynamic computed tomography of the pancreas in normal dogs and in a dog with pancreatic insulinoma. Vet Radiol Ultrasound 2007;48:328–31.

[24] Kishimoto M, Tsuji Y, Katabami N, et al. Measurement of canine pancreatic perfusion using dynamic computed tomography: influence of input-output vessels on deconvolution and maximum slope methods. Eur J Radiol 2011;77:175–81.

[25] Kloer TB, Rao S, Twedt DC, et al. Computed tomographic evaluation of pancreatic perfusion in healthy dogs. Am J Vet Res 2020;81(2):131–8.

[26] Lell MM, Wildberger JE, Alkadhi H, et al. Evolution in computed tomography: the battle for speed and dose. Invest Radiol 2015;50(9):629–44. https://doi.org/10.1097/RLI.0000000000000172.

[27] Buls N, Van Gompel G, Van Cauteren T, et al. Contrast agent and radiation dose reduction in abdominal CT by a combination of low tube voltage and advanced image reconstruction algorithms. Eur Radiol 2015;25:1023–31.

[28] Le Pommellet HM, Scansen BA, Mathys DA, et al. Arterial anomalies of the celiac trunk and median arcuate ligament compression in dogs and cats assessed by computed tomography angiography. Vet Surg 2018;47: 252–60.

[29] Vititoe KP, Fries RC, Joslyn S, et al. Detection of intra-cardiac thrombi and congestive heart failure in cats using computed tomographic angiography. Vet Radiol Ultrasound 2018;59:412–22.

[30] Labrès-Diaz FJ, Brissot H, Ibarrola P. Imaging diagnosis-celiac artery pseudoaneurysm associated with a migrating grass awn. Vet Radiol Ultrasound 2010;51:508–11.

[31] Specchi S, d'Anjou M-A. Diagnostic imaging for the assessment of acquired abdominal vascular diseases in small animals: A pictorial review. Vet Radiol Ultrasound 2019;60:613–32.

[32] Kanasaki S, Furukawa A, Fumoto K, et al. Acute Mesenteric Ischemia: Multidetector CT Findings and Endovascular Management. Radiographics 2018;38:3, 945-961.

[33] Hamilton TR, Thacher CW, Forsee KM, et al. Trauma-associated acute mesenteric ischemia in a dog. J Vet Emerg Crit Care (San Antonio) 2010;20(6):595–600.

[34] Lee M, Park N, Kim J, et al. Imaging diagnosis—acute mesenteric ischemia associated with hypertrophic cardiomyopathy in a cat. Vet Radiol Ultrasound 2015;56: E44–7.

[35] Rautala EK, Björkenheim PS, Laitinen MR, et al. Radiographic and ultrasonographic findings in three surgically confirmed cases of small intestinal ischemia related to mesenteric volvulus or intestinal torsion in dogs. Open Journal of Veterinary Medicine (OJVM) 2017;7(9). https://doi.org/10.4236/ojvm.2017.79010.

[36] Lerman O, Israeli I, Weingram T, et al. Acute mesenteric ischemia-like syndrome associated with suspected Spirocerca lupi aberrant migration in dogs. J Vet Emerg Crit Care (San Antonio) 2019;29:668–73.

[37] Lee SK, Yoon S, Kim C, et al. Triple-phased mesenteric CT angiography using a test bolus technique for evaluation of the mesenteric vasculature and small intestinal wall contrast enhancement in dogs. Vet Radiol Ultrasound 2019;60. https://doi.org/10.1111/vru.12781.

[38] Bertolini G, Diana A, Cipone M, et al. Multidetector row computed tomography and ultrasound characteristics of caudal vena cava duplication in dogs. Vet Radiol Ultrasound 2014;55:521–30.

[39] Ryu C, Choi S, Choi H, et al. CT variants of the caudal vena cava in 121 small breed dogs. Vet Radiol Ultrasound 2019;60:680–8.

[40] Bélanger R, Shmon CL, Gilbert PJ, et al. Prevalence of circumcaval ureters and double caudal vena cava in cats. Am J Vet Res 2014;75(1):91–5.

[41] Pey P, Marcon O, Drigo M, et al. Multidetector-row computed tomographic characteristics of presumed preureteral vena cava in cats. Vet Radiol Ultrasound 2015; 56(4):359–66.
[42] Hunt GB, Bellenger CR, Borg R, et al. Congenital interruption of the portal vein and caudal vena cava in dogs: Six case reports and a review of the literature. Vet Surg 1998;2:203–15.
[43] Specchi S, d'Anjou MA, Carmel EN, et al. Computed tomographic characteristics of collateral venous pathways in dogs with caudal vena cava obstruction. Vet Radiol Ultrasound 2014;55(5):531–8.
[44] Kapur S, Paik E, Rezaei A, et al. Where there is blood, there is a way: unusual collateral vessels in superior and inferior vena cava obstruction. Radiographics 2010;30:67–78.
[45] Bertolini G. Anomalies of the Portal Venous System in Dogs and Cats as Seen on Multidetector-Row Computed Tomography: An Overview and Systematization Proposal. Vet Sci 2019;6:10.
[46] Oui H, Kim J, Bae Y, et al. Computed tomography angiography of situs inversus, portosystemic shunt and multiple vena cava anomalies in a dog. J Vet Med Sci 2013; 75:1525–8.
[47] van den Ingh TS, Rothuizen J, Meyer HP. Circulatory disorders of the liver in dogs and cats. Vet Q 1995;17: 70.
[48] Pillai S, Center SA, McDonough SP, et al. Ductal Plate Malformation in the Liver of Boxer Dogs: Clinical and Histological Features. Vet Pathol 2016; 53(3):602–13.
[49] Buob S, Johnston A, Webster C. Portal Hypertension: Pathophysiology, Diagnosis, and Treatment. J Vet Intern Med 2011;25:169–86.
[50] Sato K, Sakai M, Hayakawa S, et al. Gallbladder Agenesis in 17 Dogs: 2006–2016. J Vet Intern Med 2018;32: 188–94.
[51] Bertolini G, Caldin M. Computed tomography findings in portal vein aneurysm of dogs. Vet J 2012;193(2): 475–80.
[52] Specchi S, Pey P, Ledda G, et al. Computed tomographic and ultrasonographic characteristics of cavernous transformation of the obstructed portal vein in small animals. Vet Radiol Ultrasound 2015. https://doi.org/10.1111/Vru.12265.
[53] Specchi S, Rossi F, Weisse C, et al. Canine and feline abdominal arterioportal communications can be classified based on branching patterns in computed tomographic angiography. Vet Radiol Ultrasound 2018;59: 687–96.
[54] Lamb CR, White RN. Morphology of congenital intrahepatic portacaval shunts in dogs and cats. Vet Rec 1998; 142:55–60.
[55] D'Anjou MA, Huneault L. Imaging diagnosis - Complex intrahepatic portosystemic shunt in a dog. Vet Radiol Ultrasound 2008;49(1):51–5.
[56] Culp WTN, Zwingenberger AL, Giuffrida MA, et al. Prospective evaluation of outcome of dogs with intrahepatic portosystemic shunts treated via percutaneous transvenous coil embolization. Vet Surg 2018;47(1):74–85.
[57] Nelson NC, Nelson LL. Anatomy of extrahepatic portosystemic shunts in dogs as determined by computed tomography angiography. Vet Radiol Ultrasound 2011;52: 498–506.
[58] White RN, Parry AT. Morphology of congenital portosystemic shunts emanating from the left gastric vein in dogs and cats. J Small Anim Pract 2013;54:459–67.
[59] White RN, Parry AT. Morphology of congenital portosystemic shunts involving the right gastric vein in dogs. J Small Anim Pract 2015;56:430–40.
[60] White RN, Parry AT. Morphology of congenital portosystemic shunts involving the left colic vein in dogs and cats. J Small Anim Pract 2016;57:247–54.
[61] Specchi S, Pey P, Javard R, et al. Mesenteric-reno-caval shunt in an aged dog. J Small Anim Pract 2015;56:72.
[62] Bertolini G. Acquired portal collateral circulation in the dog and cat. Vet Radiol Ultrasound 2010;51:25–33.
[63] Bertolini G. The systemic thoracic vasculature. In: Body MDCT in small animals. Springer International Publishing AG; 2017. https://doi.org/10.1007/978-3-319-46904-1.
[64] Henjes CR, Nolte I, Wefstaedt P. Multidetector-row computed tomography of thoracic aortic anomalies in dogs and cats: patent ductus arteriosus and vascular rings. BMC Vet Res 2011;7:57.
[65] Ledda G, Caldin M, Mezzalira G, et al. Multidetector-row computed tomography patterns of bronchoesophageal artery hypertrophy and systemic-to-pulmonary fistula in dogs. Vet Radiol Ultrasound 2015;56(4):347–58.
[66] Choi SY, Song YM, Lee YW, et al. Imaging characteristics of persistent left cranial vena cava incidentally diagnosed with computed tomography in dogs. J Vet Med Sci 2016; 78(10):1601–6.
[67] Bertolini G, Lorenzi DD, Ledda G, et al. Esophageal Varices due to a Probable Arteriovenous Communication in a Dog. J Vet Intern Med 2007;21:1392–5.
[68] Randi D. The pulmonary vasculature. In: Body MDCT in small animals. Cham, Switzerland: Springer International Publishing AG; 2017. p. 265–73. https://doi.org/10.1007/978-3-319 46904-1_12.
[69] Thieme SF, Becker CR, Hacker M. Dual energy CT for the assessment of lung perfusion–correlation to scintigraphy. Eur J Radiol 2008;68(3):369–74.
[70] Angeloni L, Costa CM, Bertolini G. Abstracts of the european veterinary diagnostic imaging (EVDI) congress, Basel, Switzerland, August 21–24, 2019. Vet Radiol Ultrasound 2020;61:85–118.

Advances in Small Animal Care 1 (2020) 75–90

ADVANCES IN SMALL ANIMAL CARE

Lymph Node Evaluation with Diagnostic Imaging

Elissa Randall, DVM, MS, DACVR

Veterinary Teaching Hospital, Colorado State University, 300 West Drake Road, 135 Animal Cancer Center, Fort Collins, CO 80523, USA

KEYWORDS

• Lymph node • Sentinel lymph node • Canine • Feline • Imaging

KEY POINTS

- Evaluation of lymph nodes on diagnostic images of dogs and cats is critical in the evaluation of patients with cancer.
- Certain imaging characteristics may suggest lymph nodes are metastatic or neoplastic, but significant overlap exists between neoplastic and reactive or inflammatory lymph nodes.
- Sentinel lymph node mapping is used to determine which lymph node is the first draining lymph node so that it may be sampled by cytology or histopathology to determine if metastasis is present.

INTRODUCTION

The identification and evaluation of lymph nodes by diagnostic imaging is important for prognosis and determination of therapeutic options. Lymph node evaluation is most critical in oncology patients but is also important in infectious diseases. At least 4 million dogs and 4 million cats develop cancer each year [1]. Imaging is an important part of staging these patients, with complete primary lesion evaluation and determination of metastatic status being critically important, including lymph node detection and characterization. All diagnostic imaging modalities play a role in evaluating lymph nodes in veterinary patients and different criteria exist for lymph node evaluation according to the modality in use. This chapter will review the evaluation of lymph nodes using each imaging modality with a focus on oncologic disease. The imaging modalities that will be reviewed include radiography, contrast radiography, ultrasound, computed tomography (CT), magnetic resonance imaging (MRI), and nuclear medicine (planar scintigraphy and PET/CT.)

Lymph nodes can enlarge and change shape in response to neoplastic or inflammatory stimuli [2]. That enlargement is one major criterion used to detect abnormal lymph nodes on imaging studies. However, it is also well established that normal size lymph nodes may contain metastatic disease, and not all enlarged lymph nodes are metastatic [3]. This clinical conundrum may be better addressed by more advanced imaging techniques or modalities. With all modalities there is overlap in characteristics seen with benign and malignant lymph nodes. Ultimately, cytologic or histopathologic sampling of a lymph node is necessary to determine whether it is normal, reactive, or neoplastic.

Identification of the sentinel lymph node is of clinical importance in patients with cancer. The sentinel lymph node is defined as the lymph node that first receives draining lymph from a tumor or specific region [4]. The sentinel lymph node is not always the closest lymph node anatomically. If the sentinel lymph node is identified, cytology or histopathology of that lymph node should be pursued to determine if metastatic disease is present in the lymphatic system. Specific techniques can be used with different imaging modalities to identify the sentinel lymph node.

E-mail address: Elissa.Randall@colostate.edu

https://doi.org/10.1016/j.yasa.2020.07.006

SURVEY RADIOGRAPHY

Radiography is the most widely available modality in veterinary medicine and is typically affordable, with fast and technically easy acquisition.

A disadvantage of radiography for detecting lymph nodes is that most lymph nodes must be moderately to markedly enlarged to be identified on radiographs.

The sternal lymph nodes may be seen in some normal dogs on lateral thoracic radiographs and are better visualized on the right lateral view in large breed dogs [5]. The popliteal lymph node is often visualized on radiographs that include the stifle in dogs. However, measurements of this lymph node on radiographs overlap in cases of degenerative joint disease of the stifle and osteosarcoma of the distal femur/proximal tibia and should not be used to differentiate between those disease processes on radiographs [6]. Other intrathoracic, abdominal, and peripheral lymph nodes are not usually seen on radiographs if they are normal [7].

When lymph nodes are detected as being enlarged on radiographs, interpretation of that information depends on what structures the lymph node drains, if a single or multiple lymph nodes are enlarged, and other radiographic findings. The sternal lymph nodes drain the peritoneal cavity, the ribs, sternum, thymus, mammary glands, the diaphragm, abdominal wall, and adjacent muscles [8]. When the sternal lymph node is the only intrathoracic lymph node that is enlarged, disease of the abdomen must be considered as the reason for enlargement. This includes neoplastic and inflammatory disease and hematologic conditions [9]. When tracheobronchial lymph nodes are detected as enlarged on radiographs, traditional differential diagnoses included lymphoma and fungal infection. A retrospective study found other diseases should be considered with enlargement of these lymph nodes, including histiocytic sarcoma, carcinoma, and other neoplasms, as well as other infectious diseases (mycobacterium, nocardia.) [10] The iliosacral lymph nodes are often called "sublumbar" lymph nodes on radiographs, as specific lymph nodes cannot be distinguished. This lymph center drains the pelvic and perineal areas, hind limbs, bladder, ureters and urethra, and dorsal and ventral superficial structures of the caudal abdomen [8]. Enlargement of sublumbar lymph nodes radiographically may be due to multicentric neoplasia such as lymphoma or neoplasia of the caudal abdominal, pelvic, or perineal structures (such as transitional cell carcinoma of the bladder or urethra, anal sac adenocarcinoma, soft tissue, or bone tumors of the pelvic limbs). See Figs. 1 and 2 for radiographic examples of lymph node enlargement.

CONTRAST RADIOGRAPHY AND SENTINEL LYMPH NODE DETECTION

Radiographic contrast media use has been described to visualize lymphatic drainage patterns for the thoracic duct and mammary glands, sentinel lymph node identification, and visualization of peripheral lymph nodes for radiation therapy planning purposes [11–15].

Injection may be direct (into a lymph node or lymphatic vessel) or indirect (into tissues of a specific region or surrounding a structure or mass).

Injection may be performed with undiluted iodinated contrast material or iodized oil, lipid-soluble

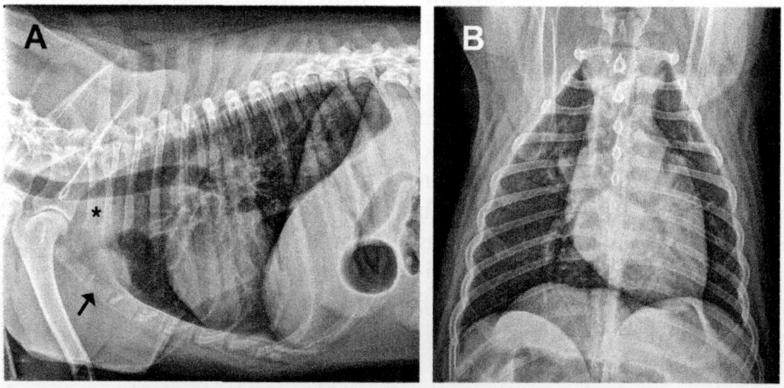

FIG. 1 Left lateral (**A**) and ventrodorsal (**B**) thoracic radiographs of a dog diagnosed with lymphoma. The sternal lymph nodes (*arrow*) and cranial mediastinal lymph nodes (*asterisk*) are enlarged and seen as masses on the lateral view as well as widening of the cranial mediastinum on the VD. The tracheobronchial lymph nodes are also enlarged and are seen as ill-defined increased soft tissue opacity surrounding the carina on the lateral view as well as increased soft tissue opacity between laterally displaced mainstem bronchi on the VD view. VD, ventrodorsal.

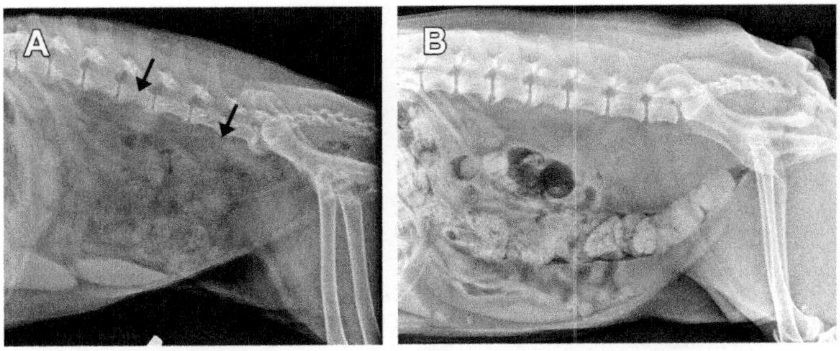

FIG. 2 (**A**) Caudal lateral abdomen radiograph of a dog with lymphoma. Sublumbar and periaortic lymph nodes are mild to moderately enlarged and seen as round soft tissue opacities ventral to the lumbar vertebrae (*arrows*). (**B**) Caudal lateral abdomen radiograph of a dog with metastatic anal gland carcinoma. The sublumbar lymph nodes are severely enlarged, seen as a soft tissue mass ventral to the caudal lumbar vertebrae and causing ventral displacement of the colon.

iodinated contrast. Iodinated contrast may be seen in draining lymphatics immediately after a 2.5- to 5-minute injection, with decreasing visibility over 20 minutes [11]. Iodized oil may be visualized in lymphatics and draining lymph nodes on immediate postcontrast images with direct injection, but visualization after indirect injection is more variable and may be anywhere from several minutes to 24 hours [13,15]. Iodized oil may be retained in lymph nodes for weeks to months [15] (Fig. 3).

ULTRASOUND

Ultrasound is another imaging modality that is widely available and affordable. Ultrasound provides the ability to visualize and evaluate more lymph nodes than radiography. Many peripheral and abdominal lymph nodes can be visualized. Sternal lymph nodes can sometimes be seen when normal and can often be seen when enlarged. Other intrathoracic lymph nodes are rarely seen unless markedly enlarged and intrapelvic lymph nodes are difficult to visualize in many patients. Smaller lymph nodes throughout the body and deeper abdominal lymph nodes can be difficult to visualize.

Normal lymph node echogenicity is described as homogenous and isoechoic or slightly hypoechoic to surrounding tissues. Normal lymph nodes are often elongated, being greater in length than thickness, and have distinct margins. Normal lymph nodes have a hilar

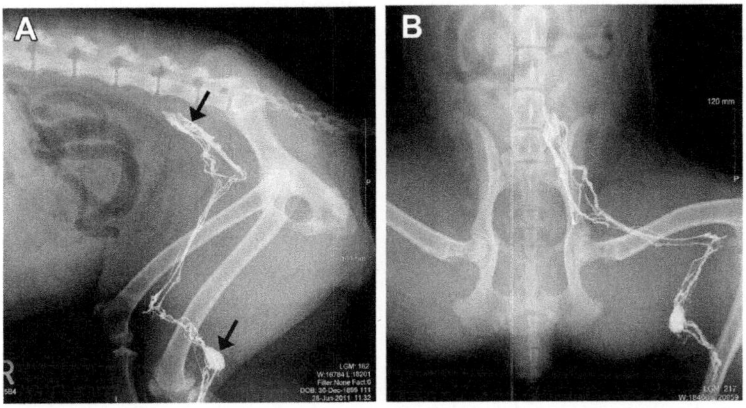

FIG. 3 Lateral (**A**) and ventrodorsal (**B**) images of a normal dog taken immediately after injection of iodized oil directly into lymphatic vessels of the dorsal aspect of the metatarsal region. Contrast is seen in draining lymphatic vessels as well as in the popliteal lymph node and medial iliac lymph nodes (*arrows*). (*Courtesy of* Dr. Monique Mayer, Western College of Veterinary Medicine, University of Saskatchewan, Saskatoon, Canada.)

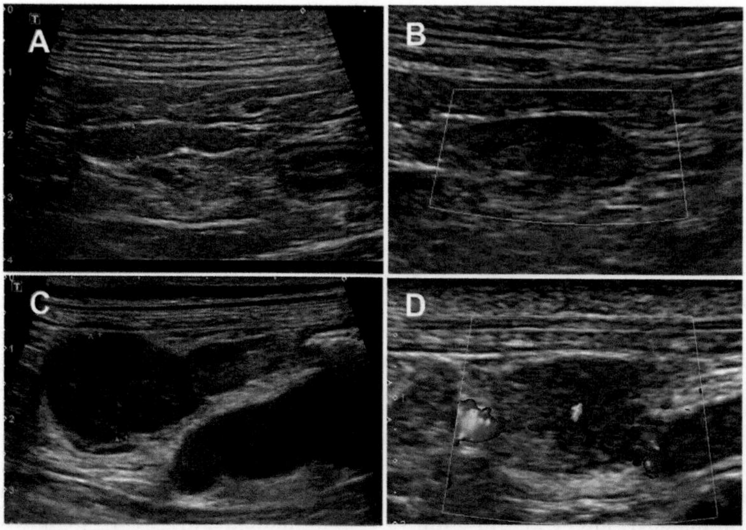

FIG. 4 (**A**) B-mode ultrasound image of a normal jejunal lymph node, which measured 5.1 mm in thickness. (**B**) Color Doppler image of a medial iliac lymph node with hilar blood flow. The lymph node was considered mildly hypoechoic but normal in size. The entire length of the lymph node was not imaged in order to obtain the best Doppler image. (**C**) B-mode ultrasound image of abnormal mesenteric lymph nodes that are enlarged and hypoechoic with hyperechoic surrounding mesentery. The lymph node with calipers measured 15 mm in thickness. A concentric jejunal mass was also found, and lymphoma or adenocarcinoma was suspected. (**D**) Color Doppler image of a medial iliac lymph node that was considered abnormal in size and had hyperechoic surrounding mesentery. The lymph node measured 10 mm in width, which was 2 times the width of the contralateral lymph node. The Doppler flow pattern is mixed, with hilar and peripheral blood flow. Metastatic mast cell tumor was diagnosed.

pattern of blood flow on Doppler examination or appear avascular [2] (Fig. 4).

Characteristics of lymph nodes on B mode and Doppler examination that may indicate malignancy have been described. There is discrepancy between study findings, leading to a lack of consensus of features that indicate malignancy (Tables 1 and 2). Criteria that are generally agreed on are size and shape. Lymph nodes that are neoplastic are more round in shape and are enlarged [2,16–18].

Benign, inflamed lymph nodes tend to enlarge symmetrically but maintain their fusiform shape, whereas malignant lymph nodes tend to enlarge more in width and become more round in shape [2,18].

Some studies found that malignant lymph nodes tend to be hypoechoic, whereas others found malignant and benign lymph nodes to be hypoechoic [17–20].

Heterogeneity has been found to be associated with malignancy in some studies but not useful for determining malignancy in other studies [16,18,21–23].

Hyperechoic perinodal fat may increase the suspicion for malignancy, as normal or benign lymph nodes typically have normal perinodal fat [18,20].

An increased number of lymph nodes found on ultrasound may indicate malignancy [16,20].

Color Doppler evaluation of lymph nodes is similarly controversial. Some studies suggest that hilar blood flow or minimal/absent flow indicates normal lymph nodes and a prominent hilar pattern indicates reactive lymph nodes, whereas peripheral or mixed peripheral and hilar blood flow increases suspicion for malignancy [2,19]. However, other studies did not find color Doppler useful in determining malignancy [18,23] (see Fig. 4).

Pulsed wave Doppler techniques, such as resistive index and pulsatility index, are slightly more challenging to acquire but have shown promise in predicting malignancy: resistive index (RI) = (peak systolic velocity–end diastolic velocity)/peak systolic velocity and pulsatility index (PI) = (peak systolic velocity–end diastolic velocity)/time averaged maximum velocity. One study of superficial lymph nodes found it better to use PI to differentiate between nonmalignant (normal and reactive) lymph nodes and malignant (lymphoma and metastatic) lymph nodes in dogs. Suggested cutoff values were 0.68 for RI and 1.49

TABLE 1
Ultrasound Characteristics of Malignant Lymph Nodes

Characteristic	Feature/Measurement	Literature Support	Reference
Round shape	Short/long axis >0.7 (superficial LN) Short/long axis > 0.5 (MILN) Short/long axis >0.48 (mandibular LN)	Nyman Llabres-Diaz Choi	[16,19,30]
Size	Short axis > 1.73 cm (superficial LN)	Belotta	[29]
Echogenicity	Hypoechoic	Nyman	[19]
Echotexture	Heterogenous	Kinns, Llabres-Diaz	[16,21]
Number	Increased # in cats Increased # in dogs	Dave Llabres-Diaz	[16,20]
Doppler pattern	Peripheral or mixed	Nyman, Belotta	[19,29]
Doppler evaluation	Increased # vessels	Nyman 06	[22]
Vascular pattern	Displaced hilar vessel, aberrant, pericapsular, or subcapsular vessels	Salwei	[26]
Perinodal fat	Hyperechoic with round cell neoplasia	Dave	[20]
Resistive index	>0.67(MILN) >0.76(mesent LN) >0.68–0.69 (superficial LN)	Prieto Belotta Nyman	[19,24,29]
Pulsatility index	>1.02(MILN), >1.23(mesent LN) >1.49 (superficial LN)	Prieto Belotta Nyman	[19,24,29]
Stiffness	Elastography—mean vue histogram, pattern, stiffness area ratio	Choi	[30]
Stiffness	Qualitative score >2.5	Belotta	[29]
Stiffness	ARFI-elastography (acoustic radiation force impulse)	Silva	[23]

Abbreviations: ARFI, acoustic radiation force impulse; LN, lymph node; MILN, medial iliac lymph node.

for PI [19]. Another study found a significant difference in RI and PI in nonneoplastic versus neoplastic abdominal lymph nodes in dogs. Suggested cutoff values for the medial iliac lymph node were 0.67 for RI and 1.02 for PI. Cutoff values for mesenteric lymph nodes were 0.76 for RI and1.23 for PI. Higher values are found in neoplastic lymph nodes [24] (Fig. 5).

Contrast-enhanced ultrasound using intravenous microbubble ultrasound contrast allows for better depiction of vascular architecture than color or power Doppler. This has been shown in normal canine lymph nodes and lymphomatous canine lymph nodes [25,26]. Use of contrast-enhanced ultrasound has led to a better depiction of normal and abnormal vascular patterns in lymph nodes. Normal lymph nodes tend to have hilar blood flow, and reactive lymph nodes may have pronounced hilar blood flow. Patterns of blood flow seen in malignant lymph nodes include displacement of the central hilar vessel, aberrant vessels, pericapsular vessels, and subcapsular vessels [26]. Ultrasound contrast media is not readily available at all veterinary institutions, and the cost had been prohibitive, although decreasing. The US Food and Drug Administration approved Sonovue (Bracco Imaging) for use in human patients in 2016.

Elastography is an advanced ultrasound imaging technique that measures tissue stiffness, which increases with malignancy and other chronic disease processes. Methods can be strain based (external tissue pressure) or shear wave–based (using induced acoustic waves.) Patient- and operator-based factors as well as pathology affect the accuracy and reliability of elastography [27]. Qualitative elastography in dogs and cats has shown some promise for determining malignancy in abdominal and superficial lymph nodes, although there is overlap in stiffness scores between benign and

TABLE 2
Ultrasound Characteristics that Do Not Reliably Differentiate Between Benign and Malignant Lymph Nodes

Characteristic	Feature/Measurement	Literature Support	Reference
Doppler	Presence of Flow	De Swarte	[18]
Doppler	Distribution of vessels	De Swarte, Silva	[18,23]
Doppler	# of vessels	De Swarte	[18]
Echotexture	Heterogeneity	De Swarte, Dave, Belotta, Silva	[18,20,23,29]
Echogenicity	Hypoechoic	De Swarte, Dave, Llabres-Diaz, Choi, Silva	[16,18,20,23,30]
Cavitations	Present	De Swarte	[18]
Hilus	Defined/Present	De Swarte, Choi, Belotta	[18,29,30]
Round shape	Subjective	De Swarte	[18]
Surrounding mesentery	Hyperechoic	De Swarte, Belotta	[18,29]
Echotexture cats	Heterogenous	Kinns	[21]
Stiffness	Elastography—qualitative and quantitative score	Seiler	[28]
Size	Width	Choi	[30]

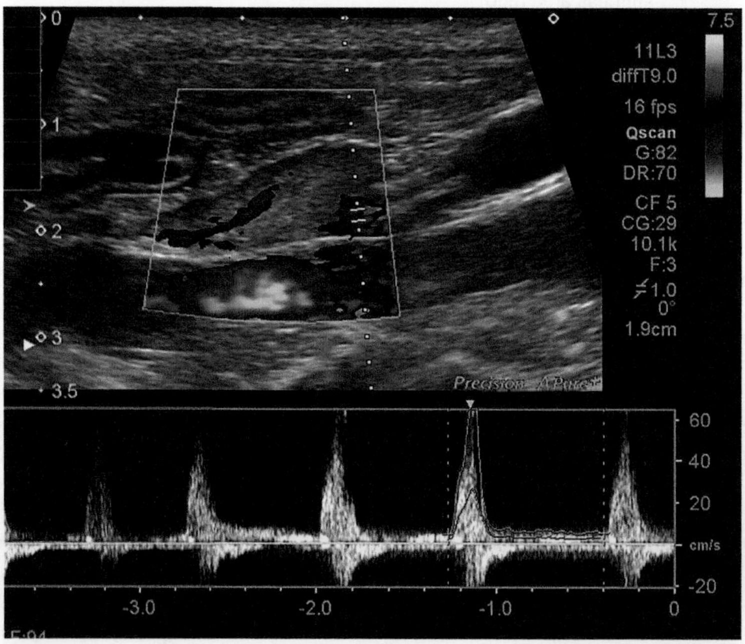

FIG. 5 A medial iliac lymph node in a large breed juvenile patient that was considered normal for the age and breed. Normal hilar blood flow is noted. A spectral tracing was obtained to measure resistive index (RI) and pulsatility index (PI).

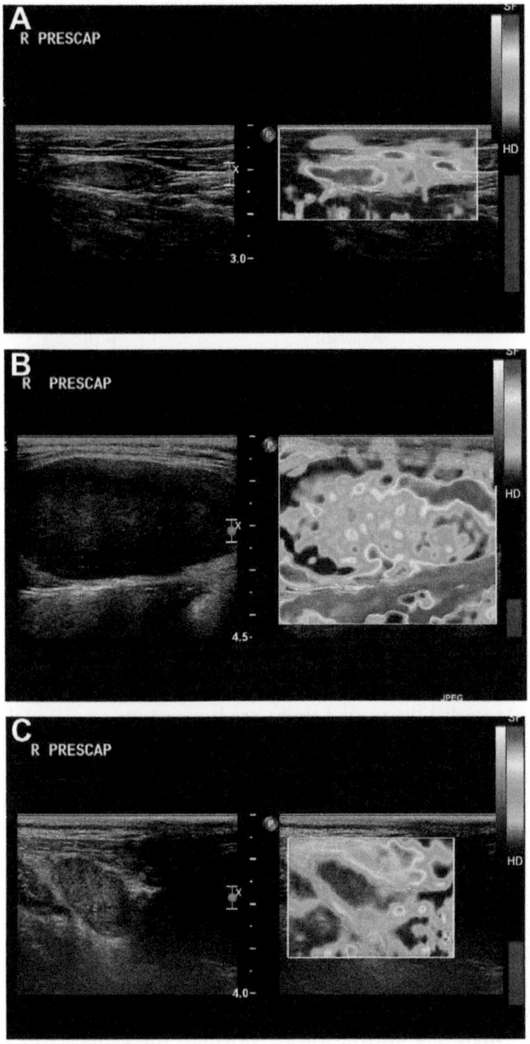

FIG. 6 Qualitative strain elastography images of lymph nodes with B-mode images on the left and corresponding elastography images on the right. (**A**) Normal prescapular, or superficial cervical, lymph node. The lymph node is mostly red and yellow on elastography, which is considered normal and "soft" on the scale, which is on the right side of the image. Soft is red and stiff is blue. (**B, C**) Two different neoplastic prescapular, or superficial cervical, lymph nodes, both diagnosed as metastatic mast cell tumor. The lymph node in B is mostly green with some blue at the periphery and was considered abnormal and stiff. The lymph node in C is mostly blue and graded as increasingly stiff compared with B. (*Courtesy of* Dr. Nathalie Rademacher, School of Veterinary Medicine, Louisiana State University, Baton Rouge, LA.)

malignant lymph nodes [28,29]. Qualitative elastography involves a subjective analysis of tissue stiffness based on color mapping of a structure. See Fig. 6. A study using acoustic radiation force impulse elastography was highly sensitive and specific in detecting metastasis in inguinal and axillary lymph nodes in dogs with mammary neoplasia [23]. Another study found that semiquantitative strain elastography using computer-aided histogram analysis and stiffness area ratios had high sensitivity and specificity for detecting malignancy in mandibular lymph nodes and was reproducible and repeatable [30].

ULTRASOUND AND SENTINEL LYMPH NODE DETECTION

Contrast-enhanced ultrasound has been used to successfully identify the sentinel lymph node draining mammary glands and dorsal metatarsal region in normal dogs and in dogs with head and neck tumors [31–33]. Contrast media is injected into or around a structure or mass, and local lymphatic vessels and lymph nodes are imaged for presence of contrast media uptake. Contrast can be seen in afferent lymphatic vessels, which can be followed from the area of injection to the draining lymph node [31,32]. In some regions, such as the tarsus, afferent vessels can be difficult to visualize due to superficial location and close proximity of bone [33]. The range of time to visible nodal contrast was 2 to 30 minutes in dogs with tumors, within 2 minutes in one study of normal dogs and an average of 3 minutes in another study of normal dogs [31–33].

COMPUTED TOMOGRAPHY

CT is an advanced imaging modality that provides better visualization of structures by eliminating the superimposition of anatomy that can be problematic on radiographs and alleviates the problems of patient size and gastrointestinal and pulmonary gas that can make ultrasound imaging of lymph nodes difficult. Intrapelvic lymph nodes are better evaluated with CT as well. Small structures are also much better delineated on CT.

On CT images, normal lymph nodes are soft tissue attenuating, mildly contrast enhancing, homogenous pre- and postcontrast administration. A hypoattenuating hilus is often seen. Lymph nodes may be elongated, ovoid, rounded, or miscellaneous in shape [34,35]. See Tables 3 and 4 for normal attenuation criteria.

TABLE 3
Computed Tomographic Attenuation Characteristics of Normal Canine Lymph Nodes

Lymph Node	Characteristic	Feature/Measurement	Literature Support	Reference
Abdominal	Precontrast	37 HU (range 20–52)	Beukers	[35]
Abdominal	Postcontrast	109 HU (range 36–223)	Beukers	[35]
Sternal	Precontrast	18.3 (4.4–36.9) HU 30.2 ± 10.4 HU	Milovancev Iwasaki	[34,36]
Sternal	Postcontrast	41.3 (24.0–77.4) HU 61.7 ± 5.2	Milovancev Iwasaki	[34,36]
Upper cervical	Precontrast	36.6 ± 13.3 HU	Kneissl	[49]
Upper cervical	Postcontrast	110.3 ± 3.3 HU	Kneissl	[49]

A percentage of normal lymph nodes may be mildly heterogenous pre- or postcontrast administration [34–37].

Size of lymph nodes can be measured directly or evaluated using ratios of lymph node to other anatomy. There is some evidence for increasing lymph node size with increasing body size, which may make a ratio a better evaluation of lymph node size [34,36].

Normal sternal lymph node HU is 30.2 ± 10.4 HU precontrast and 61.7 ± 5.2 HU postcontrast. Normal sternal LN mean 18.3 (range 4.4–36.9 HU), postcontrast mean 41.3 (range 24.0–77.4 HU) [34]. Normal abdominal LN precontrast 22 to 52 HU (mean 37), postcontrast 36 to 223 (mean 109) [35]. Normal cat abdomen LN precontrast 27 to 36 HU and postcontrast 106 to 157 HU [37].

ABNORMAL LYMPH NODES ON COMPUTED TOMOGRAPHY

Several imaging characteristics have been suggested to differentiate between malignant and nonmalignant lymph nodes on CT. These include absolute size, ratio size, and postcontrast enhancement pattern [38,39]. Malignant lymph nodes are larger than nonmalignant lymph nodes and may have rim or heterogenous contrast enhancement.

Precontrast attenuation (HU) has been shown to be higher in metastatic lymph nodes and the combination of size ratio cutoff of greater than 1.0 (lymph node height to second sternebra height) and precontrast attenuation cutoff of greater than 37.5 HU had a specificity and PPV of 100% for sternal lymph nodes in dogs [39].

As with ultrasound there are limitations to CT evaluation of lymph nodes. A study of contrast-enhanced CT to evaluate mandibular and medial retropharyngeal lymph nodes in dogs with oral and nasal cancer found no individual CT findings that were predictive of metastasis and concluded that CT alone cannot be used for assessment of metastasis in those lymph nodes [40]. Another study found no difference in size between metastatic and nonmetastatic mandibular lymph nodes in cats with oral squamous cell carcinoma [41]. A comparison study found that, although CT found more normal iliosacral lymph nodes than ultrasound in dogs with anal gland carcinoma, ultrasound detected more abnormal lymph nodes, theorized to be related to ultrasound being better able to detect subtle architecture changes [42] (Fig. 7).

TABLE 4
Computed Tomographic Attenuation Characteristics of Normal Feline Lymph Nodes

Lymph Node	Characteristic	Feature/Measurement	Literature Support	Reference
All feline LNs	Precontrast	37–36 HU	Perlini	[37]
All feline LNs	Postcontrast	106–157 HU	Perlini	[37]
Medial retropharyngeal	Precontrast	40.2 HU ± 5.3	Nemanic	[77]

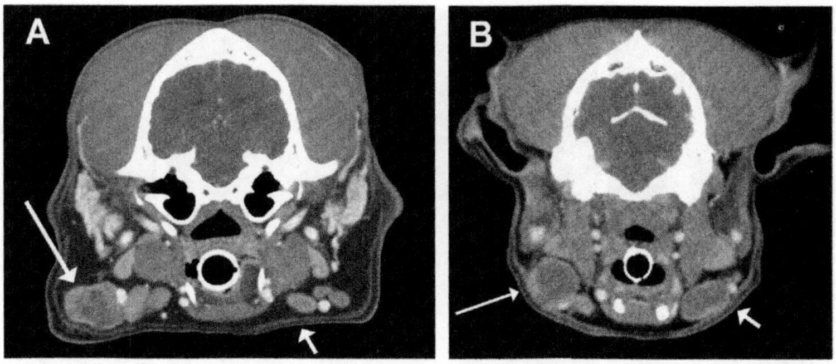

FIG. 7 Postcontrast transverse CT images of 2 different patients. (**A**) Dog with an oral carcinoma, diagnosed as metastatic to the right mandibular lymph node (*long arrow*). This lymph node is round, enlarged, and heterogeneously contrast enhancing. Normal mandibular lymph nodes are seen on the left (*short arrow*) and are small, elongated, and have a normal fatty hilus. (**B**) Dog with a tonsillar squamous cell carcinoma diagnosed as metastatic to the left and right mandibular lymph nodes. The right mandibular lymph node is rounded, enlarged, and rim contrast enhancing (*long arrow*). The left mandibular lymph node is enlarged, ovoid, and rim contrast enhancing (*short arrow*).

COMPUTED TOMORAPHIC SENTINEL LYMPH NODE IDENTIFICATION

Because CT cannot reliably detect lymph node metastasis based on imaging characteristics alone, indirect CT lymphography has been investigated to identify the sentinel lymph node.

Aqueous iodinated contrast material injected around tumors, postoperative scars, and normal structures is a feasible technique for detecting draining lymphatic vessels and lymph nodes [12,43–45]. A total of 1 to 2 mL of contrast injected peritumorally typically allows identification of the sentinel lymph node within 3 minutes [43–47].

The typical procedure for indirect CT lymphography involves the injection of 0.25 mL aliquots of aqueous iodinated contrast material at 4 quadrants around a mass (12, 3, 6, and 9 o'clock). CT scans are acquired starting at 1 minute postinjection, then continued every 2 to 3 minutes for up to 5 to 6 minutes. Contrast is often seen in the first draining lymph node on the 1-minute scan.

Although one study found postlymphography lymph node characteristics to have significant diagnostic value for predicting metastasis to the lymph node in dogs with mammary tumors, another study of dogs with melanoma or mast cell tumor did not find any CT lymphography findings that correlated with the metastatic status of the sentinel lymph node [46,48] (Fig. 8).

MAGNETIC RESONANCE IMAGING

Normal lymph nodes have a homogenous, isointense signal on T1-weighted images compared with muscle and are hyperintense on T2-weighted images. When compared with fat, normal lymph nodes are hypointense on T1-weighted images, isointense after contrast on T1-weighted images, and slightly hypointense on T2-weighted images [49,50] (Fig. 9).

Lymph nodes containing metastatic disease may be larger than their contralateral lymph node [50]. Other characteristics described for malignant lymph nodes include heterogenous signal on STIR sequences, a heterogenous contrast enhancement pattern, a round shape, and irregular or undulating margination [51] (Fig. 10).

Diffusion-weighted MRI and apparent diffucion coefficient maps have been able to differentiate between metastatic and benign lymph nodes in humans [52,53]. A study in veterinary medicine found the method feasible in dogs with head and neck disease but did not find a significant difference between benign and metastatic lymph nodes [54].

MAGNETIC RESONANCE IMAGING SENTINEL LYMPH NODE DETECTION

A pilot study evaluated indirect MR lymphography in normal dogs using a conventional contrast agent (gadolinium) and a lymphotropic contrast agent (gadofluorine). Following intradermal injection, the sentinel lymph node was identified 15 to 20 minutes after gadolinium and 60 minutes after gadofluorine in all imaged dogs [55].

NUCLEAR MEDICINE

Conventional nuclear medicine and PET-CT have been used in veterinary medicine for the evaluation of lymph

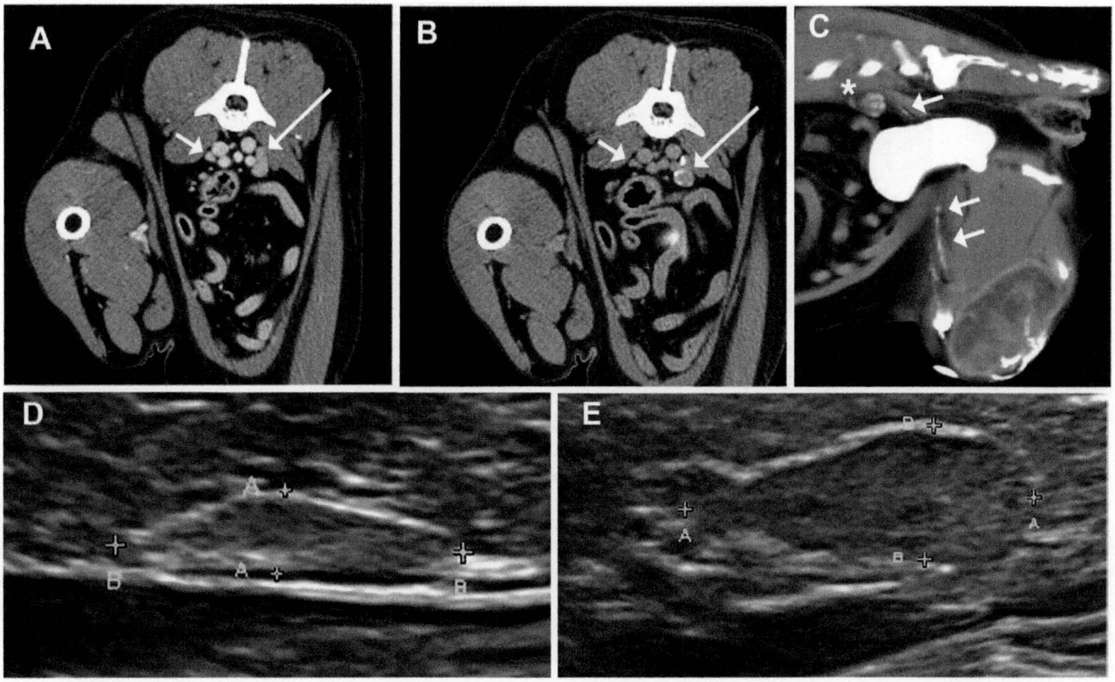

FIG. 8 Images of a dog with a mast cell tumor of the left medial proximal pelvic limb. (**A**) Postintravenous contrast transverse CT image. The right medial iliac lymph node (*short arrow*) is normal. The left medial iliac lymph node (*long arrow*) is mildly enlarged and homogenously contrast enhancing. (**B**) CT lymphography images of the same patient after 4-quadrant peripheral injection of iohexol around the mast cell tumor. Contrast is seen in the left medial iliac lymph node, identifying it as the sentinel lymph node. (**C**) Sagittal reconstruct after 4-quadrant peripheral injection of iohexol around the mast cell tumor. The tumor is seen at the bottom of the image with focal areas of peritumoral contrast, secondary to the procedure. Contrast is seen in draining lymphatic vessels (*arrows*) and in the left medial iliac lymph node (*asterisk*). (**D**) Ultrasound image of the right medial iliac lymph node, which was 4.3 mm in thickness and was elongated. (**E**) Ultrasound image of the left medial iliac lymph node, which measured up to 9.3 mm in thickness and was elongated but asymmetric. The left medial iliac was diagnosed as metastatic mast cell tumor on cytology.

nodes. Nuclear medicine provides the advantage of functional imaging and complements traditional anatomic imaging.

Lymphoscintigraphy with Tc99m-dextran and Tc99m-sulfur colloid has been used to identify the sentinel lymph node in mammary glands, lungs, and anal sacs of normal dogs and in dogs with neoplasia [45,56–59]. Lymphatic drainage and sentinel lymph node identification can be done with a gamma camera or hand-held gamma probe. Either method requires a nuclear medicine service with a "hot lab" and license to use radioactive materials.

Preoperative lymphoscintigraphy with Tc99m-sulfur colloid uses a low dose (125 μCi) that enables the patient to reach releasable levels immediately after injection so that lymphoscintigraphy and surgery can occur in one anesthetic event [45].

Image-based lymphoscintigraphy requires the use of a gamma camera, and images can be challenging to interpret anatomically.

Intraoperative lymphoscintigraphy with a hand-held gamma probe performed better than image-based scintigraphy in one study and better than blue dye injection and CT lymphography in another study [45].

POSITRON EMISSION TOMOGRAPHY–COMPUTED TOMOGRAPHY

PET is a nuclear medicine modality that uses different radiopharmaceuticals than traditional nuclear medicine. When emitted positrons interact with electrons, a pair of 511 keV gamma rays are given off in 180° opposite directions, and these gamma rays are detected by a

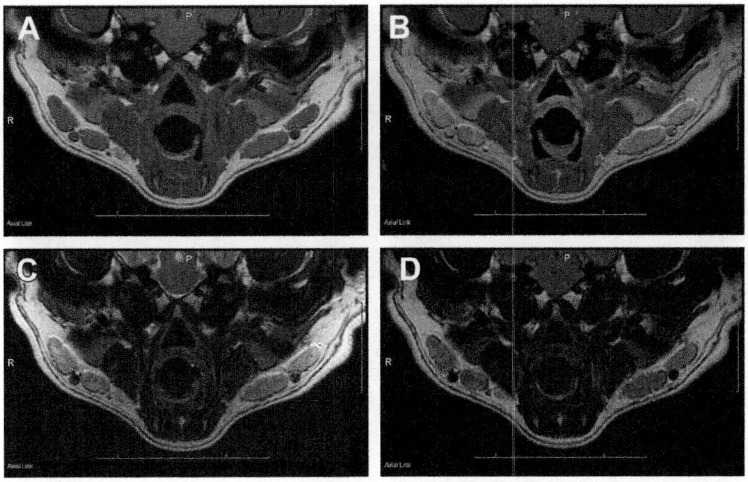

FIG. 9 MRI transverse images of a dog with 2 mandibular lymph nodes on each side. Pulse sequences are: T1, (*A*) top left, T1 post contrast, (*B*) top right, T2, (*C*) bottom left, FLAIR, (*D*) bottom right. Note the lymph nodes are isointense signal on T1-weighted images compared to muscle and are hyperintense on T2-weighted images. When compared to fat, normal lymph nodes are hypointense on T1-weighted images, isointense after contrast on T1-weighted images, and slightly hypointense on T2-weighted images.

ring of detectors. PET images lack anatomic specificity so are often fused with CT images acquired at the same time.

The most commonly used PET radiopharmaceutical is (^{18}F)-fluoro-2-deoxy-D-glucose (FDG). FDG has uptake in areas of glucose metabolism and can detect metabolic/functional abnormalities before there are anatomic abnormalities. One limitation of FDG is that it is not specific for neoplasia, and some normal tissue as well as inflammatory tissues will have increased FDG uptake.

Lymph nodes are suspected to be abnormal based on subjective increased avidity or FDG uptake in comparison to other lymph nodes and surrounding soft tissues. Avidity can also be measured as standardized uptake value (SUV), which is a region of interest computer-aided analysis that compares activity concentration in the region measured with activity in the whole body [60]. The SUV value that is commonly reported is SUVmax.

PET or PET-CT have detected lymphoma or metastatic disease in lymph nodes of dogs and cats, including lymph nodes that were not suspected to be malignant before PET or PET-CT [61,62]. Malignant lymph nodes have been reported to have a SUVmax of 0.56 to 19.59 [62–65]. The SUVmax of normal lymph nodes is not well reported but is approximately 1 to 3 at the author's institution. There is obvious overlap between normal and malignant lymph nodes, and reactive or inflamed lymph nodes also overlap with both groups (Fig. 11).

With FDG PET/CT analysis of lymph nodes both false positives (due to inflammatory disease) and false negatives (due to spatial resolution and small size of abnormality) are possible.

EMERGING LYMPH NODE IMAGING

There are no characteristics that reliably detect malignancy in lymph nodes using the standard and just reviewed modalities. In human medicine and veterinary medicine, new imaging techniques are being investigated to better detect lymph node malignancy.

Superparamagnetic iron oxide nanoparticles can be used as a contrast agent with MRI. The nanoparticles are readily taken up by macrophages, and normal lymph nodes appear dark on postinjection images, whereas metastatic lymph nodes appear bright or heterogenous [66]. Research with human patients has shown promise, with this technique being effective in identifying metastases in nonenlarged lymph nodes and lymph nodes only partially replaced by neoplastic cells [67]. A pilot study in dogs with head and neck tumors showed promising results in a small group of dogs, with subjective assessment being 100% sensitive and

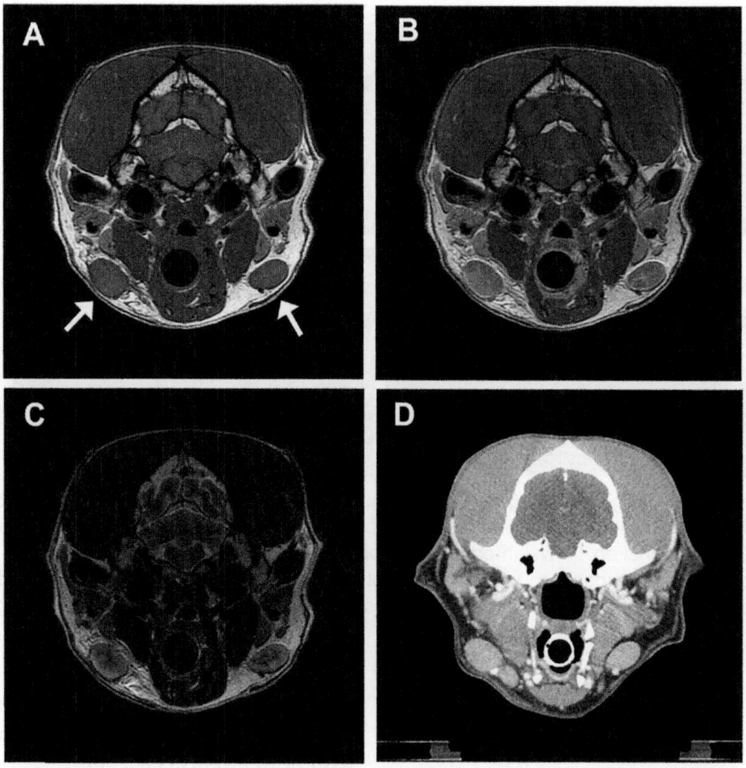

FIG. 10 Transverse Images of a dog with nasal adenocarcinoma. (**A**) Precontrast T1-weighted MRI. Right and left mandibular lymph nodes are enlarged, rounded, and homogenous (*arrows*). (**B**) Postcontrast T1-weighted MRI. The lymph nodes are mildly heterogeneously contrast enhancing. (**C**) T2-weighted MRI image. The lymph nodes are heterogenous. (**D**) Postcontrast CT images. The lymph nodes are enlarged, rounded, and homogenously contrast enhancing. Both lymph nodes were diagnosed as metastatic carcinoma on cytology.

88% specific for identifying metastasis in 24 lymph nodes in 5 dogs. A calculated value, percentage signal intensity loss, was also significantly different between metastatic and nonmetastatic lymph nodes [68] (Fig. 12).

Specific PET tracers may be more diagnostic than FDG. F-18 Fluorothymidine (FLT) is a thymidine analogue that reflects DNA synthesis and accumulates in proliferating tissues, including malignant masses. One study evaluated F18-FLT in dogs with lymphoma and found it useful for detecting disease sites during staging and detecting early response and early recrudescence of disease in lymph nodes [60]. PET tracers for specific human tumor types, such as prostate specific membrane antigen for detecting lymph node metastases in prostatic carcinoma can improve detection of metastasis in lymph nodes with high sensitivity and specificity in some studies [66]. Developing tracers specific for veterinary neoplasms is not common due to cost of development compared with potential financial reward.

Near infrared (NIR) fluorescence is a relatively new sentinel lymph node mapping technique in human medicine. Fluorescent probes, such as indocyanine green, are excited and fluoresce in the infrared spectrum. Specific imaging systems are used to detect the fluorescent probes, which can be detected to about 10 mm. This technique can be used for preoperative and intraoperative imaging [69]. Transcutaneous NIR fluorescence has been evaluated in normal dogs and successfully identified the sentinel lymph node in 17 of 18 locations in a median time of 5 minutes (range 2–25 minutes). [33] Dogs have also been used in

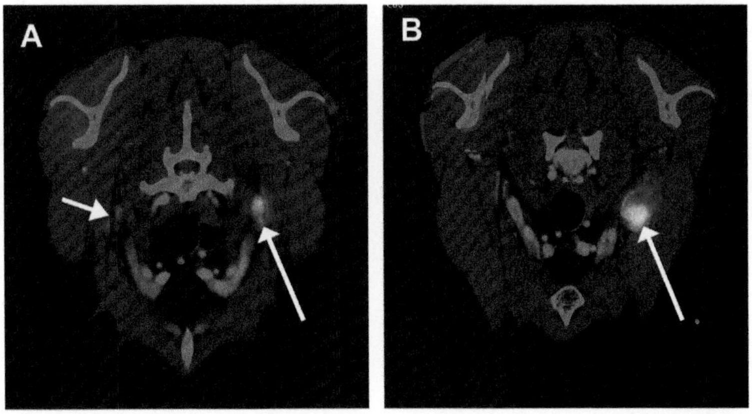

FIG. 11 PET/CT images of a dog with osteosarcoma of the distal left radius. (**A**) Fused FDG-PET/CT image at the time of initial staging. The left axillary lymph node is mildly enlarged compared with the right and has increased avidity, with an SUVmax of 4.7 (*long arrow*). The right axillary lymph node is normal in size and similar in avidity to surrounding soft tissues (*arrow*). The left axillary lymph node was diagnosed as either reactive or metastatic on PET/CT. Fine-needle aspirates were attempted but were nondiagnostic. (**B**) Fused FDG-PET/CT image obtained 7 weeks later. The left axillary lymph node is increased in size, is heterogeneously contrast enhancing, and has further increased avidity with an SUV max of 6.6 (*long arrow*.) The diagnosis based on PET/CT was metastasis. Histopathology showed metastatic osteosarcoma. The right axillary is not well visualized on this image.

research settings as translational models for NIR fluorescence [70–72].

Radiomics is a newer field of investigation that evaluates images by extracting a large number of quantitative features using data characterization algorithms. Regions of interest or volumes of interest are identified and can be evaluated on most imaging modalities, including ultrasound, CT, MRI, and PET. Information produced can be used to assist in diagnosis, prognosis, and prediction of response to therapy [73]. The human medical literature suggests favorable results for detecting lymph node metastasis using radiomics [74,75]. In veterinary medicine, CT radiomics has been investigated to evaluate sinonasal pathology, but lymph node analysis had not been reported [76].

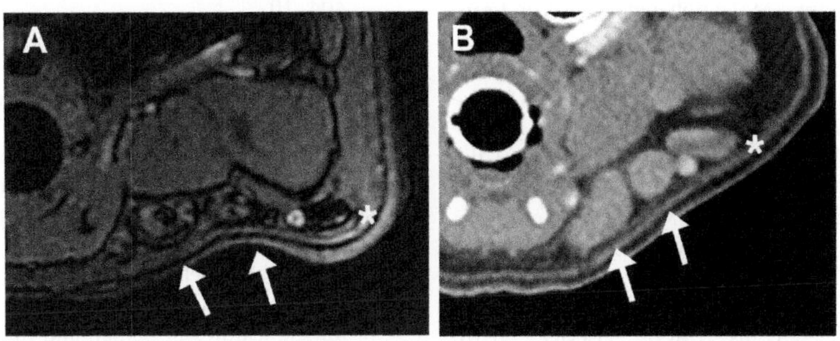

FIG. 12 Images of a dog with a mast cell tumor of the rostral mandibular lip. (**A**) T2* GRE MRI image acquired 48 hours after intravenous injection of superparamagnetic iron oxide nanoparticles. The medial and middle left mandibular lymph nodes (*arrows*) are heterogenous and did not exhibit complete negative enhancement, therefore were considered metastatic. The lateral left mandibular lymph node (*asterisk*) did exhibit complete negative enhancement and was considered normal. (**B**) Postcontrast CT image obtained 2 days prior. The medial and middle left mandibular lymph nodes (*arrows*) are homogenous to minimally heterogeneously contrast enhancing and are mildly enlarged and the middle lymph node is rounded. The lateral lymph node is normal in size and shape and has a normal fatty hilus. The characteristics of the middle and medial lymph nodes were not considered conclusive for metastasis. (*Images with permission* of Lynn Griffin, College of Veterinary Medicine and Biomedical Sciences, Colorado State University.)

SUMMARY

Lymph nodes can be evaluated on multiple imaging modalities. However, there is no consensus as to what characteristics can be used to reliably diagnose metastasis in any modality. This drives continued research in human and veterinary medicine. Until more precise imaging tests are created and validated, sampling by cytology or histopathology is warranted for sentinel lymph nodes and lymph nodes with abnormalities on palpation or imaging studies.

ACKNOWLEDGMENTS

The author would like to thank Ray Parham, LVT for his assistance in finding and acquiring images.

DISCLOSURE

The author has nothing to disclose.

REFERENCES

[1] Vail DM, Thamm DH, Liptak JM. Withrow and MacEwen's small animal clinical oncology. 6th edition. Edinburgh (Scotland): Elsevier; 2020. p. XIX.
[2] Nyman HT, O'Brien RT. The sonographic evaluation of lymph nodes. Clin Tech Small Anim Pract 2007;22(3): 128–37.
[3] Langenbach A, McManus PM, Hendrick MJ, et al. Sensitivity and specificity of methods of assessing the regional lymph nodes for evidence of metastasis in dogs and cats with solid tumors. J Am Vet Med Assoc 2001;218(9): 1424–8.
[4] Christiansen A, Detmar M. Lymphangiogenesis and cancer. Genes Cancer 2011;2(12):1146–58.
[5] Kirberger RM, Avner A. The effect of positioning on the appearance of selected cranial thoracic structures in the dog. Vet Radiol Ultrasound 2006;47(1):61–8.
[6] Fiorini T, Hostnik ET. Radiographic Assessment of the Popliteal Lymph Node to Aid the Differentiation of Canine Stifle Osteosarcoma From Moderate to Severe Stifle Degenerative Joint Disease. Top companion Anim Med 2018;33(4):136–40.
[7] Thrall DE. Textbook of veterinary diagnostic radiology. Seventh edition. St.Louis (MO): Elsevier; 2018. p. 649–775.
[8] Evans HE, Miller ME. Miller's anatomy of the dog. Fifth edition. St Louis (MO): Elsevier; 2020. p. 628–30, 635-636.
[9] Smith K, O'Brien R. Radiographic characterization of enlarged sternal lymph nodes in 71 dogs and 13 cats. J Am Anim Hosp Assoc 2012;48(3):176–81.
[10] Jones BG, Pollard RE. Relationship between radiographic evidence of tracheobronchial lymph node enlargement and definitive or presumptive diagnosis. Vet Radiol Ultrasound 2012;53(5):486–91.
[11] Naganobu K, Ohigashi Y, Akiyoshi T, et al. Lymphography of the thoracic duct by percutaneous injection of iohexol into the popliteal lymph node of dogs: experimental study and clinical application. Vet Surg 2006; 35(4):377–81.
[12] Papadopoulou PL, Patsikas MN, Charitanti A, et al. The lymph drainage pattern of the mammary glands in the cat: a lymphographic and computerized tomography lymphographic study. Anat Histol Embryol 2009;38(4):292–9.
[13] Patsikas MN, Karayannopoulou M, Kaldrymidoy E, et al. The lymph drainage of the neoplastic mammary glands in the bitch: a lymphographic study. Anat Histol Embryol 2006;35(4):228–34.
[14] Brissot HN, Edery EG. Use of indirect lymphography to identify sentinel lymph node in dogs: a pilot study in 30 tumours. Vet Comp Oncol 2017;15(3):740–53.
[15] Mayer MN, Silver TI, Lowe CK, et al. Radiographic lymphangiography in the dog using iodized oil. Vet Comp Oncol 2013;11(2):151–61.
[16] Llabres-Diaz FJ. Ultrasonography of the medial iliac lymph nodes in the dog. Vet Radiol Ultrasound 2004; 45(2):156–65.
[17] Cruz-Arambulo R, Wrigley R, Powers B. Sonographic features of histiocytic neoplasms in the canine abdomen. Vet Radiol Ultrasound 2004;45(6):554–8.
[18] De Swarte M, Alexander K, Rannou B, et al. Comparison of sonographic features of benign and neoplastic deep lymph nodes in dogs. Vet Radiol Ultrasound 2011; 52(4):451–6.
[19] Nyman HT, Kristensen AT, Skovgaard IM, et al. Characterization of normal and abnormal canine superficial lymph nodes using gray-scale B-mode, color flow mapping, power, and spectral Doppler ultrasonography: a multivariate study. Vet Radiol Ultrasound 2005;46(5): 404–10.
[20] Dave AC, Zekas LJ, Auld DM. Correlation of cytologic and histopathologic findings with perinodal echogenicity of abdominal lymph nodes in dogs and cats. Vet Radiol Ultrasound 2017;58(4):463–70.
[21] Kinns J, Mai W. Association between malignancy and sonographic heterogeneity in canine and feline abdominal lymph nodes. Vet Radiol Ultrasound 2007;48(6): 565–9.
[22] Nyman HT, Nielsen OL, McEvoy FJ, et al. Comparison of B-mode and Doppler ultrasonographic findings with histologic features of benign and malignant mammary tumors in dogs. Am J Vet Res 2006;67(6):985–91.
[23] Silva P, Uscategui RAR, Maronezi MC, et al. Ultrasonography for lymph nodes metastasis identification in bitches with mammary neoplasms. Sci. Rep 2018;8(1): 17708.
[24] Prieto S, Gomez-Ochoa P, De Blas I, et al. Pathologic correlation of resistive and pulsatility indices in canine abdominal lymph nodes. Vet Radiol Ultrasound 2009; 50(5):525–9.

[25] Gaschen L, Angelette N, Stout R. Contrast-enhanced harmonic ultrasonography of medial iliac lymph nodes in healthy dogs. Vet Radiol Ultrasound 2010;51(6):634–7.
[26] Salwei RM, O'Brien RT, Matheson JS. Characterization of lymphomatous lymph nodes in dogs using contrast harmonic and Power Doppler ultrasound. Vet Radiol Ultrasound 2005;46(5):411–6.
[27] Ozturk A, Grajo JR, Dhyani M, et al. Principles of ultrasound elastography. Abdom Radiol (N Y) 2018;43(4): 773–85.
[28] Seiler GS, Griffith E. Comparisons between elastographic stiffness scores for benign versus malignant lymph nodes in dogs and cats. Vet Radiol Ultrasound 2018;59(1): 79–88.
[29] Belotta AF, Gomes MC, Rocha NS, et al. Sonography and sonoelastography in the detection of malignancy in superficial lymph nodes of dogs. J Vet Intern Med 2019; 33(3):1403–13.
[30] Choi M, Yoon J, Choi M. Semi-quantitative strain elastography may facilitate pre-surgical prediction of mandibular lymph nodes malignancy in dogs. J Vet Sci 2019;20(6):e62.
[31] Gelb HR, Freeman LJ, Rohleder JJ, et al. Feasibility of contrast-enhanced ultrasound-guided biopsy of sentinel lymph nodes in dogs. Vet Radiol Ultrasound 2010; 51(6):628–33.
[32] Lurie DM, Seguin B, Schneider PD, et al. Contrast-assisted ultrasound for sentinel lymph node detection in spontaneously arising canine head and neck tumors. Invest Radiol 2006;41(4):415–21.
[33] Favril S, Stock E, Hernot S, et al. Sentinel lymph node mapping by near-infrared fluorescence imaging and contrast-enhanced ultrasound in healthy dogs. Vet Comp Oncol 2019;17(1):89–98.
[34] Milovancev M, Nemanic S, Bobe G. Computed tomographic assessment of sternal lymph node dimensions and attenuation in healthy dogs. Am J Vet Res 2017; 78(3):289–94.
[35] Beukers M, Grosso FV, Voorhout G. Computed tomographic characteristics of presumed normal canine abdominal lymph nodes. Vet Radiol Ultrasound 2013; 54(6):610–7.
[36] Iwasaki R, Mori T, Ito Y, et al. Computed Tomographic Evaluation of Presumptively Normal Canine Sternal Lymph Nodes. J Am Anim Hosp Assoc 2016;52(6): 371–7.
[37] Perlini M, Bugbee A, Secrest S. Computed tomographic appearance of abdominal lymph nodes in healthy cats. J Vet Intern Med 2018;32(3):1070–6.
[38] Ballegeer EA, Adams WM, Dubielzig RR, et al. Computed tomography characteristics of canine tracheobronchial lymph node metastasis. Vet Radiol Ultrasound 2010; 51(4):397–403.
[39] Iwasaki R, Murakami M, Kawabe M, et al. Metastatic diagnosis of canine sternal lymph nodes using computed tomography characteristics: A retrospective cross-sectional study. Vet Comp Oncol 2018;16(1):140–7.
[40] Skinner OT, Boston SE, Giglio RF, et al. Diagnostic accuracy of contrast-enhanced computed tomography for assessment of mandibular and medial retropharyngeal lymph node metastasis in dogs with oral and nasal cancer. Vet Comp Oncol 2018;16(4):562–70.
[41] Gendler A, Lewis JR, Reetz JA, et al. Computed tomographic features of oral squamous cell carcinoma in cats: 18 cases (2002-2008). J Am Vet Med Assoc 2010; 236(3):319–25.
[42] Pollard RE, Fuller MC, Steffey MA. Ultrasound and computed tomography of the iliosacral lymphatic centre in dogs with anal sac gland carcinoma. Vet Comp Oncol 2017;15(2):299–306.
[43] Rossi F, Korner M, Suarez J, et al. Computed tomographic-lymphography as a complementary technique for lymph node staging in dogs with malignant tumors of various sites. Vet Radiol Ultrasound 2018;59(2): 155–62.
[44] Grimes JA, Secrest SA, Northrup NC, et al. Indirect computed tomography lymphangiography with aqueous contrast for evaluation of sentinel lymph nodes in dogs with tumors of the head. Vet Radiol Ultrasound 2017; 58(5):559–64.
[45] Randall EK, Jones MD, Kraft SL, et al. The development of an indirect computed tomography lymphography protocol for sentinel lymph node detection in head and neck cancer and comparison to other sentinel lymph node mapping techniques. Vet Comp Oncol 2020 [Online ahead of print].
[46] Soultani C, Patsikas MN, Karayannopoulou M, et al. Assessment of Sentinel Lymph Node Metastasis in Canine Mammary Gland Tumors Using Computed Tomographic Indirect Lymphography. Vet Radiol Ultrasound 2017;58(2):186–96.
[47] Majeski SA, Steffey MA, Fuller M, et al. Indirect Computed Tomographic Lymphography for Iliosacral Lymphatic Mapping in a Cohort of Dogs with Anal Sac Gland Adenocarcinoma: Technique Description. Vet Radiol Ultrasound 2017;58(3):295–303.
[48] Grimes JA, Secrest SA, Wallace ML, et al. Use of indirect computed tomography lymphangiography to determine metastatic status of sentinel lymph nodes in dogs with a pre-operative diagnosis of melanoma or mast cell tumour. Vet Comp Oncol 2020 [Online ahead of print].
[49] Kneissl S, Probst A. Magnetic resonance imaging features of presumed normal head and neck lymph nodes in dogs. Vet Radiol Ultrasound 2006;47(6):538–41.
[50] Pokorny E, Hecht S, Sura PA, et al. Magnetic resonance imaging of canine mast cell tumors. Vet Radiol Ultrasound 2012;53(2):167–73.
[51] Anderson CL, MacKay CS, Roberts GD, et al. Comparison of abdominal ultrasound and magnetic resonance imaging for detection of abdominal lymphadenopathy in dogs with metastatic apocrine gland adenocarcinoma of the anal sac. Vet Comp Oncol 2015;13(2):98–105.
[52] Wu LM, Xu JR, Hua J, et al. Value of diffusion-weighted MR imaging performed with quantitative apparent

diffusion coefficient values for cervical lymphadenopathy. J Magn Reson Imaging 2013;38(3):663–70.
[53] He XQ, Wei LN. Diagnostic value of lymph node metastasis by diffusion-weighted magnetic resonance imaging in cervical cancer. J Cancer Res Ther 2016;12(1):77–83.
[54] Stahle JA, Larson MM, Rossmeisl JH, et al. Diffusion weighted magnetic resonance imaging is a feasible method for characterizing regional lymph nodes in canine patients with head and neck disease. Vet Radiol Ultrasound 2019;60(2):176–83.
[55] Mayer MN, Kraft SL, Bucy DS, et al. Indirect magnetic resonance lymphography of the head and neck of dogs using Gadofluorine M and a conventional gadolinium contrast agent: a pilot study. Can Vet J 2012;53(10): 1085–90.
[56] Pereira CT, Luiz Navarro Marques F, Williams J, et al. 99mTc-labeled dextran for mammary lymphoscintigraphy in dogs. Vet Radiol Ultrasound 2008;49(5):487–91.
[57] Worley DR. Incorporation of sentinel lymph node mapping in dogs with mast cell tumours: 20 consecutive procedures. Vet Comp Oncol 2014;12(3):215–26.
[58] Tuohy JL, Worley DR. Pulmonary lymph node charting in normal dogs with blue dye and scintigraphic lymphatic mapping. Res Vet Sci 2014;97(1):148–55.
[59] Linden DS, Cole R, Tillson DM, et al. Sentinel lymph node mapping of the canine anal sac using lymphoscintigraphy: A pilot study. Vet Radiol Ultrasound 2019; 60(3):346–50.
[60] Lawrence J, Vanderhoek M, Barbee D, et al. Use of 3′-deoxy-3′-[18F]fluorothymidine PET/CT for evaluating response to cytotoxic chemotherapy in dogs with non-Hodgkin's lymphoma. Vet Radiol Ultrasound 2009; 50(6):660–8.
[61] LeBlanc AK, Jakoby BW, Townsend DW, et al. 18FDG-PET imaging in canine lymphoma and cutaneous mast cell tumor. Vet Radiol Ultrasound 2009;50(2):215–23.
[62] Ballegeer EA, Hollinger C, Kunst CM. Imaging diagnosis-multicentric lymphoma of granular lymphocytes imaged with FDG PET/CT in a dog. Vet Radiol Ultrasound 2013; 54(1):75–80.
[63] Seiler SM, Baumgartner C, Hirschberger J, et al. Comparative Oncology: Evaluation of 2-Deoxy-2-[18F]fluoro-D-glucose (FDG) Positron Emission Tomography/Computed Tomography (PET/CT) for the Staging of Dogs with Malignant Tumors. PloS one 2015;10(6): e0127800.
[64] Randall EK, Kraft SL, Yoshikawa H, et al. Evaluation of 18F-FDG PET/CT as a diagnostic imaging and staging tool for feline oral squamous cell carcinoma. Vet Comp Oncol 2016;14(1):28–38.
[65] Griffin LR, Thamm DH, Selmic LE, et al. Pilot study utilizing Fluorine-18 fluorodeoxyglucose-positron emission tomography/computed tomography for glycolytic phenotyping of canine mast cell tumors. Vet Radiol Ultrasound 2018;59(4):461–8.
[66] Muteganya R, Goldman S, Aoun F, et al. Current Imaging Techniques for Lymph Node Staging in Prostate Cancer: A Review. Front Surg 2018;5:74.
[67] Saksena MA, Saokar A, Harisinghani MG. Lymphotropic nanoparticle enhanced MR imaging (LNMRI) technique for lymph node imaging. Eur J Radiol 2006;58(3): 367–74.
[68] Griffin L, Frank CB, Seguin B. Pilot study to evaluate the efficacy of lymphotropic nanoparticle enhanced MRI for diagnosis of metastatic disease in canine head and neck tumours. Vet Comp Oncol 2019;18(2):176–83.
[69] Schaafsma BE, Mieog JS, Hutteman M, et al. The clinical use of indocyanine green as a near-infrared fluorescent contrast agent for image-guided oncologic surgery. J Surg Oncol 2011;104(3):323–32.
[70] Knapp DW, Adams LG, Degrand AM, et al. Sentinel lymph node mapping of invasive urinary bladder cancer in animal models using invisible light. Eur Urol 2007; 52(6):1700–8.
[71] Liss MA, Stroup SP, Qin Z, et al. Robotic-assisted fluorescence sentinel lymph node mapping using multimodal image guidance in an animal model. Urology 2014; 84(4):982.e9-14.
[72] Kong SH, Noh YW, Suh YS, et al. Evaluation of the novel near-infrared fluorescence tracers pullulan polymer nanogel and indocyanine green/gamma-glutamic acid complex for sentinel lymph node navigation surgery in large animal models. Gastric Cancer 2015;18(1):55–64.
[73] Liu Z, Wang S, Dong D, et al. The Applications of Radiomics in Precision Diagnosis and Treatment of Oncology: Opportunities and Challenges. Theranostics 2019;9(5): 1303–22.
[74] Gu Y, She Y, Xie D, et al. A texture analysis-based prediction model for lymph node metastasis in stage IA lung adenocarcinoma. Ann Thorac Surg 2018;106(1):214–20.
[75] Ji GW, Zhang YD, Zhang H, et al. Biliary tract cancer at CT: a radiomics-based model to predict lymph node metastasis and survival outcomes. Radiology 2019; 290(1):90–8.
[76] Loeber S, Schimek M, Dreyfus J, et al. Textural Radiomics characteristics and computed tomography findings as preditors of canine sinonasal pathology. Abstracts, Amer College Vet Radiol Intern Vet Rad Assoc Joint Scientific Conf, Fort Worth, TX, October 14–19, 2018.
[77] Nemanic S, Nelson N. Ultrasonography and noncontrast computed tomography of medial retropharyngeal lymph nodes in healthy cats. Am J Vet Res 2012;73:1377–85.

Gastroenterology

Advances in Small Animal Care 1 (2020) 91–100
ADVANCES IN SMALL ANIMAL CARE

Genetics and Immunopathogenesis of Chronic Inflammatory Enteropathies in Dogs

Karin Allenspach, DVM, PhD, DECVIM[a,*], Jonathan P. Mochel, DVM, MS, PhD, DECVPT[b]
[a]Iowa State University College of Veterinary Medicine, Veterinary Clinical Sciences, 1809 South Riverside Drive, Ames, IA 50010, USA; [b]Iowa State University College of Veterinary Medicine, Biomedical Sciences, 1809 South Riverside Drive, Ames, IA 50010, USA

KEYWORDS
• Innate immunity • Adaptive immunity • Macrophages • Toll-like receptors • Genetics • Immunopathogenesis

KEY POINTS

- The pathogenesis of lymphoplasmacytic chronic inflammatory enteropathies (CIE) involves several genetic defects, a severe dysbiosis of the intestinal microbiome, and innate and adaptive immunity hyperresponsiveness.
- The cytokine profile in lymphoplasmacytic CIE is defined by an increase in mucosal interleukin 1β.
- Cellular infiltrates of lymphocytes and plasma cells are less important than architectural changes of the epithelial cells in lymphoplasmacytic CIE.
- Granulomatous colitis develops from a genetic defect that renders dogs unable to kill intracellular bacteria.
- Overgrowth of adherent-invasive *Escherichia coli* is pathognomonic of granulomatous colitis.

INTRODUCTION AND DEFINITION OF CHRONIC INFLAMMATORY ENTEROPATHIES

Chronic inflammatory enteropathies (CIE) in dogs describe a group of idiopathic disorders characterized by chronic persistent or recurrent gastrointestinal (GI) signs, with histologic evidence of inflammation in the lamina propria of the small intestine, large intestine, or both. The diagnosis of CIE is one of exclusion, and a full diagnostic workup needs to be done to rule out all known causes of GI inflammation. Currently, endoscopic evaluation and histopathology of intestinal biopsies is the only way to definitively diagnose CIE. Although the exact cause of CIE is unknown, it is widely accepted that the pathogenesis involves a complex interplay among host genetics, the intestinal mucosal immune system, the environment, and the intestinal microbiota [1]. In this article, the authors focus on the most frequently seen form of CIE, which is characterized by lymphoplasmacytic inflammation (also called lymphoplasmacytic enteritis [LPE]) and granulomatous colitis (GC), which—even though much rarer—is a severe form of CIE mostly seen in young Boxers and French Bulldogs [2] with an interesting pathogenesis involving the interplay of genetics and mucosal immunology.

ETIOPATHOGENESIS OF CHRONIC INFLAMMATORY ENTEROPATHIES

Over the last 15 years, studies have shown that the pathogenesis of canine CIE is complex and involves an overly aggressive cell-mediated response due to the loss of tolerance to antigens found in the food and the complex commensal microbiome in genetically susceptible hosts.

*Corresponding author, *E-mail address:* allek@iastate.edu

https://doi.org/10.1016/j.yasa.2020.07.007
2666-4518/20/ Published by Elsevier Inc.

Genetic Predisposition in German Shepherd Dog

Lymphoplasmacytic (LP) enteritis is the most common form of CIE in dogs and is a polygenic disease, similar to inflammatory bowel disease (IBD) in people. In humans, mutations in innate immunity pattern recognition receptors, such as NOD2 and toll-like receptor (TLR) 4, and others have all been associated with the development of IBD [3]. In dogs, it has always been obvious to clinicians that CIE seems to have a genetic component, because many breeds are predisposed to developing CIE. German Shepherd dogs (GSDs), in particular, are predisposed to developing LP CIE in the United Kingdom [4]. Extensive genetic investigations into the pathogenesis of CIE have accumulated over the last 10 years and are a representative example of how genetics influence the pathogenesis in CIE. In a candidate gene analysis study, single nucleotide polymorphisms (SNPs) in canine TLR2, TLR4, and TLR5 were found to be associated with CE in GSDs [5]. The polymorphisms that were identified in the TLR5 and TLR4 genes have been further evaluated in a case-control study with more than 50 cases and GSD breed controls. The G22A SNP in TLR5 was significantly associated with CE in GSDs, whereas the remaining 2 SNPs were found to be significantly protective for CE. Furthermore, the 2 SNPs in TLR4 (A1571T and G1807A) were in complete linkage disequilibrium and were also significantly associated with IBD [5]. The results for the TLR5 risk-associated genotype were also mirrored in non-GSD breeds: the heterozygote genotype for all 4 SNPs was significantly more frequently found in a population of 96 dogs of different breeds with IBD compared with the non-GSD control population [6]. To follow-up on this finding, the functional significance of the canine TLR5 SNPs was determined by transfecting the identified risk-protective and risk-associated haplotype into human embryonic kidney cells and assessed nuclear factor-kappa B (NF-κB) activation and CXCL8 production after stimulation. In addition, a whole-blood assay for TLR5 activation was developed using blood derived from carrier dogs of either haplotype. There was a significant increase in NF-kB activity when cells transfected with the risk-associated TLR5 haplotype were stimulated with flagellin compared with the cells expressing the risk-protective TLR5 haplotype [7]. This difference in NF-κB activation correlated with CXCL8 expression in the supernatant measured by enzyme-linked immunosorbent assay (ELISA). Furthermore, whole blood taken from carrier dogs of the risk-associated TLR5 haplotype produced significantly more tumor necrosis factor after stimulation with flagellin compared with that taken from carriers of the risk-protective haplotype. This study therefore showed, for the first time, a direct functional impact of the canine CIE risk-associated TLR5 haplotype, which results in hyperresponsiveness to flagellin compared with the CIE risk-protective TLR5 haplotype [7]. In another recent study, the association of major histocompatibility complex class II locus (Dog Leukocyte Antigen, DLA) mutations with disease was assessed. Sequence-based genotyping of the 3 polymorphic DLA genes—DLA-DRB1, -DQA1, and -DQB1—was performed in 56 GSDs affected by IBD (defined as steroid-responsive CIE) and in 50 breed-matched controls without any history of GI signs. The haplotype DLA-DRB1*015:02–DQA1*006:01–DQB1*023:01 was found to be present only in the control population and was associated with a reduced risk of IBD (P<.001). In contrast, the haplotype DLA-DRB1*015:01–DQA1*006:01–DQB1*003:01 was associated with IBD (odds ratio [OR] = 1.93, 95% confidence interval [CI] = 1.02 to 3.67, P = .05). The findings of this study therefore lend additional support to the immunogenetic cause and immunopathogenesis of this disease. In a follow-up genome-wide association study (GWAS), 98 cases and 98 controls were genotyped [8]. GWAS identified an additional 16 genes to be associated with CIE in GSDs, with many of them associated with classic Th2-type cytokine responses, such as interleukin 13 (IL-13), IL-4, and IL-5 [8]. This finding could have important implications for investigations of novel treatment options, as GSDs (especially in Europe) express a severe clinical phenotype of CIE/IBD that is difficult to control with conventional treatment options [9,10].

The Role of Intestinal Microbiota in the Immunopathogenesis of Chronic Inflammatory Enteropathies

Dogs with CIE exhibit a typical dysbiosis of the intestinal microbiome, which can be assessed using molecular methods to investigate the genome of bacterial DNA found in biopsies and feces. This dysbiosis is thought to be a sequelae as well as a potential perpetuating factor of the disease [11–15]. A decrease in microbial diversity along with an increased abundance of members belonging to the *Enterobacteriaceae* family (and specifically, *E coli*), significantly higher number of clones belonging to *Proteobacteria*, and a significantly lower abundance of *Clostridia* have been found to be the most consistent changes of the microbiome in dogs with CIE. In general, these changes can be characterized as an increase in proinflammatory bacterial phyla, along with decreased abundance of antiinflammatory phyla and decreased diversity, all of which have been shown to also be associated with IBD in humans [16].

However, there is evidence that some of these microbiome changes could be breed-associated. In the duodenum of GSDs with CIE, bacterial clones within the order *Lactobacillales* were significantly more frequently found than in the duodenum of healthy dogs [9]. GSDs with CIE have a distinctly different microbiome than that from healthy dogs, as well as from other breeds of dogs presenting with CIE, with overrepresentation of certain traditionally labeled "beneficial" bacteria in the duodenum, specifically sequences of the order of *Lactobacillales*. Furthermore, novel studies have investigated the functional significance of this dysbiosis, that is, those metabolites produced by the dysbiotic microbiome and what systemic effects this may have [15,17]. It seems that the fecal metabolome in CIE cases displays overrepresented bacterial secretion systems and transcription factors and underrepresented amino acid metabolism [18]. The serum metabolites 3-hydroxybutyrate, hexuronic acid, ribose, and gluconic acid lactone were significantly more abundant in dogs with CIE than in healthy controls. These data suggest the presence of oxidative stress in the intestinal epithelium and a functional alteration of the GI microbiota in dogs with CE, which can persist even in the face of a clinical response to medical therapy [17]. Another recent study also clearly showed that the lipid metabolism in dogs with CIE is disturbed, again indicating increased oxidative stress and membrane damage in the intestinal epithelium [19]. Encouragingly, in dogs with food-responsive enteropathy (FRE), these changes were minimized after treatment, suggesting that FRE dogs revert to a more normal metabolism after successful treatment. Just as with antibiotic treatment of antibiotic-responsive enteropathy (ARE), colonic commensals are the main groups of bacteria that are diminished in the microbiome of dogs with CIE.

Evidence of Innate Immunity Hyper-Responsiveness in Chronic Inflammatory Enteropathies

TLRs have been shown to be upregulated in the intestine of human beings with Crohn disease (CD) and ulcerative colitis. This may be either a consequence of the ongoing stimulation of TLRs by an altered microbiota or it may be a causal factor contributing to the pathogenesis of disease. Most human studies show that the mRNA and protein expression of TLR2 as well as TLR4 are increased in the intestine of people with active IBD. In canine studies, dogs of different breeds with clinically severe, active IBD express higher levels of TLR2 receptors in the duodenum compared with healthy dogs when measured by real-time polymerase chain reaction in whole endoscopic biopsies [20]. Furthermore, TLR2 expression was correlated with the clinical severity of IBD using the Canine Chronic Enteropathy Clinical Activity Index. In further studies looking at German Shepherd dogs with IBD in the investigator's laboratory, it was found that TLR4 expression was 60-fold higher in the duodenum, ileum, and colon of dogs with IBD compared with samples from healthy dogs; however, TLR2 and TLR9 were similarly expressed as in healthy dogs [2]. These data show that it is important to look at similar phenotypes of dogs when choosing cases for such studies, as the results will vary depending on the severity of disease, the treatment response in the cases, and the specific breed of dogs. To the contrary, TLR5 expression was seen to be consistently downregulated in the intestine of German Shepherd dogs with IBD as compared with healthy dogs. The upregulation of TLRs in the mucosa of dogs with CIE is thought to be a sign of consistent activation of innate immunity by the luminal bacteria. Specifically, the dysbiosis associated with CIE, which is characterized by a decrease in microbial diversity and an increase in *Enterobacteriaceae*, probably plays a role in this. In the healthy intestine, TLRs will consistently sample diverse bacterial antigens, which overall will downregulate excessive inflammation. In the case of CIE, however, the increased binding of LPS from mostly gram-negative bacteria will signal through TLR4 and result in a hyperresponsiveness of the innate immune system in the mucosa. This sets off an alarm response, switching the mucosal homeostasis to a proinflammatory state.

The Role of the Adaptive Immune System in Chronic Inflammatory Enteropathies

The concept of impaired immunoregulation in CIE is supported by observations of increased numbers of immunoglobulin-producing plasma cells as well as cytokine-producing T-cell subsets in canine IBD [4,21]. The inflammation seen in IBD is thought to result from inappropriate cytokine production by these different T-cell subsets. In dogs, there is a mixed Th1 and Th2 profile, which has been demonstrated in several case series [21]. Most of the studies have shown an increased IL-12 and Il-23 production in the mucosa of dogs with IBD [22,23], although the associations are not as strong as those seen in patients with human IBD. However, nuclear factor-kappa B activation has been confirmed in at least 2 studies in dogs in IBD, which points to an important role of cytokines in the pathogenesis of the disease [24,25].

A new concept stems from macrophages and T-helper lymphocyte cells (T cells) infiltrating the lamina propria, producing large amounts of interleukin (IL) 1β [26,27] in response to an overactive immune activation to commensal bacteria (Fig. 1). One recent study showed IL-β overexpression in FRE dogs before treatment, which declined after successful clinical treatment [28]. IL-1β overexpression in the mucosa of dogs with IBD could therefore represent a good target for novel treatment options, which has not been widely investigated so far. There is also direct evidence that humoral antibodies are produced in dogs with CIE, similar to what occurs in people with IBD. Antibodies elevated in the peripheral blood of CIE dogs are either autoimmune antibodies, antibodies against bacterial proteins, such as flagellins, or *E coli* in outer membrane proteins. Perinuclear antineutrophilic cytoplasmic antibodies (pANCA) belong to the group of autoimmune antibodies and have previously been found to be useful in the diagnosis of human IBD for decades [29]. These antibodies are serum autoantibodies similar to antinuclear antibodies (ANA), which are much more specific for intestinal disease than ANA in dogs. They are detected by indirect immunofluorescence assays, where a typical pattern of perinuclear staining of canine granulocytes can be seen, or by ELISA. In the first study assessing the possible clinical usefulness of pANCA in dogs with IBD, sensitivity was 0.51 and specificity ranged between 0.56 and 0.95 [30]. pANCA proved to be a highly specific marker for CIE in dogs when the group of dogs with chronic diarrhea of other causes were tested against the group of dogs with CIE (specificity 0.95). This is in agreement with reports from human medicine that show a specificity of up to 94% for pANCA when distinguishing between IBD and patients with non-IBD–related diarrhea. Furthermore, when pANCA were measured in a group of dogs with FRE versus IBD, positive pANCA titers were signifcantly more frequently found in the group of dogs with FRE than in in dogs with steroid-responsive CIE.. The pANCA assay could therefore provide valuable help to the veterinarian presented with the clinical picture of a dog with chronic diarrhea and possible CIE: if the result is positive, an FRE is highly likely; however, if the result is negative, CIE cannot be excluded. pANCA also seem to be associated with the syndrome of familial protein-losing enteropathy in Soft Coated Wheaten Terriers (SCWT): pANCA were detectable in the serum of dogs on average 1 to 2 years before the onset of clinical disease and were highly correlated with hypoalbuminemia [31]. This test could serve as a useful adjunct for this specific disease in SCWT as an early screening test.

Care must be taken in interpreting a positive pANCA test result if other inflammatory or immune-mediated diseases are present in the dog. A recent study showed that many dogs with various vector-borne diseases or immune-mediated hemolytic anemia were positive for pANCA [32]. A commercially available indirect immunofluorescence assay developed for human beings has been used successfully to identify pANCA in dogs, which should be useful for further clinical research in this area [33]. A recent publication also identified other serum antibodies to be elevated in dogs with CIE as opposed to dogs presenting acute diarrhea, such as antibodies against flagellin, antibodies against outer membrane protein of *E coli*, and gliadin antibodies [34]. However, the clinical usefulness in the setting of differentiating dogs with CIE from dogs with other causes of chronic diarrhea still needs to be determined.

Evidence of Intestinal Epithelial Damage in Chronic Inflammatory Enteropathies

Immune cell dysfunction, as described earlier, has been identified in CIE in dogs; however, it is difficult to link these findings directly with evidence of immune cell infiltrates in histologic samples of CIE, specifically LPE. This is highlighted by the fact that the degree of lymphoplasmacellular infiltration in the intestinal lamina propria is not associated with clinical activity [2,35] or outcome [35]. It is therefore reasonable to assume that other components of the mucosa, namely the intestinal epithelial cell (IEC) membrane, are also critically involved in the pathogenesis of the disease. Recognizing the disparity between histologic infiltrates and clinical disease, a task force has tackled the development of a new histologic grading system for CIE, called the World Small Animal Veterinary Association (WSAVA) histologic scoring system [36]. This system puts particular weight on architectural changes of the mucosa and especially, epithelial changes. This is an important finding, as it indicates that in many cases of canine CIE, the inflammatory infiltrate *per se* may not be of as much importance as previously thought. In a recent study, the original WSAVA scoring was modified in order to achieve better correlation with clinical activity scores, pinpointing that architectural changes seem to be more important if a correlation with clinical activity score is desired [37]. In a recent study on FRE cases, an in-depth pathologic and ultrastructural investigation was performed on biopsies of the same dogs before and after elimination diet treatment [38]. This study showed that light microscopy does not implicate any changes in these dogs' WSAVA scores; however, on transmission electron

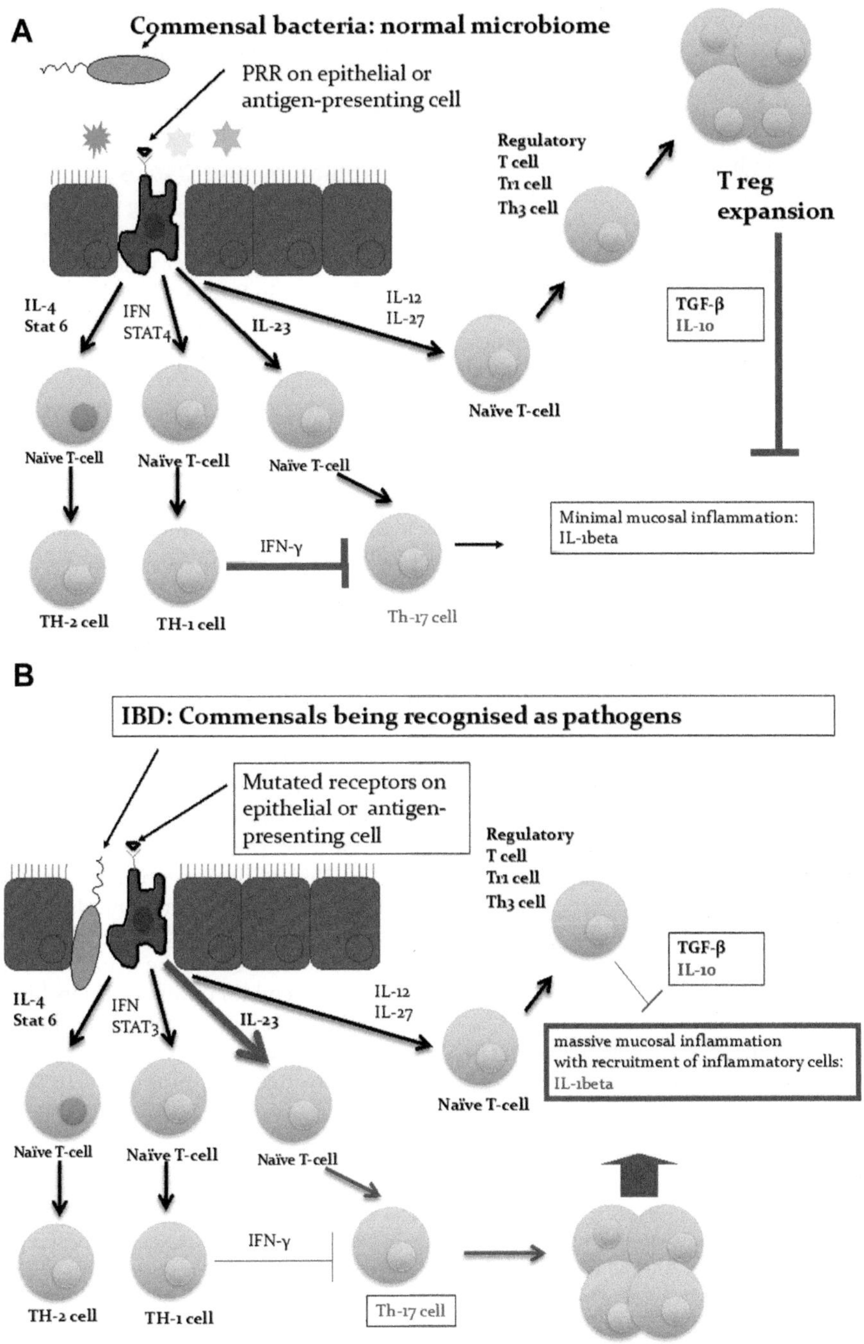
A
Commensal bacteria: normal microbiome
PRR on epithelial or antigen-presenting cell
Regulatory T cell
Tr1 cell
Th3 cell
T reg expansion
IL-4
Stat 6
IFN
STAT4
IL-23
IL-12
IL-27
TGF-β
IL-10
Naïve T-cell
Naïve T-cell
Naïve T-cell
Naïve T-cell
IFN-γ
Minimal mucosal inflammation:
IL-1beta
TH-2 cell
TH-1 cell
Th-17 cell
B
IBD: Commensals being recognised as pathogens
Mutated receptors on epithelial or antigen-presenting cell
Regulatory T cell
Tr1 cell
Th3 cell
TGF-β
IL-10
IL-4
Stat 6
IFN
STAT3
IL-23
IL-12
IL-27
massive mucosal inflammation
with recruitment of inflammatory cells:
IL-1beta
Naïve T-cell
Naïve T-cell
Naïve T-cell
Naïve T-cell
IFN-γ
TH-2 cell
TH-1 cell
Th-17 cell

microscopy (EM), ultrastructural changes in epithelial cells become obvious. Before treatment, these dogs showed blunted and sparse microvilli, along with vacuolization of the cytoplasm and mitochondrial changes, which all normalized after treatment [38]. Similar effects have been noted in children diagnosed with celiac disease, where biopsies after 6 months of elimination diet did not show much change; however, on EM, microarchitectural changes of the IECs had normalized [39]. Architectural changes of the IECs in dogs with CIE also seem to go along with an increase in epithelial permeability. Recent work in the investigator's laboratory using biopsies and organoids from dogs with CIE has demonstrated similar findings. Canine organoids are 3-dimensional cultures derived from the epithelial cell layer and faithfully reproduce structural and functional changes of the epithelium of the individual dog [40]. The authors found that the percentage of intestinal stem cells is increased in the epithelium of CIE dogs as compared with healthy dogs. This in turn results in a lesser percentage of absorptive IECs, which may be one of the factors leading to diarrhea in these dogs. Tight junctional expression of zonulin-1 is also increased in dogs with CIE compared with healthy dogs [41]. Zonulin-1 protein loosens interepithelial cell junctions and therefore results in leakage of fluid into the intestinal lumen [42,43]. These findings are promising, as organoids from dogs with CIE could be used to investigate novel drugs that affect tight junctional regulation ex vivo, before being used in clinical trials. However, at this point, more research needs to be performed in order to evaluate the epithelial changes in dogs with CIE in more detail.

GRANULOMATOUS COLITIS IN DOGS

Introduction

GC is a rare form of CIE that occurs most frequently in young Boxer dogs. It was first described 30 years ago and has since been reported in other breeds, such as Mastiffs, Alaskan Malamutes, French Bulldogs, English Bulldogs, and one cat. This article describes the pathophysiology, diagnosis, and approach to treatment of GC.

Pathobiology and Cause

In a publication investigating the possibility of an infectious cause for canine GC, large numbers of coccobacilli were found in the colonic mucosa by fluorescent in-situ hybridization in Boxers affected with GC but not in histologically normal tissues or in the mucosa of dogs with other types of colitis. Further studies using culture, cloning, and sequencing of the colonic microbiome from Boxers with GC identified the bacteria to be *E coli*. EM of GC lesions allowed identification and localization of the bacteria to the intracellular compartment of Periodic Acid Schiff (PAS)-positive macrophages [44]. In addition, the intracellular material found in PAS-positive macrophages from dogs with granulomatous colitis stains positive for polyclonal antibodies against *E coli*. Altogether these findings are exciting, particularly because further classification of the virulence genes and biological behavior of these bacteria in coculture with epithelial cells and macrophages revealed specific adhesive and invasive properties [44]. The *E coli* strains associated with GC have a similar phenotype with the adhesive and invasive behavior of *E coli* isolates associated with CD in people. In several studies, a particular strain of *E coli* (LF82) could be detected in biopsies of 20% to 35% of ileal lesions in CD but only in 6% of ileal samples from healthy controls or other colonic inflammatory diseases [45]. CD affects primarily the mucosa and submucosa of the ileum and colon in human beings. It resembles canine GC in its histologic appearance, as granulomas are the main feature of the disease. As in canine GC, some cases of CD seem to be susceptible to treatment with antibiotics. The *E coli* strains

FIG. 1 (**A** [*top*] and **B** [*bottom*]): current hypothesis of the pathogenesis of canine CIE. In the normal intestinal mucosa, TLRs sample pathogen-associated molecular patterns (PAMPs) from commensals in the intestinal lumen, which send signals to naïve T cells to differentiate primarily into T regulatory cells, which produce antiinflammatory cytokines, such as tissue growth factor (TGF)-β and IL-10. In the case of canine CIE, microbiome dysbiosis drives the messaging toward a proinflammatory pathway of T helper cell differentiation, resulting in the production of proinflammatory cytokines, mainly IL-1β. In addition, mutations in pattern recognition receptors, such as TLR5, result in hyperresponsiveness to flagellin. Since the dysbiosis in canine CIE is characterized by an increase in *Enterobacteriaceae* (which express flagellin), this will further increase proinflammatory responses of the mucosa. Moreover, the inflammatory cytokines will lead to architectural changes in epithelial cells, such as increased leakage through tight junctions, and therefore increased permeability. This in turn will result in more bacteria breaching the mucosal barrier, therefore leading to a vicious cycle of inflammation.

such as LF82 that have increasingly been associated with CD are unusual because they adhere to and invade intestinal epithelial cells in culture and have been shown to replicate within the phagolysosomes of macrophages in the granulomatous lesions instead of being cleared by the adaptive immune system. There is evidence that the adhesive and invasive *E coli* (AIEC) associated with GC are taken up by endosomes and persist in the macrophages instead of being cleared [44] (Fig. 2). These findings support the hypothesis that genetics play a major role in the pathogenesis of CD and possibly of canine GC. A genetic predisposition for GC is suspected due to the preponderance of cases in young Boxer dogs and French Bullterriers. In the first report of the disease in 1967, most of the affected dogs could be traced back to a single ancestor [46]. Definite confirmation of the exact identification of mutations in Boxers or French Bulldogs with GC is still lacking. However, it seems likely that a defect in innate immunity and in particular, mutated proteins of the oxidative burst render dogs with GC more susceptible to infections with specific bacteria, such as the AIEC strains described earlier.

Clinical Presentation and Differential Diagnosis

Differential diagnoses include extra-GI as well as infectious GI diseases such as parasites, diet-responsive diseases such as food intolerance, food allergy, or other forms of CIE, such as FRE, ARE, or IBD (steroid-responsive enteropathy). Rectal and colonic polyps as well as neoplastic disorders, such as lymphoma or adenocarcinoma, are less likely to occur in younger animals. The onset of disease occurs predominantly before 4 years of age. Clinical signs are those of severe chronic large intestinal inflammation (colitis) and comprise diarrhea, hematochezia, increased frequency of defecation, tenesmus, and presence of excessive mucus in the feces. Physical examination findings are normal in many cases of GC; however, weight loss and inappetence can be seen. Typically, colonoscopy reveals sites of severe colonic hemorrhage and ulcerations interspersed with stretches of normal-appearing mucosa. Early lesions can consist of a mixed inflammatory infiltrate in the lamina propria, which are subjacent to degenerative epithelium. With more extensive lesions and chronic disease, the ulcerations become more visible on histology with severe infiltration of the lamina propria and the submucosal regions with predominantly neutrophils and macrophages. There is also usually severe loss of the epithelial surface in biopsies from lesions and loss of goblet cells in the entire colon. Accumulation of large PAS-positive macrophages is pathognomonic for GC [47] and remains the best way to confirm the diagnosis.

Treatment

The prognosis for GC was guarded to poor until approximately 10 years ago. In recent years, several reports have sparked hope for treatment of GC: cases have shown a dramatic response to treatment with enrofloxacin (5 mg/kg po once daily) or a combination protocol

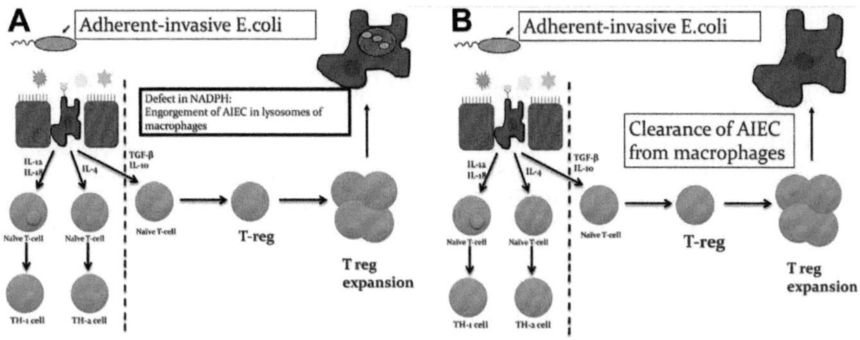

FIG. 2 (**A** [*left*] and **B** [*right*]): Granulomatous colitis (GC) is thought to be caused by the overgrowth of a pathogenic adherent-invasive *E coli* (AIEC) in a genetically susceptible host (Boxers, French Bulldogs). (**A**) In the normal case scenario, occasional *E coli* cross the intestinal barrier but will swiftly be destroyed by lysosomes in the cytoplasm of macrophages, therefore causing only minimal inflammation. (**B**) In the case of GC, AIEC overgrow and become more virulent, cross the intestinal barrier, and infect IECs and macrophages in the lamina propria. The (unknown) genetic defect in Boxers and French Bulldogs results in a defective oxidative burst reaction within the macrophages, impairing intracellular bacterial killing. The resulting granulomatous inflammation is characterized by PAS-positive macrophages.

with enrofloxacin (5 mg/kg po twice daily), amoxicillin (20 mg/kg po twice daily), and metronidazole (10–15 mg/kg po twice daily) [48]. Very early reports of the disease almost 30 years ago have also occasionally described a good response to treatment to antibiotics, namely chloramphenicol and tetracycline [46]. The response to treatment with enrofloxacin is dramatic, with all dogs responding within 3 to 12 days of initiating therapy. It is particularly encouraging that several dogs were reportedly disease-free after the drug had been discontinued following a 4- to 6-week course of enrofloxacin treatment [48]. This implies that GC may be cured in some cases. Five dogs were rebiopsied when they were in clinical remission after completion of the antibiotic treatment. A dramatic improvement in the histologic lesions was evident in all cases, with disappearance of PAS-positive macrophages in 3 dogs and marked reduction in the number of macrophages in the other 2 cases [48]. However, there is emerging evidence that long-term remission in dogs with GC is difficult to achieve, because most dogs eventually develop severe multidrug resistance to all available antibiotics [49]. Therefore, it is important to send intestinal biopsies for culture and sensitivity at the time of diagnosis, that is, before starting treatment, so that the use of antibiotics can be tailored to the specific sensitivity profile of the cultured *E coli*. It is recommended to treat dogs with GC for at least 8 weeks with antibiotics and to rebiopsy before discontinuing the treatment, in order to ascertain that histologic remission has occurred.

SUMMARY

CIE is a polygenetic disease, which develops in dogs through environmental influences over time, therefore typically presenting for the first time in middle-aged dogs. Dysbiosis of the microbiome, with particular overgrowth of gram-negative *Enterobacteriaceae*, perpetuates an overstimulation of the innate immune system (likely via TLRs and other receptors), culminating in increased secretion of IL-1β and other cytokines as well as dysregulation of the adaptive immune response.

In GC, a more precise genetic defect in oxidative burst proteins, rather than many mutations in innate immunity receptors, can be found. This defect, in conjunction with an overgrowth of a specific pathogen (AIEC), leads to severe granulomatous inflammation of the colon, predominantly in young Boxers and French Bulldogs. Although most cases of GC respond quickly to antibiotic treatment, recent evidence suggests that many of these dogs eventually succumb to the disease following development of severe antibiotic resistance.

DISCLOSURE

The authors have nothing to disclose.

REFERENCES

[1] Allenspach K. Clinical immunology and immunopathology of the canine and feline intestine. Vet Clin North Am Small Anim Pract 2011;41:345–60.

[2] Allenspach K, Wieland B, Grone A, et al. Chronic enteropathies in dogs: evaluation of risk factors for negative outcome. J Vet Intern Med 2007;21:700–8.

[3] Kaser A, Pasaniuc B. IBD genetics: focus on (dys) regulation in immune cells and the epithelium. Gastroenterology 2014;146:896–9.

[4] Kathrani A, Werling D, Allenspach K. Canine breeds at high risk of developing inflammatory bowel disease in the south-eastern UK. Vet Rec 2011;169:635.

[5] Kathrani A, House A, Catchpole B, et al. Polymorphisms in the TLR4 and TLR5 gene are significantly associated with inflammatory bowel disease in German shepherd dogs. PLoS One 2010;5:e15740.

[6] Kathrani A, House A, Catchpole B, et al. Breed-independent toll-like receptor 5 polymorphisms show association with canine inflammatory bowel disease. Tissue Antigens 2011;78(2):94–101.

[7] Kathrani A, Holder A, Catchpole B, et al. TLR5 Risk-Associated Haplotype for Canine Inflammatory Bowel Disease Confers Hyper-Responsiveness to Flagellin. PLoS One 2012;7:e30117.

[8] Peiravan A, Bertolini F, Rothschild MF, et al. Genome-wide association studies of inflammatory bowel disease in German shepherd dogs. PLoS One 2018;13(7):e0200685.

[9] Allenspach K, House A, Smith K, et al. Evaluation of mucosal bacteria and histopathology, clinical disease activity and expression of Toll-like receptors in German shepherd dogs with chronic enteropathies. Vet Microbiol 2010;146:326–35.

[10] Allenspach K, Culverwell C, Chan D. Long-term outcome in dogs with chronic enteropathies: 203 cases. Vet Rec 2016;178:368.

[11] Suchodolski JS. Intestinal microbiota of dogs and cats: a bigger world than we thought. Vet Clin North Am Small Anim Pract 2011;41:261–72.

[12] Suchodolski JS, Markel ME, Garcia-Mazcorro JF, et al. The fecal microbiome in dogs with acute diarrhea and idiopathic inflammatory bowel disease. PLoS One 2012;7:e51907.

[13] Suchodolski JS. Molecular analysis of the bacterial microbiota in duodenal biopsies from dogs with idiopathic inflammatory bowel disease. Vet Microbiol 2010;142(3–4):394–400.

[14] Kalenyak K, Isaiah A, Heilmann RM, et al. Comparison of the intestinal mucosal microbiota in dogs diagnosed with idiopathic inflammatory bowel disease and dogs with food-responsive diarrhea before and after treatment. FEMS Microbiology Ecology, Volume 94, Issue 2,

February 2018, fix173, https://doi.org/10.1093/femsec/fix173.
[15] AlShawaqfeh MK, Wajid B, Minamoto Y, et al. A dysbiosis index to assess microbial changes in fecal samples of dogs with chronic inflammatory enteropathy. FEMS Microbiology Ecology, Volume 93, Issue 11, November 2017, fix136, https://doi.org/10.1093/femsec/fix136.
[16] Vázquez-Baeza Y, Hyde ER, Suchodolski JS, et al. Dog and human inflammatory bowel disease rely on overlapping yet distinct dysbiosis networks. Nat Microbiol 2016; 1:16177.
[17] Minamoto Y, Otoni CC, Steelman SM, et al. Alteration of the fecal microbiota and serum metabolite profiles in dogs with idiopathic inflammatory bowel disease. Gut Microbes 2015;6:33–47.
[18] Guard BC, Honneffer JB, Jergens AE, et al. Longitudinal assessment of microbial dysbiosis, fecal unconjugated bile acid concentrations, and disease activity in dogs with steroid-responsive chronic inflammatory enteropathy. J Vet Intern Med 2019;33(3):1295–305.
[19] Ambrosini YM, Park Y, Jergens AE, et al. Recapitulation of the accessible interface of biopsy-derived canine intestinal organoids to study epithelial-luminal interactions. Published: April 17, 2020. https://doi.org/10.1371/journal.pone.0231423.
[20] McMahon LA, House AK, Catchpole B, et al. Expression of Toll-like receptor 2 in duodenal biopsies from dogs with inflammatory bowel disease is associated with severity of disease. Vet Immunol Immunopathol 2010; 135:158–63.
[21] Schmitz S, Garden OA, Werling D, et al. Gene expression of selected signature cytokines of T cell subsets in duodenal tissues of dogs with and without inflammatory bowel disease. Vet Immunol Immunopathol 2012;146: 87–91.
[22] Tamura Y, Ohta H, Yokoyama N, et al. Evaluation of selected cytokine gene expression in colonic mucosa from dogs with idiopathic lymphocytic-plasmacytic colitis. J Vet Med Sci 2014;76(10):1407–10.
[23] Rychlik A, Nieradka R, Kander M, et al. The effectiveness of natural and synthetic immunomodulators in the treatment of inflammatory bowel disease in dogs. Acta Vet Hung 2013;61(3):297–308.
[24] Okanishi H, Kabeya H, Maruyama S, et al. Activation of nuclear factor-kappa B and cell adhesion molecule mRNA expression in duodenal mucosa of dogs with lymphocytic-plasmacytic enteritis. Vet Immunol Immunopathol 2013;154(3–4):145–52.
[25] Luckschander N, Hall JA, Gaschen F, et al. Activation of nuclear factor-kappaB in dogs with chronic enteropathies. Vet Immunol Immunopathol 2010;133(2–4): 228–36.
[26] Hawes M, Riddle A, Kirk J, et al. Interleukin-1β expression is increased in the duodenum of dogs with idiopathic inflammatory bowel disease. Vet Rec 2018; 183(17):536.
[27] Maeda S, Ohno K, Nakamura K, et al. Mucosal imbalance of interleukin-1beta and interleukin-1 receptor antagonist in canine inflammatory bowel disease. Vet J 2012; 194:66–70.
[28] Schmitz S, Werling D, Allenspach K. Effects of ex-vivo and in-vivo treatment with probiotics on the inflammasome in dogs with chronic enteropathy. PLoS One 2015; 10(3):e0120779.
[29] Falk RJ, Hogan SL, Wilkman AS, et al. Myeloperoxidase specific anti-neutrophil cytoplasmic autoantibodies (MPO-ANCA). Neth J Med 1990;36:121–5.
[30] Luckschander N, Allenspach K, Hall J, et al. Perinuclear Antineutrophilic Cytoplasmic Antibody and Response to Treatment in Diarrheic Dogs with Food Responsive Disease or Inflammatory Bowel Disease. First published: 05 February 2008 https://doi.org/10.1111/j.1939-1676.2006.tb02849.x.
[31] Allenspach K, Lomas B, Wieland B, et al. Evaluation of perinuclear anti-neutrophilic cytoplasmic autoantibodies as an early marker of protein-losing enteropathy and protein-losing nephropathy in Soft Coated Wheaten Terriers. American Journal of Veterinary Research. October 2008, Vol. 69, No. 10, Pages 1301-1304. https://doi.org/10.2460/ajvr.69.10.1301.
[32] Karagianni AE, Solano-Gallego L, Breitschwerdt EB, et al. Perinuclear antineutrophil cytoplasmic autoantibodies in dogs infected with various vector-borne pathogens and in dogs with immune-mediated hemolytic anemia. Am J Vet Res 2012;73:1403–9.
[33] Florey J, Viall A, Streu S, et al. Use of a Granulocyte Immunofluorescence Assay Designed for Humans for Detection of Antineutrophil Cytoplasmic Antibodies in Dogs with Chronic Enteropathies. J Vet Intern Med 2017;31(4):1062–6.
[34] Estruch JJ, Barken D, Bennett N, et al. Evaluation of novel serological markers and autoantibodies in dogs with inflammatory bowel disease. J Vet Intern Med 2020; 34(3):1177–86. Available at: https://onlinelibrary.wiley.com/doi/abs/10.1111/jvim.15761.
[35] Schreiner NM, Gaschen F, Grone A, et al. Clinical signs, histology, and CD3-positive cells before and after treatment of dogs with chronic enteropathies. J Vet Intern Med 2008;22:1079–83.
[36] Day MJ, Bilzer T, Mansell J, et al. Histopathological standards for the diagnosis of gastrointestinal inflammation in endoscopic biopsy samples from the dog and cat: a report from the World Small Animal Veterinary Association Gastrointestinal Standardization Group. J Comp Pathol 2008;138(Suppl 1):S1–43.
[37] Allenspach KA, Mochel JP, Du Y, et al. Correlating Gastrointestinal Histopathologic Changes to Clinical Disease Activity in Dogs With Idiopathic Inflammatory Bowel Disease. Vet Pathol 2019;56(3):435–43.
[38] Walker D. A comprehensive pathological survey of duodenal biopsies from dogs with diet-responsive chronic inflammatory enteropathy. J Vet Intern Med 2013;27(4):862–74.

[39] Morroni M, Sbarbati A, D'Angelo G, et al. Scanning electron microscopy of the small intestine mucosa in children with celiac disease after long-term dietary treatment. Scanning Microsc 1989;3(4):1161–6 [discussion: 1166–7].
[40] Chandra L, Borcherding DC, Kingsbury D, et al. Derivation of adult canine intestinal organoids for translational research in gastroenterology. BMC Biol 2019;17(1):33.
[41] Mao S, Iennarella-Servantez C, Atherly T, et al. Phenotypic and functional characterization of adult intestinal organoids from dogs with inflammatory bowel disease. Report No.: Iowa State Research Day, August 2019, Ames, IA.
[42] Sturgeon C, Fasano A. Zonulin, a regulator of epithelial and endothelial barrier functions, and its involvement in chronic inflammatory diseases. Tissue Barriers 2016;4(4):e1251384.
[43] Tripathi A, Lammers KM, Goldblum S, et al. Identification of human zonulin, a physiological modulator of tight junctions, as prehaptoglobin-2. Proc Natl Acad Sci U S A 2009;106(39):16799–804.
[44] Simpson KW, Dogan B, Rishniw M, et al. Adherent and invasive Escherichia coli is associated with granulomatous colitis in boxer dogs. Infect Immun 2006;74:4778–92.
[45] Darfeuille-Michaud A, Colombel JF. Pathogenic Escherichia coli in inflammatory bowel diseases Proceedings of the 1st International Meeting on E. coli and IBD, June 2007, Lille, France. J Crohns Colitis 2008;2:255–62.
[46] Van Kruiningen HJ. Granulomatous colitis of boxer dogs: comparative aspects. Gastroenterology 1967;53:114–22.
[47] Craven M, Mansfield CS, Simpson KW. Granulomatous colitis of boxer dogs. Vet Clin North Am Small Anim Pract 2011;41:433–45.
[48] Davies DR, O'Hara AJ, Irwin PJ, et al. Successful management of histiocytic ulcerative colitis with enrofloxacin in two Boxer dogs. Aust Vet J 2004;82:58–61.
[49] Craven M, Dogan B, Schukken A, et al. Antimicrobial resistance impacts clinical outcome of granulomatous colitis in boxer dogs. J Vet Intern Med 2010;24:819–24.

Advances in Small Animal Care 1 (2020) 101–110

ADVANCES IN SMALL ANIMAL CARE

The Intestinal Microbiome in Canine Chronic Enteropathy and Implications for Extraintestinal Disorders

Jan S. Suchodolski, MedVet, DrMedVet, PhD, DACVM

Gastrointestinal Laboratory, Department of Small Animal Clinical Sciences, Texas A&M University, 4474 TAMU, College Station, TX 77843-4474, USA

KEYWORDS

• Microbiome • Bile acids • Short-chain fatty acids • Dysbiosis • Metabolism

KEY POINTS

- Gut microbiome (GM) plays important role in health and disease in intestinal and extraintestinal diseases.
- The GM is a metabolic organ, with bacteria producing various metabolites that influence various organ systems.
- Dysbiosis includes changes in bacterial taxa but also functional changes in the microbiota (eg, altered production of metabolites).
- Manipulation of GM likely is an important adjunct treatment of various intestinal and extraintestinal disorders.

INTRODUCTION—IMPORTANCE AND FUNCTION OF THE INTESTINAL MICROBIOME

- The gut harbors a complex ecosystem consisting of various microorganisms (viruses, bacteria, fungi, and protozoa). This collective of microbes is called intestinal microbiota when referring to the taxonomy (ie, "Who is there?") and as microbiome when referring to their gene content and function (ie, "What are they doing?")
- Bacteria are by far the largest component of the intestinal microbiome [1,2]. A balanced bacterial gut microbiome (GM) has an important influence on host health, because it modulates the immune system, helps in the defense against enteropathogens, and provides many metabolic and nutritional benefits. Interactions between the GM and the immune system are mediated either through direct contact (eg, dendritic cells and Toll-like receptors) or through microbiota-derived metabolites.
- The GM consists mostly of strict or facultative anaerobic bacteria, such as *Ruminococcus, Faecalibacterium, Lachnospiraceae,* and *Clostridiales* [3]. These bacteria produce metabolites that have direct beneficial effects on the host, and the GM now is considered an important metabolic organ. For example, dietary carbohydrates (eg, starch, cellulose, and pectin) are fermented and metabolized by bacteria into short-chain fatty acids (SCFAs). These act as energy sources for the host, regulate intestinal motility, and are important growth factors for epithelial cells. SCFAs also have direct anti-inflammatory properties through expansion of immunoregulatory T cells [4]. Other bacterially derived metabolites, such as indole [5], a byproduct of tryptophan degradation, or secondary bile acids (BAs) [6], also have immunomodulatory properties and/or strengthen the intestinal barrier.
- Drugs and other xenobiotics are metabolized by intestinal microbes, and the produced intermediates

E-mail address: JSuchodolski@cvm.tamu.edu

https://doi.org/10.1016/j.yasa.2020.07.008
2666-4518/20/

then are absorbed by the host. Antimicrobials [7–9] and major changes in macronutrient content [10–13] have been shown to affect the intestinal microbiome to some extent, and these changes in the microbiota may influence metabolic host pathways directly or indirectly (Table 1).

- These effects of the normal or abnormal gut microbiota reach beyond the gastrointestinal (GI) tract. Recent research has shown that alterations in the GM are associated with intestinal disease [14,15] and also with various extraintestinal disorders, such as diabetes mellitus [16–18], obesity [19], and chronic kidney disease (CKD) [20], and also neurologic disorders [21]. At this point, however, the underlying mechanisms and whether these associations are cause or effect of the disease and how they are applicable to clinical practice are unclear. Nevertheless, much progress has been made in understanding the intricate relationship between the host and the GM and the important contributions of a balanced GM to health.

ASSESSMENT OF THE INTESTINAL MICROBIOME

- Due to the complexity of the intestinal microbiota, differences in intestinal physiology along the upper and lower GI tract, and differences in luminal versus mucosa-adherent bacterial populations, currently it is not possible to provide a comprehensive clinical assessment of the entire GM. Furthermore, the same bacterial taxa may express, depending on the surrounding intestinal environment, different genes and, therefore, different virulence factors and metabolic functions. For example, the stress hormone norepinephrine [22] and SCFAs [23] alter virulence expression of *Salmonella enterica*. The germination of *Clostridium difficile* spores is regulated by the proper ratio of primary BAs to secondary BAs in the colon [24]. Therefore, more mechanistic studies are needed to understand how specific bacterial taxa are modulated by the microenvironment within the gut, and under which situations they contribute to health and disease.
- Because a majority of intestinal bacteria are anaerobes, using traditional bacterial culture as performed in diagnostic laboratories, only between 5% and 20% of bacteria can be grown. Hence, the actual number of bacterial taxa is vastly underestimated by bacterial culture, and, consequently, species that are cultured often are erroneously considered as clinically more significant. Therefore, bacterial culture has limited value when describing the intestinal microbiota. Bacterial culture remains very important, however, to test for antibiotic susceptibility of those few cultivable organisms that are known to be associated with intestinal infections (ie, *Campylobacter jejuni* and *Salmonella* spp).
- Culture-independent methods, such as broad sequencing of the bacterial 16S rRNA gene, allow for a more comprehensive characterization of the intestinal microbial ecosystem, but these methods are not widely available or have not been proper validated for diagnostic use in dogs and cats.
- A rapid quantitative polymerase chain reaction assay, that measures the abundances of key bacterial taxa within canine fecal samples and expresses the data as a dysbiosis index, has been validated for use in dogs [25]. This assay allows for assessment of normal microbiota versus abnormal microbiota [9,26]. It can be used to track how the fecal microbiota changes during the clinical treatment of

TABLE 1
Examples of Metabolic and Physiologic Mechanisms Carried Out By the Intestinal Microbiome

Action or Metabolic Function	Consequence
Surface colonization	Competition with potential pathogens for binding sites
Fermentation of carbohydrates	Formation of butyrate, an energetic substrate for enterocytes
Antigenic challenge	Promotion of Peyer patch formation, stimulates production of IgA
Production of antibacterial compounds	Suppression of potential pathogens
BA metabolism	Inhibit the growth of transients and potential pathogens
Synthesis of folic acid/folates	Source of folates for host animal and other commensal bacteria

chronic enteropathies [27,28], after therapeutic interventions with probiotics [29], fecal microbiota transplantation [9], and after antibiotic usage in dogs with acute diarrhea [9,30] or healthy dogs [7]. The dysbiosis index also allows, based on measuring the abundance of the BA 7α-dehydroxylating bacterium *C hiranonis*, predicting the ability of the intestinal microbiota to convert primary BAs to secondary BAs [26,27]. This now is considered an important pathway, because the proper physiologic level of secondary BAs in the intestine is associated with intestinal health [9,31] and control of potential enteropathogens, such as *C difficile*, *Escherichia coli*, and *C perfringens* in humans and dogs [24,32,33].

- There are limitations when assessing the fecal microbiota only. It does not allow proper assessment of the mucosa-adherent/invasive bacteria or the composition and, more importantly, the quantity of the small intestinal microbiota. An abnormal small intestinal GM can contribute to clinical signs, either through production of toxins or through abnormal metabolization of increased luminal food substrates that are not properly absorbed by the host. The latter can be the case either through feeding of diets that are not highly digestible or in diseases like exocrine pancreatic insufficiency (EPI) (lack of digestive enzymes) [34] or small intestinal inflammation (due to destruction of transporters and/or digestive enzyme producing epithelial cells in the brush border) [26,35]. In such cases, an empirical trial with antimicrobials may lead to decrease of luminal bacteria and improvement of diarrhea [34,36]. The long-term success of this antibiotic treatment approach may depend, however, on the resolution of the underlying disease process, and recent studies have shown that most of these dogs relapse when antimicrobials are withdrawn [37,38]. Another reason for responsiveness to antimicrobials are mucosa-adherent or invasive bacterial populations. The prime example is granulomatous colitis associated with invasive *E coli*, most commonly observed in boxer dogs and French bulldogs [39,40]. For diagnosis, colonic biopsies need to be obtained, which can be stained using fluorescence in situ hybridization and the localization of bacteria within the intestinal tissue can be confirmed, but this technique currently is offered only through few specialized laboratories.
- An emerging area for assessment of abnormal microbiota is to measure concentrations of microbial-derived metabolites as markers of dysbiosis rather than changes in bacterial taxonomy. Because these metabolites have biological function, their changes may correlate with the pathophysiology of disease. For example, an increase in serum trimethylamine N-oxide (TMAO), a bacterial product of microbial metabolism of dietary compounds (ie, choline and L-carnitine), is associated with atherosclerosis and cardiovascular disease in humans [20] and with chronic heart failure in dogs [41]. Bacterial metabolites, such as p-cresol (microbial breakdown of tyrosine and phenylalanine) and indoxyl sulfate (microbial breakdown of tryptophan), can act as uremic toxins and their increase in serum correlates with progression of CKD [42].
- Alterations in the intestinal microbiota are defined as dysbiosis. This can include changes in the total amount of bacteria and changes in composition and/or number of bacterial species. The term, dysbiosis, is an evolving concept, as more understanding is gained about the interactions between microbiota and the host. Although currently not well described in literature, dysbiosis also should be understood as a potential change in microbiota function, with alterations in microbial-derived metabolites. These metabolite changes can be associated with or without measurable shifts in microbiota composition. For example, reductions in bacterial taxa known to produce SCFAs have been correlated with a reduction in total amounts of SCFAs in dogs with chronic enteropathies [43]. In contrast, although there was an increase in serum concentrations of the bacterial metabolites p-cresol and indoxyl sulfate in cats with CKD, this was not linked with measurable shifts in the fecal microbiota composition [42].

ALTERATIONS IN THE INTESTINAL MICROBIOME IN INTESTINAL DISEASE

- The commensal GM is of importance for the development and homeostasis of gut structure and function. For example, germ-free raised mice exhibit an altered epithelial architecture (eg, decreased number of lymphoid follicles) and an underdeveloped immune system [44,45]. The microbiota in early life is important for establishing oral tolerance in order to prevent onset of an inappropriate immune responses against luminal bacteria and food antigens, which have been associated with chronic GI inflammation [46].

- The communication between GM and the host immune system is mediated through a combination of microbiota-derived metabolites and microbial surface molecules that activate receptors of the innate immune system (eg, Toll-like receptors) [47]. Some of these metabolic pathways are discussed in more detail later. Of importance is that this often is a 2-way communication, and microbiota may influence the host but also changes in the host immune system (eg, increased inflammatory responses) affect the mucosal environment, leading to changes in microbiota. Therefore, dysbiosis is present in most dogs with intestinal inflammation [26,43,48], but the contributions of dysbiosis to clinical signs vary depending on the type and the magnitude of metabolic changes, which are difficult to assess clinically. To increase treatment success, therapy should aim at the underlying GI pathology as well as restoration of the microbiota.
- Dysbiosis can be present both in the small intestine or large intestine, but, when present, it is likely to be in both. Based on pathophysiology, presence of dysbiosis in the small intestine may be clinically more relevant, because the upper intestine typically is populated only by small number of bacteria and, therefore, has fewer defense mechanisms.
- Small intestinal dysbiosis, also often termed antibiotic-responsive diarrhea, due to empirical improvement of clinical signs in response to broad spectrum antibiotics, is suspected to be caused by an unspecific alteration in composition or an increase in numbers [49]. Although historically it was considered due to increases in total bacterial populations alone (small intestinal bacterial overgrowth) without detectable underlying GI pathology [50], recent data in humans suggest that this syndrome often is associated with intestinal inflammation, and this is likely the case also in dogs and cats [51]. Other reasons for small intestinal dysbiosis are alterations in intestinal motility, anatomic changes (ie, blind intestinal loops, short bowel syndrome, and resection of the ileocolic valve), and malabsorption/maldigestion due to EPI but also due to feeding of less digestible diets. The dysbiosis has a negative impact on the function of the GI tract through changes in various metabolic pathways, as best illustrated in dogs with EPI that show increase in duodenal bacterial populations [52] and increased fecal lactate and altered fecal BA profiles, both of which may stimulate mucosal irritation and diarrhea [48,53]. Dysbiosis may lead to increased intestinal permeability, competition for vitamins such as cobalamin, and additional damages to the intestinal brush border and enterocytes. Treatment of small intestinal dysbiosis depends on the underlying disease. In EPI, pancreatic enzyme replacement leads to gradual improvement of dysbiosis in most dogs [48,54], but some dogs may require additional antibiotic administration. Because bacteria drive on undigested food within the small intestinal lumen, dietary modification to a highly digestible diet always should be considered when small intestinal dysbiosis or disease is suspected.
- Reasons for dysbiosis in the large intestine include changes in the small intestine, as shown in dogs with EPI, which also have altered fecal microbiota populations [48,53] and colonic inflammation. Large intestinal dysbiosis often is characterized in decreases in the major anaerobic bacterial groups, such as *Blautia*, *Faecalibacterium*, *Ruminococcaceae*, *Turicibacter*, and *Clostridia*. These bacterial groups are producers of many immunomodulatory metabolites, such as SCFAs, indoles, and secondary BAs. Consequently, changes in fecal SCFAs have been reported in dogs with chronic enteropathies [43,55].
- Dysbiosis also can be induced trough medications, such as use of broad-spectrum antibiotics (eg, metronidazole and tylosin) and proton-pump inhibitors [7,9,56]. But this dysbiosis does not always correlate with development of clinical signs, especially in healthy dogs. For example, metronidazole administered to healthy dogs [8] but also dogs with acute diarrhea [9] induced major dysbiosis, with reductions in the normal commensal microbiota and substantial increases in *E coli*. Furthermore, the microbiota dysbiosis was associated with extensive changes in fecal bacterial metabolites (eg, increase in oxidative stress and reductions in secondary BAs) [9,57]. Nine out of 16 healthy dogs receiving metronidazole developed loose stools while on antibiotics, but the remaining dogs did not exhibit any clinical signs, despite having similar microbial and biochemical changes [58]. This suggests that an interplay of multiple microbial and host factors needs to occur for clinical signs to develop (eg, underlying genetic susceptibility of the host and dietary and environmental triggers). Nevertheless, antibiotic-induced dysbiosis is an example of how changes in microbial composition and metabolism can affect host health in some patients. Recent epidemiologic studies in humans have linked antibiotic-induced dysbiosis in early

childhood or repeated pulse therapy to the development onset of Crohn disease and obesity [59,60]. These emerging epidemiologic data in humans and evolving understanding of the immunomodulatory and metabolic properties of the gut microbiota suggest that proper diagnosis and correction of dysbiosis will be important therapeutic goals in various diseases.

INTESTINAL MICROBIOME AS METABOLIC ORGAN AND THE IMPACT ON EXTRAINTESTINAL SYSTEMS

- Recent studies have described links between dysbiosis and changes in various biochemical pathways (eg, dysmetabolism in BAs, SCFAs, and tryptophan pathways) that affect the host immune system and metabolism. Because these changes in microbial-derived metabolites can affect the overall health of the host, some examples of important microbial-derived metabolic pathways are discussed.

Short-Chain Fatty Acids

- Major nutrient sources of bacteria are dietary fibers, such as cellulose, pectin, and inulin. Fermentation of these fibers by bacteria results in production of SCFAs and other metabolites. SCFAs, primarily acetate, propionate, and butyrate, are produced through multiple pathways and various bacteria, again highlighting the need for a diverse bacterial population in the gut capable of performing multiple functions through mutual relationships. For example, the primary fermenters Bacteroidetes are able to transform simple sugars derived from the breakdown of complex carbohydrates to acetate. Then, butyrate-producing bacteria (eg, *Clostridium* spp) further utilize acetate to generate butyrate. Propionate can be produced by Bacteroidetes and some Firmicutes (eg, Lachnospiraceae) from lactate or succinate through the acetylate or succinate pathway, respectively.
- Approximately 95% of intestinal SCFAs are absorbed rapidly from the gut lumen either by directly crossing the epithelial barrier or by uptake through specialized transporters. SCFA absorption stimulates water absorption, which provides an antidiarrheic effect [61]. Butyrate is preferentially utilized as an energy source by intestinal epithelial cells, and only small amounts (<10%) of butyrate reach the portal circulation. In contrast, up to 70% of acetate and propionate enter portal circulation, are metabolized by the liver, and are utilized for lipid metabolism (acetate) and gluconeogenesis (propionate). Acetate reaches the systemic circulation and provides energy for muscle, heart, adipose tissue, and kidney. Receptors for SCFAs (G-protein–coupled receptors) are located on many cell types, including epithelial cells, various immune cells, adipocytes, endocrine and smooth muscle cells; thereby, activations of these cells by SCFAs has various health functions [62,63]. Butyrate can reduce oxidative damage to DNA, whereas acetate modulates intestinal permeability [4,64]. SCFAs decrease proinflammatory cytokines, such as interleukin (IL)-6, IL-8, and tumor necrosis factor α, and modulate colonic regulatory T cells [65].

Bile Acid Metabolism

- BA metabolism involves multiple steps. The primary BAs, cholic acid and chenodeoxycholic acid, are synthesized in the liver from cholesterol via 7α-hydroxylase (CYP7A1) and conjugated with taurine and to a lesser extent glycine. Meal intake leads to release of BA into the intestinal lumen. In proper gut homeostasis, active reabsorption of BA takes place in the ileum through the apical sodium–BA transporter (ASBT), leading to enterohepatic circulation [26]. A small proportion of BAs enters the large intestine, where bacterial species (eg, *C hiranonis* in dogs) with 7α-dehydroxylation activity are able to convert the primary BA to the secondary BAs, deoxycholic acid and lithocholic acid.
- Altered BA metabolism leads to BA malabsorption and therefore is a frequent cause of diarrhea in humans [31]. BA diarrhea can be due to various causes, such as malabsorption, that are secondary to ileal resection or inflammation (type I), idiopathic (type 2), or intestinal dysbiosis due to lack of bacteria with 7α-dehydroxylation activity (type 3). It has been suggested that approximately 30% to 40% of human patients with irritable bowel syndrome or Crohn disease suffer from BA diarrhea [31]. In humans with irritable bowel syndrome, the destruction of ASBT in the ileum leads to decreased reabsorption of BAs in the small intestine, leading to increases in primary BAs in the colon that cause secretory diarrhea [66]. The use of glucocorticoids induces the expression of ASBT in the small intestine [67], potentially reducing BAs malabsorption and improving diarrhea.
- Altered BA metabolism also is present in dogs with chronic enteropathies, with primary BAs increased and secondary BAs decreased, suggesting impaired

bacterial conversion from primary BAs to secondary BAs and/or lack of absorption in the ileum [26,27]. A significant negative correlation exist between secondary BAs and *C hiranonis*, a bacterial species with 7α-dehydroxylation activity [26,48]. This suggests that lack of *C hiranonis* in the canine intestine leads to the inability of the animal to convert primary BAs to secondary BAs. Broad-spectrum antibiotics reduce *C hiranonis*, thereby preventing the conversion of primary BAs to secondary BAs [7].

- The lack of secondary BA has significant implications on the entire organism. BAs now are recognized as important regulator of host health, because they are agonists for various receptors across the body. Binding activates various transcriptional factors, which lead to the expression of genes involved in cholesterol and carbohydrate metabolism [68]. Activation of the TGR5 receptor through secondary BAs, which is present on many cell types and various organs, results in down-regulation of inflammation and secretion of glucagon-like peptide 1, which helps in the regulation of insulin [69]. BAs also can activate nuclear receptors, such as pregnane X receptor and the vitamin D receptor. It is suggested that various forms of liver disorders and metabolic diseases may benefit from targeting these BA receptors, highlighting the important link between gut dysbiosis, dysregulation of BA metabolism, and various metabolic disorders [70–72].

Tryptophan-Indole Metabolism

- An emerging pathway, important for intestinal disease is the serotonin-tryptophan pathway. Tryptophan and its degradation products (eg, serotonin, tryptamine, indoles, and kynurenines) are important in the regulation of T-cell response within the intestine as well as intestinal motility. Indole compounds are synthesized exclusively by bacteria and serve as signaling molecules, activating pathways locally and systemically. Indole, a metabolite produced by many gut bacteria, is anti-inflammatory and decreases IL-8 expression, induces expression of mucin genes, and also increases gene expression that strengthens tight junction resistance [5]. Alterations in tryptophan metabolism are associated with irritable bowel syndrome in humans and dogs [73], and dietary supplementation with tryptophan have been shown to have anti-inflammatory effects in experimental colitis models [74].

EXAMPLES OF EXTRAINTESTINAL DISORDERS THAT ARE LINKED TO GUT DYSBIOSIS

Chronic Kidney Disease

- Various studies have reported an altered intestinal microbiota in human patients as well as animal models with CKD. Because an altered microbiota contributes to inflammation and abnormal clearance of uremic toxins derived from the intestine, microbiota dysbiosis may add to systemic complications of CKD [42,75].
- The term kidney-gut axis refers to these bidirectional interactions between gut microbiota and the kidney in human patients with CKD [76]. The metabolic changes caused by CKD (eg, uremia) affect the GI tract through intestinal hypoperfusion, changes in pH, and changes in intestinal motility [77]. These, in turn, affect the intestinal barrier system, leading to increased intestinal permeability and potential translocation of bacterial endotoxin, leading to systemic low-grade inflammation [78]. Furthermore, dietary changes (low fiber intake) and/or drugs or treatment regimens (eg, antibiotics and phosphate binders), as commonly used in humans or animals during treatment periods of CKD, can cause changes in the intestinal microbiota (ie, dysbiosis) [10,79]. The increased systemic levels of uremic toxins also may cause intestinal dysbiosis [80,81]. The dysbiosis together with increased intestinal permeability potentiates endotoxemia and low-grade systemic inflammation, which in turn may affect the progression of CKD [76].
- Examples of microbiota-derived metabolic changes in humans is for example, TMAO, a gut microbial-dependent metabolite of dietary choline. TMAO is increased in CKD and is associated with poorer prognosis [20]. In animal models, an increase in dietary choline led to increased TMAO, which in turn led to progressive renal tubulointerstitial fibrosis [20].
- Data in cats with CKD showed changes in bacteria metabolites, with increases in serum concentrations of p-cresol and indoxyl sulfate [42] and increases in some branched-chain fatty acids [75].
- These important changes in the kidney-gut axis are raising the therapeutic interest in modulating the intestinal microbiota using either dietary fibers (eg, prebiotics) or probiotics, but initial clinical trials are needed.

Gut-Brain Axis

- Gut microbiota composition is associated with changes in cognition, behavior, stress, and other disorders of the nervous system [82,83]. Pathways thought to be involved include direct cell-to-cell interaction between the enteric nervous and/or immune system and secretion of endocrine metabolites by the GM that in turn stimulate the nervous system.

- Some bacteria produce neurotransmitters, such as γ-aminobutyric acid or acetylcholine, at least under in vitro conditions [84]. Under periods of stress, the host also can produce neuroendocrine substances, which may modulate the virulence of some enteropathogens in vivo [22]. Intestinal colonization with enteropathogens (eg, *C jejuni*) alters behavior, with the infected animals showing increased anxiety [85].
- Global changes in the GM are associated with multiple sclerosis in humans [86]. Dogs with meningoencephalomyelitis of unknown origin, an immune-mediated condition of similar pathophysiology as multiple sclerosis, also had decreases in specific bacterial taxa that are associated with reduced risk for developing immune-mediated brain disease [87].
- Human patients with autism spectrum disorders exhibit neurologic and often GI disorders, associated with alterations in gut microbiota [88,89]. Therapeutic GM manipulation in children with autism spectrum disorders lead to improved GI and behavioral symptoms [90].
- Nutrition affects cognition and behavior by modulating gut microbiota. Mice fed resistant starches developed anxiety-like behavior [91]. Mood disorders have been associated with dietary sensitivities, suspected through increased gut permeability after infection with *Toxoplasma gondii* [92].

DISCLOSURE

The author is employee of the Gastrointestinal Laboratory at Texas A&M University, which offer diagnostic microbiome testing on a fee-for-service basis.

REFERENCES

[1] Swanson KS, Dowd SE, Suchodolski JS, et al. Phylogenetic and gene-centric metagenomics of the canine intestinal microbiome reveals similarities with humans and mice. ISME J 2011;5(4):639–49.

[2] Barry KA, Middelbos IS, Vester Boler BM, et al. Effects of dietary fiber on the feline gastrointestinal metagenome. J Proteome Res 2012;11(12):5924–33.

[3] Honneffer JB, Steiner JM, Lidbury JA, et al. Variation of the microbiota and metabolome along the canine gastrointestinal tract. Metabolomics 2017;13(26). https://doi.org/10.1007/s11306-11017-11165-11303.

[4] Arpaia N, Campbell C, Fan X, et al. Metabolites produced by commensal bacteria promote peripheral regulatory T-cell generation. Nature 2013;504(7480):451–5.

[5] Bansal T, Alaniz RC, Wood TK, et al. The bacterial signal indole increases epithelial-cell tight-junction resistance and attenuates indicators of inflammation. Proc Natl Acad Sci U S A 2010;107(1):228–33.

[6] Hang S, Paik D, Yao L, et al. Bile acid metabolites control TH17 and Treg cell differentiation. Nature 2019; 576(7785):143–8.

[7] Manchester AC, Webb CB, Blake AB, et al. Long-term impact of tylosin on fecal microbiota and fecal bile acids of healthy dogs. J Vet Intern Med 2019;33(6): 2605–17.

[8] Igarashi H, Maeda S, Ohno K, et al. Effect of oral administration of metronidazole or prednisolone on fecal microbiota in dogs. PLoS One 2014;9(9):e107909.

[9] Chaitman J, Ziese AL, Pilla R, et al. Fecal microbial and metabolic profiles in dogs with acute diarrhea receiving either fecal microbiota transplantation or oral metronidazole. Front Vet Sci 2020;7:192.

[10] Schmidt M, Unterer S, Suchodolski JS, et al. The fecal microbiome and metabolome differs between dogs fed Bones and Raw Food (BARF) diets and dogs fed commercial diets. PLoS One 2018;13(8):e0201279.

[11] Beloshapka AN, Dowd SE, Suchodolski JS, et al. Fecal microbial communities of healthy adult dogs fed raw meat-based diets with or without inulin or yeast cell wall extracts as assessed by 454 pyrosequencing. FEMS Microbiol Ecol 2013;84(3):532–41.

[12] Li Q, Lauber CL, Czarnecki-Maulden G, et al. Effects of the dietary protein and carbohydrate ratio on gut microbiomes in dogs of different body conditions. mBio 2017; 8(1):e01703-16.

[13] Bermingham EN, Young W, Kittelmann S, et al. Dietary format alters fecal bacterial populations in the domestic cat (Felis catus). Microbiologyopen 2013;2(1):173–81.

[14] Honneffer JB, Minamoto Y, Suchodolski JS. Microbiota alterations in acute and chronic gastrointestinal inflammation of cats and dogs. World J Gastroenterol 2014; 20(44):16489–97.

[15] Pilla R, Suchodolski JS. The role of the canine gut microbiome and metabolome in health and gastrointestinal disease. Front Vet Sci 2019;6:498.

[16] Jergens AE, Guard BC, Redfern A, et al. Microbiota-related changes in unconjugated fecal bile acids are associated with naturally occurring, insulin-dependent diabetes mellitus in dogs. Front Vet Sci 2019;6:199.

[17] Vrieze A, Out C, Fuentes S, et al. Impact of oral vancomycin on gut microbiota, bile acid metabolism, and insulin sensitivity. J Hepatol 2014;60(4):824–31.

[18] Kootte RS, Levin E, Salojarvi J, et al. Improvement of insulin sensitivity after lean donor feces in metabolic syndrome is driven by baseline intestinal microbiota composition. Cell Metab 2017;26(4):611–9.e6.

[19] Turnbaugh PJ, Ley RE, Mahowald MA, et al. An obesity-associated gut microbiome with increased capacity for energy harvest. Nature 2006;444(7122):1027–31.
[20] Tang WH, Wang Z, Kennedy DJ, et al. Gut microbiota-dependent trimethylamine N-oxide (TMAO) pathway contributes to both development of renal insufficiency and mortality risk in chronic kidney disease. Circ Res 2015;116(3):448–55.
[21] Larroya-Garcia A, Navas-Carrillo D, Orenes-Pinero E. Impact of gut microbiota on neurological diseases: Diet composition and novel treatments. Crit Rev Food Sci Nutr 2019;59(19):3102–16.
[22] Pullinger GD, Carnell SC, Sharaff FF, et al. Norepinephrine augments Salmonella enterica-induced enteritis in a manner associated with increased net replication but independent of the putative adrenergic sensor kinases QseC and QseE. Infect Immun 2010;78(1):372–80.
[23] Lawhon SD, Maurer R, Suyemoto M, et al. Intestinal short-chain fatty acids alter Salmonella typhimurium invasion gene expression and virulence through BarA/SirA. Mol Microbiol 2002;46(5):1451–64.
[24] Weingarden AR, Chen C, Bobr A, et al. Microbiota transplantation restores normal fecal bile acid composition in recurrent Clostridium difficile infection. Am J Physiol Gastrointest Liver Physiol 2014;306(4):G310–9.
[25] AlShawaqfeh MK, Wajid B, Minamoto Y, et al. A dysbiosis index to assess microbial changes in fecal samples of dogs with chronic inflammatory enteropathy. FEMS Microbiol Ecol 2017;93(11). https://doi.org/10.1093/femsec/fix136.
[26] Giaretta PR, Rech RR, Guard BC, et al. Comparison of intestinal expression of the apical sodium-dependent bile acid transporter between dogs with and without chronic inflammatory enteropathy. J Vet Intern Med 2018;32(6):1918–26.
[27] Guard BC, Honneffer JB, Jergens AE, et al. Longitudinal assessment of microbial dysbiosis, fecal unconjugated bile acid concentrations, and disease activity in dogs with steroid-responsive chronic inflammatory enteropathy. J Vet Intern Med 2019;33(3):1295–305.
[28] Bresciani F, Minamoto Y, Suchodolski JS, et al. Effect of an extruded animal protein-free diet on fecal microbiota of dogs with food-responsive enteropathy. J Vet Intern Med 2018;32(6):1903–10.
[29] Ziese AL, Suchodolski JS, Hartmann K, et al. Effect of probiotic treatment on the clinical course, intestinal microbiome, and toxigenic Clostridium perfringens in dogs with acute hemorrhagic diarrhea. PLoS One 2018;13(9):e0204691.
[30] Werner M, Suchodolski JS, Straubinger RK, et al. Effect of amoxicillin-clavulanic acid on clinical scores, intestinal microbiome, and amoxicillin-resistant Escherichia coli in dogs with uncomplicated acute diarrhea. J Vet Intern Med 2020;34(3):1166–76.
[31] Duboc H, Rajca S, Rainteau D, et al. Connecting dysbiosis, bile-acid dysmetabolism and gut inflammation in inflammatory bowel diseases. Gut 2013;62(4):531–9.
[32] Berry ASF, Kelly BJ, Barnhart D, et al. Gut microbiota features associated with Clostridioides difficile colonization in puppies. PLoS One 2019;14(8):e0215497.
[33] Wang S, Martins R, Sullivan MC, et al. Diet-induced remission in chronic enteropathy is associated with altered microbial community structure and synthesis of secondary bile acids. Microbiome 2019;7(1):126.
[34] Westermarck E, Myllys V, Aho M. Effect of treatment on the jejunal and colonic bacterial flora of dogs with exocrine pancreatic insufficiency. Pancreas 1993;8:559–62.
[35] Honneffer J, Guard B, Steiner JM, et al. Mo1805 untargeted metabolomics reveals disruption within bile acid, cholesterol, and tryptophan metabolic pathways in dogs with idiopathic inflammatory bowel disease. Gastroenterology 2015;148(4):S-715.
[36] Westermarck E, Frias R, Skrzypczak T. Effect of diet and tylosin on chronic diarrhea in beagles. J Vet Intern Med 2005;19(6):822–7.
[37] Kilpinen S, Spillmann T, Syrja P, et al. Effect of tylosin on dogs with suspected tylosin-responsive diarrhea: a placebo-controlled, randomized, double-blinded, prospective clinical trial. Acta Vet Scand 2011;53:26.
[38] Allenspach K, Culverwell C, Chan D. Long-term outcome in dogs with chronic enteropathies: 203 cases. Vet Rec 2016;178(15):368.
[39] Mansfield CS, James FE, Craven M, et al. Remission of histiocytic ulcerative colitis in boxer dogs correlates with eradication of invasive intramucosal Escherichia coli. J Vet Intern Med 2009;23(5):964–9.
[40] Simpson KW, Dogan B, Rishniw M, et al. Adherent and invasive Escherichia coli is associated with granulomatous colitis in boxer dogs. Infect Immun 2006;74(8):4778–92.
[41] Karlin ET, Rush JE, Freeman LM. A pilot study investigating circulating trimethylamine N-oxide and its precursors in dogs with degenerative mitral valve disease with or without congestive heart failure. J Vet Intern Med 2019;33(1):46–53.
[42] Summers SC, Quimby JM, Isaiah A, et al. The fecal microbiome and serum concentrations of indoxyl sulfate and p-cresol sulfate in cats with chronic kidney disease. J Vet Intern Med 2019;33(2):662–9.
[43] Minamoto Y, Minamoto T, Isaiah A, et al. Fecal short-chain fatty acid concentrations and dysbiosis in dogs with chronic enteropathy. J Vet Intern Med 2019;33(4):1608–18.
[44] Abrams GD, Bishop JE. Effect of the normal microbial flora on gastrointestinal motility. Proc Soc Exp Biol Med 1967;126(1):301–4.
[45] Thompson GR, Trexler PC. Gastrointestinal structure and function in germ-free or gnotobiotic animals. Gut 1971;12(3):230–5.
[46] Wambre E, Jeong D. Oral tolerance development and maintenance. Immunol Allergy Clin North Am 2018;38(1):27–37.

[47] Kathrani A, House A, Catchpole B, et al. Polymorphisms in the Tlr4 and Tlr5 gene are significantly associated with inflammatory bowel disease in german shepherd dogs. PLoS One 2010;5(12):1–10.
[48] Blake AB, Guard BC, Honneffer JB, et al. Altered microbiota, fecal lactate, and fecal bile acids in dogs with gastrointestinal disease. PLoS One 2019;14(10):e0224454.
[49] Hall EJ. Antibiotic-responsive diarrhea in small animals. Vet Clin North Am Small Anim Pract 2011;41:273–86.
[50] Rutgers HC, Batt RM, Elwood CM, et al. Small intestinal bacterial overgrowth in dogs with chronic intestinal disease. J Am Vet Med Assoc 1995;206:187–93.
[51] Ricci JERJ, Chebli LA, Ribeiro T, et al. Small-intestinal bacterial overgrowth is associated with concurrent intestinal inflammation but not with systemic inflammation in crohn's disease patients. J Clin Gastroenterol 2018;52(6):530–6.
[52] Westermarck E, Myllys V, Aho M. Intestinal bacterial overgrowth in dogs with exocrine pancreatic insufficiency: Effect of enzyme replacement and antibiotic therapy. J Vet Intern Med 1991;5:131.
[53] Isaiah A, Parambeth JC, Steiner JM, et al. The fecal microbiome of dogs with exocrine pancreatic insufficiency. Anaerobe 2017;45:50–8.
[54] Wiberg ME, Lautala HM, Westermarck E. Response to long-term enzyme replacement treatment in dogs with exocrine pancreatic insufficiency. J Am Vet Med Assoc 1998;213(1):86–90.
[55] Xu J, Verbrugghe A, Lourenco M, et al. Does canine inflammatory bowel disease influence gut microbial profile and host metabolism? BMC Vet Res 2016;12(1):114.
[56] Garcia-Mazcorro JF, Suchodolski JS, Jones KR, et al. Effect of the proton pump inhibitor omeprazole on the gastrointestinal bacterial microbiota of healthy dogs. FEMS Microbiol Ecol 2012;80(3):624–36.
[57] Pilla R, Gaschen FP, Barr JW, et al. Effects of metronidazole on the fecal microbiome and metabolome in healthy dogs. J Vet Intern Med 2020 in press.
[58] Olson EHJ, Waddle M, Steiner JM, et al. Evaluation of the effects of a 2-week treatment with metronidazole on the fecal microbiome of healthy dogs. J Vet Intern Med 2015;29(4):1184–5.
[59] Ungaro R, Bernstein CN, Gearry R, et al. Antibiotics associated with increased risk of new-onset Crohn's disease but not ulcerative colitis: a meta-analysis. Am J Gastroenterol 2014;109(11):1728–38.
[60] Saari A, Virta LJ, Sankilampi U, et al. Antibiotic exposure in infancy and risk of being overweight in the first 24 months of life. Pediatrics 2015;135(4):617–26.
[61] Binder HJ. Fecal fatty acids - mediators of diarrhea. Gastroenerology 1973;65:847–50.
[62] Kim MH, Kang SG, Park JH, et al. Short-chain fatty acids activate GPR41 and GPR43 on intestinal epithelial cells to promote inflammatory responses in mice. Gastroenterology 2013;145(2):396–406.e1-\10.
[63] Yang G, Chen S, Deng B, et al. Implication of G protein-coupled receptor 43 in intestinal inflammation: a mini-review. Front Immunol 2018;9:1434.
[64] Rondeau MP, Meltzer K, Michel KE, et al. Short chain fatty acids stimulate feline colonic smooth muscle contraction. J Feline Med Surg 2003;5(3):167–73.
[65] Smith PM, Howitt MR, Panikov N, et al. The microbial metabolites, short-chain fatty acids, regulate colonic Treg cell homeostasis. Science 2013;341(6145):569–73.
[66] Duboc H, Rainteau D, Rajca S, et al. Increase in fecal primary bile acids and dysbiosis in patients with diarrhea-predominant irritable bowel syndrome. Neurogastroenterol Motil 2012;24(6):513–e247.
[67] Jung D, Fantin AC, Scheurer U, et al. Human ileal bile acid transporter gene ASBT (SLC10A2) is transactivated by the glucocorticoid receptor. Gut 2004;53(1):78–84.
[68] Sayin SI, Wahlstrom A, Felin J, et al. Gut microbiota regulates bile acid metabolism by reducing the levels of tauro beta-muricholic acid, a naturally occurring FXR antagonist. Cell Metab 2013;17(2):225–35.
[69] Giaretta PR, Suchodolski JS, Blick AK, et al. Distribution of bile acid receptor TGR5 in the gastrointestinal tract of dogs. Histol Histopathol 2019;34(1):69–79.
[70] Austad WI, Lack L, Tyor MP. Importance of bile acids and of an intact distal small intestine for fat absorption. Gastroenterology 1967;52(4):638–46.
[71] Cummings JH, Macfarlane GT. Role of intestinal bacteria in nutrient metabolism. JPEN J Parenter Enteral Nutr 1997;21(6):357–65.
[72] Pavlidis P, Powell N, Vincent RP, et al. Systematic review: bile acids and intestinal inflammation-luminal aggressors or regulators of mucosal defence? Aliment Pharmacol Ther 2015;42(7):802–17.
[73] Kathrani A, Lezcano V, Hall EJ, et al. Indoleamine-pyrrole 2,3-dioxygenase-1 (IDO-1) mRNA is overexpressed in the duodenal mucosa and is negatively correlated with serum tryptophan concentrations in dogs with protein-losing enteropathy. PLoS One 2019;14(6):e0218218.
[74] Cervenka I, Agudelo LZ, Ruas JL. Kynurenines: Tryptophan's metabolites in exercise, inflammation, and mental health. Science 2017;357(6349).
[75] Summers S, Quimby JM, Phillips RK, et al. Preliminary evaluation of fecal fatty acid concentrations in cats with chronic kidney disease and correlation with indoxyl sulfate and p-cresol sulfate. J Vet Intern Med 2020;34(1):206–15.
[76] Sabatino A, Regolisti G, Brusasco I, et al. Alterations of intestinal barrier and microbiota in chronic kidney disease. Nephrol Dial Transplant 2015;30(6):924–33.
[77] Vaziri ND, Yuan J, Norris K. Role of urea in intestinal barrier dysfunction and disruption of epithelial tight junction in chronic kidney disease. Am J Nephrol 2013;37(1):1–6.

[78] Vaziri ND, Yuan J, Nazertehrani S, et al. Chronic kidney disease causes disruption of gastric and small intestinal epithelial tight junction. Am J Nephrol 2013;38(2):99–103.
[79] Rahbar Saadat Y, Niknafs B, Hosseiniyan Khatibi SM, et al. Gut microbiota; an overlooked effect of phosphate binders. Eur J Pharmacol 2020;868:172892.
[80] Chaves LD, McSkimming DI, Bryniarski MA, et al. Chronic kidney disease, uremic milieu, and its effects on gut bacterial microbiota dysbiosis. Am J Physiol Renal Physiol 2018;315(3):F487–502.
[81] Vaziri ND, Wong J, Pahl M, et al. Chronic kidney disease alters intestinal microbial flora. Kidney Int 2013;83(2):308–15.
[82] Montiel-Castro AJ, Gonzalez-Cervantes RM, Bravo-Ruiseco G, et al. The microbiota-gut-brain axis: neurobehavioral correlates, health and sociality. Front Integr Neurosci 2013;7:70.
[83] Martin CR, Mayer EA. Gut-brain axis and behavior. Nestle Nutr Inst Workshop Ser 2017;88:45–53.
[84] Barrett E, Ross RP, O'Toole PW, et al. gamma-Aminobutyric acid production by culturable bacteria from the human intestine. J Appl Microbiol 2012;113(2):411–7.
[85] Lyte M, Varcoe JJ, Bailey MT. Anxiogenic effect of subclinical bacterial infection in mice in the absence of overt immune activation. Physiol Behav 1998;65(1):63–8.
[86] Jangi S, Gandhi R, Cox LM, et al. Alterations of the human gut microbiome in multiple sclerosis. Nat Commun 2016;7:12015.
[87] Jeffery ND, Barker AK, Alcott CJ, et al. The association of specific constituents of the fecal microbiota with immune-mediated brain disease in dogs. PLoS One 2017;12(1):e0170589.
[88] Strati F, Cavalieri D, Albanese D, et al. New evidences on the altered gut microbiota in autism spectrum disorders. Microbiome 2017;5(1):24.
[89] Berding K, Donovan SM. Microbiome and nutrition in autism spectrum disorder: current knowledge and research needs. Nutr Rev 2016;74(12):723–36.
[90] Kang DW, Adams JB, Gregory AC, et al. Microbiota Transfer Therapy alters gut ecosystem and improves gastrointestinal and autism symptoms: an open-label study. Microbiome 2017;5(1):10.
[91] Lyte M, Chapel A, Lyte JM, et al. Resistant starch alters the microbiota-gut brain axis: implications for dietary modulation of behavior. PLoS One 2016;11(1):e0146406.
[92] Casella G, Pozzi R, Cigognetti M, et al. Mood disorders and non-celiac gluten sensitivity. Minerva Gastroenterol Dietol 2017;63(1):32–7.

Advances in Small Animal Care 1 (2020) 111–125
ADVANCES IN SMALL ANIMAL CARE

Important and Novel Laboratory Parameters and Biomarkers for Canine Chronic Enteropathy

Romy M. Heilmann, Dr med vet, Dipl ACVIM (SAIM), Dipl ECVIM-CA (SAIM), MANZCVS (Small Animal Medicine), PhD
Small Animal Internal Medicine, Department for Small Animals, Veterinary Teaching Hospital, College of Veterinary Medicine, An den Tierkliniken 23, DE-04103 Leipzig, SN, Germany

KEYWORDS
• Calprotectin • Cobalamin • C-reactive protein • Fecal dysbiosis index • Folate
• Food-responsive enteropathy • Serum • Steroid-responsive enteropathy

KEY POINTS

- Routine clinicopathologic parameters, fecal parasitology, and diagnostic imaging are essential to assess the overall patient condition but are not specific for diagnosing chronic enteropathies.
- Surrogate biomarkers that are more organ specific and/or disease specific offer additional information about the disease and can be useful in the management of canine chronic enteropathy.
- Several functional, biochemical, and microbiomic biomarkers have been studied in dogs with chronic enteropathies and have expanded the diagnostic toolbox of the small animal clinician.
- The search for novel biomarkers continues, and more studies are needed to evaluate further the clinical usefulness of established biomarker assays for the management of canine chronic inflammatory enteropathies.

INTRODUCTION

- Chronic enteropathies in dogs comprise several different disease entities (Fig. 1).
- Chronic inflammatory enteropathies (CIE) in dogs are an important group of disorders and are defined by:
  1. Chronic recurrent or persistent clinical signs of gastrointestinal disease (vomiting, diarrhea, weight loss) [1,2].
  2. Histologic evidence of mucosal inflammation [2,3].
  3. Exclusion of other underlying gastrointestinal or extragastrointestinal conditions, and
  4. Measurable responses—or the lack thereof—to a sequentially implemented treatment plan consisting of elimination dietary trials and, if needed, anti-inflammatory and/or immunosuppressive medication [1,4–6].
- Based on the response to empirical treatment trials, CIEs are retrospectively classified as either food-responsive enteropathy (FRE) or steroid-/immunosuppressant-responsive enteropathy (SRE/IRE). Refractoriness to immunomodulatory treatment is called a nonresponsive enteropathy (NRE). Dogs with CIE and intestinal protein loss are said to have protein-losing enteropathy (PLE) [1,4,5].
  - Histologically and also clinicopathologically, the different groups of canine CIEs are indistinguishable, except for some characteristics that can indicate a PLE [2,3,5].

E-mail address: romy.heilmann@kleintierklinik.uni-leipzig.de

https://doi.org/10.1016/j.yasa.2020.07.009
2666-4518/20/

Chronic enteropathy		
Inflammatory		Neoplastic
Primary inflammatory *= chronic inflammatory enteropathy*	Secondary inflammatory	• Lymphoma • Adenocarcinoma • Mast cell tumor • Gastrointestinal stroma tumor • Leiomyosarcoma etc.
• FRE • (ARE) • SRE/IRE, NRE	• Helminths • Protozoa • Fungi/algae	

FIG. 1 Classification of chronic enteropathies in dogs. A diagnosis of a chronic inflammatory enteropathy requires that causes of secondary inflammation and a neoplastic etiology have been ruled out. ARE, antibiotic-responsive enteropathy.

- ○ The existence of antibiotic-responsive enteropathy, another previously proposed subgroup of CIE, in which affected dogs show a marked and lasting improvement in clinical signs during and after antibiotic administration, is currently being questioned [6].
- Routine clinicopathologic parameters (minimum database [MDB]), fecal parasitology, and diagnostic imaging are essential to assess the overall health of the patient with suspected chronic enteropathy and to rule out other etiologies with a clinical picture that can mimic CIE.
  - ○ Further special diagnostic tests to confirm a diagnosis of CIE are usually more invasive (endoscopy or laparotomy) (Fig. 2).
  - ○ More organ-specific or even disease-specific biomarkers can be useful additional tools for the diagnosis and management of canine CIE (Fig. 3).

LABORATORY PARAMETERS IN DOGS WITH CHRONIC ENTEROPATHY

- Routine laboratory parameters (MDB, fecal parasitology) and diagnostic imaging are necessary to evaluate the dog's overall health status and also to rule out other extragastrointestinal etiologies. However, these diagnostics are usually not specific for a diagnosis of CIE in dogs.

Routine Clinical Pathology Parameters in Dogs with Chronic Enteropathy

- Routine clinicopathologic parameters obtained as part of the MDB (hematology, clinical chemistry, and urinalysis) generally are not specific for diagnosing dogs with CIE.
  - ○ The MDB is, however, critical in the diagnostic evaluation of dogs with suspected CIE.
  - ○ The MDB can help to rule out other diseases that also cause gastrointestinal signs and to assess the overall health status of the patient [4–6].
- Routine hematology
  - ○ A mild nonregenerative, normocytic, and normochromic anemia (anemia of chronic disease) can be detected in dogs with CIE.
  - ○ A nonregenerative, microcytic (normochromic or hypochromic) anemia and/or decreased reticulocyte hemoglobin content as indicators of iron deficiency together with a mild (reactive) thrombocytosis (or robust platelet count) and an increased blood urea nitrogen concentration might signal a chronic gastrointestinal blood loss [5].
  - ○ A mild leukocytosis with neutrophilia is often seen in dogs with CIE and is reflective of a stress leukogram [5,7]. Lymphopenia can be part of the stress leukogram but is also a frequent finding in dogs with PLE [8].
  - ○ Lack of a stress leukogram (or trends for a stress leukogram), particularly a lymphocyte count of 750/μL or greater and an eosinophil count of 570/μL or greater, or a neutrophil-to-lymphocyte ratio of 2.3 or less might indicate hypoadrenocorticism [9].
  - ○ The neutrophil-to-lymphocyte ratio can also aid in the subclassification of dogs with CIE. A neutrophil-to-lymphocyte ratio of 4.6 or greater can distinguish dogs with SRE/IRE from FRE with moderate sensitivity (77%) and specificity (69%) [10].
  - ○ Peripheral eosinophilia can reflect endoparasites, eosinophilic gastritis and/or enteritis, fungal

Laparotomy	Endoscopy
✓ transmural (*full thickness*) biopsies	✓ minimal-invasive procedure
✓ tissue biopsies also from other organs (eg, liver)	✓ visualization of the mucosa for evaluation and collection of biopsies
⊗ lack of visualization of the mucosa	✓ collection of multiple biopsies per segment
⊗ limited number of tissue biopsies per segment	⊗ mucosal (*partial thickness*) biopsies
⊗ invasive procedure	⊗ intubation of the ileum can be challenging
⊗ possible delay of treatment (eg, immuno-suppressive medication, chemotherapy)	⊗ colonic preparation necessary prior to procedure
⊗ risk of suture dehiscence	⊗ very small risk of gastrointestinal perforation

FIG. 2 Advantages and disadvantages of surgical versus endoscopic gastrointestinal tissue biopsies in dogs. ✓ = advantages of the procedure; ⊗ = disadvantages of the procedure.

Biomarkers for canine chronic enteropathy

Currently available biomarkers	Currently a research tool
Functional biomarkers	
• Serum cobalamin (vitamin B_{12}), folate (vitamin B_9) • Fecal alpha$_1$-proteinase inhibitor (α_1PI)	• Serum or urine methylmalonic acid (MMA) • Fecal Immunoglobulin A (IgA)
Biochemical biomarkers	
• Serum C-reactive protein (CRP) • Fecal calprotectin (S100A8/A9)	• Serum, urine, or fecal N-methylhistamine (NMH) • Perinuclear anti-neutrophilic cytoplasmic antibodies • Fecal S100A12 (calgranulin C) • Fecal intestinal alkaline phosphatase (iAP) • Serum soluble receptor of advanced glycation end products • Serum or fecal 3-bromotyrosine • Serum cytokines and chemokines
Microbiomic biomarkers	
• Fecal dysbiosis index (fDI)	• Fecal (or intestinal) microbiome
Metabolomic biomarkers	
–	• Serum metabolome (eg, plasma amino acid profiles)
Cellular biomarkers	
–	• Peripheral blood (circulating) regulatory T cells (T_{reg})
Genetic biomarkers	
–	• Genomic markers (eg, single nucleotide polymorphisms) • Alterations in gene expression (eg, profiles, microRNA)
Proteomic biomarkers	
–	–

FIG. 3 Groups of biomarkers in dogs with chronic enteropathy. The figure summarizes the functional, biochemical, microbiomic, metabolomic, cellular, and genomic biomarkers that have been evaluated in dogs with chronic enteropathies. Proteomic studies have not been studied or reported in dogs with this condition.

enteritis, or paraneoplastic eosinophilia (eg, lymphoma, mast cell tumor).
  - Normal hematology does not rule out the diagnosis of a significant disease process.
- Serum biochemistry
  - Hypoalbuminemia can be detected in dogs with PLE and is also of relevance for the patient prognosis [11,12]. Differentials for hypoalbuminemia include hepatic disease and renal causes of protein loss (protein-losing nephropathy).
  - Hypocalcemia (as well as hypomagnesemia) and hypocholesterolemia can also be detected in dogs with PLE [13].
    - Fasting hypercholesterolemia might indicate a protein-losing nephropathy.
    - Hypercalcemia (confirmed by ionized calcium) can be a paraneoplastic syndrome in dogs with lymphoma, particularly T-cell lymphoma, and is a negative prognostic factor [14]. Differentials include hypoadrenocorticism and granulomatous disease (eg, *Heterobilharzia americana* infection).
  - Serum liver enzyme activities, particularly serum alanine aminotransferase and alkaline phosphatase activity can be mildly increased owing to a reactive hepatopathy. Serum bile acid concentrations and the liver substrates can help to further evaluate the dog for a chronic hepatopathy [5].
  - Increased serum blood urea nitrogen concentrations (which might indicate gastrointestinal bleeding) are also a negative prognostic factor in dogs with PLE [15].
- Serum or plasma electrolytes
  - Na^+, K^+, and Cl^- should be evaluated for characteristic electrolyte changes (hypokalemia, hyponatremia).
- Urinalysis
  - The MDB in dogs with CIE should also include a urinalysis with a urine sediment examination and, if needed, bacterial culture and antimicrobial susceptibility testing.
  - A urine protein-to-creatinine ratio can help to diagnose or rule out a renal loss of protein (protein-losing nephropathy) in hypoalbuminemic dogs.
- Fecal examination
  - Fecal consistency can be assessed by a semiobjective standard fecal scoring system (www.proplanveterinarydiets.ca).
  - A fecal parasite examination (direct smear or fecal wet mount and fecal flotation technique) should be performed to rule out an endoparasite infection [5].
  - *Giardia spp.* can be detected by a combination of centrifugal flotation and fecal *Giardia* spp. antigen by enzyme-linked immunosorbent assay (standard format or patient-side test). Direct immunofluorescence assay for *Giardia* spp. is considered the gold standard test.
    - Analysis of 3 fecal samples collected within 5 days can help to maximize the sensitivity of both tests.
    - Prevalences are similar in healthy and diarrheic dogs, but clinical giardiasis is more likely in immunocompromised patients or with an underlying chronic gastrointestinal disease (eg, chronic enteropathy).
  - Fecal bacteriology is often challenging to interpret, particularly with chronic diarrhea. The most common pathogens cultured from feces in dogs are *Salmonella* spp., *Campylobacter* spp., *Clostridium perfringens,* and *Clostridium difficile* [16]. Still, these bacteria are also isolated in healthy dogs, and shedding might be transient. Fecal bacteriology might be warranted in specific situations (eg, zoonotic concern, raw meat-based diet).
    - Diagnosis of *Salmonella* spp., *C perfringens, Campylobacter* spp., or *C difficile* requires fecal culture, polymerase chain reaction (organism or toxin gene), and/or toxin enzyme-linked immunosorbent assay.
    - *Escherichia coli* is a commensal organism in dogs but can be pathogenic with certain virulence factors and impaired host immunity. Adherent-invasive *E coli* strains can cause granulomatous (histiocytic ulcerative) colitis [17]. Diagnosis is by the typical histopathologic features in colonic biopsies (periodic acid-Schiff-positive macrophages, loss of goblet cells, and mucosal ulceration) and intracellular adherent-invasive *E coli* by fluorescence *in-situ* hybridization (and adherent-invasive *E coli* isolation with antibiotic susceptibility testing) [17]. Isolation of *E coli* from fecal samples does not prove a diagnosis of granulomatous colitis.
  - *H americana* infection (endemic in the coastal areas of the Gulf of Mexico and the southern Atlantic) can be diagnosed by fecal sedimentation, fecal *H americana* polymerase chain

reaction, and/or fine-needle aspirate cytology or histopathology (liver and/or intestines).

- Gastrointestinal panel
  - Serum canine specific pancreatic lipase concentration should be determined to assess dogs with suspected CIE for concurrent pancreatitis.
    - Serum canine specific pancreatic lipase concentrations of 400 μg/L or greater are consistent with a diagnosis of pancreatitis in dogs with compatible clinical signs and/or ultrasound findings.
    - An increased serum canine specific pancreatic lipase concentration is also a negative prognostic factor in canine CIE [18].
  - Serum canine trypsin-like immunoreactivity concentration should be measured (on a 12-hour fasted sample) to rule out a diagnosis of exocrine pancreatic insufficiency (EPI).
    - A serum canine trypsin-like immunoreactivity concentration of less than 2.5 μg/L is consistent with a diagnosis of EPI in dogs [19].
- Adrenal cortical function tests
  - A baseline serum cortisol concentration (>2 μg/dL, >55 nmol/L) or an adrenocorticotrophic hormone stimulation test (stimulated serum cortisol concentration of >6 μg/dL or >165 nmol/L) can exclude a diagnosis of (atypical) hypoadrenocorticism [20].
- Other specific diagnostic tests
  - A blood gas analysis can help to detect acid–base disturbances, the most common of which in dogs with chronic gastrointestinal disease is metabolic acidosis.
  - Fluid analysis after diagnostic abdominocentesis and/or thoracocentesis should be performed in any dog with evidence of peritoneal and/or pleural effusion.
    - Diagnostic evaluation of the fluid should include macroscopic and routine laboratory assessment (specific gravity, protein concentration, total and nucleated cell counts), cytologic examination (direct smear or centrifugation), and—if appropriate—bacterial culture and antibiotic susceptibility testing.
  - Routine coagulation testing is currently not recommended in all dogs suspected or known to have CIE, unless a thromboembolic complication is suspected [21].
    - The hypercoagulability in dogs with PLE requires thromboelastography to be confirmed [22].
  - Measurement of serum 25-hydroxyvitamin D concentrations in dogs with CIE is currently not routinely performed, but can help to detect hypovitaminosis D [13,23].
    - Hypovitaminosis D occurs commonly in dogs with CIE, particularly those dogs with PLE, and is an independent predictor of mortality [13,23,24].
  - *Histoplasma capsulatum* infections (in dogs from the southern United States) can be diagnosed by cytology (eg, fine-needle aspirate from a lymph node, rectal scrape), histopathology (eg, intestinal biopsies), and/or detection and quantification of *H capsulatum* antigen in serum and/or urine [25].
  - *Pythium insidiosum* infection (in dogs from states lining the Gulf of Mexico) is diagnosed by histopathology (hematoxylin and eosin and Gomori methenamine silver staining), immunohistochemistry, culture and polymerase chain reaction, or *P insidiosum*-antigen enzyme-linked immunosorbent assay [26].
  - Serum gastrin concentration can be measured for the (rare) suspicion of gastric hyperacidity owing to a gastrinoma in dogs with chronic gastrointestinal signs (particularly vomiting, hematemesis, and weight loss).
    - Serum gastrin concentrations can be increased up to 3-fold above the reference interval in dogs with CIE, particularly when receiving a gastric acid suppressant [27].
    - Gastrinoma should be considered as a (rare) cause of gastrointestinal signs in dogs if serum gastrin is increased more than 10-fold above the normal reference interval [27].

BIOMARKERS IN CHRONIC ENTEROPATHIES OF DOGS

- Clinically useful surrogate biomarkers can help to evaluate organ function, disease risk, specific disease processes, disease severity, treatment response, or individual outcome.
  - Biomarkers used in clinical practice should be easy to evaluate, affordable, and minimally invasive (ie, measurable in routine clinical specimens).
  - Several functional, biochemical, and microbiomic biomarkers are currently routinely available in canine gastroenterology (see Fig. 3).
- The correct interpretation of any diagnostic test (routine parameters and also specific biomarkers)

requires consideration of the test performance characteristics.
- The incorporation of a specific biomarker should add value to existing clinical algorithms.

BIOMARKERS THAT ARE CURRENTLY AVAILABLE FOR CLINICAL USE IN SMALL ANIMAL MEDICINE

Food Antigen Testing

- Detection of food-specific IgG and IgE titers in serum or food-specific IgA and IgM in saliva are not reliable tests to diagnose adverse food reactions or FRE [28,29].
  - Increased immunoglobulin titers indicate responses to individual food components, but do not prove an antigenic effect as a cause of adverse food reactions or FRE.
  - Healthy dogs can also have increased food-specific immunoglobulin titers owing to exposure [29], and immunologic cross-reactivity can also occur.
- Lymphocyte proliferation assays are more reliable to detect allergenic food components in dogs [30] but are not readily available.

Serum Cobalamin and Methylmalonic Acid Concentrations

- Cobalamin (vitamin B_{12}) is a water-soluble vitamin that is absorbed in the distal small intestine (ileum) via specific cobalamin-intrinsic factor receptors [31].
- Hypocobalaminemia can indicate the presence of CIE (prevalence of hypocobalaminemia: 19%–54% [32]) or also EPI (prevalence of hypocobalaminemia: >80% [33]).
  - CIE: hypocobalaminemia can result from ileal cobalamin malabsorption, dysregulated transport proteins, and/or secondary intestinal dysbiosis.
    - Hypocobalaminemia is a negative prognostic factor in canine CIE [12,34].
    - Normocobalaminemia does not rule out a diagnosis of CIE, and dogs with CIE can also be hypercobalaminemic [35].
  - EPI: hypocobalaminemia is likely due to a combination of intrinsic factor deficiency (causing cobalamin malabsorption) and secondary intestinal dysbiosis.
  - Hypocobalaminemia or a low-normal serum cobalamin concentration (<400 ng/L) indicates the need for parenteral (subcutaneous) or oral supplementation with cyanocobalamin [31].
- Accumulation of methylmalonic acid (MMA) occurs with a decreased activity of the cobalamin-dependent enzyme methylmalonyl-coenzyme A mutase owing to a lack of intracellular cobalamin [31].
  - Increased serum or urine MMA indicates cobalamin deficiency at the cellular level. Thus, paired cobalamin and MMA measurement is a superior marker for cobalamin status in dogs. However, MMA assays are currently not routinely offered in veterinary medicine.
  - Renal insufficiency can affect serum and urine MMA concentrations.

Serum Folate Concentration

- Folate (vitamin B_9) is also a water-soluble vitamin that is absorbed in the proximal small intestine (duodenum and proximal jejunum) by folate carriers.
- Hypofolatemia (14% prevalence in canine CIE [32]) likely results from chronic malabsorption in the proximal small intestine, but is not specific for CIE.
- Hyperfolatemia (or a falsely normal serum folate concentration) can indicate a small intestinal dysbiosis and can also be seen with hypocobalaminemia [36].

Fecal and Serum Alpha$_1$-Proteinase Inhibitor

- As a major proteinase inhibitor, alpha$_1$-proteinase inhibitor (α_1PI) is primarily synthesized in the liver and resists degradation by proteases. Its role as an acute phase reactant is controversial.
- Owing to their similar molecular weight, α_1PI and albumin are lost through the gastrointestinal tract (with a PLE) at about the same rate (Fig. 4) [37]. Thus, increased fecal α_1PI levels (measured in samples from 3 consecutive days) can detect diseases with gastrointestinal protein loss and even before clinical or clinicopathologic evidence (hypoalbuminemia or panhypoproteinemia) is seen [38,39].
  - Normal reference intervals: less than 13.9 μg/g (3-day mean fecal α_1PI concentration) and less than 21.0 μg/g (3-day maximum fecal α_1PI concentration) [40].
  - The 3-day mean fecal α_1PI concentrations of 19.0 μg/g or greater indicate the presence of typical histologic lesions of PLE (lacteal dilatation, crypt abscesses) in dogs with SRE/IRE or NRE [39].
  - The 3-day mean fecal α_1PI concentrations of less than 4.0 μg/g exclude a PLE in dogs with CIE (negative predictive value >90%) [39].

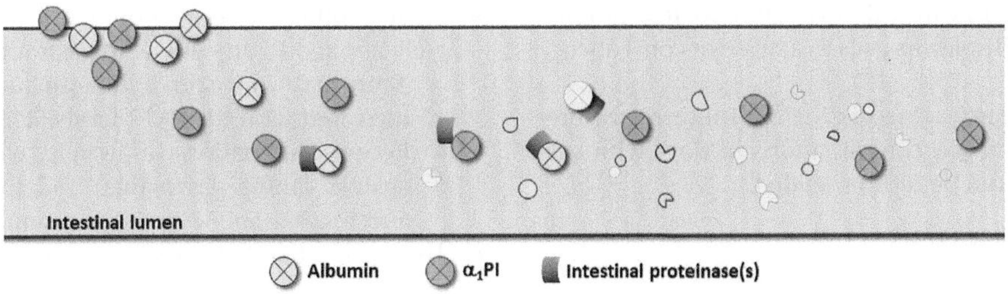

FIG. 4 Fecal α_1-proteinase inhibitor (α_1-PI) test. Canine α_1-PI and canine albumin are of similar molecular weight. Thus, with gastrointestinal protein loss, these 2 proteins should reach similar high concentrations within the intestinal lumen. Although albumin succumbs to degradation by intestinal proteinases, α_1-PI as a proteinase inhibitor resists proteolysis and can be measured in fecal samples.

  - Serum-to-fecal α_1PI ratio improves the diagnostic accuracy for PLE in hypoalbuminemic dogs naïve to corticosteroid treatment [39].
- Fecal α_1PI concentrations can be higher in dogs less than 6 to 12 months old and, if increased, should be retested (at $\geq$1 year of age) [40].

Serum C-Reactive Protein

- C-Reactive protein (CRP)—a positive acute phase protein produced in the liver—is a nonspecific marker of systemic inflammation, infection, or cancer [32]. Several assay formats can routinely measure serum CRP (reference interval: $\leq$8 mg/L) [32].
- Serum CRP concentrations of 9.1 mg/L or greater can distinguish dogs with SRE/IRE or NRE from dogs with FRE/antibiotic-responsive enteropathy with moderate to high sensitivity (72%) and specificity (100%) (positive predictive value for SRE/IRE or NRE: approximately 100%) [41].
- Serum CRP concentrations are even more useful for monitoring canine CIE during treatment [42], but only changes in serum CRP concentrations of at least 2.7-fold are clinically relevant [43].

Fecal Calprotectin

- Calprotectin (S100A8/A9) is primarily released by activated macrophages and neutrophils [32]. Calprotectin accumulates at sites of inflammation and plays a central role in acute and chronic inflammatory processes [32].
- Hypercalprotectinemia is seen in dogs with CIE but is not specific for the gastrointestinal tract and has even less diagnostic value in corticosteroid-treated dogs [44].
- Increased fecal calprotectin concentrations are useful to detect intestinal inflammation in dogs [41,45,46].
  - Fecal calprotectin concentrations of 50 μg/g or greater are associated with severe clinical disease [45].
  - Fecal calprotectin concentrations of 15.2 μg/g or greater are predictive of only partial or no response to treatment in dogs with SRE/IRE (sensitivity: 80%, specificity: 75%) [41].
- Fecal calprotectin levels should not be indiscriminately tested in any dog with gastrointestinal signs.
  - Acute gastrointestinal inflammation can also cause increased fecal calprotectin levels [47].
  - Breed size also affects fecal calprotectin concentrations in dogs.
- A canine calprotectin assay is currently not widely available, but a human assay using polyclonal antibodies looks promising for use with canine samples [48].

Fecal Dysbiosis Index

- Fecal microbiome changes in dogs with CIE include a reduced number of the short chain fatty acid producers *Faecalibacterium* spp. and Fusobacteria [49–51].
- The Fecal Dysbiosis Index is a biomarker that can quantify intestinal dysbiosis by evaluating 8 bacterial groups that are commonly altered in canine CIE (*Blautia, Clostridium hiranonis, E coli, Faecalibacterium, Fusobacterium, Streptococcus, Turicibacter*, and total bacteria) [52].
  - Bacterial microbiome changes as assessed by Fecal Dysbiosis Index can diagnose SRE/IRE in dogs with moderate to high sensitivity (74%) and specificity (95%) [51,52].

BIOMARKERS THAT ARE CURRENTLY PRIMARILY A RESEARCH TOOL IN SMALL ANIMAL GASTROENTEROLOGY

Fecal IgA Concentration

- Fecal IgA concentrations reflect the production of secretory IgA by the intestinal mucosa.
- Fecal IgA concentrations can be decreased (relative or absolute "IgA deficiency") mainly in German

Shepherd dogs with CIE owing to impaired production of IgA by plasma cells as a cause or consequence of CIE [53].

- Further research is needed before routine measurement of fecal IgA concentrations in dogs with suspected CIE can be recommended.

N-Methylhistamine

- A stabile histamine metabolite, *N*-methylhistamine is a marker of mast cell activation and degranulation.
- Increased urine or fecal *N*-methylhistamine levels (measurement in serum is also possible) indicate a mast cell component of the inflammatory infiltrate in some dogs (<50%) with CIE [54,55].
- Further research is needed before routine measurement of urine or fecal *N*-methylhistamine concentrations in dogs with suspected CIE can be recommended.

Perinuclear Antineutrophilic Cytoplasmic Antibodies

- Serum perinuclear antineutrophilic cytoplasmic antibodies are autoantibodies against components of neutrophil granules that cross-react with a gastrointestinal bacterial antigen and are detected by immunofluorescence assay.
- Serum perinuclear antineutrophilic cytoplasmic antibodies positivity and higher titers can point to a diagnosis of FRE in dogs with CIE [46,56].
- Seropositivity for perinuclear antineutrophilic cytoplasmic antibodies, however, is not specific for CIE and can also be detected with other primary or secondary inflammatory conditions [57].

Fecal S100A12

- S100A12 (calgranulin C) is involved in the immune response and has a cellular distribution similar to calprotectin [32].
- Serum S100A12 concentrations increase with various inflammatory disorders but are not affected by corticosteroid treatment.
- Increased fecal S100A12 concentrations are an indicator of gastrointestinal inflammation in dogs [32].
    - Fecal S100A12 levels correlate with clinical and endoscopic disease severity.
    - A fecal S100A12 concentration less than 490 ng/g indicates a high chance for a dog with CIE to have FRE (or antibiotic-responsive enteropathy) (negative predictive value >80%) [58].
    - Fecal S100A12 concentrations less than 2700 ng/g are predictive of at least a partial response in dogs with SRE/IRE (negative predictive value approximately 100%) [58].
- Fecal S100A12 testing should not be indiscriminately applied to any dog with gastrointestinal signs.
    - Acute gastrointestinal inflammation can cause increased fecal S100A12 levels [47].
    - Recent vaccination (especially with a vaccine against canine parvovirus) and breed size also affect fecal S100A12 concentrations in dogs.
- The canine S100A12 assay is currently not readily available yet.

Intestinal Alkaline Phosphatase

- Fecal intestinal alkaline phosphatase levels are decreased in dogs with CIE, especially with moderate or severe disease [59].
- Further study is needed to determine if fecal intestinal alkaline phosphatase levels are a useful biomarker in canine CIE.

Soluble Receptor for Advanced Glycation End Products

- Serum soluble receptor for advanced glycation end products is a nonspecific anti-inflammatory decoy receptor that can sequester proinflammatory ligands of RAGE (Fig. 5) [60].
- Serum soluble receptor for advanced glycation end products concentrations are significantly decreased in dogs with CIE, correlate with histologic duodenal lesions, and normalize in dogs that achieve clinical remission [60,61].
- Further research is needed to determine the potential of serum soluble receptor for advanced glycation end products as a clinical biomarker in canine CIE.

Serum and Fecal 3-bromotyrosine

- Serum 3-bromotyrosine (3-BrY), a stable substance indicating activation and degranulation of eosinophils, is a marker of eosinophilic inflammation [62].
- Serum and also fecal 3-BrY concentrations are increased in dogs with CIE, particularly those with SRE/IRE [62,63].
- Further research is needed before routine measurement of serum 3-BrY levels in dogs with suspected CIE can be recommended.

Cytokines and Chemokines

- Cytokine (IL-1β, IL-2, IL-4, IL-5, IL-6, IL-8, IL-10, IL-12p40, IL-17, IL-18, IL-23, IL-25, IL-33, interferon-γ, tumor necrosis factor-α, and transforming growth factor-β1) studies in dogs with CIE do not support a Th1, Th2, or Th17 signature [64,65].
- Chemokine (CC chemokine ligand [CCL]2, CCL20, CCL25, CCL28, and CXC chemokine ligand [CXCL]

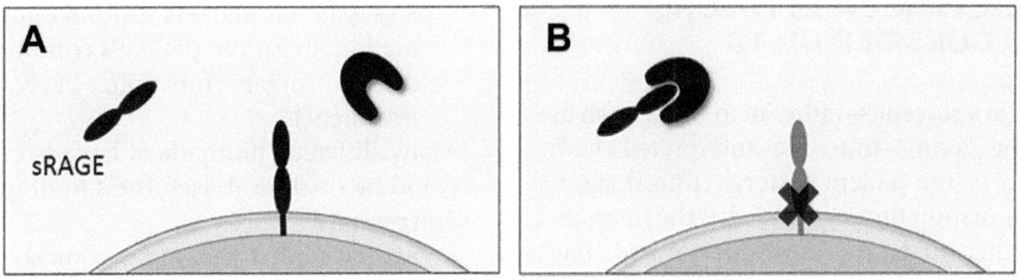

FIG. 5 Soluble receptor for advanced glycation end products (sRAGE) as an anti-inflammatory decoy receptor. (*A*) sRAGE is a truncated variant of transmembrane (full-length) RAGE (depicted in *blue*) and (*B*) acts as an anti-inflammatory decoy receptor by sequestering RAGE ligands such as damage-associated molecular pattern molecules (presented in *red*) leading to an abrogation of proinflammatory signaling downstream of transmembrane RAGE (depicted in *light blue*) activation. (*Modified from* Heilmann RM. PhD thesis, Texas A&M University, TX, USA, 2015.)

8) studies in canine CIE show increases in T and B lymphocyte chemotaxins [66].

- Further research is needed to determine the potential of certain cytokines or chemokines as a clinical biomarker in canine CIE.

Metabolome

- Serum and fecal metabolite profiles in dogs with CIE are indicative of nutritional changes, oxidative stress, and alterations in the function of the intestinal microbiome [50,67–69].
  - Changes in the plasma amino acid profile in dogs with CIE (particularly the amino acids methionine, tryptophan, proline, and serine—but not citrulline) might be a good nutritional biomarker [70–72].
  - Fecal metabolome changes in dogs with CIE include altered fecal short chain fatty acid (particularly acetate and propionate), fecal lactate, and also fecal bile acid concentrations (particularly unconjugated bile acids indicating bile acid dysmetabolism) [67–69].
- Routine assessment of the serum and/or fecal metabolome is currently not feasible in dogs, and further research is needed to determine the clinical usefulness of plasma amino acid concentrations and other serum and/or fecal metabolites as biomarkers in dogs with CIE.

Cellular Biomarkers

- Numbers of circulating regulatory T cells are decreased in dogs with SRE/IRE (and PLE) and might be useful to monitor disease progression and response to treatment [73].
- Further studies need to determine the potential of regulatory T cells numbers as a biomarker in canine CIE.

Genomic Biomarkers

- Several genetic (single nucleotide) polymorphisms in genes encoding innate immune receptors, reduced diversity of the T-cell receptor repertoire, and alterations in the mucosal expression of several other genes are associated with canine CIE [74].
- Expression patterns of mucosal and serum microRNAs (miR) are dysregulated in canine CIE (upregulation of miR-16, miR-21, miR-122, and miR-147; downregulation of miR-185, miR-192, and miR-223) and have potential clinical usefulness as a diagnostic biomarker [75]. Fecal miRs also hold promise as a diagnostic marker for gastrointestinal disease in dogs [76], but further study is needed to characterize miR expression profiles in dogs with gastrointestinal disease.
- Genomic markers are primarily research tools for the further pathogenetic study of canine CIE and are currently not yet of relevance in routine clinical practice.

Other Functional Biomarkers

- The absorption of ^{51}Cr-EDTA or iohexol can test the gastrointestinal absorptive function, and gastrointestinal permeability can be tested using simple sugar probes (urine sucrose for gastric permeability, serum or urine lactulose/rhamnose or xylose/methylglucose ratio for intestinal permeability). Because these tests are impractical, they are not used routinely in dogs.
- The ^{13}C-octanoic acid breath test can noninvasively assess gastric emptying time. This technique is also impractical and invasive, and with the availability of newer methods to assess gastric emptying, the ^{13}C-octanoic acid breath test is no longer used in small animal medicine.

PRESENT RELEVANCE AND FUTURE AVENUES TO CONSIDER OR TO INVESTIGATE

- Any diagnostic test result—rather than being seen as a stand-alone result—must be interpreted with consideration of the patient history, clinical signs, physical examination findings, and also the interpretation of other diagnostic tests performed (eg, routine clinicopathologic parameters, diagnostic imaging findings) (Fig. 6).
  - Routine laboratory parameters and diagnostic imaging are not specific for a diagnosis of CIE, but these tests are essential to evaluate the overall health status of the dog and rule out extragastrointestinal diseases.
  - Surrogate biomarkers can offer additional information about the patient's condition (eg, risk of disease, organ function, likely response to treatment).
- Many different biomarkers have been studied and could be of clinical usefulness in dogs with chronic enteropathy.
  - Several biomarkers can be quickly and noninvasively determined in serum, urine, and—even more specific for the gastrointestinal tract—in fecal samples. Some biomarkers can also be measured in a combination of biological specimens.
  - Other biomarkers, however, seem to be of limited clinical usefulness because of a current

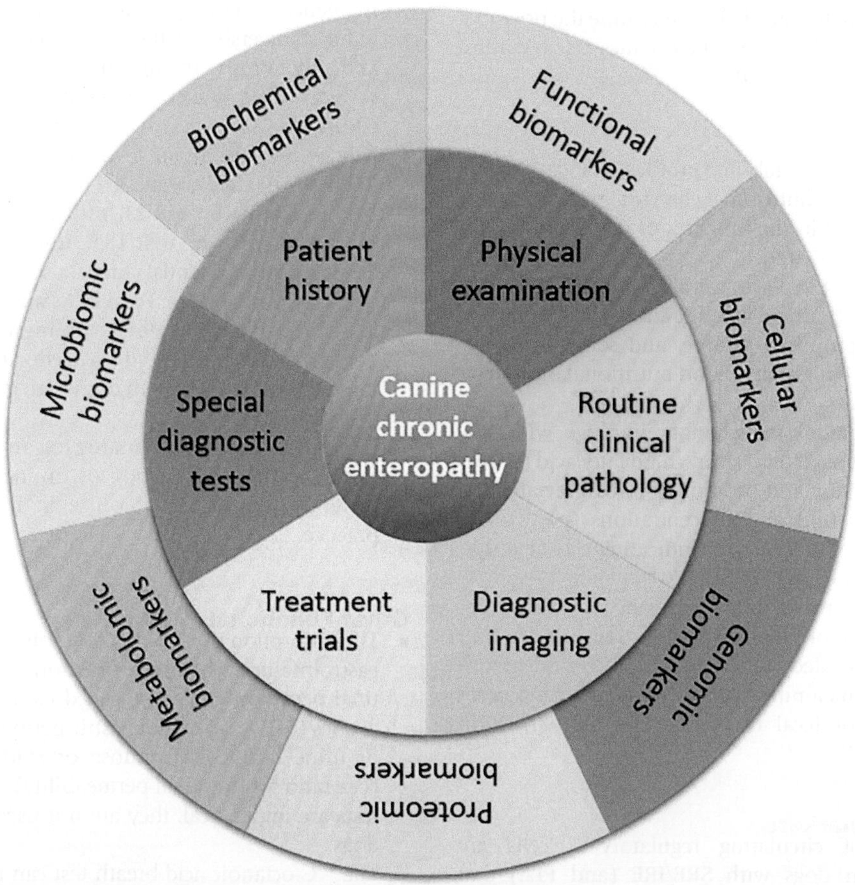

FIG. 6 Integrative diagnostic approach to chronic enteropathy in dogs. This figure illustrates the interdependency of the different modalities for the diagnosis and subclassification of chronic enteropathies in dogs. No single diagnostic modality can function as a stand-alone diagnostic test and needs to be interpreted in light of other diagnostic test results. Biomarkers can be clinically useful surrogate parameters in the management of canine chronic enteropathy.

lack of wide or routine availability (eg, sophisticated technique), expense, and/or low stability in routine biological specimens (eg, small molecules such as cytokines and chemokines).

- Several functional, biochemical, and microbiomic biomarkers that were shown to be useful surrogate biomarkers are currently routinely available and are frequently used in the diagnostic evaluation of dogs with chronic enteropathies.
  - Functional biomarkers: Measurement of serum cobalamin and folate can help to detect vitamin deficiencies as an indicator of chronic gastrointestinal disease, and fecal α_1PI can help to identify gastrointestinal protein loss in dogs.
  - Inflammatory biomarkers: Assays for measurement of serum CRP and fecal calprotectin concentrations are routinely available, allowing for their use in the clinical setting.
  - Microbiomic biomarkers: The fecal dysbiosis index is available as a diagnostic test to assess dogs for the presence of intestinal dysbiosis.
- Correct interpretation and integration of biomarker results in the clinical setting require an understanding of the general clinical usefulness and the limitations of individual biomarkers to prevent any potential pitfalls in the interpretation of biomarker data.
  - Beyond the sensitivity and specificity of a biomarker assay, the diagnostic performance of a biomarker test depends on the prevalence of the disease in the clinical setting in which the test is being applied (Fig. 7).
    - Given the diagnostic accuracy and disease prevalence, some biomarker assays are useful diagnostic tests, whereas other assays are better confirmatory (diagnostic) tests (Fig. 8).
    - Study prevalences rarely mirror disease prevalence in the general dog population, and the actual prevalence (pretest probability) is not known for most diseases in dogs.
  - Preanalytical factors (eg, sample handling, storage) can affect the performance of a biomarker assay.
  - Biological variability (intraindividual and interindividual variation) is an inherent characteristic of all biomarkers and needs to be considered in the interpretation of biomarker data.
    - Biological variability determines the usefulness of a population-based reference interval for a quantitative biomarker and whether the marker performs better for diagnosing a disease ("event marker") or monitoring of a condition ("chronic disease marker"). For some biomarkers, stratification of the reference population is needed.
    - Biological variability also determines the reference change value (minimum critical difference) of a quantitative biomarker assay.
- Future avenues to consider for the laboratory approach to chronic enteropathies in dogs include

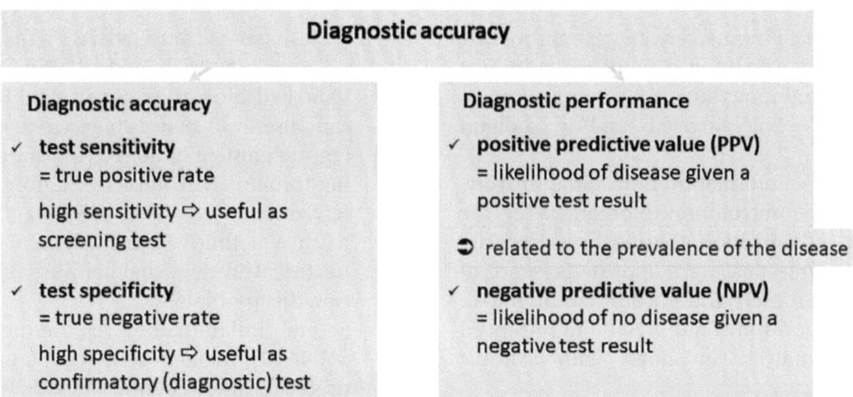

Diagnostic accuracy
Diagnostic accuracy
✓ test sensitivity
= true positive rate
high sensitivity ⇨ useful as screening test
✓ test specificity
= true negative rate
high specificity ⇨ useful as confirmatory (diagnostic) test
Diagnostic performance
✓ positive predictive value (PPV)
= likelihood of disease given a positive test result
related to the prevalence of the disease
✓ negative predictive value (NPV)
= likelihood of no disease given a negative test result

FIG. 7 Individual components that determine the diagnostic accuracy of a biomarker. The diagnostic accuracy of a biomarker is determined by the diagnostic accuracy of the test format as well as the diagnostic performance of this test in a given population of individual dogs to be tested. The predictive values of the assay strongly depend on the prevalence of the disease, condition, or characteristic individuals are being tested for.

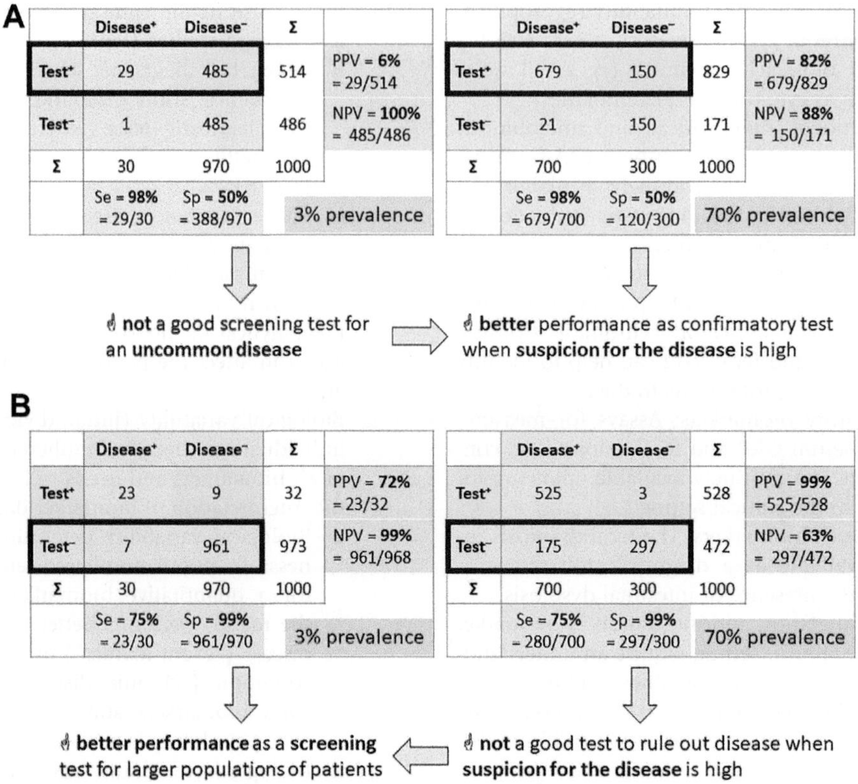

FIG. 8 Clinical usefulness of a biomarker as determined by the overall diagnostic accuracy of the test. The 2 examples (*A*, *B*) in this figure illustrate how (i) sensitivity and specificity of a test and (ii) the prevalence of the disease in which the test is used can affect the predictive values and the performance of the biomarker as either a screening test or confirmatory test. NPV, negative predictive value; PPV, positive predictive value; Se, sensitivity; Sp, specificity; Σ, sum (of all row or column values).

the development of biomarkers panels followed by their inclusion into existing diagnostic algorithms alongside the continuous search for novel noninvasive biomarkers (via targeted and/or shotgun approach).

- Combining the information from inflammatory, functional, and microbiomic biomarkers (eg, the severity of inflammation, the absorptive capacity of the gastrointestinal tract, and the presence of intestinal dysbiosis) and incorporation into a diagnostic algorithm could present an improved diagnostic strategy in dogs with chronic enteropathy.
  - Combining the results of several biomarkers within the same marker category (eg, the inflammatory biomarkers serum CRP and fecal calprotectin, paired measurement of serum cobalamin and MMA concentrations) can also have additive effects on the diagnostic accuracy of the individual biomarkers.
- Validated biomarker panels could also be clinically useful to better characterize dogs with CIE (eg, assignment of dogs to CIE subgroups) allowing for an earlier implementation of specific interventions (eg, more invasive diagnostics to reach a definitive diagnosis, anti-inflammatory treatment in dogs that are likely to fail elimination dietary trials).
- Several inflammatory (eg, serum 3-BrY, fecal S100A12), metabolomic (eg, plasma metabolite profiles), and genomic markers (eg, fecal miRNAs) are currently not readily available but hold promise as useful surrogate biomarkers for canine CIE management and could represent future avenues to individualized treatment and monitoring.

SUMMARY

Routine laboratory parameters are essential to assess the overall patient condition but are usually not specific for diagnosing dogs with chronic enteropathy. Surrogate biomarkers offer additional information about the disease and play an essential role in the management of canine chronic enteropathy. Several biomarkers have been studied in dogs with chronic enteropathies and have expanded the diagnostic toolbox of the small animal clinician. The search for novel biomarkers continues, and more studies are needed to evaluate further the clinical usefulness of established biomarker assays for canine CIE management.

DISCLOSURE

The author has nothing to disclose.

REFERENCES

[1] Allenspach K, Culverwell C, Chan D. Long-term outcome in dogs with chronic enteropathies: 203 cases. Vet Rec 2016;178:368.

[2] Washabau RJ, Day MJ, Willard MD, et al. Endoscopic, biopsy, and histopathologic guidelines for the evaluation of gastrointestinal inflammation in companion animals. J Vet Intern Med 2010;24:10–26.

[3] Day MJ, Bilzer T, Mansell J, et al. Histopathological standards for the diagnosis of gastrointestinal inflammation in endoscopic biopsy samples from the dog and cat: a report from the World Small Animal Veterinary Association Gastrointestinal Standardization Group. J Comp Pathol 2008;138:S1–43.

[4] Dandrieux JR. Inflammatory bowel disease versus chronic enteropathy in dogs: are they one and the same? J Small Anim Pract 2016;57:589–99.

[5] Erdmann C, Heilmann RM. Diagnostic and therapeutic approach to chronic inflammatory enteropathies in dogs. Tierarztl Prax Ausg K Kleintiere Heimtiere 2017;45:317–27.

[6] Cerquetella M, Rossi G, Suchodolski JS, et al. Proposal for rational antibacterial use in the diagnosis and treatment of dogs with chronic diarrhoea. J Small Anim Pract 2020;61:211–5.

[7] Craven M, Simpson JW, Ridyard AE, et al. Canine inflammatory bowel disease: retrospective analysis of diagnosis and outcome in 80 cases (1995–2002). J Small Anim Pract 2004;45:336–42.

[8] Kull PA, Hess RS, Craig LE, et al. Clinical, clinicopathologic, radiographic, and ultrasonographic characteristics of intestinal lymphangiectasia in dogs: 17 cases (1996–1998). J Am Vet Med Assoc 2001;219:197–202.

[9] Zeugswetter FK, Schwendenwein I. Diagnostic efficacy of the leukogram and the chemiluminometric ACTH measurement to diagnose canine hypoadrenocorticism. Tierarztl Prax Ausg K Kleintiere Heimtiere 2014;42:223–30.

[10] Becher A, Suchodolski JS, Steiner JM, et al. Neutrophil-to-lymphocyte ratio (NLR) as a biomarker in dogs with chronic inflammatory enteropathies. J Vet Intern Med 2020;34:386.

[11] Wennogle SA, Priestnall SL, Webb CB. Histopathologic characteristics of intestinal biopsy samples from dogs with chronic inflammatory enteropathy with and without hypoalbuminemia. J Vet Intern Med 2017;31:371–6.

[12] Allenspach K, Wieland B, Gröne A, et al. Chronic enteropathies in dogs: evaluation of risk factors for negative outcome. J Vet Intern Med 2007;21:700–8.

[13] Titmarsh H, Gow AG, Kilpatrick S, et al. Association of vitamin D status and clinical outcome in dogs with a chronic enteropathy. J Vet Intern Med 2015;29:1473–8.

[14] Zandvliet M. Canine lymphoma: a review. Vet Q 2016;36:76–104.

[15] Kathrani A, Sánchez-Vizcaíno F, Hall EJ. Association of chronic enteropathy activity index, blood urea concentration, and risk of death in dogs with protein-losing enteropathy. J Vet Intern Med 2019;33:536–43.

[16] Marks SL, Rankin SC, Byrne BA, et al. Enteropathogenic bacteria in dogs and cats: diagnosis, epidemiology, treatment, and control. J Vet Intern Med 2001;25:1195–208.

[17] Manchester AC, Hills S, Sabatino B, et al. Association between granulomatous colitis in French Bulldogs and invasive Escherichia coli and response to fluoroquinolone antimicrobials. J Vet Intern Med 2013;27:56–61.

[18] Kathrani A, Steiner JM, Suchodolski JS, et al. Elevated canine pancreatic lipase immunoreactivity concentration in dogs with inflammatory bowel disease is associated with a negative outcome. J Small Anim Pract 2009;50:126–32.

[19] Heilmann RM, Steiner JM. Laboratory testing for the exocrine pancreas. In: Bonagura JD, Twedt DC, editors. Kirk's current veterinary therapy XV. St Louis (MO): Saunders Elsevier; 2014. p. 554–7.

[20] Bovens C, Tennant K, Reeve J, et al. Basal serum cortisol concentration as a screening test for hypoadrenocorticism in dogs. J Vet Intern Med 2014;28:1541–5.

[21] Jacinto AML, Ridyard AE, Aroch I, et al. Thromboembolism in dogs with protein-losing enteropathy with non-neoplastic chronic small intestinal disease. J Am Anim Hosp Assoc 2017;53:185–92.

[22] Goodwin LV, Goggs R, Chan DL, et al. Hypercoagulability in dogs with protein-losing enteropathy. J Vet Intern Med 2011;25:273–7.

[23] Allenspach K, Rizzo J, Jergens AE, et al. Hypovitaminosis D is associated with negative outcome in dogs with protein losing enteropathy: a retrospective study of 43 cases. BMC Vet Res 2017;13:96.

[24] Wennogle SA, Priestnall SL, Suárez-Bonnet A, et al. Comparison of clinical, clinicopathologic, and histologic variables in dogs with chronic inflammatory enteropathy

and low or normal serum 25-hydroxycholecalciferol concentrations. J Vet Intern Med 2019;33:1995–2004.
[25] Cunningham L, Cook A, Hanzlicek A, et al. Sensitivity and specificity of Histoplasma antigen detection by enzyme immunoassay. J Am Anim Hosp Assoc 2015; 51:306–10.
[26] Grooters AM, Leise BS, Lopez MK, et al. Development and evaluation of an enzyme-linked immunosorbent assay for the serodiagnosis of pythiosis in dogs. J Vet Intern Med 2002;16:142–6.
[27] Heilmann RM, Berghoff N, Grützner N, et al. Effect of gastric acid-suppressive therapy and biological variation of serum gastrin concentrations in dogs with chronic enteropathies. BMC Vet Res 2017;13:321.
[28] Mueller RS, Olivry T. Critically appraised topic on adverse food reactions of companion animals (4): can we diagnose adverse food reactions in dogs and cats with in vivo or in vitro tests? BMC Vet Res 2017;13:275.
[29] Udraite Vovk L, Watson A, Dodds WJ, et al. Testing for food-specific antibodies in saliva and blood of food allergenic and healthy dogs. Vet J 2019;245:1–6.
[30] Fujimura M, Masuda M, Okayama T. Flow cytometric analysis of lymphocyte proliferative responses to food allergens in dogs with food allergy. J Vet Med Sci 2011;73: 1309–17.
[31] Kather S, Grützner N, Kook PH, et al. Review of cobalamin status and disorders of cobalamin metabolism in dogs. J Vet Intern Med 2020;34:13–28.
[32] Heilmann RM, Steiner JS. Clinical utility of currently available biomarkers in inflammatory enteropathies of dogs. J Vet Intern Med 2018;32:1495–508.
[33] Batchelor DJ, Noble PJ, Taylor RH, et al. Prognostic factors in canine exocrine pancreatic insufficiency: prolonged survival is likely if clinical remission is achieved. J Vet Intern Med 2007;21:54–60.
[34] Volkmann M, Steiner JM, Fosgate GT, et al. Chronic diarrhea in dogs—retrospective study in 136 cases. J Vet Intern Med 2017;31:1043–55.
[35] Sielski L, Kather S, Dengler F, et al. Association of hypercobalaminemia with pathological findings in dogs and cats. J Vet Intern Med, in press.
[36] Ruaux CG. Laboratory testing for the diagnosis of intestinal disorders. In: Steiner JM, editor. Small animal gastroenterology. Hannover (Germany): Schlütersche; 2008. p. 50–5.
[37] Melgarejo T, Williams DA, Griffith G. Isolation and characterization of alpha2-protease inhibitor from canine plasma. Am J Vet Res 1996;57:258–63.
[38] Vaden SL, Vidaurri A, Levine JF, et al. Fecal α_1-proteinase inhibitor activity in soft coated wheaten terriers. J Vet Intern Med 2002;16:382.
[39] Heilmann RM, Parnell NK, Grützner N, et al. Serum and fecal canine alpha$_1$-proteinase inhibitor concentrations reflect the severity of intestinal crypt abscesses and/or lacteal dilation in dogs. Vet J 2016;207:131–9.
[40] Heilmann RM, Paddock CG, Ruhnke I, et al. Development and analytical validation of a radioimmunoassay for the measurement of α1-proteinase inhibitor concentrations in feces from healthy puppies and adult dogs. J Vet Diagn Invest 2011;23:476–85.
[41] Heilmann RM, Berghoff N, Mansell J, et al. Association of fecal calprotectin concentrations with disease severity, response to treatment, and other biomarkers in dogs with chronic inflammatory enteropathies. J Vet Intern Med 2018;32:679–92.
[42] Jergens AE, Crandell J, Morrison JA, et al. Comparison of oral prednisone and prednisone combined with metronidazole for induction therapy of canine inflammatory bowel disease: a randomized-controlled trial. J Vet Intern Med 2010;24:269–77.
[43] Carney PC, Ruaux CG, Suchodolski JS, et al. Biological variability of C-reactive protein and specific pancreatic lipase immunoreactivity (Spec cPL) in apparently healthy dogs. J Vet Intern Med 2011;25:825–30.
[44] Heilmann RM, Jergens AE, Ackermann MR, et al. Serum calprotectin concentrations in dogs with idiopathic inflammatory bowel disease. Am J Vet Res 2012;73: 1900–7.
[45] Grellet A, Heilmann RM, Lecoindre P, et al. Fecal calprotectin concentrations in adult dogs with chronic diarrhea. Am J Vet Res 2013;74:706–11.
[46] Otoni CC, Heilmann RM, García-Sancho M, et al. Serologic and fecal markers to predict response to induction therapy in dogs with idiopathic inflammatory bowel disease. J Vet Intern Med 2018;32:999–1008.
[47] Heilmann RM, Guard MM, Steiner JM, et al. Fecal inflammatory biomarkers and microbial changes in dogs with acute hemorrhagic diarrhea syndrome (AHDS). J Vet Emerg Crit Care 2017;27:586–9.
[48] Truar K, Nestler J, Schwarz J, et al. Feasibility of measuring fecal calprotectin concentrations in dogs and cats by the fCAL® turbo immunoassay. J Vet Intern Med 2018;32:580.
[49] Suchodolski JS, Markel ME, Garcia-Mazcorro JF, et al. The fecal microbiome in dogs with acute diarrhea and idiopathic inflammatory bowel disease. PLoS One 2012;7:e51907.
[50] Minamoto Y, Otoni CC, Steelman SM, et al. Alteration of the fecal microbiota and serum metabolite profiles in dogs with idiopathic inflammatory bowel disease. Gut Microbes 2015;6:33–47.
[51] Suchodolski JS. Diagnosis and interpretation of intestinal dysbiosis in dogs and cats. Vet J 2016;215:30–7.
[52] AlShawaqfeh MK, Wajid B, Minamoto Y, et al. A dysbiosis index to assess microbial changes in fecal samples of dogs with chronic inflammatory enteropathy. FEMS Microbiol Ecol 2017;93:136.
[53] Littler RM, Batt RM, Lloyd DH. Total and relative deficiency of gut mucosal IgA in German Shepherd dogs demonstrated by faecal analysis. Vet Rec 2006;158: 334–41.
[54] Anfinsen KP, Berghoff N, Priestnall SL, et al. Urinary and faecal N-methylhistamine concentrations do not serve as markers for mast cell activation or clinical disease activity

in dogs with chronic enteropathies. Acta Vet Scand 2014;56:90.

[55] Berghoff N, Hill S, Parnell NK, et al. Fecal and urinary N-methylhistamine concentrations in dogs with chronic gastrointestinal disease. Vet J 2014;201:289–94.

[56] Luckschander N, Allenspach K, Hall J, et al. Perinuclear antineutrophilic cytoplasmic antibody and response to treatment in diarrheic dogs with food responsive disease or inflammatory bowel disease. J Vet Intern Med 2006;20:221–7.

[57] Karagianni AE, Solano-Gallego L, Breitschwerdt EB, et al. Perinuclear antineutrophil cytoplasmic autoantibodies in dogs infected with various vector-borne pathogens and in dogs with immune-mediated hemolytic anemia. Am J Vet Res 2012;73:1403–9.

[58] Heilmann RM, Volkmann M, Otoni CC, et al. Fecal S100A12 concentration predicts a lack of response to treatment in dogs affected with chronic enteropathy. Vet J 2016;215:96–100.

[59] Ide K, Kato K, Sawa Y, et al. Comparison of the expression, activity, and fecal concentration of intestinal alkaline phosphatase between healthy dogs and dogs with chronic enteropathy. Am J Vet Res 2016;77:721–9.

[60] Heilmann RM, Otoni CC, Jergens AE, et al. Systemic levels of the anti-inflammatory decoy receptor sRAGE (soluble receptor for advanced glycation end products) are decreased in dogs with inflammatory bowel disease. Vet Immunol Immunopathol 2014;161:184–92.

[61] Cabrera-García IA, Suchodolski JS, Steiner JM, et al. Decreased serum soluble RAGE concentrations correlate with the severity of histologic lesions in dogs with chronic inflammatory enteropathies. J Vet Intern Med 2019;33:1029.

[62] Sattasathuchana P, Allenspach K, Lopes R, et al. Evaluation of serum 3-bromotyrosine concentrations in dogs with steroid-responsive diarrhea and food-responsive diarrhea. J Vet Intern Med 2017;31:1056–61.

[63] Sattasathuchana P, Thengchaisri N, Suchodolski JS, et al. Analytical validation of fecal 3-bromotyrosine concentrations in healthy dogs and dogs with chronic enteropathy. J Vet Diagn Invest 2019;31:434–9.

[64] Heilmann RM, Suchodolski JS. Is inflammatory bowel disease in dogs and cats associated with a Th1 or Th2 polarization? Vet Immunol Immunopathol 2015;168:131–4.

[65] Schmitz S, Garden OA, Werling D, et al. Gene expression of selected signature cytokines of T cell subsets in duodenal tissues of dogs with and without inflammatory bowel disease. Vet Immunol Immunopathol 2012;146:87–91.

[66] Maeda S, Ohno K, Nakamura K, et al. Quantification of chemokine and chemokine receptor gene expression in duodenal mucosa of dogs with inflammatory bowel disease. Vet Immunol Immunopathol 2011;144:290–8.

[67] Minamoto Y, Minamoto T, Isaiah A, et al. Fecal short-chain fatty acid concentrations and dysbiosis in dogs with chronic enteropathy. J Vet Intern Med 2019;33:1608–18.

[68] Blake AB, Guard BC, Honneffer JB, et al. Altered microbiota, fecal lactate, and fecal bile acids in dogs with gastrointestinal disease. PLoS One 2019;14:e0224454.

[69] Guard BC, Honneffer JB, Jergens AE, et al. Longitudinal assessment of microbial dysbiosis, fecal unconjugated bile acid concentrations, and disease activity in dogs with steroid-responsive chronic inflammatory enteropathy. J Vet Intern Med 2019;33:1295–305.

[70] Kathrani A, Allenspach K, Fascetti AJ, et al. Alterations in serum amino acid concentrations in dogs with protein-losing enteropathy. J Vet Intern Med 2018;32:1026–32.

[71] Gerou-Ferriani M, Allen R, Noble PM, et al. Determining optimal therapy of dogs with chronic enteropathy by measurement of serum citrulline. J Vet Intern Med 2018;32:993–8.

[72] Tamura Y, Ohta H, Kagawa Y, et al. Plasma amino acid profiles in dogs with inflammatory bowel disease. J Vet Intern Med 2019;33:1602–7.

[73] Volkmann M, Hepworth MR, Ebner F, et al. Frequencies of regulatory T cells in the peripheral blood of dogs with primary immune-mediated thrombocytopenia and chronic enteropathy: a pilot study. Vet J 2014;202:630–3.

[74] Heilmann RM, Allenspach K. Pattern recognition receptors: signaling pathways and dysregulation in canine chronic enteropathies—brief review. J Vet Diagn Invest 2017;29:781–7.

[75] Konstantinidis AO, Pardali D, Adamama-Moraitou KK, et al. Colonic mucosal and serum expression of microRNAs in canine large intestinal inflammatory bowel disease. BMC Vet Res 2020;16:69.

[76] Cirera S, Willumsen LM, Johansen TT, et al. Evaluation of microRNA stability in feces from healthy dogs. Vet Clin Pathol 2018;47:115–21.

Advances in Small Animal Care 1 (2020) 127–141

ADVANCES IN SMALL ANIMAL CARE

Inflammatory Bowel Disease, Food-Responsive, Antibiotic-Responsive Diarrhoea, Protein Losing Enteropathy

Acronyms, Clinical Staging, and Treatment of Chronic Inflammatory Enteropathy in Dogs

Fabio Procoli, DMV, MVetMed, DipACVIM, DipECVIM-CA, MRCVS

Unità Operativa di Medicina Interna, Ospedale Veterinario I Portoni Rossi, Via Roma 57/A, Zola Predosa, Bologna 40069, Italy

KEYWORDS

• IBD • FRE • ARD • PLE • Clinical activity index • Diet • Immunosuppressive drugs • Probiotics

KEY POINTS

- Canine CIE is currently classified as food-responsive enteropathy (FRE), antibiotic-responsive enteropathy (ARE), and immunosuppressive-responsive enteropathy (IRE), the latter also referred to as steroid-responsive enteropathy (SRE) or inflammatory bowel disease (IBD).
- Whether FRE, ARE, and IRE are three distinct disease entities or whether they represent three phenotypes of the same disease remains to be ascertained but significant overlap exists in clinical, endoscopic, and histopathologic findings among them.
- Therapeutic diets are the mainstay of CIE treatment, with recent evidence supporting their role also in protein-losing enteropathy (PLE), a severe phenotype of CIE.
- The use of antibiotics in CIE management is currently under scrutiny and considered controversial.
- Immunosuppressive drugs (ISDs) are used for induction and maintenance therapy for CIE cases when dietary and alternative treatment trials have failed.

INTRODUCTION

Definition and Classification of Canine Chronic Inflammatory Enteropathy

- Chronic inflammatory enteropathy (CIE) broadly refers to a group of idiopathic disorders of dogs characterized by persistent or recurrent gastrointestinal (GI) signs of more than 3 weeks' duration associated with varying degrees and types of intestinal mucosal inflammatory infiltrates and/or ultrastructural changes [1].
- Based on the response to sequential treatment trials, canine CIE is classified as food-responsive (FRE), antibiotic-responsive (ARE), and immunosuppressive-responsive enteropathies (IRE). ARE was formerly also often termed antibiotic-responsive diarrhea (ARD), but enteropathy is preferred in the light of the other classifications. IRE is preferred over steroid-responsive enteropathy (SRE) or inflammatory bowel disease (IBD), because these conditions do not fully

E-mail address: Fabio.Procoli@portonirossi.it

https://doi.org/10.1016/j.yasa.2020.07.010

resemble IBD in people and might not respond to steroids alone. A small proportion of cases are refractory to all treatment trials and are referred to as nonresponsive enteropathy (NRE) [2].

- Protein-losing enteropathy (PLE) is characterized by excessive enteric protein loss and subsequent development of hypoalbuminemia [3], but does not allow speculation about the underlying intestinal cause.
- It remains to be ascertained whether FRE, ARE, IRE, and PLE represent different disease entities with different etiologies or whether they are a phenotypic variation of the same complex multifactorial disease.
- A prevailing hypothesis is that CIE is a multifactorial disease that involves a complex interaction of host genome, intestinal barrier function, intestinal microbiota, dietary antigens, and the intestinal immune system [4], in which each factor might play a role in individual subgroups of CIE (Fig. 1).
- The reader is referred to the Karin Allenspach and Jon P. Mochel's article, "Genetics and Immunopathogenesis of Chronic Inflammatory Enteropathies in Dogs," in this issue for more detailed information on the immunopathogenesis of CIE.

INSIGHT INTO CHRONIC INFLAMMATORY ENTEROPATHY ACRONYMS

Food-Responsive Enteropathy

- Strictly speaking, FRE should be reserved for idiopathic CIE cases that have: (1) failed antibiotic trials, (2) undergone GI biopsies with histopathologic evidence of intestinal mucosal inflammation, and most importantly (3) have achieved swift clinical remission following a trial with a therapeutic (selected antigen, hydrolyzed or highly digestible) diet [1].
- It is unknown whether all cases of FRE truly suffer from a complex multifactorial disease, such CIE, or whether they encompass cases of adverse food reactions of food intolerance.
- Irrespective of the exact pathophysiology behind FRE, 55% to 66% of CIE cases are food responsive [1,5–7].

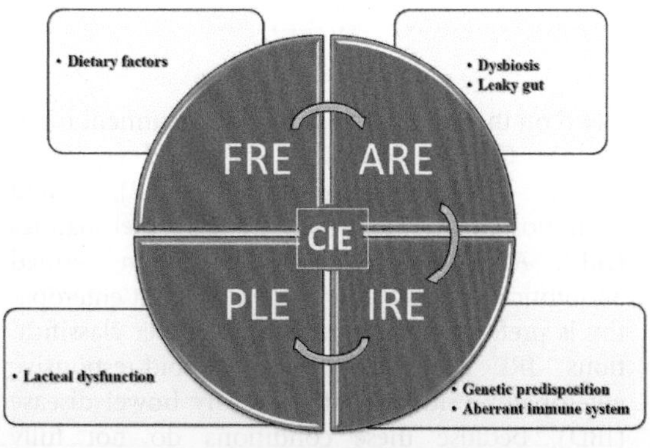

FIG. 1 Pathogenesis of canine CIE. Canine CIE is a multifactorial disease: an aberrant immune system response, luminal antigens (commensal bacteria, dietary antigen), host genetics, dysbiotic microbiota composition, intestinal barrier function, and environmental triggers all contribute to development of inflammatory and morphologic changes.

Antibiotic-Responsive Enteropathy

- The term ARE refers to dogs with unexplained chronic GI signs, mostly diarrhea, that will: (1) achieve clinical remission following antibiotic trial, (2) experience a relapse when treatment is discontinued, and most importantly (3) achieve remission when the antibiotic is reintroduced.
- ARE was originally described as a syndrome of malabsorption affecting young German Shepherd dogs responsive to antibiotics [8]. It was believed to be caused by an overgrowth of aerobic and/or anaerobe bacteria in the proximal small intestine and initially was termed "small bacterial intestinal overgrowth."
- Subsequent studies questioned the existence of primary small bacterial intestinal overgrowth, because similar or higher bacterial numbers were found in the duodenum of healthy dogs and dogs with other chronic GI disorders [9]. The term "ARE" replaced small bacterial intestinal overgrowth because of the largely unknown pathogenesis of the disease.
- The occurrence of ARE among CIE cases is modest with large retrospective studies revealing a prevalence of 10% and 16%, respectively [6,7].

Immunosuppressive-Responsive Enteropathies

- In this review the term "IRE" refers to dogs with CIE that have failed to respond to therapeutic diet and antibiotic trials but show some responsiveness to glucocorticoids and/or other immunosuppressive drugs (ISDs) [10].
- A prevalence of 19% to 22% for SRE/IRE has been reported [6,7].

Protein-Losing Enteropathy

- PLE refers to a syndrome characterized by excessive nonselective enteric protein loss with ensuing hypoalbuminemia for which specific breed associations are known [3].

- Several GI diseases can cause PLE: primary intestinal lymphangiectasia (IL), idiopathic CIE, and intestinal neoplasia (ie, small and large cell lymphoma) [8].
- Pathogenesis of "inflammatory" PLE includes a combination of severe epithelial injury, severe mucosal inflammation (erosive or nonerosive), lacteal obstruction with subsequent dilation and rupture, and increased vascular permeability [11].
- The true prevalence of PLE among canine CIE is not known, but significant hypoalbuminemia (<2.0 g/dL) is found in up to 21% [1].

CLINICAL STAGING OF CHRONIC INFLAMMATORY ENTEROPATHY: ASSESSING DISEASE ACTIVITY AND SEVERITY

Background

- Clinical staging is fundamental to defining disease localization and severity, and evaluating the presence of complications and factors associated with negative outcome.
- Clinical staging is based on the integration of signalment and clinical presentation with findings from physical examination, clinical pathology, and abdominal ultrasound.
- Disease-specific clinical activity indices (CAIs) or scores have been validated across all subtypes of canine CIE. They allow a reliable assessment of disease severity and response to treatment and are used to predict short- and long-term outcome [1,12].

Signalment

- Although CIE can affect dogs of any age, sex and breed, specific breed associations have been reported for some subtypes (Table 1) [3,8,13–22].
- Dogs with FRE (median age, 2 years) and ARE (median age, 3 years) are typically younger than those diagnosed with IBD (median, 6 years) and PLE.
- Dogs with FRE are often larger (>10 kg body weight) than dogs with IRE (<10 kg body weight) [23].

Clinical Presentation

- Clinical signs in dogs with CIE are attributed to mucosal cellular infiltrates, inflammatory mediators, inflammation-associated enterocyte dysfunction, and intestinal dysmotility [10].
- The most common presenting clinical signs are chronic (>3 weeks) diarrhea, vomiting, weight loss, and inappetence.
- Clinical signs can be persistent or, more often, intermittent with periods of clinical activity ("flare") intercalated by periods of spontaneous remission [12].
- By carefully evaluating fecal characteristics, clinicians should attempt to localize the disease to the upper (small intestinal CIE), or lower GI tract (large intestinal CIE), or both (diffuse CIE), because disease localization varies across phenotypes.

TABLE 1
Known Breed Predispositions in Canine Chronic Inflammatory Enteropathy

Breed	CE Phenotype	Reference
German Shepherd Dog	ARE	Batt et al [8], 1983
Chinese Shar-pei	PLE, hypocobalaminemia	Peterson & Willard [3], 2003, Kather et al [22], 2020
Basenji	Lymphoproliferative	Breitschwerdt et al [13], 1984
Norwegian Lundehund	PLE	Kolbjørnsen et al [14], 1994
Soft Coated Wheaten Terrier	PLE and PLN	Littman et al [15], 2000
Yorkshire terrier	PLE	Simmerson et al [16], 2014
Rottweiler	PLE/eosinophilic	Dijkstra et al [17], 2010
Boxer	GC	Simpson et al [18], 2006
French Bulldog	GC	Manchester et al [19], 2013
Irish Setter	Gluten sensitivity	Hall and Batt [20], 1992
Border Terrier	Gluten sensitivity	Black et al [21], 2014

Abbreviations: GC, granulomatous colitis; PLN, protein-losing nephropathy.

- Large intestinal disease is more frequently reported in dogs with FRE compared with those with IRE and PLE, as shown by a large cohort study: 86% of dogs with FRE had large intestinal involvement compared with only 10% and 0% in dogs with SRE and PLE, respectively [1]. Large intestinal disease is also common in dogs with ARE [24].
- Abdominal distention (peritoneal effusion), peripheral edema, and dyspnea/tachypnea (pleural effusion or pulmonary thromboembolism), are variably associated with severe hypoalbuminemia in PLE and are present with or without concurrent GI signs [3,25].
- The frequency of thromboembolism in dogs with PLE is unknown. Soft Coated Wheaten Terriers with PLE showed thromboembolism events in 18% of cases [15], whereas in a study of various breeds, thromboembolism was detected in 7.5% of cases [3]. Dogs with PLE occasionally present with acute paraparesis or paraplegia because of distal aortic thromboembolism [16].
- Rarely, dogs with PLE show seizures secondary to severe hypocalcemia [26].

Laboratory Work-up

- Thorough clinicopathologic testing is essential and helps to exclude other common causes of chronic GI signs (Table 2) including extraintestinal diseases.

Differences in Clinicopathologic Variables Between Chronic Inflammatory Enteropathy Phenotypes

- Hypoalbuminemia and hypocobalaminemia have been associated with disease severity and negative outcome.
- When comparing serum albumin and cobalamin concentrations across CIE subgroups, consistently, dogs with IRE have been found with significantly

TABLE 2
Differential Diagnoses (Rule-Outs) for Chronic Gastrointestinal Signs and Their Matching Diagnostic Test

Disease	Diagnostic Test
EPI	cTLI
Atypical hypoadrenocorticism	Basal cortisol, ACTHst
Chronic endoparasite infestation (eg, *Giardia* spp, *Cryptosporidium*)	Fecal flotation, ELISA, IFA, PCR
Adverse reaction to food (eg, food allergy, food intolerance)	Elimination diet trial and challenge
Gastrointestinal obstruction (eg, mechanical obstruction)	Abdominal radiography, abdominal ultrasonography, endoscopy, histopathology
Gastrointestinal neoplasia (eg, lymphoma)	Abdominal ultrasonography, cytology, histopathology, IHC, PARR
Granulomatous colitis	PAS staining, FISH, culture and antimicrobial sensitivity testing
Protothecosis (*Prototheca zopfii*)	Rectal scraping cytology, PAS staining, urine microscopy and/or culture, histopathology, PCR
Fungal granulomatous enterocolitis (histoplasmosis, pythiosis)	Cytology, GMS staining, histopathology, PCR, urinary antigen EIA
Hepatic functional impairment or failure[a]	Serum bile acid stimulation test, fecal α-1 protease inhibitor (possibly useful to confirm intestinal protein loss in dogs with concurrent hepatopathy), cystatin C, miRNA

Abbreviations: ACTHst, adrenocorticotropic hormone stimulation test; cTLI, canine trypsin like immunoreactivity; EIA, enzyme immunoassay; ELISA, enzyme-linked immunosorbent assay; EPI, exocrine pancreatic insufficiency; FISH, fluorescence in situ hybridization; GMS, Grocott methenamine silver; IFA, indirect immunofluorescence assay; IHC, immunohistochemistry; PARR, PCR for antigen receptor rearrangement; PAS, periodic acid–Schiff; PCR, polymerase chain reaction.

[a] If hypoalbuminemia with normal globulins, and/or hypocholesterolemia and/or low urea are present.

lower concentrations compared with dogs with FRE/ARE [1].

- In a recent abstract, the diagnostic value of serum folate alterations in 321 dogs with GI disorders was evaluated. Hypofolatemia was present in 30% and hyperfolatemia in 27% of dogs. However, serum folate did not differentiate between CIE and other GI conditions. In addition, when dogs were divided in CIE subgroups, no difference in folate was observed, and it was not associated with response to treatment and outcome [34].
- The reader is referred to the Romy M. Heilmann's article, "Important and Novel Laboratory Parameters and Biomarkers for Canine Chronic Enteropathy," in this issue for more details on laboratory and biologic markers in canine CIE.

Clinical Activity Indices in Canine Chronic Inflammatory Enteropathy

- In 2003, a Canine IBD Activity Index (CIBDAI) was validated in a population of 58 dogs and found to correlate well with markers of systemic inflammation before and after treatment [12].
- The score consists of six clinical variables (attitude/activity, appetite, vomiting, fecal consistency, frequency of defecation, and weight loss) that receive a numerical score from 0 (normal/absent) to 3 (severe). The cumulative score of the individual parameters reflects disease severity, ranging from insignificant (CIBDAI score 0–3), mild (score 4–5), moderate (score 6–8), to severe (score >9) [15].
- In 2007, the Canine Chronic Enteropathy Clinical Activity Index (CCECAI) was established in a population of 70 dogs [1]. This score is based on the CIBDAI but added two clinical parameters (pruritus and ascites/edema) and serum albumin values (>2.0 g/dL, score of 0; 15–19.9 g/L, score of 1; 1.2–1.49 g/dL, score of 2; <1.2 g/dL, score of 3). The total cumulative CCECAI score ranges from insignificant (score 0–3), mild (score 4–5), moderate (score 6–8), severe (score 9–11), to very severe (score >12).
- Median CCECAI correlates with disease phenotype (lower in dogs with FRE compared with IRE and PLE), and with negative outcome [1].
- Several clinical studies have used both CAIs to assess disease activity before and after treatment finding differences across CIE subgroups.
- They indicate that dogs with FRE and ARE are more likely to have mild disease (median CCECAI 5–8), whereas dogs with IRE or NRE have higher scores (median CCECAI 9–11).
- CAIs were able to retrospectively distinguish FRE (median CIBDAI 3, range 0–8; median CCECAI 5, range 2–10) from IRE and NRE PLE cases (median CIBDAI 10, range 4–17; median CCECAI 11, range 6–18) [35].

Abdominal Ultrasonography for Staging of Dogs with Chronic Inflammatory Enteropathy

- Although its diagnostic utility in dogs with chronic GI signs has recently been questioned [36,37], abdominal ultrasonography remains a useful tool to exclude other conditions and further characterize CIE.
- Despite low sensitivity for CIE, the finding of normal mucosal echogenicity in young dogs with mild clinical activity/severity makes FRE more likely, whereas finding of mucosal hyperechoic striation is highly predictive of intestinal lacteal dilation and PLE.
- Ultrasonography should be performed before GI endoscopy to rule out the presence of selective submucosal or muscular involvement or jejunal and proximal ileal regional disease, which can guide the recommended type of sampling.
- Most commonly, mild to moderate diffuse, transmural wall thickening with preservation of wall layering, increased mucosal echogenicity, and mild reactive lymphadenomegaly are reported with CIE [38].
- Selective thickening of the muscularis layer is believed to represent reactive hypertrophy. Loss of layering is seen with erosive disease, severe inflammatory infiltration, or neoplasia [38].
- Abdominal effusion, intestinal wall thickening, hyperechoic radial mucosal striations of the small intestine ("tiger stripes") (Fig. 2), and mesenteric lymphadenomegaly have all been associated with IL and PLE [38].
- Rule-outs for a focal intestinal mass with loss of layering (with or without mucosal changes) in dogs with hypoalbuminemia are lipogranulomatous lymphangitis, a rare form of primary IL, or neoplasia [39].
- In one study, a normal (hypoechoic) intestinal mucosa had a sensitivity of 80% and specificity of 81% for the diagnosis of FRE [40]. Hyperechoic mucosal striations had a sensitivity of 75% but a specificity of 96% for PLE, whereas hyperechoic speckles were nonspecific. There was a significant correlation between ultrasound score and CIBDAI before, but not following therapy [40].

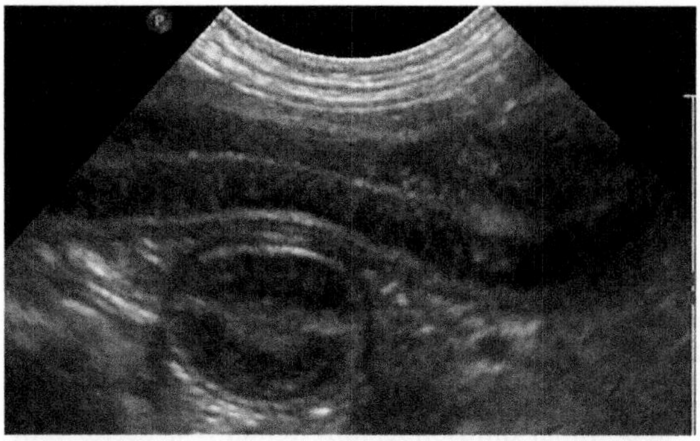

FIG. 2 Ultrasonographic image of hyperechoic mucosal striations. Several radial hyperechoic mucosal striations indicative of villous lymphangiectasia are visible, indicative of lacteal dilation (dog was diagnosed with PLE). (*Courtesy of* Prof. Alessia Diana, Department of Veterinary Medical Sciences, University of Bologna, Italy.)

Role of Endoscopy in Canine Chronic Inflammatory Enteropathy

- Endoscopy is an important diagnostic tool in dogs with idiopathic chronic GI signs, because it allows noninvasive assessment of the GI mucosa and targeted collection of mucosal biopsies for histopathologic examination.
- Endoscopy is not indicated immediately but should be reserved for dogs with severe CAI or those that have failed appropriate trials with therapeutic diets, but before immunosuppression is attempted.
- When evaluating endoscopic findings with CAI scores, clinicopathologic variables, and disease subgroups, a lack of correlation has been shown by several studies, with the exception of white mucosal spots correlating with lymphangiectasia [41].
- A qualitative endoscopic score has been validated in a population of 58 dogs with histologically moderate-to-severe CIE and achieved an excellent level of agreement among experienced operators [42].

Histopathology in Canine Chronic Inflammatory Enteropathy

- Histopathology is considered the diagnostic gold standard for canine CIE [10]. However, the accuracy and reliability of histopathology for the diagnosis of canine CIE seems to be hampered by several intrinsic and extrinsic factors including the lack of standardized and universally accepted diagnostic criteria; the subjectivity of histopathologic interpretation leading to an unacceptably poor agreement among different pathologists; and finally the negative impact of poor sampling and, postsampling processing standards on the diagnostic adequacy of biopsies [43–45].
- Several studies have shown a consistent lack of correlation of histopathology to CAIs, clinicopathologic variables, response to treatment, and outcome [1,12,46–48].
- In 2008, the World Small Animal Veterinary Association (WSAVA) GI Standardization Group developed pictorial and textual guidelines to standardize the evaluation of inflammatory and morphologic features in endoscopic biopsies obtained from the stomach, duodenum, and colon [49].
- However, these guidelines have not been universally accepted in subsequent studies and excessive interobserver variability persists.
- Recently, a simplified histopathologic model for defining GI inflammation in dogs and cats has been designed from additional analysis of the original WSAVA GI histopathologic templates [50].
- The model is based on those parameters for which the pathologists involved with the WSAVA GI group had strongest agreement. The parameters for the stomach are intraepithelial lymphocytes (IELs), lamina propria [LP] infiltrates, and mucosal fibrosis. The parameters for the duodenum are villus atrophy, epithelial injury, IELs, crypt changes, and LP infiltrates. The parameters for the colon are epithelial injury, crypt dilation, fibrosis, LP infiltrates, and goblet cell depletion [50].
- When tested (15 CIE dogs, 5 control animals), excellent agreement between different pathologists was achieved [50], and confirmed subsequently in a larger study (42 CIE dogs, 19 control animals) [51].
- In light of the current state of knowledge, the author performs endoscopy with GI mucosal biopsies only after antihelminthic, dietary, and probiotic trials have failed unless severe clinical disease or significant hypoalbuminemia are present.

Histopathologic Findings in Dogs with Hypoalbuminemia

- Several histopathologic findings have been variably reported to be associated with PLE. They include villus stunting, lacteal dilation, and crypt abscesses (Fig. 3) [52,53]. The latter has been found to be predictive of more severe hypoalbuminemia and negative outcome [53].
- A recent study evaluated histopathologic lesions predictive of hypoalbuminemia. Dilated lacteals were present in a high proportion of dogs overall (44/83; 53%), but they were more likely to be present

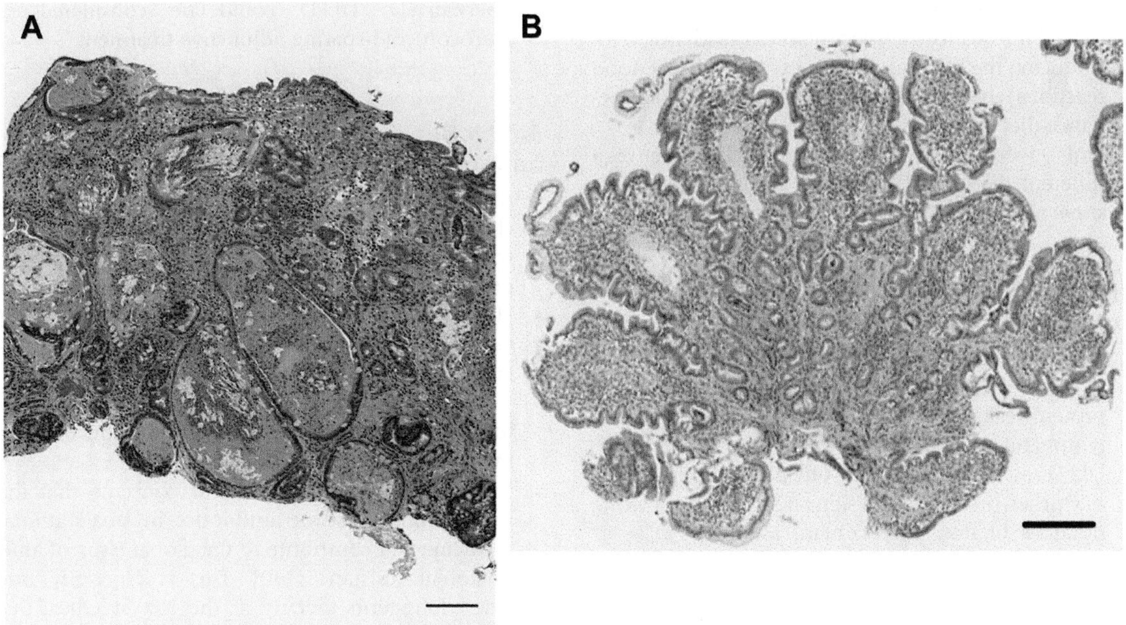

FIG. 3 Typical histologic findings in dogs with protein-losing enteropathy. (**A**) Multiple crypt abscesses with severely dilated intestinal crypts filled with mucus, sloughed epithelial cells, and inflammatory cells (hematoxylin and eosin, original magnification ×200; bar 100 μm). (**B**) villus blunting with mild to moderate villous lacteal dilation (hematoxylin and eosin, original magnification ×100; bar 250 μm). (*Courtesy of* Prof. Simon Priestnall, The Royal Veterinary College, London, UK.)

in hypoalbuminemic (76%) compared with normoalbuminemic dogs (35%). Crypt distention was found more often in dogs with hypoalbuminemia (65%) than normoalbuminemic dogs (10%), as was villous stunting, epithelial injury, number of IEL, and LP neutrophils. No differences in lymphoplasmacytic or eosinophilic infiltrates were found between the two groups [54].

- Morphologic abnormalities on histopathology, such as villus atrophy, lacteal dilation, and crypt disease, show superior correlation to disease severity than inflammatory infiltrates.

TREATMENT OF CANINE CHRONIC INFLAMMATORY ENTEROPATHY

General Considerations

- Sequential treatment trials with therapeutic diets, antibiotics, and ISDs used to be the standard of care in dogs with CIE (provided other conditions have been suitably ruled out) [1], and with the exception of antibiotics still are.
- This "step up" approach is perceived to be safer, because treatment modalities with a higher propensity for adverse reactions are given later.
- This is also supported by the evidence that most dogs with CIE (55%–67%) have FRE [1,6,7].
- Deviations from this strategy might be considered in severe clinical disease or the presence of negative prognostic indicators.

Therapeutic Diets

- Diets that have shown efficacy in canine CIE include (1) single (often novel) selected protein and carbohydrate diets, (2) hydrolyzed protein diets, (3) highly digestible diets (4) low-fat diets, and (5) home cooked ultralow-fat diet (ULFD) [55].
- The exact mechanisms by which therapeutic diets induce clinical remission are unknown, but are thought to include reduced immunogenicity, elimination of dietary allergens, improved digestibility, and modulation of intestinal microbiota.
- Clinical remission is achieved swiftly with most FRE cases improving within 7 to 14 days [1,6,56].

- When improvement is achieved, it is recommended to feed the diet for 12 weeks before considering reintroducing the original diet (to exclude adverse food reactions) or switching to a commercial maintenance diet [1].
- Only a few studies allow comparison between different diets in CIE. Overall, single protein diets show similar response rates to hydrolyzed diets.

Dietary Management of Protein-Losing Enteropathy

- ULFDs and low-fat diets are typically recommended in cases of PLE. Fat-restricted diets reduce intestinal protein leakage decreasing lymph production and lymphatic pressure.
- ULFDs are usually made by one part of white turkey or chicken breast without skin and two parts of white potatoes or rice. They contain as low as 0.36 g/100 kcal and are nutritionally complete if formulated by a qualified veterinary nutritionist [3,55], which is recommended.
- Theoretically, a restricted antigen or hydrolyzed diet could be equally appropriate, because increased mucosal permeability could increase the immunogenicity of dietary antigens [3]. However, this distinction cannot be made in individual cases. Because particularly hydrolyzed diets are often high in fat content, empirical diet choice is sometimes required.
- Traditionally, concurrent use of glucocorticoids and second-line agents (azathioprine, cyclosporine, chlorambucil) has been advocated in dogs with PLE [3,25]. However, recent evidence seems to refute these recommendations [57].
- In a substantial number of dogs (Yorkshire terriers, but also other breeds) with PLE, clinical remission and significant improvement of serum albumin values are achieved with sole dietary intervention (80% of cases) [58], to the point that prednisolone dosage could be decreased after introduction of a ULFD [57].
- In a recent retrospective cohort study [35], dogs with food-responsive PLE were significantly younger (mean age, 7.5 vs 10.4 years), had lower CIBDAI (median score, 3 vs 10) and CCECAI (median, 5 vs 11) scores, and a better prognosis than dogs needing immunosuppressants [35].
- In light of these studies it seems reasonable to offer a trial with a ULFD as a first treatment step or even as a rescue treatment in refractory PLE and to expect a significant improvement within 1 to 2 weeks.
- Alternatively, ULFD could be considered as glucocorticoid-sparing adjunctive treatment.

Antibiotics and Canine Chronic Inflammatory Enteropathy

- Antibiotics have been used to manage idiopathic chronic GI signs in dogs for decades [9,10], and traditionally included metronidazole, tylosin, oxytetracycline, or rifaximin.
- However, recent and mounting evidence shows that use of antibiotics can induce a pattern of dysbiosis largely comparable with the one found in dogs with CIE and that such dysbiotic effect can persist for several weeks beyond the interruption of treatment [59].
- In addition, there are justified concerns that the indiscriminate use of antibiotics in small animal medicine will contribute to the global issue of antimicrobial resistance [60]. This is especially true when long-term therapy at the lowest efficacious dose is recommended [24,61].
- Given the modest prevalence of 10% to 16% for ARE among all CIE cases [6,7], the frequency of relapses as soon as antibiotics are discontinued, and that one study reported none of the 32 dogs diagnosed with ARE to be in remission at 12 months after the diagnosis [6], antibiotic trials should probably not remain part of the diagnostic and treatment strategy of canine CIE [62], but only be considered if all other treatment options have been explored (Fig. 4).
- No studies have evaluated a superior efficacy of antibiotics compared with other treatment modalities by means of randomized clinical trials (RCT), whereas one RCT comparing metronidazole + prednisolone versus prednisolone alone found no difference in short-term clinical remission [63,64].

Antibiotics and Protein-Losing Enteropathy

- Antibiotics are almost always present in the treatment protocols in published studies of canine PLE, but there is no evidence regarding their contribution to clinical remission and survival.
- Although one rationale for use of antibiotics could be to reduce the risks of bacteremia and sepsis from translocation of luminal bacteria across a severely impaired and permeable intestinal mucosa, one study demonstrated that crypt abscesses are sterile (using fluorescence in situ hybridization) [65].

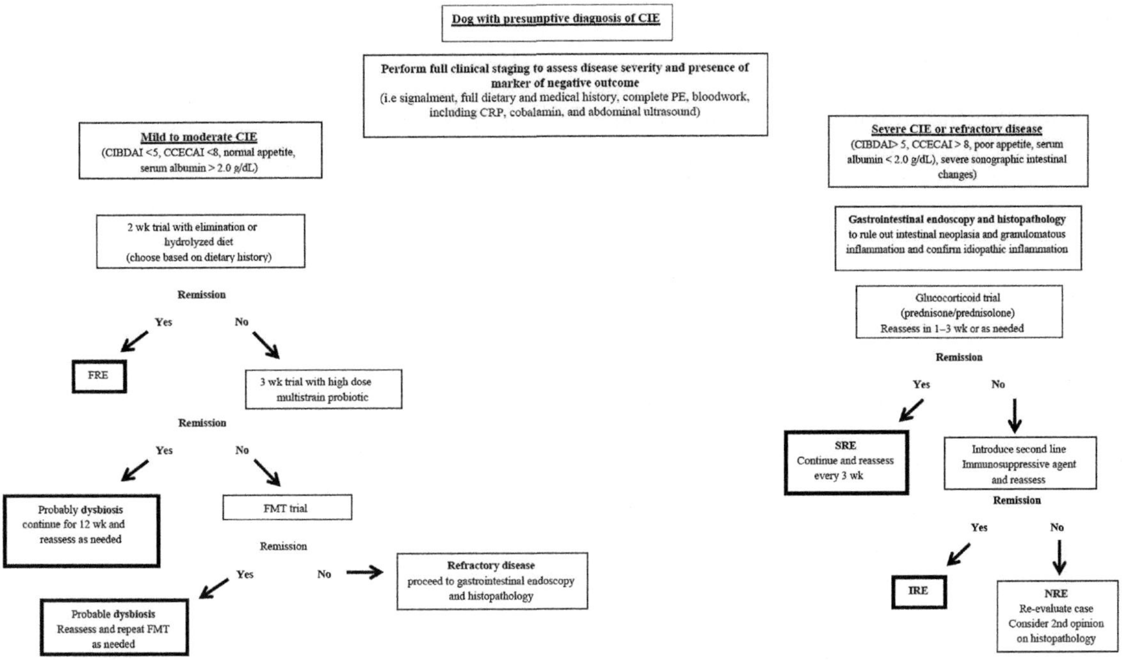

FIG. 4 Proposed treatment approach for dogs with CIE without hypoalbuminemia. Dogs with mild to moderate disease undergo sequential trials with therapeutic diet, alternative treatments (eg, probiotics), and immunosuppressives (endoscopy with biopsies should be performed before the latter). CRP, C-reactive protein; FMT, fecal microbiota transplantation; PE, physical examination.

Immunosuppressive Drugs and Chronic Inflammatory Enteropathy

- ISDs are the mainstay therapy with human IBD and are used for induction and maintenance of remission in canine IRE. They include glucocorticoids (prednisone, prednisolone, budesonide), cyclosporine, azathioprine, chlorambucil, mycophenolate mofetil, and others.
- ISDs should only be used after trials with therapeutic diets or alternative treatments have failed and GI biopsies have been histologically assessed.
- ISDs used include glucocorticoids and second-line agents, the latter used as alternative or in addition to glucocorticoids. Guidelines for the use of second-line agents are not available for dogs, but they are often used empirically in severe or refractory cases or as "glucocorticoid-sparing" drugs.
- Assessing true efficacy of glucocorticoids in canine CIE is difficult because of the paucity of well-conducted RCTs and the lack of treatment standardization across studies [29]. Overall, efficacy of glucocorticoids alone seems to be around 20%, whereas 10% to 18% of dogs with CIE have intractable disease (NRE).
- When comparing prednisone with budesonide, no significant difference in remission rate (69% with prednisone, 78% in the budesonide group) is reported [66].
- Evidence regarding the efficacy of second-line ISD in canine IRE is scarce. An older study reported improvement of clinical signs in 12 of 14 steroid-refractory dogs (85%) with cyclosporine [67].
- However, in a later study, only 2 of 8 steroid-refractory dogs receiving cyclosporine achieved remission, whereas the other 6 were euthanized [1].

Immunosuppressive Drugs and Protein-Losing Enteropathy

- Because of the severity of the clinical presentation and the notoriously poor prognosis, dogs with PLE are often treated aggressively with a combination of diet and either glucocorticoids alone or with the addition of one or more second-line ISDs as mentioned previously [3,25].

- No RCTs have compared efficacy of single ISDs in dogs with PLE. However, early studies suggest that cyclosporine could be superior to prednisone alone [1], whereas a more recent study found no difference in remission rate or duration between PLE dogs treated with glucocorticoids alone versus the addition of cyclosporine.
- A significantly greater survival rate was found in a retrospective cohort study comparing the combination of chlorambucil/prednisolone (10/14 dogs) with azathioprine/prednisolone (2/13 dogs) [68].
- Based on the available evidence, it seems reasonable to adopt a staged approach for PLE (Fig. 5), similar to treating CIE without hypoalbuminemia, where the respective decision to introduce glucocorticoids or a second-line ISD is made after an appropriate time (ie, 1–2 weeks) to assess treatment response.

ASSESSING TREATMENT RESPONSE IN CANINE CHRONIC INFLAMMATORY ENTEROPATHY: TREAT TO TARGET

- Clinical remission remains the universally accepted goal of therapy. Most studies have shown a lack of correlation between clinical signs and endoscopic and histopathologic scores 6 to 12 weeks after treatment. It remains to be ascertained whether this indicates ongoing subclinical disease and has implications on long-term outcome.
- Since their validation, CAIs have become the preferred means of measuring disease remission. Complete remission is usually defined as a reduction in CAIs score of greater than 75% from pretreatment to post-treatment, partial remission as a decline between 75% and 50% of baseline, and treatment failure a reduction of less than 25% [1,12].

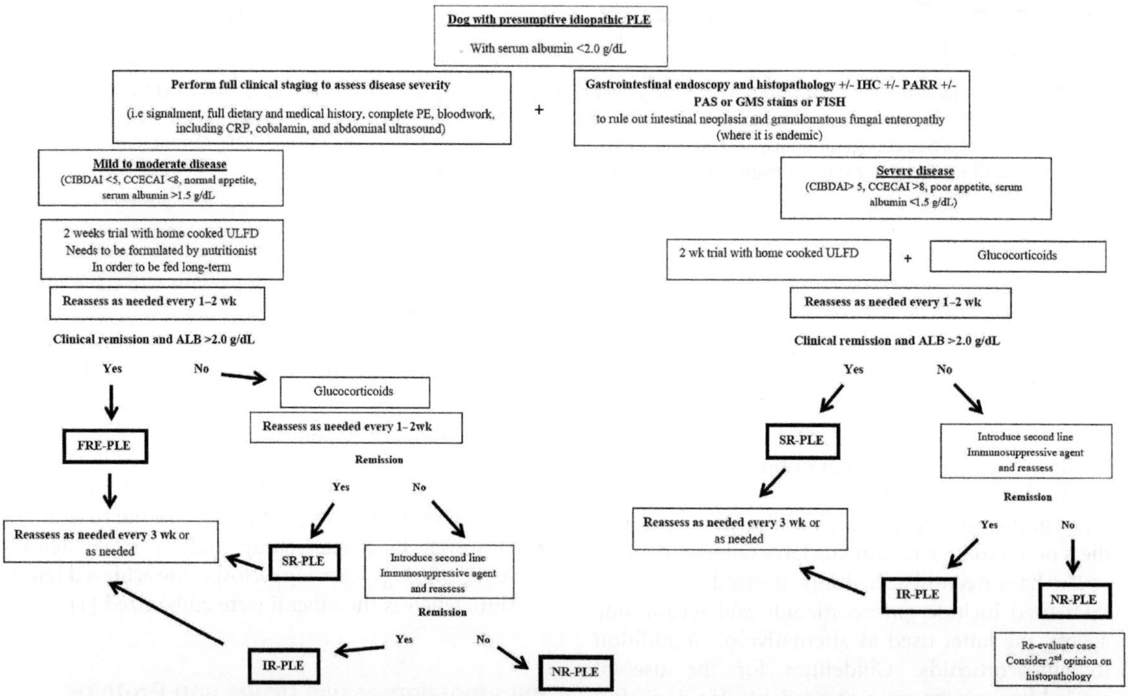

FIG. 5 Proposed treatment approach for dogs with PLE. Dogs with mild PLE undergo sequential treatment with a balanced home-cooked ULFD or commercial low-fat diet, followed by immunosuppression (glucocorticoids followed by a second-line ISD). Dogs with severe PLE should receive ULFD and glucocorticoids concurrently, with second-line ISD introduced in the absence of clinical or biochemical remission. ALB, serum albumin; FISH, fluorescence in situ hybridization; FR, food responsive; GMS, Grocott methenamine silver; IHC, immunohistochemistry; IR, immunosuppressive-responsive; NR, nonresponsive; PARR, polymerase chain reaction for antigen receptor rearrangement; PAS, periodic acid–Schiff; SR, steroid-responsive.

- For PLE, remission is typically defined as biochemical improvement: serum albumin within the reference range, although values at or just less than the lower end of the reference interval, are considered acceptable, especially if complete clinical remission is present.

PROGNOSIS AND LONG-TERM OUTCOME IN CANINE CHRONIC INFLAMMATORY ENTEROPATHY

- One study indicated that 3 years after start of treatment 38/39 dogs with FRE were in remission (97%) compared with 12/21 (53%) dogs with IRE. The overall mortality rate was 13/70 (18%) [1]. A subsequent study found 66% of dogs with FRE were in remission at 12 months compared with 20% of dogs with IRE [7].
- One study followed up 203 dogs with CIE (131 FRE, 39 IRE, and 33 ARE) and revealed that none of the ARE dogs were in remission at 12 months from starting antibiotic treatment and they had all been transitioned onto ISDs [6].
- When looking at IRE dogs only, 26% were reported in full remission after 14 to 19 months, 50% of dogs had intermittent clinical signs, and 4% had uncontrolled disease in a recent study. Ten dogs (13%) were euthanized because of refractory disease [29].
- Several markers have been associated to negative outcome in CIE (Table 3).
- Decreased 25 hydroxyvitamin D (25-[OH]D_3) has been shown to predict negative outcome in dogs with CIE with or without hypoalbuminemia [32,33], and to correlate with higher CCECAI scores, higher serum C-reactive protein, and lower serum albumin concentrations [69].
- However, causality between low serum 25-(OH)D_3 and severity of mucosal disease has not been established. Hence it remains unclear if vitamin D supplementation will influence CIE or PLE outcome positively.

Long-Term Outcome in Protein-Losing Enteropathy

- Even though there are breed-associated variations, response rates in PLE overall range between 35% and 60%, whereas median survival times between 45 days and 5 months have been reported.
- Serum C-reactive protein, urea, and α1-proteinase inhibitor concentrations are associated to negative outcome, as is clonality of T-cell receptors on PCR for antigen-receptor rearrangement, and increased CIBDAI [27,28,30].
- PLE has a poor long-term prognosis because of severity of disease, refractoriness to treatment, and

TABLE 3
Negative Prognostic Indicators in Dogs with CIE ± PLE

Variable	CE Subgroup	Reference
CIBDAI	CIE, PLE	Allenspach et al [1], 2007, Nakashima et al [27], 2015
CCECAI	CIE, PLE	Allenspach et al [1], 2007, Kathrani et al [28], 2019
Hct	CIE	Volkmann et al [7], 2017
Hypoalbuminemia	CIE, PLE	Allenspach et al [1], 2007, Volkmann et al [7], 2017, Simmerson et al [16], 2014
Hypocobalaminemia	CIE	Allenspach et al [1], 2007
CRP	CIE, PLE	Craven et al [29], 2004, Equilino et al [30], 2015
Spec cPL	CIE	Kathrani et al [31], 2009
Increased urea	PLE	Nakashima et al [27], 2015, Kathrani et al [28], 2019
Decreased urea	PLE	Simmerson et al [16], 2014
Decreased 25(OH)D_3	CIE, PLE	Titmarsh et al [32], 2015, Allenspach et al [33], 2017

Abbreviations: 25(OH)D_3, 25-hydroxy vitamin D; CRP, C-reactive protein; Hct, hematocrit.

high rate of complications [3], but some dogs experience long-term survival.

ALTERNATIVE AND NOVEL TREATMENT OPTIONS

- The role of intestinal microbiota in the pathogenesis of canine CIE has been established. (See Jan S. Suchodolski's article, "The Intestinal Microbiome in Canine Chronic Enteropathy and Implications for Extra-Intestinal Disorders," in this issue.) In addition, considering the detrimental effects of antibiotics on intestinal microbiota, alternative treatment options have been sought.
- Despite the widespread use of probiotics in small animals with gut disease, scientific evidence of their beneficial effects in canine CIE is scarce and contrasting.
- Some evidence exists that high-dose multistrain probiotics are equally able than glucocorticoids to induce short-term remission in dogs with IRE, whereas the use of single-strain probiotics is not supported [70–73].
- The overall effect on microbiota composition and function from probiotics is negligible; however, there might be some improvement of intestinal barrier function [71].
- Fecal microbiota transplantation has been used anecdotally for the management of canine CIE, but results are variable and evidence-based data are lacking.[74–76]
- Mesenchymal stem cells have been used in small cohort studies, and their intravenous application led to clinical remission in 9/11 dogs, but histologic remission was not achieved [77].
- Larger sized RCTs are needed to confirm efficacy and best application of alternative and novel treatments in CIE.

SUMMARY

- Although FRE, ARE, and IRE carry a good to excellent short-term prognosis, response to treatment seems to be sustained only in FRE cases, indicating the need of alternative or improved treatment strategies for ARE, IRE, and NRE.
- A food-responsive phenotype of PLE has been described, supporting the use of sequential treatment strategies in this form of CIE.
- Validated CAIs allow reliable assessment of disease severity and response to treatment, and seem to correlate with long-term outcome.
- The clinical utility of GI endoscopy and histopathology has been questioned, but recent progress has been made in standardization of these diagnostic tools.
- Several clinical and laboratory prognostic markers have been described in the literature of which decreased 25(OH)D_3 merits further attention.
- Use of antibiotics in canine CIE is controversial and no longer recommended before anti-inflammatory treatment.
- Alternative treatment options could include multistrain probiotics, whereas data on fecal microbiota transplantation and the use of mesenchymal stem cells are patchier and require further assessment.

DISCLOSURE

The author has nothing to disclose.

REFERENCES

[1] Allenspach K, Wieland B, Grone A, et al. Chronic enteropathies in dogs: evaluation of risk factors for negative outcome. J Vet Intern Med 2007;21(4):700–8.

[2] Dandrieux JRS. Inflammatory bowel disease versus chronic enteropathy in dogs: are they one and the same? J Small Anim Pract 2016;57(11):589–99.

[3] Peterson PB, Willard MD. Protein-losing enteropathies. Vet Clin North Am Small Anim Pract 2003;33(5):1061–82.

[4] Allenspach K. Clinical immunology and immunopathology of the canine and feline intestine. Vet Clin North Am Small Anim Pract 2011;41(2):345–60.

[5] Mandigers PJ, Biourge V, Van Den Ingh TS, et al. A randomized, open-label, positively controlled field trial of a hydrolyzed protein diet in dogs with chronic small bowel enteropathy. J Vet Intern Med 2010;24(6):1350–7.

[6] Allenspach K, Culverwell C, Chan D. Long-term outcome in dogs with chronic enteropathies: 203 cases. Vet Rec 2016;178(15):362–8.

[7] Volkmann M, Steiner JM, Fosgate GT, et al. Chronic diarrhea in dogs: retrospective study in 136 cases. J Vet Intern Med 2017;31(4):1043–55.

[8] Batt RM, Needham JR, Carter MW. Bacterial overgrowth associated with a naturally occurring enteropathy in the German shepherd dog. Res Vet Sci 1983;35(1):42–6.

[9] German AJ, Day MJ, Ruaux CG, et al. Comparison of direct and indirect tests for small intestinal bacterial overgrowth and antibiotic-responsive diarrhea in dogs. J Vet Intern Med 2003;17(1):33–43.

[10] Simpson KW, Jergens AE. Pitfalls and progress in the diagnosis and management of canine inflammatory

bowel disease. Vet Clin North Am Small Anim Pract 2011;41(2):381–98.
[11] Craven MD, Washabau RJ. Comparative pathophysiology and management of protein-losing enteropathy. J Vet Intern Med 2019;33(2):383–402.
[12] Jergens AE, Schreiner CA, Frank DE, et al. A scoring index for disease activity in canine inflammatory bowel disease. J Vet Intern Med 2003;17(3):291–7.
[13] Breitschwerdt EB, Ochoa R, Barta M, et al. Clinical and laboratory characterization of Basenjis with immunoproliferative small intestinal disease. Am J Vet Res 1984; 45(2):267–73.
[14] Kolbjørnsen O, Press CM, Landsverk T. Gastropathies in the Lundehund. I. Gastritis and gastric neoplasia associated with intestinal lymphangiectasia. APMIS 1994; 102(9):647–61.
[15] Littman MP, Dambach DM, Vaden SL, et al. Familial protein-losing enteropathy and protein-losing nephropathy in Soft Coated Wheaten Terriers: 222 cases (1983-1997). J Vet Intern Med 2000;14(1):68–80.
[16] Simmerson SM, Armstrong PJ, Wünschmann A, et al. Clinical features, intestinal histopathology, and outcome in protein-losing enteropathy in Yorkshire Terrier dogs. J Vet Intern Med 2014;28(2):331–7.
[17] Dijkstra M, Kraus JS, Bosje JT, et al. Protein-losing enteropathy in Rottweilers. Tijdschr Diergeneeskd 2010; 135(10):406–12.
[18] Simpson KW, Dogan B, Rishniw M, et al. Adherent and invasive *Escherichia coli* is associated with granulomatous colitis in boxer dogs. Infect Immun 2006;74(8): 4778–92.
[19] Manchester AC, Hill S, Sabatino B, et al. Association between granulomatous colitis in French Bulldogs and invasive *Escherichia coli* and response to fluoroquinolone antimicrobials. J Vet Intern Med 2013;27(1): 56–61.
[20] Hall EJ, Batt RM. Dietary modulation of gluten sensitivity in a naturally occurring enteropathy of Irish setter dogs. Gut 1992;33(2):198–205.
[21] Black V, Garosi L, Lowrie M, et al. Phenotypic characterisation of canine epileptoid cramping syndrome in the Border terrier. J Small Anim Pract 2014;55(2): 102–7.
[22] Kather S, Grützner N, Kook PH, et al. Review of cobalamin status and disorders of cobalamin metabolism in dogs. J Vet Intern Med 2020;34(1):13–28.
[23] Luckschander N, Allenspach K, Hall J, et al. Perinuclear antineutrophilic cytoplasmic antibody and response to treatment in diarrheic dogs with food responsive disease or inflammatory bowel disease. J Vet Intern Med 2006; 20(2):221–7.
[24] Hall EJ. Antibiotic-responsive diarrhea in small animals. Vet Clin North Am Small Anim Pract 2011;41(2): 273–86.
[25] Dossin O, Lavoué R. Protein-losing enteropathies in dogs. Vet Clin North Am Small Anim Pract 2011;41(2): 399–418.
[26] Whitehead J, Quimby J, Bayliss D. Seizures associated with hypocalcemia in a Yorkshire Terrier with protein-losing enteropathy. J Am Anim Hosp Assoc 2015; 51(6):380–4.
[27] Nakashima K, Hiyoshi S, Ohno K, et al. Prognostic factors in dogs with protein-losing enteropathy. Vet J 2015;205(1):28–32.
[28] Kathrani A, Sánchez-Vizcaíno F, Hall EJ. Association of chronic enteropathy activity index, blood urea concentration, and risk of death in dogs with protein-losing enteropathy. J Vet Intern Med 2019;33(2):536–43.
[29] Craven M, Simpson JW, Ridyard AE, et al. Canine inflammatory bowel disease: retrospective analysis of diagnosis and outcome in 80 cases (1995-2002). J Small Anim Pract 2004;45(7):336–42.
[30] Equilino M, Theodoloz V, Gorgas D, et al. Evaluation of serum biochemical marker concentrations and survival time in dogs with protein-losing enteropathy. J Am Vet Med Assoc 2015;246(1):91–9.
[31] Kathrani A, Steiner JM, Suchodolski J, et al. Elevated canine pancreatic lipase immunoreactivity concentration in dogs with inflammatory bowel disease is associated with a negative outcome. J Small Anim Pract 2009; 50(3):126–32.
[32] Titmarsh H, Gow AG, Kilpatrick S, et al. Association of Vitamin D status and clinical outcome in dogs with a chronic enteropathy. J Vet Intern Med 2015;29(6): 1473–8.
[33] Allenspach K, Rizzo J, Jergens AE, et al. Hypovitaminosis D is associated with negative outcome in dogs with protein losing enteropathy: a retrospective study of 43 cases. BMC Vet Res 2017;13(1):96.
[34] Petrelli A, Salavati-Schmitz S. Is measuring serum folate pointless? Retrospective analysis of prevalence and clinical significance of hypo- or hyperfolataemia in dogs with chronic enteropathies. J Vet Intern Med 2020;34: 341.
[35] Nagata N, Ohta H, Yokoyama N, et al. Clinical characteristics of dogs with food-responsive protein-losing enteropathy. J Vet Intern Med 2020;34(2):659–68.
[36] Leib MS, Larson MM, Grant DC, et al. Diagnostic utility of abdominal ultrasonography in dogs with chronic diarrhea. J Vet Intern Med 2012;26(6):1288–94.
[37] Mapletoft EK, Allenspach K, Lamb CR. How useful is abdominal ultrasonography in dogs with diarrhoea? J Small Anim Pract 2018;59(1):32–7.
[38] Gaschen L. Ultrasonography of small intestinal inflammatory and neoplastic diseases in dogs and cats. Vet Clin North Am Small Anim Pract 2011; 41(2):329–44.
[39] Watson VE, Hobday MM, Durham AC. Focal intestinal lipogranulomatous lymphangitis in 6 dogs (2008-2011). J Vet Intern Med 2014;28(1):48–51.
[40] Gaschen L, Kircher P, Stüssi A, et al. Comparison of ultrasonographic findings with clinical activity index (CIBDAI) and diagnosis in dogs with chronic enteropathies. Vet Radiol Ultrasound 2008;49(1):56–64.

[41] Larson RNN, Ginn JAA, Bell CMM, et al. Duodenal endoscopic findings and histopathologic confirmation of intestinal lymphangiectasia in dogs. J Vet Intern Med 2012;26(5):1087–92.
[42] Slovak JE, Wang C, Sun Y, et al. Development and validation of an endoscopic activity score for canine inflammatory bowel disease. Vet J 2015;203(3):290–5.
[43] Willard MD, Jergens AE, Duncan RB, et al. Interobserver variation among histopathologic evaluations of intestinal tissues from dogs and cats. J Am Vet Med Assoc 2002;220(8):1177–82.
[44] Willard MD, Moore GE, Denton BD, et al. Effect of tissue processing on assessment of endoscopic intestinal biopsies in dogs and cats. J Vet Intern Med 2010; 24(1):84–9.
[45] Willard MD, Mansell J, Fosgate GT, et al. Effect of sample quality on the sensitivity of endoscopic biopsy for detecting gastric and duodenal lesions in dogs and cats. J Vet Intern Med 2008;22(5):1084–9.
[46] Willard M, Mansell J. Correlating clinical activity and histopathologic assessment of gastrointestinal lesion severity: current challenges. Vet Clin North Am Small Anim Pract 2011;41(2):457–63.
[47] Roth L, Leib MS, Davenport DJ, et al. Comparisons between endoscopic and histologic evaluation of the gastrointestinal tract in dogs and cats: 75 cases (1984-1987). J Am Vet Med Assoc 1990;196(4):635–8.
[48] García-Sancho M, Rodríguez-Franco F, Sainz A, et al. Evaluation of clinical, macroscopic, and histopathologic response to treatment in non-hypoproteinemic dogs with lymphocytic-plasmacytic enteritis. J Vet Intern Med 2007;21(1):11–7.
[49] Day MJ, Bilzer T, Mansell J, et al. Histopathological standards for the diagnosis of gastrointestinal inflammation in endoscopic biopsy samples from the dog and cat: a report from the World Small Animal Veterinary Association Gastrointestinal Standardization Group. J Comp Pathol 2008;138(Suppl 1):S1–43.
[50] Jergens AE, Evans RB, Ackermann M, et al. Design of a simplified histopathologic model for gastrointestinal inflammation in dogs. Vet Pathol 2014;51(5):946–50.
[51] Allenspach KA, Mochel JP, Du Y, et al. Correlating gastrointestinal histopathologic changes to clinical disease activity in dogs with idiopathic inflammatory bowel disease. Vet Pathol 2019;56(3):435–43.
[52] Willard MD, Helman G, Franking JM, et al. Intestinal crypt lesions associated with protein-losing enteropathy in the dog. J Vet Intern Med 2000;14:298–307.
[53] Stroda K, Wakamatsu N, Gaschen L, et al. Histopathological, clinical, endoscopic, and ultrasound features of dogs with chronic enteropathies and small intestinal crypt lesions. J Vet Intern Med 2012;26:767–8.
[54] Wennogle SA, Priestnall SL, Webb CB. Histopathologic characteristics of intestinal biopsy samples from dogs with chronic inflammatory enteropathy with and without hypoalbuminemia. J Vet Intern Med 2017; 31(2):371–6.
[55] Rudinsky AJ, Rowe JC, Parker VJ. Nutritional management of chronic enteropathies in dogs and cats. J Am Vet Med Assoc 2018;253(5):570–8.
[56] Heilmann RM, Berghoff N, Mansell J, et al. Association of fecal calprotectin concentrations with disease severity, response to treatment, and other biomarkers in dogs with chronic inflammatory enteropathies. J Vet Intern Med 2018;32(2):679–92.
[57] Okanishi H, Yoshioka R, Kagawa Y, et al. The clinical efficacy of dietary fat restriction in treatment of dogs with intestinal lymphangiectasia. J Vet Intern Med 2014; 28(3):809–17.
[58] Rudinsky AJ, Howard JP, Bishop MA, et al. Dietary management of presumptive protein-losing enteropathy in Yorkshire terriers. J Small Anim Pract 2017;58(2):103–8.
[59] Manchester AC, Webb CB, Blake AB, et al. Long-term impact of tylosin on fecal microbiota and fecal bile acids of healthy dogs. J Vet Intern Med 2019;33(6):2605–17.
[60] Nguyen GC. Tip of the iceberg?: the emergence of antibiotic-resistant organisms in the IBD population. Gut Microbes 2012;3(5):434–6.
[61] Kilpinen S, Spillmann T, Westermarck E. Efficacy of two low-dose oral tylosin regimens in controlling the relapse of diarrhea in dogs with tylosin-responsive diarrhea: a prospective, single-blinded, two arm parallel, clinical field trial. Acta Vet Scand 2014;56:43.
[62] Cerquetella M, Rossi G, Suchodolski JS, et al. Proposal for rational antibacterial use in the diagnosis and treatment of dogs with chronic diarrhoea. J Small Anim Pract 2020;61:211–5.
[63] Jergens AE, Crandell J, Morrison JA, et al. Comparison of oral prednisone and prednisone combined with metronidazole for induction therapy of canine inflammatory bowel disease: a randomized controlled trial. J Vet Intern Med 2010;24(2):269–77.
[64] Menozzi A, Dall'Aglio M, Quintavalla F, et al. Rifaximin is an effective alternative to metronidazole for the treatment of chronic enteropathy in dogs: a randomised trial. BMC Vet Res 2016;12(1):217.
[65] Craven MD, Duhamel GE, Sutter NB, et al. Absence of bacterial association in Yorkshire terriers with protein losing enteropathy and cystic intestinal crypts. J Vet Intern Med 2009;23:757.
[66] Dye TL, Diehl KJ, Wheeler SL, et al. Randomized, controlled trial of budesonide and prednisone for the treatment of idiopathic inflammatory bowel disease in dogs. J Vet Intern Med 2013;27(6):1385–91.
[67] Allenspach K, Rufenacht S, Sauter S, et al. Pharmacokinetics and clinical efficacy of cyclosporine treatment of dogs with steroid-refractory inflammatory bowel disease. J Vet Intern Med 2006;20(2):239–44.
[68] Dandrieux JR, Noble PJ, Scase TJ, et al. Comparison of a chlorambucil-prednisolone combination with an azathioprine-prednisolone combination for treatment of chronic enteropathy with concurrent protein-losing enteropathy in dogs: 27 cases (2007-2010). J Am Vet Med Assoc 2013;242(12):1705–14.

[69] Wennogle SA, Priestnall SL, Suárez-Bonnet A, et al. Comparison of clinical, clinicopathologic, and histologic variables in dogs with chronic inflammatory enteropathy and low or normal serum 25-hydroxycholecalciferol concentrations. J Vet Intern Med 2019; 33(5):1995–2004.
[70] Rossi G, Pengo G, Caldin M, et al. Comparison of microbiological, histological, and immunomodulatory parameters in response to treatment with either combination therapy with prednisone and metronidazole or probiotic VSL#3 strains in dogs with idiopathic inflammatory bowel disease. PLoS One 2014;9:e94699.
[71] White R, Atherly T, Guard B, et al. Randomized, controlled trial evaluating the effect of multi-strain probiotic on the mucosal microbiota in canine idiopathic inflammatory bowel disease. Gut Microbes 2017;3(8): 451–66.
[72] Sauter SN, Benyacoub J, Allenspach K, et al. Effects of probiotic bacteria in dogs with food responsive diarrhoea treated with an elimination diet. J Anim Physiol Anim Nutr (Berl) 2006;90(7–8):269–77.
[73] Schmitz S, Glanemann B, Garden OA, et al. A prospective, randomized, blinded, placebo-controlled pilot study on the effect of *Enterococcus faecium* on clinical activity and intestinal gene expression in canine food-responsive chronic enteropathy. J Vet Intern Med 2015;29(2):533–43.
[74] Burton EN, O'Connor E, Ericsson AC, et al. Evaluation of fecal microbiota transfer as treatment for postweaning diarrhea in research-colony puppies. J Am Assoc Lab Anim Sci 2016;55(5):582–7.
[75] Pereira GQ, Gomes LA, Santos IS, et al. Fecal microbiota transplantation in puppies with canine parvovirus infection. J Vet Intern Med 2018;32(2):707–11.
[76] Murphy T, Chaitman J, Han E. Use of fecal transplant in eight dogs with refractory *Clostridium perfringens* associated diarrhea. J Vet Intern Med 2014;28:976.
[77] Pérez-Merino EM, Usón-Casaús JM, Hermida-Prieto M, et al. Correlation between canine inflammatory bowel disease activity indices after stem cell therapy. Vet Rec 2016;179(18):464, 2–464.

Infectious Disease

Advances in Small Animal Care 1 (2020) 143–160
ADVANCES IN SMALL ANIMAL CARE

Enteric Viruses of Dogs

Nicola Decaro, DVM, PhD, DipECVM
Department of Veterinary Medicine, University of Bari, Strada Prov. per Casamassima Km 3, 70010 Valenzano, Bari, Italy

KEYWORDS
• Dogs • Viral enteritis • Causal agents • Clinical signs • Diagnosis • Prophylaxis

KEY POINTS

- Several viruses are involved in the occurrence of acute enteritis in dogs, which is a very common disease in juvenile puppies.
- The role of traditional viral agents, such as canine parvovirus, canine coronavirus, and canine rotaviruses, in viral enteritis of dogs is well known.
- Emerging viruses have been discovered in recent decades, mainly thanks to advanced molecular methods, including next-generation sequencing.
- Antiviral drugs have not been developed against any enteric virus, so treatment of canine viral enteritis is mainly supportive, aiming to restore fluids and electrolytic balance and to prevent concurrent infections by opportunistic bacteria.
- Vaccines are available only against canine parvovirus because most other enteric viruses lack firm evidence for their involvement in canine enteritis or are only sporadically associated with acute diarrhea in dogs.

INTRODUCTION

Canine infectious enteritis is a common cause of dogs' presentation to veterinary clinics and hospitalization. Although different microbial agents are involved in the occurrence of enteritis in dogs, viruses represent the most frequently detected pathogens. In addition to well-recognized viruses, including canine parvovirus, canine coronavirus, and canine rotaviruses, emerging viral agents have been tentatively associated with canine acute diarrhea in recent decades. These viral agents include caliciviruses (noroviruses, sapoviruses, vesiviruses), astroviruses, circoviruses, kobuviruses, and other recently discovered viruses whose pathogenic potential is still largely unknown. Other viruses, such as canine distemper virus and canine adenovirus type 1, usually lead to the onset of severe gastroenteritis, but the involvement of the gastroenteric tract is a consequence of systemic infections involving complex pathogenetic mechanisms and multiorgan failure. Therefore, these viral agents are not discussed in the present article.

Clinical presentation of canine viral enteritis may vary among infections caused by different enteric viruses, with the most severe forms observed during canine parvovirus infections. The causal diagnosis can take advantage of rapid in-clinic assay only for a few of these viruses, but highly sensitive and specific molecular tools invariably represent the gold standard. Treatment of canine viral enteritis is mainly supportive because no specific antiviral drugs are available. Effective vaccines have been licensed only for canine parvovirus, considering that the other viral enteropathogens are only sporadically involved in the occurrence of canine enteritis or do not have a universally recognized pathogenetic role.

CANINE PARVOVIRUS

Virus and Host

- Canine parvovirus (CPV) emerged as a canine pathogen in the late 1970s, likely as a consequence of a

E-mail address: nicola.decaro@uniba.it

https://doi.org/10.1016/j.yasa.2020.07.012
2666-4518/20/

spillover from cats of the closely related feline parvovirus (FPV). At present, CPV, FPV and related parvoviruses form a unique viral species, referred to as *Carnivore protoparvovirus 1* (genus *Protoparvovirus*, subfamily *Parvovirinae*, family *Parvoviridae*) [1,2].

- CPV is a nonenveloped, single-stranded DNA virus (Table 1, Fig. 1A), showing exceptional stability (up to several months) in the environment. The viral DNA, about 5000 nucleotides (nt) in length, is composed of only 2 genes, NS and VP, each encoding for 2 proteins through alternative splicing of the same messenger RNA. The 4 encoded viral products are 2 nonstructural (NS1, NS2) and 2 structural (VP1, VP2) proteins, the latter 2 forming the icosahedral capsid of the virus [1].
- Three CPV antigenic variants are circulating worldwide, namely CPV-2a, CPV-2b, and CPV-2c, which mainly differ in 1 amino acid (aa), showing asparagine, aspartic acid, or glutamic acid, respectively, at position 426 of the VP2 protein. These variants are variously distributed in the different continents [3,4], with the current epidemiologic scenario being influenced by intercontinental and intracontinental migrations of strains with different geographic and temporal origins [5–7].
- Domestic dogs and wild canids are susceptible to CPV infection [1]. The old-type CPV-2, no longer circulating in the field, was unable to infect cats, whereas the 3 antigenic variants, which differ from the original strain in 5 or 6 VP2 aa residues, may sporadically infect cats, causing clinical signs overlapping with feline panleukopenia [8,9] or asymptomatic infections [10]. There are some reports of CPV infection in other carnivores [11–13] and in noncarnivore mammals [14].
- CPV is mainly transmitted through the oronasal route by direct or indirect contact with biological fluids of infected animals. Feces are the main source of infection, containing very high viral titers. Because of the virus's environmental resistance, contaminated fomites play a significant epidemiologic role [15].
- The virus replicates primarily in the lymphoid tissues and then spreads to the bloodstream through infected leukocytes, mainly lymphocytes, colonizing the crypts of the small intestine, where active virus replication induces rapid necrosis of the germinal epithelium [15].

Disease

- The incubation period of the infection caused by the antigenic variants is usually 3 to 4 days.
- Puppies less than 6 months of age are more susceptible to more severe forms of disease, with subsequent death, although overt disease has also been reported in adult dogs [16].
- Different forms of CPV disease are observed:
  - Intestinal form

    This form is characterized by loss of appetite, depression, vomiting, hemorrhagic or watery diarrhea with feces being streaked or darkened by blood (Fig. 1B), fever (inconsistent), leukopenia, anemia, dehydration, metabolic acidosis (or alkalosis), septicemia and endotoxemia, systemic inflammatory response syndrome, hypercoagulability, multiorgan dysfunction, and death. Nonhemorrhagic (catarrhal or mucoid) diarrhea is often observed. Leukocyte counts commonly decrease to less than 2000 to 3000 cells/μL of blood. Sometimes total whole blood cells (WBC) counts are within normal ranges, showing lymphopenia caused by the virus-induced necrosis of lymphoid tissues and neutrophilia consequent to infections by opportunistic bacteria. Changes in serum biochemistry are nonspecific and include hypoproteinemia (hypoalbuminemia), hypoglycemia (or mild hyperglycemia), hypocholesterolemia or hypercholesterolemia, hypocalcemia and electrolyte abnormalities, increased liver enzyme activity, and hyperbilirubinemia [15,17]. Gross lesions are characterized by hemorrhagic gastroenteritis (Fig. 1C) with thickening of the intestinal wall; repletion of the gut with dark, often bloody, material or hemorrhagic fluid; enlargement and congestions of mesenteric lymph nodes (Fig. 1D), and Peyer patches. At the histopathologic level, there is lymphocyte depletion in the lymphoid tissues and extensive necrosis of intestinal crypts with presence of intranuclear inclusion bodies in the infected cells (Fig. 1E) [15].
  - Myocardial form

    At present, the CPV involvement of myocardium is sporadic, because this is more frequent during the first 2 to 3 weeks of age, when puppies are consistently protected by maternally derived antibodies (MDAs). Puppies that develop CPV myocarditis may undergo sudden death or develop the intestinal form of disease followed by myocarditis. These puppies may present short episodes of dyspnea, crying, and retching before dying or they may develop degenerative heart disease followed by myocardial fibrosis. The typical

TABLE 1
Enteric Viruses of Dogs and Their Characteristics

Virus	Species	Genus	Family	Genome	Structure	Size (nm)	Association with Enteritis
Canine parvovirus	*Carnivore protoparvovirus 1*	*Protoparvovirus*	*Parvoviridae*	ssDNA(–), 5 kb	Nonenveloped, icosahedral	18–26	P
Canine enteric coronavirus	*Alphacoronavirus 1*	*Alphacoronavirus*	*Coronaviridae*	ssRNA(+), 30 kb	Enveloped, pleomorphic	120	P
Canine rotavirus	*Rotavirus A*	*Rotavirus*	*Reoviridae*	11-segmented dsRNA, 18.5 kb	Nonenveloped, trilaminar, icosahedral	80	P
Canine norovirus	*Norwalk virus*	*Norovirus*	*Caliciviridae*	ssRNA(+), 7.5–7.7 kb	Nonenveloped, icosahedral	38–40	S
Canine sapovirus	*Sapporo virus*	*Sapovirus*	*Caliciviridae*	ssRNA(+), 7.1–7.7 kb	Nonenveloped, icosahedral	27–40	S
Canine vesivirus	*Canine vesivirus (proposed)*	*Vesivirus*	*Caliciviridae*	ssRNA(+), 8.5 kb	Nonenveloped, icosahedral	27–40	S
Canine astrovirus	*Mamastrovirus 5*	*Mamastrovirus*	*Astroviridae*	ssRNA(+), 6.5–6.6 kb	Nonenveloped, icosahedral	38–40	S
Canine circovirus	*Canine circovirus*	*Circovirus*	*Circoviridae*	ssDNA(–), 2 kb	Nonenveloped, icosahedral	17–20	S
Canine kobuvirus	*Aichivirus A*	*Kobuvirus*	*Picornaviridae*	ssRNA(+), 8.2 kb	Nonenveloped, icosahedral	30	S
Canine bocavirus 2	*Carnivore bocaparvovirus 2*	*Bocaparvovirus*	*Parvoviridae*	ssDNA(–), 5.4 kb	Nonenveloped, icosahedral	21–22	S
Canine bufavirus	*Carnivore protoparvovirus 2*	*Protoparvovirus*	*Parvoviridae*	ssDNA(–), 4.2 kb	Nonenveloped, icosahedral	18–26	S
Canine chapparvovirus	*Carnivore chaphamaparvovirus 1*	*Chaphamaparvovirus*	*Parvoviridae*	ssDNA(–), 4.1 kb	Nonenveloped, icosahedral	18–20	S
Mammalian orthoreovirus type 3	*Mammalian orthoreovirus*	*Orthoreovirus*	*Reoviridae*	10-segmented dsRNA, 23.5 kb	Nonenveloped, trilaminar, icosahedral	80	S

The symbol (–) indicates negative sense; (+) indicates positive sense.
Abbreviations: ds, double stranded; P, proved; S, suspected; ss, single stranded.

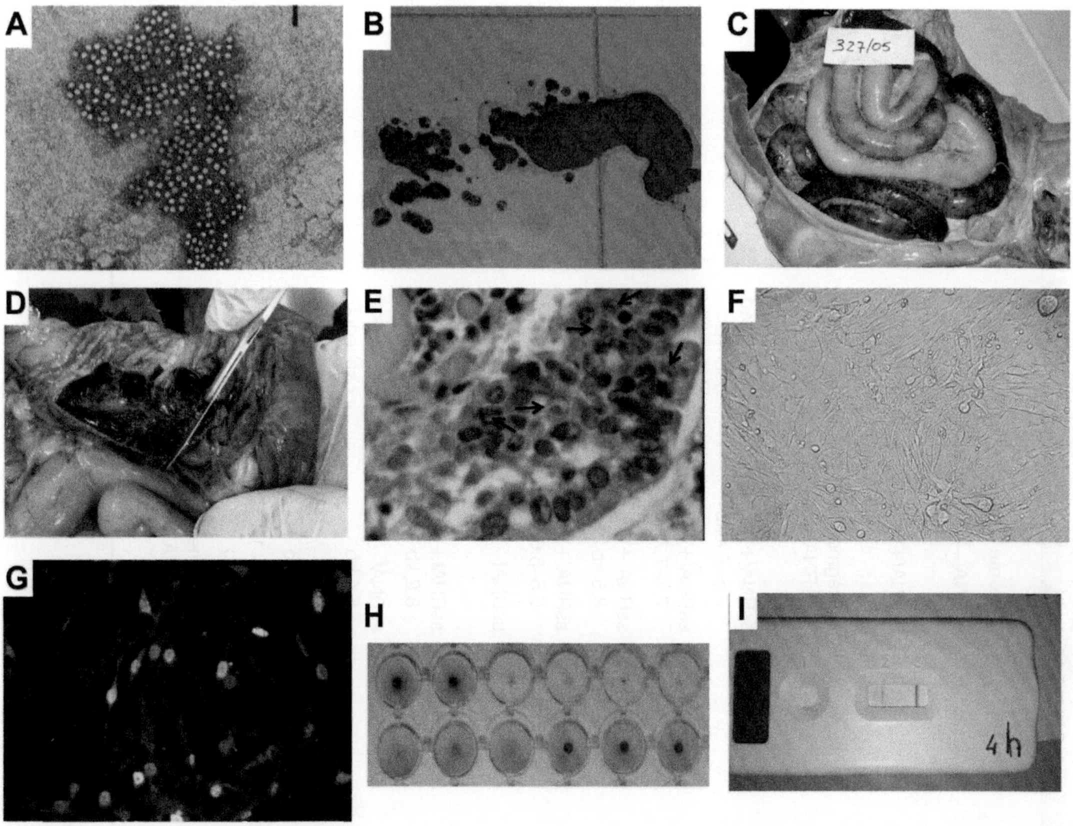

FIG. 1 Canine parvovirus infection. (**A**) Viral particles observed by electron microscopy. (**B**) Clinical signs: watery diarrhea with feces streaked by blood. (**C**) Postmortem findings: hemorrhagic enteritis. (**D**) Postmortem findings: mesenteric lymph node with severe congestion and hemorrhage. (**E**) Histopathology: presence of intranuclear inclusion bodies (*arrows*) in infected enterocytes. (**F**) Virus isolation on canine mammary fibroma A72 cells: mild cytopathic effect. (**G**) Immunofluorescence assay on infected A72 cells: nuclear fluorescence. (**H**) Hemagglutination (HA) using swine erythrocytes: canine parvovirus–positive feces with an HA titer of 1:8. (**I**) In-clinic assay with fecal positive result.

lesions of the myocardial form are pale areas of necrosis on the heart surface, which are histologically characterized by nonsuppurative myocarditis with infiltration of lymphocytes and plasma cells and presence of intranuclear inclusion bodies [15,17].

- Subclinical infections
  Puppies with intermediate levels of MDA (hemagglutination [HA]-inhibiting titers between 1:20 and 1:80) and adult dogs may develop mild forms of disease, showing lethargy and loss of appetite for a few days, along with transient moderate leukopenia [15]. Asymptomatic carriers of the virus have been also reported [18].

Diagnosis

- Clinical diagnosis
  - The presentation of a juvenile puppy with vomiting, hemorrhagic diarrhea, and leukopenia should always suggest a suspected diagnosis of CPV infection, although other viruses may induce overlapping clinical signs.
- Virological diagnosis
  - Samples suitable for direct detection of the virus or its parts include feces (where maximal CPV titers are observed) and blood antemortem and tissue samples from various organs (gut, spleen, lymph nodes) postmortem [19].
  - Traditional virological methods, including virus isolation on canine and feline cell cultures and

HA, are not routinely performed because they lack sensitivity, are time consuming, and require highly trained personnel and dedicated equipment [20]. Postmortem diagnosis can take advantage of immunohistochemistry [15]. CPV may not cause an evident cytopathic effect (CPE) in infected monolayers (Fig. 1F), thus requiring additional testing by HA or immunofluorescence assay (IFA) (Fig. 1G). HA on feces (Fig. 1H) requires fresh swine or feline erythrocytes and a temperature of +4°C [1,15,20].

- In-clinic assays (Fig. 1I), based on antigen detection by means of monoclonal antibodies, are poorly sensitive but have the advantage of providing a rapid diagnosis in the case of a positive result (<15 minutes). Samples having less than 10^5 DNA copies per 10 μL of template tested negative by an in-clinic assay, but negative results were also observed even in fecal samples with very high viral amounts. likely because of the presence of high levels of antibodies that sequestrated the viral antigens [21,22]. These tests are able to detect all CPV variants with the same efficiency [21,22].
- Molecular assays are the gold standard for CPV detection because they detect viral DNA and are very sensitive. Several conventional and real-time polymerase chain reaction (PCR) protocols are currently available [23–25], most targeting the VP2 gene and detecting the closely related FPV. Minor groove binder probe assays were developed to characterize the CPV variants and to discriminate between CPV vaccine and field strains and between CPV and FPV [26–29]. More recently, other molecular tools were proposed as an alternative to standard PCR-based methods for CPV detection and viral type characterization [30–36].

- Serologic diagnosis
  - Serology is not commonly used for diagnosis of CPV infection, because antibodies may derive from previous infections or vaccinations. These tests are used instead for evaluation of MDA levels in puppies in order to establish the best period for vaccine administration, to confirm seroconversion after vaccination, and for determination of vaccine-induced antibodies as an alternative to revaccination. Apart from traditional methods, namely HA inhibition and virus neutralization (VN), rapid in-clinic tests have been commercialized for determination of CPV actively induced antibody levels [37]. The presence of CPV antibodies, regardless of titer, in an actively immunized dog more than 20 weeks of age is correlated with protection [38].

Treatment

- Treatment of CPV enteritis is mainly supportive, aiming to restore fluids and electrolyte balance and to prevent concurrent infections by opportunistic bacteria. Therapeutic protocols include intravenous administration of lactated Ringer solution to correct hypoglycemia and hypokalemia and parenteral administration of antiemetic drugs, gastric protectants, and broad-spectrum antibiotics. Continuous feeding with a prepared liquid diet using a nasoesophageal or nasogastric tube has proved to be beneficial in puppies with severe anorexia. Whole-blood or plasma transfusion is helpful to correct erythrocyte and protein losses caused by severe enteritis [15,17].
- No specific drug has been shown to be effective in vivo against CPV infection. Administration of mitogens stimulating leukocyte production was able to increase WBC counts in puppies with severe leukopenia [39]. Hyperimmune plasma and purified immunoglobulins were anecdotally reported to be beneficial, but there was no experimental evidence for their efficacy in controlled clinical trials [17]. Analogously, recombinant feline interferon-ω reduced clinical signs and mortality only when treatment began very early after infection, but this was not reproducible in field conditions [40].

Prophylaxis

Direct prophylaxis

During an outbreak of CPV infection, strict isolation of infected puppies and extensive disinfections are highly recommended. Diluted sodium hypochlorite solutions have been proved to be effective in inactivating the virus even after few minutes of exposure [41]. Contact for 1 minute with a 0.75% sodium hypochlorite solution was able to reduce significantly the CPV titers, and lower concentrations efficiently inactivated the virus when the contact time was extended to 15 minutes [41].

Indirect prophylaxis

- Vaccination is the most effective prophylactic measure to control CPV infections, and, accordingly, CPV vaccines are included in core vaccines. Modified live virus (MLV) vaccines are available on the market, which are prepared with the original CPV type 2 or its variant CPV-2b [38]. Despite extensive vaccination, CPV still represents a major cause of acute gastroenteritis in dogs because of the frequent immunization failures that have been associated with high MDA levels in injected puppies, vaccination of nonresponder or low-responder animals, or immunologic escape by antigenic variants [42]. Although some field reports describe a possible lack of efficacy of CPV-2 (old type) vaccines against the antigenic variants [16], challenge studies have shown protection of those vaccines against all natural variants, including CPV-2c [42].

- Vaccination schedules include a primary course in the first year of life, with multiple vaccine administrations starting from 6 to 8 weeks and ending not before 16 weeks of age, followed by a booster at 6 months or 1 year later and revaccinations every 3 years. More stringent vaccination schedules may be implemented in the shelter environment, with first vaccine administration at the time of admission (as early as 4 weeks of age) and further injections at intervals of 2 to 3 weeks until 20 weeks of age [38].
- High-titer vaccines are now available that are able to induce active immunity in puppies having intermediate MDA titers [42]. Intranasal and oral administrations of CPV MLV vaccines have been also suggested to better overcome the MDA interference against vaccination [43,44].

CANINE CORONAVIRUS

Virus and Host

- Canine coronavirus (CCoV), also known as canine enteric coronavirus to distinguish it from the unrelated betacoronavirus canine respiratory coronavirus, was first isolated in 1971 from dogs with acute enteritis in a canine military unit in Germany [45,46]. The virus is an *Alphacoronavirus* closely related to feline coronavirus, transmissible gastroenteritis virus of swine (TGEV), and its derivative porcine respiratory coronavirus, with which it forms a unique viral species, *Alphacoronavirus-1* (genus *Alphacoronavirus*, subfamily *Orthocoronavirinae*, family *Coronaviridae*) [47].
- CCoV is an enveloped, single-stranded, positive-sense RNA virus (see Table 1, Fig. 2A), showing an exceptional genetic plasticity. The viral RNA, about 30,000 nt in length, consists in the 5′ two-thirds of the genome of 2 overlapping open reading frames (ORFs) that encode for nonstructural proteins, including the viral RNA-dependent RNA polymerase. The remaining one-third at the 3′ end contains ORFs encoding for the major structural spike (S), envelope (E), membrane (M), and nucleocapsid (M) proteins, plus some accessory genes not essential for viral replication [45,47].
- There are 2 known CCoV genotypes, CCoV types I (CCoV-I) and II (CCoV-II), the latter including 2 subgenotypes, CCoV-IIa and CCoV-IIb, which consist of classic and recombinant (TGEV-like) strains [48,49]. CCoV-II, the ancestor of TGEV, is likely derived from CCoV-I [50]. Apart from the enteric biotype, CCoV-IIa also comprises a hypervirulent strain, referred to as pantropic CCoV, which causes systemic disease [51].
- Juvenile puppies at the decline of MDA immunity are most frequently infected by CCoV. In addition to domestic dogs, wild canids and other carnivores may be susceptible to CCoV infection, frequently developing subclinical infections [52–55].
- Feces are the main source of the virus, because CCoV has a typical fecal-oral route of transmission; after ingestion, the virus colonizes enterocytes in intestinal villus tips, causing shortening, distortion, and loss of microvilli of the brush border, as well as sloughing of necrotic cells into the lumen. The lost epithelium is replaced by immature enterocytes, resulting in the loss of normal digestive and absorptive functions of the gut and in the appearance of diarrhea [15,56,57].

Disease

- Puppies less than 12 weeks of age are most susceptible to CCoV infection, although overt disease has also been reported in adult dogs [15,57].
- The incubation period is short and clinical signs may be first seen by 1 to 3 days after infection [56].

CCoV infection may occur in 2 different forms:

- Intestinal form
  - This variant is the form that is most commonly observed, and it is usually characterized by rapid recovery of the infected animals [45]. The role of CCoV as the primary enteropathogen has been questioned, but recent studies have shown that there is a clear association between the virus and the occurrence of acute gastroenteritis in dogs [58,59].
  - Clinical signs usually include inappetence, depression, vomiting, and nonhemorrhagic diarrhea. Feces may be mucoid or watery (Fig. 2B) and rarely are streaked with blood. No specific hematological and biochemical abnormalities are observed and mortality is very low [15,56,57]. More severe enteric forms have been

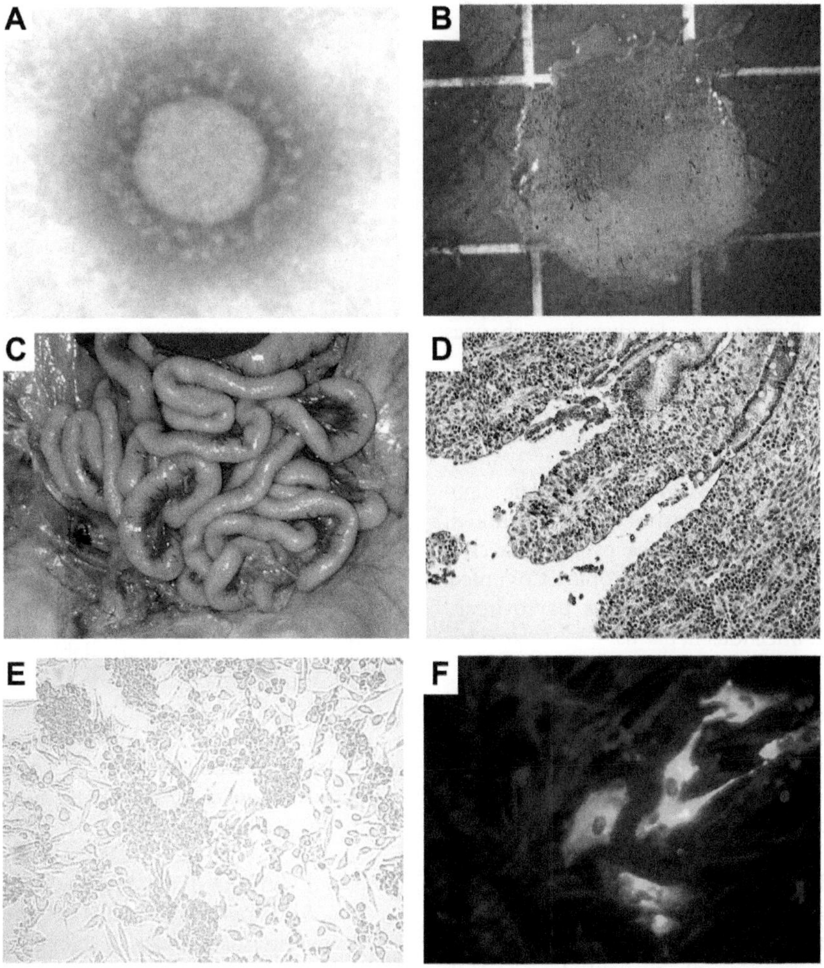

FIG. 2 CCoV infection. (**A**) Viral particles observed by electron microscopy. (**B**) Clinical signs: watery diarrhea. (**C**) Postmortem findings: mild enteritis. (**D**) Immunohistochemistry on a section of jejunum: desquamation of intestinal villi and inflammatory cell infiltration in the lamina propria; coronavirus antigens (brown stained) in epithelial cells. (**E**) Virus isolation on canine mammary fibroma A72 cells: cytopathic effect. (**F**) Immunofluorescence assay on infected A72 cells: cytoplasmic fluorescence.

reported, characterized by hemorrhagic diarrhea and higher fatality rates [15,45].

  - No gross lesions, apart from mild enteritis (Fig. 2C), are observed in mild enteric infections, whereas, in severe cases, intestinal loops are dilated and filled with thin, watery, green-yellow fecal material. In addition, mesenteric lymph nodes are enlarged and congested. Histopathologically, there is atrophy and fusion of intestinal villi with leukocyte infiltration of the lamina propria (Fig. 2D) [15].

- Systemic form
  - This sporadic form is caused by pantropic CCoV strains that are able to spread to internal organs and induce long-lasting lymphopenia [60–63].
  - Dogs infected with these hypervirulent strains may show lethargy, loss of appetite, vomiting, hemorrhagic diarrhea, and neurologic signs. Total WBC counts may decrease to less than 50% of the baseline values [46], and long-term lymphopenia is frequently observed [60]. Mortality can be high, but milder forms of disease have also been observed after experimental infections [60].

- Gross lesions observed in pantropic CCoV infections can be severe, including hemorrhagic gastroenteritis; enlargement of the Peyer patches, spleen, and mesenteric lymph nodes; as well as bronchopneumonia, degeneration of the liver and kidneys, and meningeal hyperemia [51,54,62]. Histopathology reveals hemorrhagic or necrotic enteritis, with atrophy and fusion of microvilli, edema and congestion of mesenteric lymph nodes, diffuse congestion in the lungs or interstitial pneumonia, renal cortical infarction, and hepatocyte degenerative changes [51,62].

Diagnosis

Clinical diagnosis

- CCoV must be considered in the diagnostic algorithms for canine acute gastroenteritis, although several other pathogens can cause overlapping clinical signs. The presentation of pantropic CCoV infections may mimic those of canine parvovirosis, distemper, and infectious hepatitis.

Virological diagnosis

- Feces represent the best sample for the diagnosis of CCoV enteric infection antemortem, whereas postmortem diagnosis can be performed on gut sections. Detection of pantropic strains should be performed from internal organs, because no specific test exists that is able to discriminate between enteric and pantropic strains [15,46].
- Virus isolation on cell cultures is time consuming, poorly sensitive, and is only available for CCoV-II, because CCoV-I has not been adapted to in vitro growth. CPEs are not specific, being characterized by cell rounding and detachment from the monolayer (Fig. 2E). Thus, presence of viral antigens should be confirmed by additional testing, such as IFA (Fig. 2F). Immunohistochemistry on small intestine (or on internal orgams when a pantropic strain is suspected) is a suitable tool for postmortem diagnosis (Fig. 2D). Enzyme-linked immunosorbent assay (ELISA)–based in-clinic assays to detect viral antigen are not widely used for CCoV diagnosis, because they are much less sensitive than molecular assays [15].
- Detection of viral RNA through reverse transcription (RT)-PCR or real-time RT-PCR is the most sensitive and specific method for CCoV diagnosis [56]. TaqMan assays are available for CCoV detection, quantification, and characterization [64,65].

Serologic diagnosis

- Serologic methods for detection of CCoV antibodies are mainly based on VN and ELISA but they are not useful for diagnosis of active CCoV infection, because antibodies may derive from previous infections, and CCoV, similar to other coronaviruses [66], is not highly immunogenic, so antibodies are raised late and at low titers. Serologic tests are more suitable for epidemiologic investigations [15,56].

Treatment and Prophylaxis

- As for CPV, CCoV infection requires supportive treatment to maintain fluid and electrolyte balance [15]. There are no available antiviral drugs against CCoV, although this virus has been sometimes used as an animal model for testing the efficacy of molecules against highly pathogenic human coronaviruses [67].
- Being enveloped, CCoV is much less resistant in the environment than CPV and it is easily inactivated by most disinfectants [57,68].
- There are no vaccines available on the market for CCoV prophylaxis [56,66]. The World Small Animal Veterinary Association guidelines for the vaccination of dogs and cats include CCoV vaccines among the vaccines that are not recommended because there is no strict evidence for the pathogenicity of this virus [38]. However, more recent studies have shown that CCoV is significantly associated with the onset of acute diarrhea in puppies [58,59]. Experimental MLV vaccines, administered oronasally, have been developed that are able to induce mucosal immunity, thus providing sterilizing immunity [69,70].

CANINE ROTAVIRUSES

Virus and Host

- Rotaviruses cause gastroenteritis in neonates of many mammal and avian species and were first reported in dogs in the late 1970s [71]. They are classified in 10 species, referred to as *Rotavirus A* (RVA) to *Rotavirus J*, within the family *Reoviridae*, with a distribution according to different animal species [72]. RVA is mainly circulating in dogs, although strains belonging to other species may be sporadically detected [73,74].
- Rotaviruses are nonenveloped, multilayered viruses (Fig. 3A) with 11-segmented double-stranded RNA (dsRNA), 18.5 kb in size (see Table 1), which encodes 11 or 12 proteins, including 6 structural viral

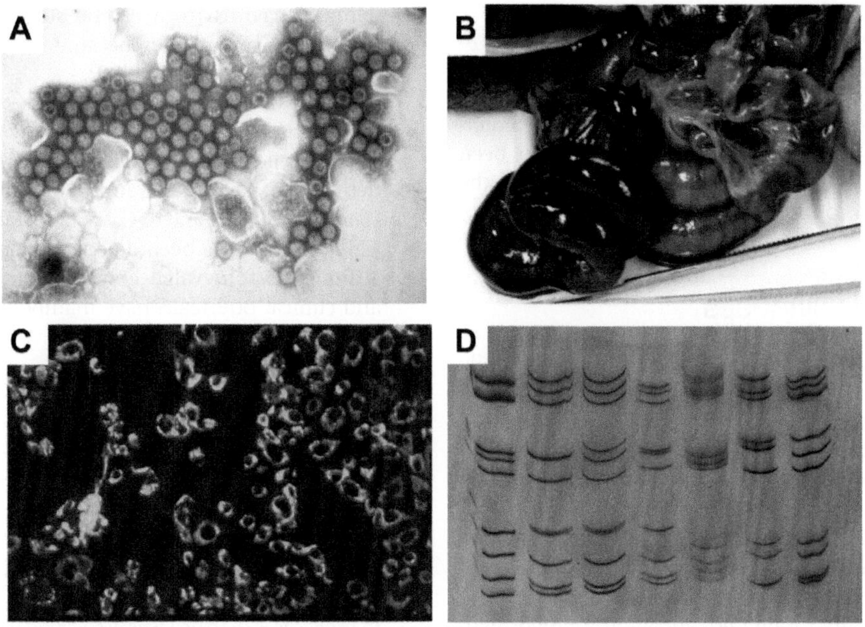

FIG. 3 Canine rotavirus infections. (**A**) Rotaviral particles observed by electron microscopy. (**B**) Postmortem findings: severe enteritis. (**C**) Immunofluorescence assay on infected MA-104 cells: cytoplasmic fluorescence. (**D**) Electrophoretic analysis of rotaviral double-stranded RNA in a silver-stained polyacrylamide gel.

proteins (VP1–VP4, VP6, and VP7) and 5 or 6 nonstructural proteins (NSP1–NSP5 or NSP6). VP7 and VP4, which are used for classification into G and P genotypes, respectively, form the outer capsid, whereas VP6, which defines the rotavirus species, is the major component of the inner capsid [72]. At present, a rotavirus strain is better defined by the complete gene constellation that takes into account its entire gene segments.

- At least 36 G and 51 P RVA genotypes have been identified by the Rotavirus Classification Working Group (https://rega.kuleuven.be/cev/viralmetagenomics/virus-classification/rcwg), with strains circulating in dogs most frequently belonging to the G3P[3] genotype and a few reports of other genotypes, including G9P[23] and G8P[1] [75–77].
- Rotavirus infection mainly occurs in puppies younger than 12 weeks [15]. Interspecies transmission is frequent and RVA strains of canine origin have been reported to cause clinical disease in humans [78].
- Rotaviruses are transmitted by fecal-oral contamination. After ingestion, the virus reaches the tips of the intestinal villi, leading to the necrosis of the epithelium and to the onset of diarrhea [15].

Disease

- Clinical signs of rotavirus infection are usually similar to those caused by enteric CCoV, with the development of watery to mucoid diarrhea that lasts for 8 to 10 days [15].
- At necropsy, only minor gross lesions of the intestine are observed in rotavirus-infected puppies. However, more severe postmortem lesions can occur (Fig. 3B).
- Histopathologic changes consist of fusion of the intestinal villi and in some circumstances of necrosis and desquamation of their epithelium [15].

Diagnosis

- Fecal antigen immunochromatographic or lateral-flow in-clinic assays available for diagnosis of human RVA can be used to detect canine RVA. Virus isolation on cell cultures is cumbersome, requiring specific cell lines and the use of trypsin. IFA is required to detect viral antigens in infected cells (Fig. 3C). HA is characterized by low specificity. Molecular methods are widely used to detect and characterize human and animal RVA strains [15,72]. By polyacrylamide gel electrophoresis of the purified nucleic acid, the classic pattern of segmented dsRNA is evident (Fig. 3D).

Treatment and Prophylaxis

- There is no specific therapy for rotavirus enteritis in dogs and the treatment is merely supportive, as in the case of CCoV enteric infection [15].
- Considering the sporadic frequency of canine enteritis caused by rotaviruses, vaccines have not been developed and prevention is only based on the adoption of common hygienic measures [15].

CANINE CALICIVIRUSES

Viruses and Host

- Caliciviruses (family *Caliciviridae*) are a large family of viruses that cause a variety of clinical manifestations in different animal species. Caliciviruses are currently classified in 11 genera (https://talk.ictvonline.org/taxonomy/) with members of 3 genera (*Norovirus, Sapovirus, Vesivirus*) being reported in dogs [79,80].
- Caliciviruses are nonenveloped virions (Fig. 4A) with a single-stranded, positive-sense RNA of 7.3 to 8.5 kb with a long ORF encoding a polyprotein consisting of 7 mostly nonstructural proteins (ORF1) and 2 to 3 structural proteins (ORF2–ORF4). In genera *Norovirus* and *Vesivirus*, ORF1 is separated from ORF2 and ORF3 near the 3′ end, whereas genus *Sapovirus* possesses a large ORF1 and a standard ORF2 (equivalent to ORF3 of norovirus). VP1 and VP2 are the major and minor capsid proteins, respectively, of caliciviruses [81].
- Based on major capsid protein sequences, genera *Norovirus and Sapovirus* (see Table 1) include a single viral species each (*Norwalk virus* and *Sapporo virus*, respectively) that is subdivided into at least 7 (GI–GVII) and 5 (GI–GV) genogroups, respectively, and variously distributed in different animal species. Numerous genotypes are recognized within each genogroup, and different variants may be included in the same genotype [79]. Recently, more sapoviruses have been detected in different animal species, and novel genogroups GVI to GXV were proposed [82]. Strains circulating in dogs belong to norovirus genogroups GIV, GVI, and GVII [79,80,83–89], and to sapovirus GXIII genogroup [88,90,91]. Human GII and GIV noroviruses have been also found to circulate in dogs [92,93], and a zoonotic transmission has been suggested for canine noroviruses (CaNoVs) [94–96].
- Genus *Vesivirus* includes 2 viral species, *Feline calicivirus* and *Vesicular exanthema of swine* (https://talk.ictvonline.org/taxonomy/), and canine vesivirus (CaVV) has been proposed as a new viral species within this genus (see Table 1) [96]. Isolation of feline calicivirus from canine stools was reported previously, but it later became evident that dogs have their own vesivirus [79].
- The host range of canine caliciviruses is largely unknown, but it likely includes not only domestic dogs but also wild and domestic felids, as suggested by the detection of CaNoV-like strains in a captive lion cub (*Panthera leo*) [97] and of CaVV-like strains in cats [98].
- Caliciviruses have been detected in dogs of all ages, although seroprevalence rates increase with age, and clinical outbreaks have mainly involved young animals [79,80,92,99].

Disease

- In humans, noroviruses are the leading cause of acute gastroenteritis worldwide, and sapoviruses have been associated with important clusters of acute diarrhea [72]. In contrast, the pathogenic potential of caliciviruses in dogs is not yet clear [79,80].
- CaNoVs have repeatedly been recovered from the stools of dogs with acute gastroenteritis (Fig. 4B), but in most cases diarrhea was associated with other infectious agents, including CPV and CCoV [80,87,88,100,101]. Healthy dogs were found to shed CaNoV [101], a circumstance that also occurs in humans infected with norovirus [72]. However, there are studies that show a clear association between CaNoV infection and acute gastroenteritis [84,101].
- Canine sapovirus (CaSaV) was first identified in the United States through metagenomic investigation of the canine fecal virome [90], but firm evidence for an association with gastroenteritis in dogs is lacking. CaSaVs have been detected in the feces of dogs with diarrhea, alone or in association with other enteric viruses [88,91]. Therefore, further studies are needed to assess their pathogenic potential and role in canine acute gastroenteritis.
- A recent study proved that CaVV has been circulating in dogs since the 1960s [102]. CaVV strains were associated with sporadic outbreaks of canine gastroenteritis worldwide [88,96,99,103–105]. However, both the presence of coinfections with other canine pathogens and CaVV detection in healthy dogs raise questions about the role of this virus in the onset of canine diarrhea [96,104,105]. Because experimental infection of dogs with a CaVV strain failed to induce any clinical signs [103], more evidence is required to elucidate the pathogenic potential of this virus.

Diagnosis

- Virus isolation on cell cultures is only available for CaVV, because noroviruses and sapoviruses are

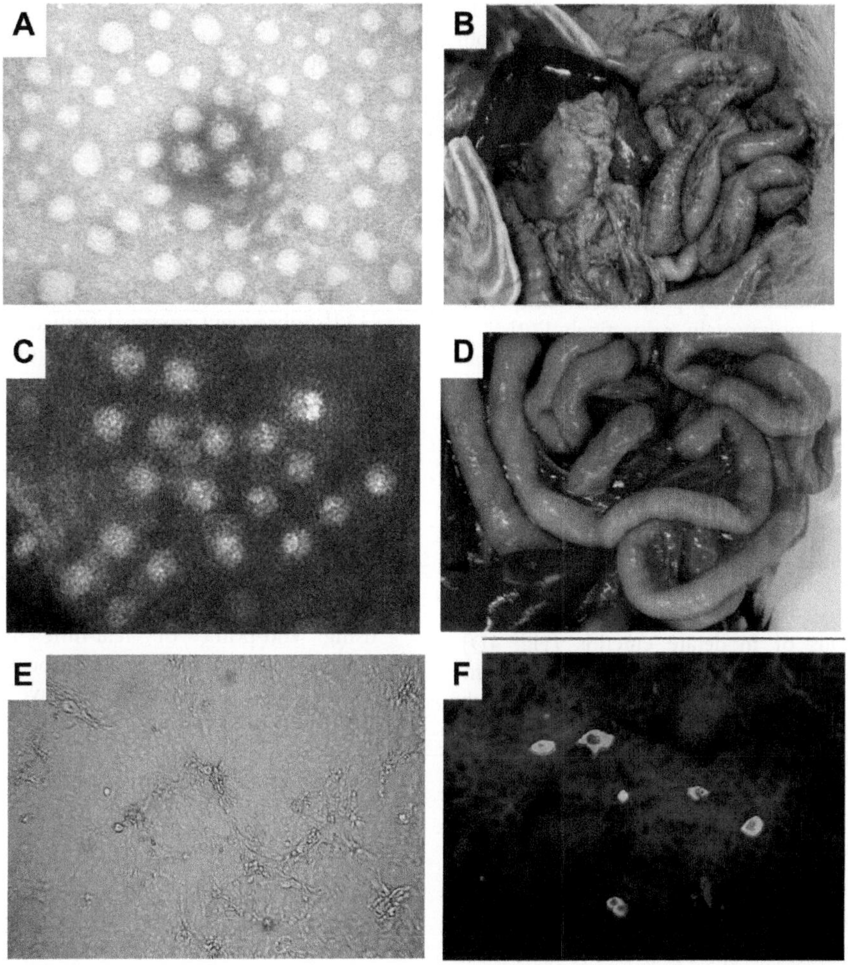

FIG. 4 Canine calicivirus (**A**, **B**) and astrovirus (**C–E**) infection. (**A**) Caliciviral particles observed by electron microscopy. (**B**) Postmortem findings: mild noroviral enteritis. (**C**) Astroviral particles observed by electron microscopy. (**D**) Postmortem findings: mild astroviral enteritis. (**E**) Astrovirus isolation on Madin-Darby canine kidney (MDCK) cells: cytopathic effect. (**F**) Immunofluorescence assay on MDCK cells infected by canine astrovirus: cytoplasmic fluorescence.

uncultivable caliciviruses. Direct virus detection, in particular viral-RNA detection methods (gel-based and real-time RT-PCR assays), are primarily used for diagnosis of canine caliciviruses. Taking into account the wide genetic variability of caliciviruses, broadly reactive molecular methods are used that target conserved genomic regions [72,80].

Treatment and Prophylaxis

- As for other enteric viral infections, the treatment of calicivirus enteritis in dogs is only supportive.
- Development of specific vaccines, currently not available, should take into account both the lack of firm evidence for an association of canine caliciviruses with enteric disease and their antigenic variability [72,80].

CANINE ASTROVIRUSES

Virus and Host

- Canine astrovirus (CaAstV), belonging to the genus *Mamastrovirus* (family *Astroviridae*), was first isolated from the stools of puppies with diarrhea in the United

States in 1980 [106]. The genus currently comprises 19 viral species (*Mamastrovirus 1–19*) (https://talk.ictvonline.org/taxonomy/), with CaAstVs belonging to *Mamastrovirus 5* including several genotypes [107,108], although divergent strains have been reported [109].

- Astroviruses are spherical, nonenveloped viruses (Fig. 4C) with a single-stranded, positive-sense RNA ranging in size from 6.8 to 7.9 kb (see Table 1). This genome contains 3 ORFs, designated as ORF1a, ORF1b, and ORF2, which encode for the viral protease, RNA-dependent RNA polymerase and viral capsid structural polyprotein, respectively [72].
- CaAstV mainly infects domestic dogs, but spillover events have been reported in wild carnivores [110] and humans [111].
- Puppies older than 2 to 3 months, when MDA tends to wane, are most susceptible to CaAstV infection [112].

Disease

- Astroviruses are the second cause of acute diarrhea in humans after rotaviruses [72]. In dogs, these viruses have been associated with acute diarrhea, with postmortem lesions of moderate enteritis (Fig. 4D). Although CaAstV has been isolated from asymptomatic dogs, its prevalence seems to be significantly higher in puppies with enteritis than in healthy dogs. In addition, the high frequency of single-pathogen infections and the peak of viral shedding at the onset of gastrointestinal signs indicate a pathogenetic role in canine enteric disease [107–109,112–118].

Diagnosis

- CaAstV can be easily isolated on various cell cultures of canine origin, causing evident CPE (Fig. 4E) and cytoplasmic fluorescence by IFA (Fig. 4F). However, the most sensitive tools for diagnosis are represented by molecular methods based on the use of broadly reactive consensus primers [112].

Treatment and Prophylaxis

- Only supportive therapy is available for astrovirus-induced enteritis in dogs.
- Vaccines against CaAstV are not available, so prevention is only based on hygienic measures.

CANINE CIRCOVIRUS

Virus and Host

- *Canine circovirus* (CaCV) is one of the 43 viral species currently forming the genus *Circovirus* within the family *Circoviridae* (https://talk.ictvonline.org/-taxonomy/). Circoviruses are small, spherical, nonenveloped viruses having a circular, single-stranded DNA genome of approximately 2 kb (see Table 1). Their genome contains only 2 main inversely arranged ORFs encoding the replicase protein and capsid protein [119].
- Domestic dogs are the natural host of CaCV, but the virus has also been detected in wild carnivores [120,121].

Disease

- CaCV was first isolated from a dog with vasculitis and hemorrhage also involving the gastroenteric tract [122]. Subsequent reports described an association of CaCV with hemorrhagic or nonhemorrhagic diarrhea [123–126], but its pathogenic potential remains controversial. There are some studies showing no correlation between CaCV infection and gastroenteritis [58,127], and others suggesting an association [122,128].

Diagnosis, Treatment, and Prophylaxis

- Although the virus has been isolated on cell cultures, diagnosis of CaCV infection is routinely performed using end-point or real-time PCR protocols [58,122–128]. As alternative tools, inverse PCR and rolling circle amplification have been proposed, which take advantage of the circular DNA of circoviruses [123,129].
- Neither specific treatments nor vaccines have been developed for CaCV.

CANINE KOBUVIRUS

Virus and Host

- Kobuviruses are small, nonenveloped RNA viruses that form a genus (*Kobuvirus*) within the large *Picornaviridae* family (see Table 1) and include 6 different viral species (*Aichivirus A–F*), with canine kobuvirus (CaKoV) belonging to the species *Aichivirus A* along with human Aichi virus, and feline and murine kobuviruses (https://talk.ictvonline.org/taxonomy/). The CaKoV genome, a single-stranded, positive-sense RNA molecule, is 8.2 kb and is composed of a single ORF encoding a polyprotein that is posttranslationally cleaved into 3 structural capsid proteins and 8 nonstructural proteins [130].
- In addition to domestic dogs, CaKoV has been isolated from wild carnivores in Africa and Europe [131–133].

Disease

- CaKoV was discovered by next-generation sequencing (NGS) in 2011 from dogs with diarrhea [90,130]. Several reports describe its involvement in acute gastroenteritis in dogs as being similar to Aichi virus in humans [134–140]. However, as for other emerging enteric viruses, the virus was frequently detected in healthy animals or in association with other canine pathogens, so further studies are needed to confirm its role in the occurrence of diarrhea [79].

Diagnosis, Treatment, and Prophylaxis

- CaKoV can be isolated on cell cultures, but molecular methods are more rapid and sensitive for its detection in the feces of infected dogs.
- There are no specific therapeutic protocols or vaccines available for CaKoV infection.

CANINE BOCAVIRUS 2

Virus and Host

- Bocaviruses are members of the genus *Bocaparvovirus* (subfamily *Parvovirinae*, family *Parvoviridae*) and currently comprise 25 different species, with 6 of them (*Carnivore bocaparvovirus 1–6*) infecting carnivores (https://talk.ictvonline.org/taxonomy/). They are structurally similar to other parvoviruses, including CPV, thus presenting a nonenveloped capsid with icosahedral symmetry and a small linear single-stranded DNA genome. Different from CPV, a third ORF encoding a highly phosphorylated nonstructural protein is located between the nonstructural and structural coding regions [141].
- In dogs, 2 canine bocaviruses (CaBoVs) are currently known, namely canine minute virus (CnMV; currently *Carnivore bocaparvovirus 1*) and CaBoV-2, previously designated as CaBoV-1 and now referred to as *Carnivore bocaparvovirus 2* (see Table 1). While CnMV has been known since the 1960s and is sporadically associated with systemic disease and mortality in neonatal puppies [142], CaBoV-2 was first recovered in 2012 from dogs with respiratory disease [141] and subsequently from puppies with fatal gastroenteritis [143].
- CaBoV-2 recognizes dogs as a primary host but has also been detected in cats [144].

Disease

- CaBoV-2 has tentatively been associated with canine acute gastroenteritis, but this virus showed high coinfection rates with other enteric viruses, such as CPV, CCoV, and CaKoV [136,145,146]. The virus has been associated with enteritis in a litter of dogs with atrophied and fused villi, severe crypt regeneration, and severe bone marrow and lymphoid atrophy [143]. CaBoV-2 respiratory and enteric disease was recently reported in a litter of puppies in Thailand, with the gut of infected animals showing eosinophilic intranuclear inclusion bodies within villous enterocytes without villous atrophy or fusion [147].

Diagnosis, Treatment, and Prophylaxis

- CaBoV-2 has not been adapted to in-vitro growth and diagnosis is obtained by means of PCR-based methods.
- No specific treatment or prophylaxis measures have been developed against CaBoV.

OTHER VIRUSES

In addition to CPV and CaBoV-2, other members of the *Parvoviridae* family have been detected in dogs with diarrhea (see Table 1). Novel protoparvoviruses (genus *Protoparvovirus*, subfamily *Parvovirinae*), genetically related to human and nonhuman primate bufaviruses, have been detected in dogs and cats. Canine bufavirus (CaBuV; species *Carnivore protoparvovirus 2*) was found in stool samples of dogs with or without enteric disease and in nasal and oropharyngeal swabs of dogs with respiratory disease [148]. Genetically closely related parvoviruses were identified in domestic cats and wild canids, suggesting limited host-species restriction among domestic carnivores [149,150]. An association of CaBuV to diarrhea in dogs has recently been suggested [151,152].

Two almost identical chapparvoviruses (species *Carnivore chaphamaparvovirus 1*, genus *Chaphamaparvovirus*, subfamily *Hamaparvovirinae*), namely cachavirus 1A and cachavirus 1B, were detected in dogs with diarrhea. Stool samples from healthy and diarrheic dogs were positive for cachavirus DNA, but the virus was statistically associated with enteric disease [153]. This virus was closely related to feline chapparvoviruses designated as fechaviruses [154].

Mammalian orthoreoviruses have traditionally been associated with asymptomatic or mild respiratory and enteric infections in animals and humans. A mammalian orthoreovirus type 3 (MRV-3) (see Table 1) was isolated on a few occasions from dogs with diarrhea, alone or with other viruses [155,156]. An Italian canine MRV-3 strain was related to strains identified in bats, pigs, and alpine chamois (*Rupicapra rupicapra*) [157].

SUMMARY

The extensive use of innovative molecular techniques, including massive sequencing, has revolutionized knowledge of the cause of canine viral enteritis. In addition to traditional enteropathogens, new viruses of the enteric tract have been discovered by means of NGS or broadly reactive PCR protocols based on consensus primers. Some of these emerging viruses have likely been circulating for decades but they were undiagnosed because they are unable to be grown on cell cultures. Whether these novel viruses are able to induce the occurrence of enteritis or they are part of the normal fecal virome has yet to be determined, so further studies, based on experimental challenge in dogs with viral isolates or contaminated feces, are needed to fulfill the Koch postulates.

FUNDING SOURCES

This study was supported by grants from the Italian Ministry of Health: Ricerca Corrente 2017 "Nuovi flussi diagnostici in sanità animale dalla NGS alla banca antigeni", recipient Alessio Lorusso, and Ricerca Corrente 2018 "Nuovi virus gastroenterici di cane e gatto: sviluppo diprotocolli NGS per la valutazione del rischio zoonosico", recipient Flora Alfano.

DISCLOSURE

The author has nothing to disclose.

REFERENCES

[1] Decaro N, Buonavoglia C. Canine parvovirus - a review of epidemiological and diagnostic aspects, with emphasis on type 2c. Vet Microbiol 2012;155:1–12.

[2] Decaro N, Buonavoglia C. Canine parvovirus post-vaccination shedding: Interference with diagnostic assays and correlation with host immune status. Vet J 2017;221:23–4.

[3] Decaro N, Desario C, Addie DD, et al. The study molecular epidemiology of canine parvovirus, Europe. Emerg Infect Dis 2007;13:1222–4.

[4] Miranda C, Thompson G. Canine parvovirus: the worldwide occurrence of antigenic variants. J Gen Virol 2016;97:2043–57.

[5] Grecco S, Iraola G, Decaro N, et al. Inter- and intracontinental migrations and local differentiation have shaped the contemporary epidemiological landscape of canine parvovirus in South America. Virus Evol 2018;4:vey011.

[6] Mira F, Dowgier G, Purpari G, et al. Molecular typing of a novel canine parvovirus type 2a mutant circulating in Italy. Infect Genet Evol 2018;61:67–73.

[7] Mira F, Purpari G, Di Bella S, et al. Spreading of canine parvovirus type 2c mutants of Asian origin in southern Italy. Transbound Emerg Dis 2019;66:2297–304.

[8] Decaro N, Buonavoglia D, Desario C, et al. Characterisation of canine parvovirus strains isolated from cats with feline panleukopenia. Res Vet Sci 2010;89:275–8.

[9] Decaro N, Desario C, Amorisco F, et al. Canine parvovirus type 2c infection in a kitten associated with intracranial abscess and convulsions. J Feline Med Surg 2011;13:231–6.

[10] Clegg SR, Coyne KP, Dawson S, et al. Canine parvovirus in asymptomatic feline carriers. Vet Microbiol 2012;157:78–85.

[11] Viscardi M, Santoro M, Clausi MT, et al. Molecular detection and characterization of carnivore parvoviruses in free-ranging Eurasian otters (*Lutra lutra*) in southern Italy. Transbound Emerg Dis 2019;66:1864–72.

[12] Spera CG, Lorenzetti E, Lavorente FLP, et al. Canine parvovirus 2b in fecal samples of asymptomatic free-living South American coatis (*Nasua nasua*, Linnaeus, 1766). Braz J Microbiol 2020. https://doi.org/10.1007/s42770-020-00293-2.

[13] Calatayud O, Esperón F, Velarde R, et al. Genetic characterization of Carnivore Parvoviruses in Spanish wildlife reveals domestic dog and cat-related sequences. Transbound Emerg Dis 2020;67:626–34.

[14] Wang SL, Tu YC, Lee MS, et al. Fatal canine parvovirus-2 (CPV-2) infection in a rescued free-ranging Taiwanese pangolin (*Manis pentadactyla pentadactyla*). Transbound Emerg Dis 2019. https://doi.org/10.1111/tbed.13469.

[15] Greene CE, Decaro N. Canine viral enteritis. In: Greene CE, editor. Infectious diseases of the dog and cat. 4th edition. St Louis (MO): Elsevier Saunders; 2012. p. 67–80.

[16] Decaro N, Desario C, Elia G, et al. Evidence for immunisation failure in vaccinated adult dogs infected with canine parvovirus type 2c. New Microbiol 2008;31:125–30.

[17] Mylonakis ME, Kalli I, Rallis TS. Canine parvoviral enteritis: an update on the clinical diagnosis, treatment, and prevention. Vet Med (Auckl) 2016;7:91–100.

[18] Marenzoni ML, Antognoni MT, Baldelli F, et al. Detection of parvovirus and herpesvirus DNA in the blood of feline and canine blood donors. Vet Microbiol 2018;224:66–9.

[19] Decaro N, Martella V, Elia G, et al. Tissue distribution of the antigenic variants of canine parvovirus type 2 in dogs. Vet Microbiol 2007;121:39–44.

[20] Desario C, Decaro N, Campolo M, et al. Canine parvovirus infection: which diagnostic test for virus? J Virol Methods 2005;121:179–85.

[21] Decaro N, Desario C, Beall MJ, et al. Detection of canine parvovirus type 2c by a commercially available in-house rapid test. Vet J 2010;184:373–5.

[22] Decaro N, Desario C, Billi M, et al. Evaluation of an in-clinic assay for the diagnosis of canine parvovirus. Vet J 2013;98:504–7.

[23] Buonavoglia C, Martella V, Pratelli A, et al. Evidence for evolution of canine parvovirus type 2 in Italy. J Gen Virol 2001;82:3021–5.

[24] Zhuang L, Ji Y, Tian P, et al. Polymerase chain reaction combined with fluorescent lateral flow immunoassay based on magnetic purification for rapid detection of canine parvovirus 2. BMC Vet Res 2019;15:30.
[25] Decaro N, Elia G, Martella V, et al. A real-time PCR assay for rapid detection and quantitation of canine parvovirus type 2 DNA in the feces of dogs. Vet Microbiol 2005;105:19–28.
[26] Decaro N, Elia G, Martella V, et al. Characterisation of the canine parvovirus type 2 variants using minor groove binder probe technology. J Virol Methods 2006;133:92–9.
[27] Decaro N, Elia G, Desario C, et al. A minor groove binder probe real-time PCR assay for discrimination between type 2-based vaccines and field strains of canine parvovirus. J Virol Methods 2006;136:65–70.
[28] Decaro N, Martella V, Elia G, et al. Diagnostic tools based on minor groove binder probe technology for rapid identification of vaccinal and field strains of canine parvovirus type 2b. J Virol Methods 2006;138: 10–6.
[29] Decaro N, Desario C, Lucente MS, et al. Specific identification of feline panleukopenia virus and its rapid differentiation from canine parvoviruses using minor groove binder probes. J Virol Methods 2008;147:67–71.
[30] Pavana JV, Akila S, Selvan MK, et al. Direct typing of Canine parvovirus (CPV) from infected dog faeces by rapid mini sequencing technique. J Virol Methods 2016;238:66–9.
[31] Chander V, Chakravarti S, Gupta V, et al. Multiplex Amplification Refractory Mutation System PCR (ARMS-PCR) provides sequencing independent typing of canine parvovirus. Infect Genet Evol 2016;46:59–64.
[32] Sun YL, Yen CH, Tu CF. Immunocapture loop-mediated isothermal amplification assays for the detection of canine parvovirus. J Virol Methods 2017;249:94–101.
[33] Geng Y, Wang J, Liu L, et al. Development of real-time recombinase polymerase amplification assay for rapid and sensitive detection of canine parvovirus 2. BMC Vet Res 2017;13:311.
[34] Liu L, Wang J, Geng Y, et al. Equipment-free recombinase polymerase amplification assay using body heat for visual and rapid point-of-need detection of canine parvovirus 2. Mol Cell Probes 2018;39:41–6.
[35] Sun Y, Cheng Y, Lin P, et al. Simultaneous detection and differentiation of canine parvovirus and feline parvovirus by high resolution melting analysis. BMC Vet Res 2019;15:141.
[36] Hoang M, Wu HY, Lien YX, et al. A SimpleProbe® real-time PCR assay for differentiating the canine parvovirus type 2 genotype. J Clin Lab Anal 2019;33:e22654.
[37] Decaro N, Elia G, Buonavoglia C. Challenge studies for registration of canine core vaccines: is it time to update the European Pharmacopeia? Vet Microbiol 2020;244: 108659.
[38] Day MJ, Horzinek MC, Schultz RD, et al. Vaccination Guidelines Group (VGG) of the World Small Animal Veterinary Association (WSAVA), 2016. WSAVA Guidelines for the vaccination of dogs and cats. J Small Anim Pract 2016;e57:4–8.
[39] Armenise A, Trerotoli P, Cirone F, et al. Use of recombinant canine granulocyte-colony stimulating factor to increase leukocyte count in dogs naturally infected by canine parvovirus. Vet Microbiol 2019;231:177–82.
[40] De Mari K, Maynard L, Eun HM, et al. Treatment of canine parvoviral enteritis with interferon-omega in a placebo-controlled field trial. Vet Rec 2003;152:105–8.
[41] Cavalli A, Marinaro M, Desario C, et al. In vitro virucidal activity of sodium hypochlorite against canine parvovirus type 2. Epidemiol Infect 2018;146:2010–3.
[42] Canine parvovirus vaccination and immunisation failures: Are we far from disease eradication?. Decaro N, Buonavoglia C and Barrsb V.R. Vet Microbiol. 2020 Aug; 247: 108760. Published online 2020 Jun 15. https://doi.org/10.1016/j.vetmic.2020.108760
[43] Martella V, Cavalli A, Decaro N, et al. Immunogenicity of an intranasally administered modified live canine parvovirus type 2b vaccine in pups with maternally derived antibodies. Clin Diagn Lab Immunol 2005; 12:1243–5.
[44] Cavalli A, Desario C, Marinaro M, et al. Oral administration of modified live canine parvovirus type 2b induces systemic immune response. Vaccine 2020;38: 115–8.
[45] Decaro N, Buonavoglia C. An update on canine coronaviruses: viral evolution and pathobiology. Vet Microbiol 2008;132:221–34.
[46] Decaro N, Buonavoglia C. Canine coronavirus: not only an enteric pathogen. Vet Clin North Am Small Anim Pract 2011;41:1121–32.
[47] Decaro N, Lorusso A. Novel human coronavirus (SARS-CoV-2): A lesson from animal coronaviruses. Vet Microbiol 2020;244:108693.
[48] Decaro N, Mari V, Campolo M, et al. Recombinant canine coronaviruses related to transmissible gastroenteritis virus of Swine are circulating in dogs. J Virol 2009;83:1532–7.
[49] Decaro N, Mari V, Elia G, et al. Recombinant canine coronaviruses in dogs, Europe. Emerg Infect Dis 2010;16: 41–7.
[50] Lorusso A, Decaro N, Schellen P. Gain, preservation, and loss of a group 1a coronavirus accessory glycoprotein. J Virol 2008;82:10312–7.
[51] Buonavoglia C, Decaro N, Martella V, et al. Canine coronavirus highly pathogenic for dogs. Emerg Infect Dis 2006;12:492–4.
[52] Wang Y, Ma G, Lu C, et al. Detection of canine coronaviruses genotype I and II in raised *Canidae* animals in China. Berl Munch Tierarztl Wochenschr 2006;119: 35–9.
[53] de Almeida Curi NH, Coelho CM, de Campos Cordeiro Malta M, et al. Pathogens of wild maned wolves (*Chrysocyon brachyurus*) in Brazil. J Wildl Dis 2012;48: 1052–6.

[54] Alfano F, Dowgier G, Valentino MP, et al. Identification of pantropic canine coronavirus in a wolf (*Canis lupus italicus*) in Italy. J Wildl Dis 2019;55:504–8.
[55] Rosa GM, Santos N, Grøndahl-Rosado R, et al. Unveiling patterns of viral pathogen infection in free-ranging carnivores of northern Portugal using a complementary methodological approach. Comp Immunol Microbiol Infect Dis 2020;69:101432.
[56] Pratelli A. Genetic evolution of canine coronavirus and recent advances in prophylaxis. Vet Res 2006;37: 191–200.
[57] Licitra BN, Duhamel GE, Whittaker GR. Canine enteric coronaviruses: emerging viral pathogens with distinct recombinant spike proteins. Viruses 2014;6: 3363–76.
[58] Dowgier G, Lorusso E, Decaro N, et al. A molecular survey for selected viral enteropathogens revealed a limited role of Canine circovirus in the development of canine acute gastroenteritis. Vet Microbiol 2017; 204:54–8.
[59] Duijvestijn M, Mughini-Gras L, Schuurman N, et al. Enteropathogen infections in canine puppies: (Co-occurrence, clinical relevance and risk factors. Vet Microbiol 2016;195:115–22.
[60] Marinaro M, Mari V, Bellacicco AL, et al. Prolonged depletion of circulating CD4+ T lymphocytes and acute monocytosis after pantropic canine coronavirus infection in dogs. Virus Res 2010;152:73–8.
[61] Decaro N, Cordonnier N, Demeter Z, et al. European surveillance for pantropic canine coronavirus. J Clin Microbiol 2013;51:83–8.
[62] Pinto LD, Barros IN, Budaszewski RF, et al. Characterization of pantropic canine coronavirus from Brazil. Vet J 2014;202:659–62.
[63] Alfano F, Fusco G, Mari V, et al. Circulation of pantropic canine coronavirus in autochthonous and imported dogs, Italy. Transbound Emerg Dis 2020. https://doi.org/10.1111/tbed.13542.
[64] Decaro N, Pratelli A, Campolo M, et al. Quantitation of canine coronavirus RNA in the faeces of dogs by TaqMan RT-PCR. J Virol Methods 2004;119: 145–50.
[65] Decaro N, Martella V, Ricci D, et al. Genotype-specific fluorogenic RT-PCR assays for the detection and quantitation of canine coronavirus type I and type II RNA in faecal samples of dogs. J Virol Methods 2005;130: 72–8.
[66] Decaro N, Martella V, Saif LJ, et al. COVID-19 from veterinary medicine and one health perspectives: What animal coronaviruses have taught us. Res Vet Sci 2020; 131:21–3.
[67] Amici C, Di Caro A, Ciucci A, et al. Indomethacin has a potent antiviral activity against SARS coronavirus. Antivir Ther 2006;11:1021–30.
[68] Pratelli A. Action of disinfectants on canine coronavirus replication in vitro. Zoonoses Public Health 2007;54: 383–6.
[69] Pratelli A, Tinelli A, Decaro N, et al. Safety and efficacy of a modified-live canine coronavirus vaccine in dogs. Vet Microbiol 2004;99:43–9.
[70] Pratelli A. High-cell-passage canine coronavirus vaccine providing sterilizing immunity. J Small Anim Pract 2007;48:574–8.
[71] Eugster AK, Sidwa T. Rotaviruses in diarrheic feces of a dog. Vet Med Small Anim Clin 1979;74:817–9.
[72] Bányai K, Estes MK, Martella V, et al. Viral gastroenteritis. Lancet 2018;392:175–86.
[73] Mihalov-Kovács E, Gellért Á, Marton S, et al. Candidate new rotavirus species in sheltered dogs, Hungary. Emerg Infect Dis 2015;21:660–3.
[74] Marton S, Mihalov-Kovács E, Dóró R, et al. Canine rotavirus C strain detected in Hungary shows marked genotype diversity. J Gen Virol 2015;96:3059–71.
[75] Martella V, Pratelli A, Elia G, et al. Isolation and genetic characterization of two G3P5A[3] canine rotavirus strains in Italy. J Virol Methods 2001;96:43–9.
[76] Sieg M, Rückner A, Köhler C, et al. A bovine G8P[1] group a rotavirus isolated from an asymptomatically infected dog. J Gen Virol 2015;96:106–14.
[77] Yan N, Tang C, Kan R, et al. Genome analysis of a G9P [23] group A rotavirus isolated from a dog with diarrhea in China. Infect Genet Evol 2019;70:67–71.
[78] Matthijnssens J, De Grazia S, Piessens J, et al. Multiple reassortment and interspecies transmission events contribute to the diversity of feline, canine and feline/canine-like human group A rotavirus strains. Infect Genet Evol 2011;11:1396–406.
[79] Caddy SL. New viruses associated with canine gastroenteritis. Vet J 2018;232:57–64.
[80] Martella V, Pinto P, Buonavoglia C. Canine noroviruses. Vet Clin North Am Small Anim Pract 2011;41:1171–81.
[81] Desselberger U. Caliciviridae other than noroviruses. Viruses 2019;11 [pii:E286].
[82] Oka T, Lu Z, Phan T, et al. Genetic characterization and classification of human and animal sapoviruses. PLoS One 2016;11:e0156373.
[83] Martella V, Lorusso E, Decaro N, et al. Detection and molecular characterization of a canine norovirus. Emerg Infect Dis 2008;14:1306–8.
[84] Martella V, Decaro N, Lorusso E, et al. Genetic heterogeneity and recombination in canine noroviruses. J Virol 2009;83:11391–6.
[85] Mesquita JR, Nascimento MS. Molecular epidemiology of canine norovirus in dogs from Portugal, 2007-2011. BMC Vet Res 2012;8:107.
[86] Tse H, Lau SK, Chan WM, et al. Complete genome sequences of novel canine noroviruses in Hong Kong. J Virol 2012;86:9531–2.
[87] Bodnar L, Lorusso E, Di Martino B, et al. Identification of a novel canine norovirus. Infect Genet Evol 2017;52: 75–81.
[88] Soma T, Nakagomi O, Nakagomi T, et al. Detection of Norovirus and Sapovirus from diarrheic dogs and cats in Japan. Microbiol Immunol 2015;59:123–8.

[89] Lyoo KS, Jung MC, Yoon SW, et al. Identification of canine norovirus in dogs in South Korea. BMC Vet Res 2018;14(1):413.
[90] Li L, Pesavento PA, Shan T, et al. Viruses in diarrhoeic dogs include novel kobuviruses and sapoviruses. J Gen Virol 2011;92:2534–41.
[91] Bodnar L, Di Martino B, Di Profio F, et al. Detection and molecular characterization of sapoviruses in dogs. Infect Genet Evol 2016;38:8–12.
[92] Di Martino B, Di Profio F, Melegari I, et al. Seroprevalence for norovirus genogroup II, IV and VI in dogs. Vet Microbiol 2017;203:268–72.
[93] Charoenkul K, Nasamran C, Janetanakit T, et al. Human norovirus infection in dogs, Thailand. Emerg Infect Dis 2020;26:350–3.
[94] Summa M, von Bonsdorff CH, Maunula L. Pet dogs–a transmission route for human noroviruses? J Clin Virol 2012;53:244–7.
[95] Di Martino B, Di Profio F, Ceci C, et al. Seroprevalence of norovirus genogroup IV antibodies among humans, Italy, 2010-2011. Emerg Infect Dis 2014;20:1828–32.
[96] Martella V, Pinto P, Lorusso E, et al. Detection and full-length genome characterization of novel canine vesiviruses. Emerg Infect Dis 2015;21:1433–6.
[97] Martella V, Campolo M, Lorusso E, et al. Norovirus in captive lion cub (*Panthera leo*). Emerg Infect Dis 2007; 13:1071–103.
[98] Mesquita JR, Delgado I, Costantini V, et al. Seroprevalence of canine norovirus in 14 European countries. Clin Vaccine Immunol 2014;21:898–900.
[99] Di Martino B, Di Profio F, Melegari I, et al. Serological and molecular investigation of 2117-like vesiviruses in cats. Arch Virol 2018;163:197–201.
[100] Ntafis V, Xylouri E, Radogna A, et al. Outbreak of canine norovirus infection in young dogs. J Clin Microbiol 2010;48:2605–8.
[101] Mesquita JR, Barclay L, Nascimento MS, et al. Novel norovirus in dogs with diarrhea. Emerg Infect Dis 2010;16:980–2.
[102] Binn LN, Norby EA, Marchwicki RH, et al. Canine caliciviruses of four serotypes from military and research dogs recovered in 1963-1978 belong to two phylogenetic clades in the *Vesivirus* genus. Virol J 2018;15:39.
[103] Schaffer FL, Soergel ME, Black JW, et al. Characterization of a new calicivirus isolated from feces of a dog. Arch Virol 1985;84:181–95.
[104] Castro TX, Cubel Garcia RC, Costa EM, et al. Molecular characterisation of calicivirus and astrovirus in puppies with enteritis. Vet Rec 2013;175:557.
[105] Renshaw RW, Griffing J, Weisman J, et al. Characterization of a vesivirus associated with an outbreak of acute hemorrhagic gastroenteritis in domestic dogs. J Clin Microbiol 2018;56 [pii:e01951-17].
[106] Williams FP Jr. Astrovirus-like, coronavirus-like, and parvovirus-like particles detected in the diarrheal stools of beagle pups. Arch Virol 1980;66(3):215–26.
[107] Zhou H, Liu L, Li R, et al. Detection and genetic characterization of canine astroviruses in pet dogs in Guangxi, China. Virol J 2017;14:156.
[108] Alves CDBT, Budaszewski RF, Torikachvili M, et al. Detection and genetic characterization of *Mamastrovirus 5* from Brazilian dogs. Braz J Microbiol 2018;49: 575–83.
[109] Mihalov-Kovács E, Martella V, Lanave G, et al. Genome analysis of canine astroviruses reveals genetic heterogeneity and suggests possible inter-species transmission. Virus Res 2017;232:162–70.
[110] Diniz Beduschi Travassos Alves C, da Fontoura Budaszewski R, Cibulski SP, et al. Mamastrovirus 5 detected in a crab-eating fox (*Cerdocyon thous*): Expanding wildlife host range of astroviruses. Comp Immunol Microbiol Infect Dis 2018;58:36–43.
[111] Japhet MO, Famurewa O, Adesina OA, et al. Viral gastroenteritis among children of 0-5 years in Nigeria: Characterization of the first Nigerian aichivirus, recombinant noroviruses and detection of a zoonotic astrovirus. J Clin Virol 2019;111:4–11.
[112] Martella V, Moschidou P, Buonavoglia C. Astroviruses in dogs. Vet Clin North Am Small Anim Pract 2011; 41:1087–95.
[113] Toffan A, Jonassen CM, De Battisti C, et al. Genetic characterization of a new astrovirus detected in dogs suffering from diarrhoea. Vet Microbiol 2009;139: 147–52.
[114] Zhu AL, Zhao W, Yin H, et al. Isolation and characterization of canine astrovirus in China. Arch Virol 2011; 156:1671–5.
[115] Martella V, Moschidou P, Catella C, et al. Enteric disease in dogs naturally infected by a novel canine astrovirus. J Clin Microbiol 2012;50:1066–9.
[116] Choi S, Lim SI, Kim YK, et al. Phylogenetic analysis of astrovirus and kobuvirus in Korean dogs. J Vet Med Sci 2014;76:1141–5.
[117] Caddy SL, Goodfellow I. Complete genome sequence of canine astrovirus with molecular and epidemiological characterisation of UK strains. Vet Microbiol 2015; 177:206–13.
[118] Takano T, Takashina M, Doki T, et al. Detection of canine astrovirus in dogs with diarrhea in Japan. Arch Virol 2015;160:1549–53.
[119] Todd D, Mcnulty MS, Adair BM, et al. Animal circoviruses. Adv Virus Res 2001;57:1–70.
[120] Zaccaria G, Malatesta D, Scipioni G, et al. Circovirus in domestic and wild carnivores: An important opportunistic agent? Virology 2016;490:69–74.
[121] De Arcangeli S, Balboni A, Kaehler E, et al. Genomic characterization of canine circovirus detected in red foxes (*Vulpes vulpes*) from Italy using a new real-time PCR assay. J Wildl Dis 2020;56:239–42.
[122] Li L, McGraw S, Zhu K, et al. Circovirus in tissues of dogs with vasculitis and hemorrhage. Emerg Infect Dis 2013;19:534–41.

[123] Thaiwong T, Wise AG, Maes RK, et al. Canine Circovirus 1 (CaCV-1) and Canine Parvovirus 2 (C9: PV-2): Recurrent dual infections in a papillon breeding colony. Vet Pathol 2016;53:1204–9.

[124] Kotsias F, Bucafusco D, Nuñez DA, et al. Genomic characterization of canine circovirus associated with fatal disease in dogs in South America. PLoS One 2019;14: e0218735.

[125] Van Kruiningen HJ, Heishima M, Kerr KM, et al. Canine circoviral hemorrhagic enteritis in a dog in Connecticut. J Vet Diagn Invest 2019;31:732–6.

[126] Anderson A, Hartmann K, Leutenegger CM, et al. Role of canine circovirus in dogs with acute haemorrhagic diarrhoea. Vet Rec 2017;180:542.

[127] Hsu HS, Lin TH, Wu HY, et al. High detection rate of dog circovirus in diarrheal dogs. BMC Vet Res 2016; 12(1):116.

[128] Gentil M, Gruber AD, Müller E. Prevalence of Dog circovirus in healthy and diarrhoeic dogs. Tierarztl Prax Ausg K Kleintiere Heimtiere 2017;45:89–94 [in German].

[129] Decaro N, Martella V, Desario C, et al. Genomic characterization of a circovirus associated with fatal hemorrhagic enteritis in dog, Italy. PLoS One 2014;9:e105909.

[130] Kapoor A, Simmonds P, Dubovi EJ, et al. Characterization of a canine homolog of human Aichivirus. J Virol 2011;85:11520–5.

[131] Di Martino B, Di Profio F, Melegari I, et al. Molecular evidence of kobuviruses in free-ranging red foxes (*Vulpes vulpes*). Arch Virol 2014;159:1803–6.

[132] Olarte-Castillo XA, Heeger F, Mazzoni CJ, et al. Molecular characterization of canine kobuvirus in wild carnivores and the domestic dog in Africa. Virology 2015; 477:89–97.

[133] Melegari I, Sarchese V, Di Profio F, et al. First molecular identification of kobuviruses in wolves (*Canis lupus*) in Italy. Arch Virol 2018;163:509–13.

[134] Carmona-Vicente N, Buesa J, Brown PA, et al. Phylogeny and prevalence of kobuviruses in dogs and cats in the UK. Vet Microbiol 2013;164:246–52.

[135] Oem JK, Choi JW, Lee MH, et al. Canine kobuvirus infections in Korean dogs. Arch Virol 2014;159:2751–5.

[136] Li C, Wei S, Guo D, et al. Prevalence and phylogenetic analysis of canine kobuviruses in diarrhoetic dogs in northeast China. J Vet Med Sci 2016;78:7–11.

[137] Soma T, Matsubayashi M, Sasai K. Detection of kobuvirus RNA in Japanese domestic dogs. J Vet Med Sci 2016; 78:1731–5.

[138] Kong N, Zuo Y, Wang Z, et al. Molecular characterization of new described kobuvirus in dogs with diarrhea in China. Springerplus 2016;5:2047.

[139] Miyabe FM, Ribeiro J, Alfieri AF, et al. Detection of canine kobuvirus RNA in diarrheic fecal samples of dogs with parvoviruses. Braz J Microbiol 2019;50: 871–4.

[140] Charoenkul K, Janetanakit T, Chaiyawong S, et al. First detection and genetic characterization of canine Kobuvirus in domestic dogs in Thailand. BMC Vet Res 2019;15:254.

[141] Kapoor A, Mehta N, Dubovi EJ, et al. Characterization of novel canine bocaviruses and their association with respiratory disease. J Gen Virol 2012;93:341–6.

[142] Decaro N, Amorisco F, Lenoci D, et al. Molecular characterization of Canine minute virus associated with neonatal mortality in a litter of Jack Russell terrier dogs. J Vet Diagn Invest 2012;24:755–8.

[143] Bodewes R, Lapp S, Hahn K, et al. Novel canine bocavirus strain associated with severe enteritis in a dog litter. Vet Microbiol 2014;174:1–8.

[144] Niu J, Yi S, Wang H, et al. Complete genome sequence analysis of canine bocavirus 1 identified for the first time in domestic cats. Arch Virol 2019;164:601–5.

[145] Choi JW, Lee KH, Lee JI, et al. Genetic characteristics of canine bocaviruses in Korean dogs. Vet Microbiol 2015; 179(3–4):177–83.

[146] Rudolf S, Neiger R, König M. [Detection of bocavirus in 4-week-old puppies with acute diarrhea]. Tierarztl Prax Ausg K Kleintiere Heimtiere 2016;44:118–22.

[147] Piewbang C, Jo WK, Puff C, et al. Canine bocavirus type 2 infection associated with intestinal lesions. Vet Pathol 2018;55:434–41.

[148] Martella V, Lanave G, Mihalov-Kovács E, et al. Novel parvovirus related to primate bufaviruses in dogs. Emerg Infect Dis 2018;24:1061–8.

[149] Diakoudi G, Lanave G, Capozza P, et al. Identification of a novel parvovirus in domestic cats. Vet Microbiol 2019;228:246–51.

[150] Melegari I, Di Profio F, Palombieri A, et al. Molecular detection of canine bufaviruses in wild canids. Arch Virol 2019;164:2315–20.

[151] Sun W, Zhang S, Huang H, et al. First identification of a novel parvovirus distantly related to human bufavirus from diarrheal dogs in China. Virus Res 2019;265: 127–31.

[152] Li J, Cui L, Deng X, et al. Canine bufavirus in faeces and plasma of dogs with diarrhoea, China. Emerg Microbes Infect 2019;8:245–7.

[153] Fahsbender E, Altan E, Seguin MA, et al. Chapparvovirus DNA found in 4% of dogs with diarrhea. Viruses 2019;11:398.

[154] Li Y, Gordon E, Idle A, et al. Virome of a feline outbreak of diarrhea and vomiting includes bocaviruses and a novel chapparvovirus. Viruses 2020;12:E506.

[155] Kokubu T, Takahashi T, Takamura K, et al. Isolation of reovirus type 3 from dogs with diarrhea. J Vet Med Sci 1993;55:453–4.

[156] Decaro N, Campolo M, Desario C, et al. Virological and molecular characterization of a mammalian orthoreovirus type 3 strain isolated from a dog in Italy. Vet Microbiol 2005;109:19–27.

[157] Besozzi M, Lauzi S, Lelli D, et al. Host range of mammalian orthoreovirus type 3 widening to alpine chamois. Vet Microbiol 2019;230:72–7.

Advances in Small Animal Care 1 (2020) 161–188
ADVANCES IN SMALL ANIMAL CARE

Advances in Molecular Diagnostics and Treatment of Feline Infectious Peritonitis

Emi N. Barker, PhD, DipECVIM-CA, MRCVS[a,b,*],
Séverine Tasker, BSc, PhD, DSAM, DipECVIM-CA, FHEA, FRCVS[b,c]
[a]Feline Centre, Langford Vets, Langford BS40 5DU, UK; [b]Bristol Veterinary School, University of Bristol, Langford BS40 5DU, UK; [c]The Linnaeus Group, Shirley, Solihull B90 1BN, UK

KEYWORDS
• Feline coronavirus • Reverse transcriptase polymerase chain reaction • Pyogranulomatous inflammation
• Effusions • Protease inhibitors • Nucleoside analogue • GS-441524

KEY POINTS

- Appreciation of the relationship between feline coronavirus (FCoV) and feline infectious peritonitis (FIP) is vital in interpreting guidance on diagnosis, treatment, and prevention.
- Presumptive diagnosis in most cases is straightforward; however, achieving confidence in a diagnosis in some cats is more complex, as is definitive confirmation of FIP.
- Molecular diagnostics (especially FCoV-targeted reverse transcriptase quantitative polymerase chain reaction on tissue or effusion samples) can increase confidence in a diagnosis of FIP.
- An appreciation of the methodology of molecular diagnostics is necessary to understand their limitations.
- Some novel therapeutics have recently been shown to be effective in the treatment of FIP (viral protease inhibitors; nucleoside analogues); however, more studies are required.

INTRODUCTION

Background

Feline coronavirus (FCoV) is ubiquitous worldwide. Infection is common among the domestic cat population, usually only causing mild enteric signs (eg, diarrhea). In a small percentage of FCoV-infected cats, viral mutations, systemic spread, and aberrant immune response results in a syndrome of serositis, vasculitis, and pyogranulomatous lesions known as feline infectious peritonitis (FIP). A presumptive diagnosis of FIP is often made in sick, particularly young, cats with the effusive disease; however, variability in presentation and test limitations can make obtaining a definitive diagnosis or even a presumptive diagnosis using noninvasive or minimally invasive approaches difficult. In the absence of treatment using novel antiviral agents, FIP is fatal in almost all cases.

Viral properties

- FCoV is an enveloped, single-stranded, positive-sense RNA coronavirus of the Alphacoronavirus genus (Fig. 1).
  - Other viral species within this genus include transmissible gastroenteritis virus (TGEV) in pigs, canine coronavirus (CCoV) in dogs, and human coronaviruses (HCoV-NL63; HCoV-229E).
  - Human pathogens include severe acute respiratory syndrome–coronavirus (SARS-CoV), Middle

*Corresponding author, *E-mail address:* emi.barker@bristol.ac.uk

https://doi.org/10.1016/j.yasa.2020.07.011
2666-4518/20/

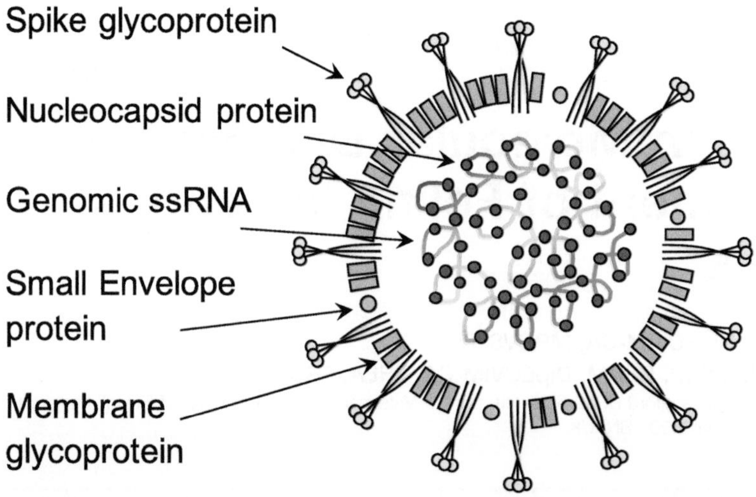

FIG. 1 A feline coronavirus virion with relative position of structural proteins and genomic single-stranded RNA (ssRNA) indicated. (*Modified from* Barker EN, Tasker S. An update on FIP. In Practice; with permission.)

East respiratory syndrome-coronavirus, and SARS-CoV-2 (the cause of COVID-19), which belong to the Betacoronavirus genus

- Coronavirus genomes are large (for an RNA virus) (Fig. 2) [1] and encode:
  - A large, nonstructural polyprotein (pp1a; pp1ab), which is cleaved into smaller proteins (including proteases and the viral RNA polymerase).
  - Spike (S) glycoprotein: a trimeric transmembrane protein involved in host-cell receptor binding and cell entry; forms part of the viral envelope.
  - Envelope (E) protein: forms part of the viral envelope.
  - Membrane (M) protein (Matrix protein): forms part of the viral envelope.
  - Nucleocapsid (N) protein: interacts with the viral genomic RNA.
  - Nonstructural proteins (3abc and 7ab): the function of these proteins is poorly understood; however, it is suspected that they play a role in viral replication and release, as well as interfering with the host cellular response to infection (eg, inhibition of apoptotic pathways).
- Like other RNA viruses, FCoV shows a high rate of mutation during replication and exist as clusters of genetically diverse populations.
- FCoV infects domestic and wild felids.
  - FCoV is not transmissible to humans.
- Two biotypes of FCoV are described [2,3]:
  - Feline enteric coronavirus (FECV): the avirulent enteric form of FCoV; replicates mainly within enterocytes; can cause enteric clinical signs; is shed in feces.
  - Feline infectious peritonitis virus (FIPV): the virulent systemic form of FCoV; replicates within monocytes and tissue macrophages, leading to systemic spread; results in the development of FIP in a minority of infected cats; shedding in feces is possible.

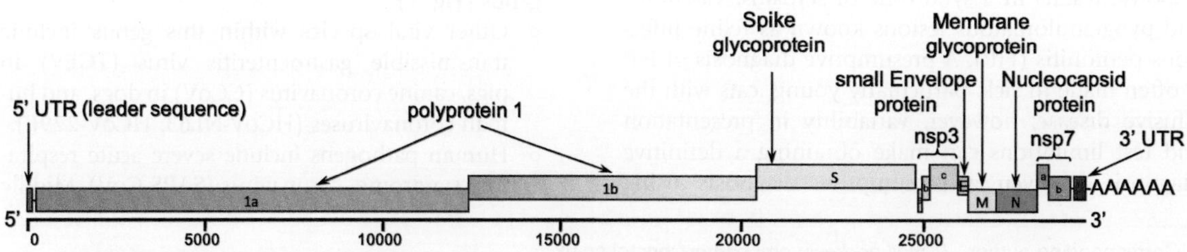

FIG. 2 The feline coronavirus genome with component genes and nucleotide scale. nsp, nonstructural protein; UTR, untranslated region.

- FIPV is considered to arise from FECV as a result of mutation within individual cats (internal-mutation hypothesis in contrast with the distinct circulating avirulent and virulent strains hypothesis).
- Genetic analysis of FIPV isolates reveal them to be most closely related to the FECV from which they arose (rather than to other FIPV isolates).

- Two serotypes of FCoV exist:
  - Type 1: predominates worldwide; difficulties in cultivation in vitro have limited research.
  - Type 2: arose following genetic recombination between FCoV and CCoV; genetic analyses have shown that this has occurred on multiple separate occasions [4–6]; extensively studied because can be cultured in vitro.
  - Serotypes are differentiated primarily based on the Spike glycoprotein, either by the immunologic response they trigger (eg, detection of virus neutralizing antibodies) [3] or, more recently, by gene amplification and sequencing (because the change in antigenicity is caused by genetic recombination detectable through this method) [7].
  - Infection with either serotype has been associated with both enteric disease and FIP; therefore, either serotype can be present as either biotype.
- Feline infection with other coronaviruses:
  - Following detection of antibody cross-reactivity between closely related coronavirus species (including FCoV serotypes 1 and 2, CCoV, and TGEV) [8,9], the potential role of cats as a vector of these infections or whether exposure to these infections conferred either protection against or enhancement of subsequent infection with FCoV was explored in early experimental studies.
  - Following exposure to TGEV cats developed transient, subclinical infection with shedding in feces [10,11]; cross-reactive antibodies were produced; protection against infection with FCoV, and subsequent development of FIP, was not documented.
  - Following exposure to CCoV, cats developed transient, subclinical infection with no fecal shedding detected [12]; cross-reactive antibodies were produced; neither protection against nor antibody-dependent enhancement (ADE) of infection with FCoV (and subsequent development of FIP) was documented.
  - Exposure to HCoV-229E did not result in clinical signs or the production of cross-reactive antibodies, although virus-specific antibodies were produced [13]; neither protection against nor ADE of infection with FCoV (and subsequent development of FIP) was documented.

Prevalence

- FCoV is found in cats worldwide, other than on a small number of isolated islands.
- FCoV frequently circulates in multicat households:
  - Seroprevalence (reviewed elsewhere [14]) is significantly greater in multicat households (26%–87%) than in single-cat households (4%–24%).
  - In environments in which FCoV is endemic, most cats experience repeated cycles of infection and subsequent viral elimination [15,16].
  - In some cats, the initial infection persists and chronic (and sometimes intermittent) shedding may occur [16,17].
- Incidence of FIP is low in comparison:
  - 1 in 5000 cats affected in 1 or 2 cat households.
  - 5% to 10% of cats affected in some catteries [18,19].
  - FIP is usually sporadic; rarely epidemics can occur, and can possibly be explained by a combination of:
    - High population density (eg, breeding catteries; rescue shelters; feral cat populations).
    - Shared genetic background.
    - Shared challenges to immune function (eg, stress; limited resources).
    - Shared viral factors.

Feline Infectious Peritonitis Risk Factors

- Some of the risk factors for the development of FIP likely relate to risk factors for FCoV infection.
- Some studies have indicated increased risk of FIP in multicat households; however, a recent study noted that most cats were living in a single-cat or 2-cat households at the time of diagnosis [20], although this would not necessarily have reflected their situation at time of exposure to FCoV.
- Male cats are at slightly higher risk of FIP [20].
- Genetic susceptibility:
  - Siblings of cats with FIP are considered to be at increased risk of developing FIP (~2× risk).
  - Some studies have indicated increased risk in specific pedigree breeds [21,22]; however, this is not borne out by every study [20] and there was geographic variation in the breeds identified as increased risk [21,22]. In addition, there may be

- a degree of reporting bias (positive and negative) from the cat-fancier community.
- There is an increased incidence of FIP in kittens and young adult cats (55% of cases ≤2 years), with a secondary peak in older cats (>10 years). However, FIP can affect cats of all ages.
  - Experimental work has shown that resistance to infection increases from 6 months of age to greater than 1 year [23].
- Stress is often a prominent historical feature; for example, recent rehoming, neutering, vaccination.

Transmission

- FECV is transmitted horizontally between cats, primarily via the feco-oral route.
  - Litter trays are the primary source of infection.
  - Contaminated fomites (eg, grooming equipment; soft furnishings) may also play a role.
- Oronasal route, via saliva and respiratory secretions, may also play a role [24,25]; however, further investigation is required to characterize this further.
- Whether fecally shed FIPV is competent of horizontal transmission is unclear [26].
- Vertical transmission in utero (ie, of FIPV from a queen with FIP to her kittens) is considered possible but rare [27,28].
- Iatrogenic transmission, via parenteral injection or aerosolization of FIPV derived from cats with FIP, has been shown experimentally [13,29].
- In large, endemically infected, multicat households, kittens commonly become infected at a young age, mostly at 5 to 6 weeks, as maternally derived antibodies (MDAs) wane below protective levels [18].
  - The queen is suspected to be the most common source of infection, followed by other breeding or nonbreeding cats (especially older litters of kittens).
- FCoV survives 1 to 2 days at room temperature, but may survive up to 7 weeks in a dry environment (eg, in feces) [30]; Fuller's earth–based cat litters seemed to be most effective at inactivating FCoV in vitro, but they failed to prevent transmission in vivo [31].
- FCoV is inactivated by most disinfectants.

Pathogenesis

- The exact pathogenesis of the development of FIP is still under investigation.
- It is suspected that FCoV strains of variable virulence, or variable potential for virulence, are circulating in the general feline population; this could, in part, account for some outbreaks.
- Ingestion of FCoV (as FECV): small intestinal villi enterocytes are the primary site of host-cell entry, with spread to colonic enterocytes.
  - Viral spike protein binds to serotype-specific cell entry receptors, leading to internalization of virus.
    - The cell receptor for serotype 1 FCoV is unknown.
    - Aminopeptidase N (APN; CD13) is the cell receptor for serotype 2 FCoV, for macrophages at least [32].
  - Replication within enterocytes:
    - Local inflammatory reaction: leads to immune response leading to infection; may be cleared or persist in chronic infections (especially in colonic enterocytes).
    - Shedding in feces within 7 days: duration of shedding is highly variable (weeks; months; lifelong) [17].
  - Intestinal macrophages acquire FCoV from infected enterocytes [33] (exact mechanism unknown) and move to regional lymph nodes (eg, mesenteric), leading to monocyte-associated viremia in most cats [34,35].
  - FCoV mutates (ie, FECV becomes FIPV), resulting in progressive acquisition of enhanced tropism for, and increased ability to replicate within, monocytes/macrophages, leading to further systemic spread (monocyte-associated viremia).
  - In an estimated 10% of cats with systemic FCoV (as FIPV) infection [36], an aberrant immune response develops whereby activated monocytes/macrophages infected with FCoV interact with endothelial cells [37] leading to granulomatous phlebitis and periphlebitis, which is FIP.
- FCoV has also been detected in conjunctival, nasal, and oropharyngeal tissue [25]; its role in upper respiratory tract disease is unknown.
- Role of the host immune response in FIP pathogenesis [38]:
  - A poor cell-mediated immune response results in vasculitis, particularly affecting serosal surfaces; this vasculitis/serositis leads to fluid accumulations in 1 or more body cavity (ie, peritoneal>-pleural>pericardial) and is termed effusive FIP.
  - A partial cell-mediated immune response leads to pyogranulomatous or granulomatous lesions in organs (often kidneys, liver, lungs, eyes, central nervous system, mesenteric lymph nodes, and gastrointestinal tract), and in the absence of effusions is termed noneffusive FIP.

- These likely reflect a continuum:
  - Some cats with initially noneffusive disease develop effusions.
  - Cats with effusive disease often have granulomas present in parenchymal organs.
- Viral factors in FIP pathogenesis:
  - Viral mutations:
    - Spike gene:
      - Functional mutations (M1058L and S1060A) within the putative fusion peptide of serotype 1 FCoV were able to differentiate 95.8% of isolates of FECV and FIPV in 1 study [39]; the FCoV isolates used were either tissue derived from cats with FIP (ie, FIPV) or feces derived from healthy cats (ie, FECV). This finding led to the suggestion that presence of either functional mutation is diagnostic for FIP (discussed later and in Table 1). A more recent study found that 12 of 45 (26.7%) cats without FIP had at least 1 tissue or effusion sample that was positive for FCoV, and, of the 18 samples from these 12 cats where Spike gene sequencing was successful, 16 (88.9%) had functional mutations consistent with FIPV [7].
      - Functional mutations within the putative furin cleavage site of serotype 1 FCoV were able to differentiate 92.7% of isolates of FECV and FIPV in another study [40]; again, the FCoV isolates used were either tissue derived from cats with FIP or feces derived from healthy cats.
    - Nonstructural protein 3c gene: mutations encoding a truncated protein are present approximately 2 in 3 cats with FIP, whereas the 3c genes are intact in cats without FIP [41–43]; again, the FCoV isolates used were either tissue derived from cats with FIP or feces derived from healthy cats. This finding has led to the conclusion that intact 3c is a requirement for enterocyte infection but not systemic spread.
    - Nonstructural protein 7b gene: mutations are present in FCoV derived from both cats with FIP and cats without FIP; their role in the development of FIP is unknown.
  - Viral mutations are thought to occur during bursts of viral replication (eg, following a period of immunosuppression).
  - Some cats experience waves of clinical disease (eg, fever and weight loss) that coincide with T-cell depletion and increased viral loads in the blood [38].
  - Acquired mutations are also suspected to have a role in tissue tropism: a functional genetic mutation in the Spike gene was only found in viral RNA extracted from the neurologic tissue of a cat with neurologic FIP but not in viral RNA extracted from other organs from the same cat [44]. The same mutation was found in FCoV purified from the neurologic tissue from another cat with neurologic FIP.

Clinical signs of enteric feline coronavirus infection

- Often subclinical.
- Replication within enterocytes may cause mild enteric-associated signs (eg, inappetence, diarrhea, vomiting); rarely causes severe enteritis.
- FCoV has been detected in conjunctival, nasal, and oropharyngeal swab samples in cats with upper respiratory tract signs [25]; however, the role of FCoV in upper respiratory tract disease requires further investigation.

Clinical signs of feline infectious peritonitis

- Two clinical variants of FIP disease are recognized:
  - Effusive (wet) form, where effusions develop in 1 or more body cavity as a result of vasculitis/serositis; accounts for ~80% of cases of FIP [20].
  - Noneffusive (dry) form, where pyogranulomatous lesions are present in 1 or more parenchymal tissue.
  - At postmortem examination, this distinction is often less clear, with many cats diagnosed with effusive disease having pyogranulomatous lesions within parenchymal tissue, and some cats diagnosed with noneffusive disease having clinically inapparent effusions present.
- The incubation period, from initial FCoV infection to development of FIP, is highly variable; clinical signs of effusive disease typically present earlier than those of noneffusive disease [45].
  - Following parenteral administration of FIPV, clinical signs of effusive disease developed after 2 to 14 days, whereas it took several weeks for clinical signs of noneffusive disease to develop.
  - In specific pathogen–free (SPF) cats, infected naturally by exposure to cats known to be shedding FCoV, the first clinical signs of FIP occurred from 6 weeks postexposure [46].

TABLE 1
Overview of Diagnostic Tests for Feline Infectious Peritonitis

Test	Sample	Target	False -Negatives	False-Positives	Comments
Rivalta test [71,72]	Effusion	Inflammatory proteins	—	Other causes of exudate; eg, bacterial peritonitis, lymphocytic cholangitis	Cheap, rapid point-of-care test Nonspecific; little advantage compared with fluid cytology and protein analysis
Histopathology [7,83]	Tissue	Inflammatory response to FIP	Tissue sampled not involved	Other causes of pyogranulomatous inflammation (consider tissue culture and IHC)	Systemic perivascular granulomatous or pyogranulomatous lesions strongly supportive of FIP in conjunction with compatible history, clinical signs, and so forth Most pathologists recommend IHC to confirm
FCoV RT-qPCR [7,99]	Effusion; CSF; aqueous humor; tissue aspirates or biopsy; (blood = very poor sensitivity)	FCoV RNA	Low cellularity or sample degradation; laboratory error (eg, strain not detected by PCR assay)	Laboratory error (contamination)	Nonspecific: should not be used as a sole diagnostic test. Positive RT-(q)PCR on tissue, CSF, aqueous humor, and effusions is strongly supportive of FIP in conjunction with compatible history, clinical signs, cytology, and so forth. Sensitivity RT-qPCR>IHC In general, samples from cats with FIP have higher viral loads than samples from cats without FIP that are also infected with FCoV

FCoV RT-LAMP [100]	Effusion, tissue, blood	FCoV RNA	Low cellularity or sample degradation; laboratory error (eg, strain not detected by PCR assay)	Laboratory error (contamination)	Poor sensitivity compared with RT-qPCR; does not require expensive equipment to perform
IHC [7,83]/ ICC [57,73,74,82]	Tissue, CSF, effusion	FCoV antigen within macrophages	Low-cellularity effusion; nonrepresentative tissue biopsy; antigen masked by patient's own FCoV antibody	Laboratory error (methodology dependent)	IHC considered reference standard for confirmation ICC of more limited specificity (laboratory dependent) can be interpreted as strongly supportive of FIP in conjunction with compatible history, clinical signs, and so forth

Abbreviations: CSF, cerebrospinal fluid; ICC, immunocytochemistry; IHC, immunohistochemistry; PCR, polymerase chain reaction; RT-LAMP, reverse transcriptase loop-mediated isothermal amplification; RT-qPCR, reverse transcriptase quantitative polymerase chain reaction.

- MDA levels against FCoV typically decline at around 4 to 8 weeks of age, allowing for FCoV infection. However, kittens as young as 2 weeks of age have been diagnosed with FIP (based on either histologic diagnosis or effusion analysis with immunostaining), although it is not known how these kittens acquired FCoV or whether they had MDA [20].

- Effusive disease typically progresses more rapidly than noneffusive disease:
  - From 6 to 42 days (average, 14 days) from onset of clinical signs to death in naturally infected SPF cats with effusive disease compared with weeks to months for noneffusive disease [34].
  - When FIP is a differential diagnosis, a careful search for cavitary effusions should be made (and likely repeated if initially unsuccessful; especially following rehydration).
  - The noneffusive form of FIP is typically more difficult to diagnose.
  - Cats with effusive disease (compared with noneffusive disease) are more likely to have pyrexia, lymphopenia, and icterus, and less likely to have ocular or neurologic signs, azotemia, and hyperproteinemia [20,45].
- The range of presenting signs and abnormalities on physical examination associated with FIP are variable because of the number and type of organs involved in individual patients [20,45].
  - Nonspecific signs, including pyrexia (nonresponsive to antibiotics), lethargy, and inappetence, are common, although some cats remain bright until the fulminant stages of disease.
  - Icterus of sclera and mucous membranes (often mild).
  - Mucous membrane pallor, caused by anemia (often mild).
  - Abdominal distention, associated with ascites and/or abdominal organomegaly (often representing mesenteric lymphadenopathy, gastrointestinal masses with focal infiltration, or renomegaly).
  - Respiratory signs (including dyspnea, tachypnea, and cough) may be associated with pleural effusion and/or pulmonary infiltration (pericardial effusions are sometimes seen, but are rarely associated with cardiac tamponade).
  - Evidence of ocular involvement: uveitis (keratic precipitate formation, anisocoria, dyscoria, and blepharospasm); chorioretinitis with perivascular cuffing; retinal detachment (leads to acute loss of vision); hyphema; hypopyon.
  - Neurologic signs, attributed to meningoencephalitis or meningomyelitis, with or without obstructive hydrocephalus, are often multifocal and can include ataxia, seizures, vestibular signs (eg, head tilt, nystagmus), cranial nerve deficits, and behavioral change (eg, obtundation).
  - Cutaneous lesions (rare), caused by perivascular pyogranulomatous dermatitis, include papular, nonpruritic lesions.

DIAGNOSTIC TESTS FOR FELINE CORONAVIRUS EXPOSURE OR SHEDDING

- Serology:
  - The uses and limitations of serologic testing of cats for coronavirus antibodies has been extensively reviewed elsewhere [47,48].
  - Antibodies may be detected in serum by enzyme-linked immunosorbent assay (ELISA; eg, FCoV/FIP Immunocomb, Biogal), immunofluorescence antibody test (IFAT; various), or immunochromatographic test (eg, Speed F-Corona, Virbac).
    - Some of these assays (eg, FCoV/FIP Immunocomb; Speed F-Corona) are point-of-care tests and give qualitative or semiquantitative results; most are very sensitive to detect even low antibody titers [49].
    - Other assays (typically offered by commercial laboratories) give quantitative results that can facilitate monitoring over time; because of potential variation between laboratories, it is important that the same laboratory is used when comparing results.
    - Coronavirus IFAT comprises virus-infected cells fixed on slides onto which test sera are applied; a secondary fluorophore-labeled antibody is then used to determine the presence of bound antibodies.
    - Coronavirus ELISAs or immunochromatographic tests comprise viral antigen bound to membranes across which test sera are washed and bound antibodies detected using a secondary labeled antibody.
    - There is marked antibody cross-reactivity between closely related coronavirus species, as detected by IFATs based on TGEV and FCoV (serotypes 1 and 2) [8,9].
      - This property has been exploited by IFATs used to investigate the serologic antibody response during the development of FIP: feline cells infected with either serotype 1

or serotype 2 FCoV can be used, or, alternatively, porcine cells infected with TGEV [50].
  - Although it is likely that seropositive cats have been exposed to FCoV rather than another coronavirus, this cannot be assumed; seropositive cats are often described as being coronavirus positive rather than FCoV positive.
- Seroconversion occurs 2 to 3 weeks following exposure to FCoV [51].
- A high antibody titer (>1:1600) is a nonspecific finding of limited value in the diagnosis of FIP, especially in cats from multicat households where the likelihood of seropositivity is high, in young cats where MDA may persist (up to 12–14 weeks), or in cats with recent exposure to others with known FCoV infection (eg, another cat with FIP in the household) [52], because most of these cats will not develop FIP.
- A high antibody titer in association with compatible clinical signs, history, and so forth can be supportive of FIP, particularly when coming from a household where the likelihood of seropositivity is low (eg, few cats resident), in that it indicates the necessary exposure to FCoV.
- Approximately 10% of cats with fulminant FIP may have negative serology caused by peracute disease (seroconversion takes 2–3 weeks), immune-complex formation, or immunosuppression [53].
- A positive antibody titer in a healthy cat does not indicate whether or not the cat is shedding FCoV in its feces [15,54]. During an 8-month observation period of 24 clinically normal cats with high FCoV antibody titers (≥1:1600), 1 frequently (>75% of samples) shed FCoV, 20 occasionally shed FCoV, and 3 did not shed [55]. Within 5 breeding catteries where FCoV was endemic, between 35% and 70% of cats were shedding at any 1 time [55].

- Fecal reverse transcriptase (RT) (quantitative [q]) polymerase chain reaction (PCR) (see also Box 1):
  - RT-PCR may be used to detect, and in some cases quantify (ie, RT-qPCR), FCoV shedding in feces.
  - Intermittent fecal shedding of FCoV or laboratory error (eg, caused by carry-over of PCR inhibitors found in feces) can produce negative results [56].
  - Repeated testing is required to identify persistent or recurrent FCoV shedders in multicat households, or whether they have stopped shedding. The optimum frequency of sample collection is unknown.
  - A positive RT-PCR result does not indicate whether a cat has, or will go on to develop, FIP.

DIAGNOSIS OF FELINE INFECTIOUS PERITONITIS

Fig. 3 shows a suggested approach to cats suspected of having FIP:

- Definitive diagnosis of FIP antemortem can be challenging, and:
  - Some investigators consider histologic colocalization of pyogranulomatous inflammation with presence of FCoV (shown by immunostaining for FCoV antigen) within monocytes/macrophages necessary to make a definitive diagnosis of FIP, and this is frequently considered the reference standard in studies evaluating diagnostic techniques [7,57]; however, this necessitates performance of procedures, of variable degrees of invasiveness, to obtain diagnostic samples.
  - In contrast, for many clinical trials and some trials of diagnostic techniques, diagnosis has been made based on a combination of signalment, clinical history, physical examination, and clinicopathologic findings (sometimes, but not always including RT-(q)PCR or immunostaining of tissue or effusions) [58–60].
- Antemortem, a clinical diagnosis of FIP is most often based on the combination of compatible signalment, history, clinical signs, typical clinical pathology changes (discussed later), analysis of effusions (if present; discussed later), and analysis of other cytologic samples (discussed later).
  - Identification of FCoV within effusions, tissue aspirates, cerebrospinal fluid (CSF) and so forth, either by immunostaining for FCoV antigen (discussed later) or by RT-(q)PCR (discussed later and also see Box 1) for genetic sequences of FCoV can be strongly supportive.
  - In some cats, tissue biopsy (discussed later) may be required to provide sufficient support for a clinical diagnosis of FIP.
  - The use of machine-learning techniques to enhance interpretation of combinations of data and indicate likelihood of disease are expected to be developed over the coming years [61].
- Imaging modalities (eg, thoracic or abdominal ultrasonography; radiography; computed tomography;

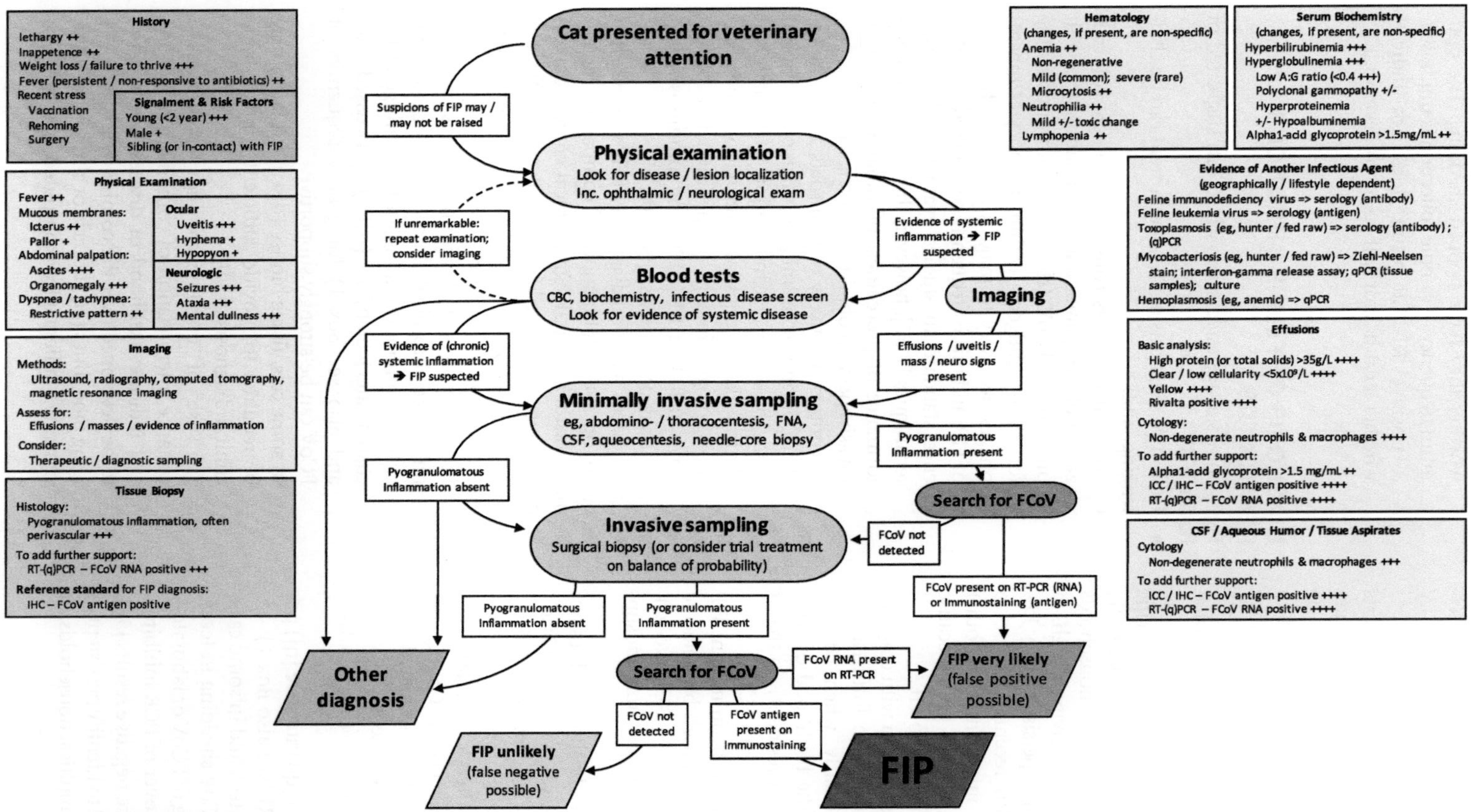

FIG. 3 Suggested diagnostic approach to cats with suspected FIP. CBC, complete blood count; CSF, cerebrospinal fluid; FNA, fine-needle aspiration; ICC, immunocytochemistry; IHC, immunohistochemistry. (*Modified from* Barker EN, Tasker S. An update on FIP. In Practice; with permission.)

MRI) can reveal evidence of fluid accumulations, mass lesions, and vasculitis/inflammation.
  - No imaging sign is pathognomonic for FIP, but imaging can facilitate exclusion of other differential diagnoses.
  - Imaging may facilitate needle sampling for further diagnostics (eg, cytology).
  - Fluid accumulations may progress over time, particularly following correction of dehydration, such that repeated imaging may be required.

Clinical pathologic changes of feline infectious peritonitis

- Hematology changes, if present, are nonspecific, but could include:
  - Mild, nonregenerative anemia (common).
  - Severe, regenerative anemia caused by immune-mediated hemolytic anemia or hemorrhage (uncommon).
  - Microcytosis in the absence of anemia (common).
  - Mild neutrophilia, with left shift or toxic changes (common); neutropenia (uncommon).
  - Lymphopenia (common); lymphocytosis (uncommon).
  - Eosinopenia (common); eosinophilia (uncommon).
  - Monocytosis (common).
  - Thrombocytopenia, caused by consumptive or immune-mediated processes (common); thrombocytosis (uncommon).
  - Increased coagulation test parameters (eg, activated partial thromboplastin time, prothrombin time) may develop caused by consumptive processes in fulminant FIP (eg, disseminated intravascular coagulation).
- Serum biochemistry changes, if present, are nonspecific, but could include:
  - Mild hyperbilirubinemia (common), attributed to systemic inflammation or vasculitis affecting hepatic parenchyma; mild increases in hepatic enzyme activities (uncommon).
  - Mild to severe hyperglobulinemia (common).
  - Serum protein electrophoresis typically shows a polyclonal gammopathy and hypoalbuminemia; less frequently, decreased beta-1 globulin (negative acute phase proteins) levels or increased alpha-2 globulin (positive acute phase proteins) levels are seen; rarely a monoclonal or restricted oligoclonal gammopathy is noted [62].
    - The frequency of electrophoretic changes seems to be decreasing over time, possibly because clinicians suspect/investigate FIP at an earlier stage in the disease, with increased numbers of cats reported with increased alpha-2 globulins without a gammopathy, and decreased numbers of cats with solely a gammopathy [63].
  - Mild hypoalbuminemia is common, attributed to a combination of a negative acute phase inflammatory response, compensation for hyperosmolarity, protein-losing enteropathy or nephropathy, and third spacing (if effusive).
  - Albumin to globulin ratio is usually low (<0.4, likely FIP; >0.8, FIP is unlikely) [64].
  - Acute phase protein measurements:
    - Alpha1-acid glycoprotein (AGP), a positive acute phase protein, is often at increased levels in cats with FIP [65–67].
      - AGP level greater than 1.5 to 2 mg/mL is considered supportive of FIP in cases where FIP is suspected [65]; however, increases are not specific to FIP, but the greater the magnitude of the increase, the more helpful it may be for cases in which there is a lower suspicion of FIP [66–69].
      - In 1 study, 85% of cats with FIP (41 of the 48) had AGP level greater than 1.5 mg/mL, whereas all cats with effusions that were subsequently shown not to have FIP (total of 21; 8 with cardiomyopathy, 6 with neoplasia, 5 with inflammatory/fibrotic disease, and 2 for which a definitive diagnosis was not achieved) had AGP less than 1.5 mg/mL, suggesting a specificity of 100% at this cutoff [65]; however, in the same study, 4 of 6 cats with terminal FIP infection had AGP level greater than 1.5 mg/mL.
      - In a second study, more than 50% of cats with inflammatory disease had AGP levels greater than 1.5 mg/mL [68]; AGP level greater than 1.5 to 2 mg/mL was also supportive of FIP where pretest probability (defined as the probability of the presence of the condition before a diagnostic test) of FIP was high (ie, signalment, clinical signs, and other clinicopathologic changes were suggestive of FIP), whereas, in cats with a low pretest probability of FIP (ie, few clinical signs and no signalment suggestive of FIP), only AGP level greater than 3 mg/mL could support a diagnosis of FIP and, even then, the probability of FIP remained less than 50%.

- In a third study, an optimal cutoff of 2.26 mg/mL achieved a sensitivity of 85% and specificity of 90% [66]; however, a definitive diagnosis (as confirmed histologically) was not made for most cats with FIP and without FIP.
- Cats with noneffusive FIP seem to have similar AGP values as those with effusive FIP [67].
- Some investigators have found AGP to be particularly useful to support a diagnosis of FIP in cases where there was a strong suspicion of FIP but where histology was equivocal [69].

▪ The utility of other positive acute phase proteins (haptoglobin, serum amyloid A) in supporting a diagnosis of FIP has been evaluated [65,66]; although levels of both were significantly increased in cats with FIP, compared with healthy cats or those with cardiac disease, neither was as accurate as AGP in differentiating cats with FIP from those with inflammatory diseases (septic processes, retroviral infection, neoplasia).

Effusion analysis

- Analysis of FIP-associated effusions (if present) can provide strong support for a diagnosis of FIP.
- Basic analysis: often FIP-associated effusions appear clear (ie, of low cellularity), straw yellow in color (reflecting the hyperbilirubinemia present), and viscous (ie, highly proteinaceous).
  - Total nucleated cell counts often less than 5×10^9/L nucleated cells, comprising predominately nondegenerate neutrophils and macrophages, with some lymphocytes.
  - Protein level often greater than 35 g/L (but can be <30 g/L, especially following repeated drainage).
  - Similar protein changes to serum [66,70,71]: often low albumin to globulin ratio.
  - Cloudy fluid is sometimes noted.
- The Rivalta test (a simple and inexpensive point-of-care test on effusions):
  - Method: mix 8 mL of distilled water with 1 drop of 98% acetic acid (or 2–3 drops of white vinegar); place 1 drop of effusion onto surface. A positive result is indicated by the effusion drop holding its shape. A negative result is indicated by the effusion drop dissipating into solution.
  - Positive results may also be obtained from other inflammatory exudates, such as those found in septic peritonitis, cholangiohepatitis, and neoplastic effusions.
  - The sensitivity of the Rivalta test in correctly identifying cats with FIP varies from 91.3% to 98% and the specificity from 65.5% to 80% [71,72].
    - ▪ In 1 study, where there was a 57% prevalence of FIP, negative and positive predictive values were 97% and 86% respectively [71]. In a larger, more recent study, where there was 34.6% prevalence of FIP, negative and positive predictive values were 93.4% and 58.4% respectively [72].
    - ▪ A recent study noted that, when the Rivalta test was combined with fluid cytology, to identify and exclude cases of lymphoma and bacterial peritonitis/pleuritis, both specificity and positive predictive value improved (73.0% and 73.4% respectively) [72].
    - ▪ These data suggest that the Rivalta test is most useful as a screening test to rule out FIP.
- Measurement of CoV antibodies in effusions: because both false-positive (specificity of 86%) and false-negative (sensitivity of 85%) results occur when used to predict the presence of FIP [71], this test is not recommended (ie, more accurate tests are available).
- Measurement of acute phase proteins [66] in effusions: using a cutoff of 1.55 mg/mL for AGP had a sensitivity and specificity of 93% in the diagnosis of FIP, based on results from 14 cats with and 53 cats without FIP; false-positive results included 3 cases of septic peritonitis and 1 retroviral-positive cat with metastatic abdominal neoplasia. Measurement of haptoglobin and serum amyloid A were both less sensitive and less specific.
- Immunostaining and molecular diagnostics of effusions are discussed later.

Analysis of cytologic samples other than effusions

- Other bodily fluids (eg, CSF, aqueous humor) and tissue aspirates (eg, lymph nodes, mass lesions) can be useful in the diagnosis of FIP.
- Cytology may provide evidence of pyogranulomatous to granulomatous inflammation: consistent with, but not diagnostic for, FIP.
  - In CSF, nonseptic pyogranulomatous (or mixed cellular, but including macrophages) inflammation compatible with FIP was present in 76% of the cats with FIP and 30% of control cats [73]. Note that 14 of the 41 cats included in the study had samples collected immediately postmortem, whereas the rest were collected during diagnostic investigations.

The influence that this would have had on results, if any, is unknown.
  - In aqueous humor, nonseptic pyogranulomatous (or mixed cellular, but including macrophages) inflammation compatible with FIP was present in 69% of the 26 cats with FIP, but in only 1 of the 12 control cats [74]. Note that all samples were collected postmortem using a larger gauge of needle (22 G) than would typically be used antemortem (27–29 G), which might have increased cellular yield.
  - On liver and kidney fine-needle aspirates (collected blind from cats with FIP at postmortem examination), cytologic sensitivity for nonseptic pyogranulomatous inflammation was 82% for liver and 42% for kidney aspirates, which is comparable with simultaneously collected needle-core biopsies [75]; however, 8 of the 50 cytologic samples were considered not of diagnostic quality and therefore were excluded from calculations. Concurrent samples processed using cytocentrifugation of aspirate material suspended in saline were even more likely to be considered nondiagnostic (21 out of 32 samples) and, of the remainder, all 6 of the liver aspirates but only 3 of the kidney aspirates revealed pyogranulomatous inflammation.
- Immunostaining and molecular diagnostics of cytologic samples other than effusions are discussed later.

Tissue biopsy analysis (histology)

- The primary disadvantage of biopsy analysis is that it requires invasive tissue collection to obtain the biopsy.
- In some cats, both with and without FIP, histologic examination is equivocal or misleading [45,69,76].
  - A small number of cats with idiopathic sterile pyogranulomatous inflammation (involving the head, neck, or mesenteric lymph nodes) have also been described in which FIP had been excluded, some of which appeared to respond to corticosteroids [77].
- The sensitivity of histology for the diagnosis of FIP in clinical cases is unknown:
  - For most studies that evaluate different diagnostic techniques for FIP, inclusion criteria use a combination of histology and immunostaining to either confirm FIP or to diagnose an alternate disorder on samples collected at postmortem examination; equivocal cases are therefore either not recruited (and not mentioned) or are excluded from further analysis [7].
  - In 1 large study, 14 of 127 recruited cats (11%) were ultimately excluded based on lack of a definitive diagnosis (including histologic examination); a further 5 cats (4%) had not had histologic examination performed and were also excluded [7].
  - In experimental FIP, of 19 cats with effusive disease examined postmortem, all had histologic lesions (histiocytic, neutrophilic, and fibrinous peritonitis) involving the omentum; mesentery; and serosal surfaces of the liver, spleen, mesenteric lymph nodes, and intestines [78]. However, not all cats had pyogranulomatous lymphadenitis or hepatitis; none had lesions within the pulmonary or cardiac tissue (excluding the pericardium); and, in the absence of clinical signs or gross evidence of disease, ocular/nervous tissue was not evaluated. Restriction of lesions to serosal surfaces would have limited biopsy were these clinical cases, despite them all presenting in a similar manner (ie, all had ascites).
  - Where blind needle-core biopsy of liver and kidneys has been evaluated in cats with FIP, possibly a better representation of what would happen clinically (compared with postmortem derived samples), sensitivity has been limited [75]. Although all liver biopsies (n = 25) were considered of diagnostic quality, only 16 (64%) had histologic changes consistent with FIP, 6 were equivocal for FIP, and 3 contained no lesions supportive of FIP; 7 out of 25 kidney biopsies were considered nondiagnostic, and, of the ones that were diagnostic, only 7 had histologic changes consistent with FIP (28% of total biopsies; 39%), 2 were equivocal for FIP, and 9 contained no lesions supportive of FIP.
- Immunostaining and molecular diagnostics of tissue are discussed later.

Immunostaining for feline coronavirus antigen

- Immunostaining is used to assess for the presence of FCoV antigen within infected macrophages.
- These assays include immunocytochemistry (ICC) [57] or immunofluorescence [71,79] of cytologic preparations (eg, centrifuge-concentrated cell preparation) or immunohistochemistry (IHC) of formalin-fixed cell pellets and tissue [46]; monoclonal or polyclonal

antibody preparations directed against FCoV antigens are used as reagents in these tests.

- Sensitivity of these assays is affected by both the cellularity of the samples being tested and the percentage of virus-infected monocytes/macrophages present, because a positive test result depends on the detection of FCoV antigen within these cells.
  - There seems to be variable geographic availability of immunostaining of cytologic samples (both effusion and noneffusion samples) as well as differences in techniques (particularly the reagents used), sensitivities, and specificities between laboratories.
- Immunostaining for FCoV applied to effusions:
  - The sensitivity for diagnosis of FIP on immunostaining varies from 57% [57,71] to 95% [80].
  - The specificity for diagnosis of FIP on immunostaining varies from to 71% to 100%.
  - False-positive results were reported for cats with neoplasia (lymphoma, adenocarcinoma) and cardiac disease [57,71,81].
  - One author described IHC on formalin-fixed cell pellets to be more sensitive than ICC [46].
- ICC for FCoV antigen on cytologic samples (both effusion and noneffusion samples) as a marker for FIP: a positive result provides support for a diagnosis of FIP, but a negative result does not rule out FIP; because false-positives occur, this should not be solely relied on to make a diagnosis.
- ICC for FCoV applied to cytologic samples other than effusions:
  - On CSF, sensitivity for FIP diagnosis was 85% and specificity was 83% [73]; however, some samples were acellular and therefore were excluded from calculations (1 out of 21 of the FIP group and 2 out of 20 of the control group). The 3 false-positive results were from a cat with lymphoma, a cat with lymphocytic meningoencephalitis, and a cat with hypertensive angiopathy (brain hemorrhage). There was no statistical difference between the sensitivities and specificities when the cats were further divided into those with or without neurologic signs.
  - On aqueous humor, sensitivity was 64% and specificity was 82% [74]; however, some samples were acellular and therefore excluded from calculations (1 out of 26 of the FIP group and 1 out of 12 of the control group). The 2 false-positive results were from a cat with lymphoma and a cat with pulmonary adenocarcinoma.
  - On mesenteric lymph node aspirates (collected under direct visualization at postmortem examination), sensitivity was 53% (16 of 30 cats with FIP were positive) and specificity was 91% (1 of 11 control cats were positive) [82], with all samples considered to be of diagnostic quality. Results of cytologic analysis alone were not reported. The 1 false-positive result was from a cat with lymphoma.
  - On liver and kidney aspirates, only 5 of the 16 (31%) liver aspirates and 2 of the 19 (11%) kidney aspirates were positive for FCoV antigen [75]. No control cats were tested for comparison.
  - However, the number of cases recruited into these studies (for both FIP and non-FIP categories) are small, and most are based on postmortem-collected samples; this increases the confidence intervals for both sensitivity and specificity calculations and limits evaluation of diagnostic utility.
    - Ideally, large prospective studies would evaluate the utility of immunostaining (and molecular diagnostics) on the antemortem diagnosis of FIP in cats suspected of having FIP.
      - IHC for FCoV antigen as a marker for FIP on tissue samples.
  - Many investigators consider the histopathologic demonstration of FCoV antigen within macrophages associated with (pyo)granulomatous lesions the reference standard for the diagnosis of FIP [46].
  - Distribution of FCoV within lesions can be variable [83,84].
  - In a large study, 62% of postmortem-collected tissue samples from cats with FIP were positive for FCoV within lesions [7]; however, because of the collection methods, not all of these tissues would have contained gross lesions.
  - The sensitivity of IHC on needle-core biopsy tissue samples was poor in the 1 study that has evaluated this: only 6 of 25 (24%) liver samples were positive and only 3 of 18 (17%) diagnostic kidney samples were FCoV antigen positive [75].

Molecular diagnostics in the diagnosis of feline infectious peritonitis

- The utility of RT-(q)PCR for FCoV (see Box 1) as a marker for FIP has been investigated for blood, effusions, other cytologic samples, and tissue samples.

- Most, but not all, RT-PCR assays used in recent studies (and available clinically) are quantitative; despite this, only qualitative (ie, positive or negative) results have been used to calculate diagnostic utility and, in some studies, only the qualitative data are reported.
  - Quantitative results (eg, copy number boundaries indicating degree of support) have not been evaluated for the diagnosis of FIP, although copy numbers are occasionally described for different samples and populations.
  - RT-qPCR for FCoV is preferable to RT-PCR for a variety of reasons, primarily related to quality control and initial assay optimization (see Box 1).
- Multiple studies (reviewed elsewhere [47]) have shown that use of FCoV RT-qPCR of blood (or blood components) for the diagnosis of FIP is often of low sensitivity, even in cats with experimental FIP [78], and that false-positives occur in cats without FIP [85].
- RT-PCR for FCoV on effusions:
  - Sensitivity for diagnosis of FIP varies from 72% to 100% [7,86,87].
  - Specificity for diagnosis of FIP varies from 83% to 100% [7,86,87]; however, numbers of samples tested in individual studies were often small.
  - Samples included in these studies were collected both antemortem, as part of the routine clinical investigation, and at postmortem examination; the numbers in these categories were not reported.
- RT-PCR for FCoV on cytologic samples other than effusions:
  - On CSF, sensitivity for diagnosis of FIP ranges from 42% to 63% for all cats [7,88,89] (combined total of 25 positive results from 49 cats); where differentiated, cats with neurologic/ocular manifestations of FIP were more likely to have a positive result (86% compared with 17%) than cats without these manifestations [88]; specificity was 100% in all studies where control cats were tested. In all studies, samples were collected postmortem.
  - On aqueous humor, sensitivity for diagnosis of FIP was 25% (4 out of 16 samples; all collected postmortem) [89]. No control cats were tested for comparison.
  - On mesenteric lymph nodes aspirates (collected under direct visualization postmortem), sensitivity for diagnosis of FIP ranges from 85% to 90% (17 of 20 cats with effusive and noneffusive FIP, and 18 of 20 cats with noneffusive FIP, respectively) [60,89] and specificity was 96% (1 out of 26 control cats was positive) [60].
  - On liver, spleen, and popliteal lymph node aspirates (20 of each from cats with either effusive or noneffusive FIP; all collected postmortem), sensitivities for diagnosis of FIP were 85%, 80%, and 65% respectively [89]. No control cats were tested for comparison.
  - However, the numbers of cases recruited into these studies (for both FIP and non-FIP categories) are small, and most are based on postmortem-collected samples; this increases the confidence intervals for both sensitivity and specificity calculations and limits evaluation of diagnostic utility.
    - Ideally, large prospective studies would evaluate the utility of molecular diagnostics (and immunostaining) on the antemortem diagnosis of FIP in cats suspected of having FIP.
- RT-PCR for FCoV on tissue samples:
  - All of these studies comprised samples collected at postmortem examination.
    - Larger volumes of tissue are often collected under these circumstances, which may increase the likelihood of achieving a definitive diagnosis and consequently the diagnostic sensitivity in cats with FIP.
    - Tissues may have been sampled that would not necessarily have been collected clinically, potentially reducing diagnostic sensitivity in cats with FIP; for example, liver and spleen biopsy in a cat with solely neurologic signs.
    - In contrast, samples may be collected from cats with more advanced clinical disease and pathologic change, potentially increasing diagnostic sensitivity in cats with FIP.
  - In studies comprising more than 20 cats with FIP, sensitivity per cat (ie, where 1 or more samples were analyzed per cat, and a single positive result considered to be diagnostic

for FIP) for diagnosis of FIP varied from 94% to 96% [7,90], whereas, when samples from individual tissues were considered, sensitivity ranged from 88% to 90% [7,91]; the tissues collected from individual cats (both FIP and non-FIP populations) varied widely.
- In studies comprising samples from more than 20 cats without FIP, specificity per cat (ie, where 1 or more samples were analyzed per cat, and a single positive result considered to be diagnostic for FIP) ranged from 39% to 90% [7,90,92], whereas, when samples from individual tissues were considered, specificity was 92% [7].
- Viral copy numbers were generally higher in cats with FIP compared with those found in cats without FIP [7,90]; viral copy numbers were also generally higher in tissue samples that were positive for FCoV antigen than for those that were negative for FCoV antigen [7].

- Overall, a positive RT-(q)PCR result on effusions, other cytologic samples, and tissue, but not blood (or its constituents) can provide strong support for a diagnosis of FIP; however:
  - Similar to immunostaining testing for FCoV antigen, sensitivity of RT-(q)PCR is affected by the number of FCoV-infected cells present in the sample under test; for cytologic samples, this is influenced by both cellularity and the disorder, whereas for tissue samples this appears to be a function of distribution of histopathological change.
  - On effusions and other cytologic samples, a negative result does not rule out FIP, particularly where cellularity was low; whereas on tissue samples where there is supportive pathology, a false-negative result is rare [7].
  - Because false-positives occur, RT-(q)PCR should not be solely relied on to make a diagnosis of FIP, particularly if multiple tissue samples are tested (because this can increase the likelihood of obtaining a single false-positive result). Fewer false-positives are documented for cytologic samples, likely reflecting their lower cellularity as well as expected distribution of potentially infected macrophages; however, caution should be used when interpreting specificities for cytologic samples because of the small sample sizes.

- FCoV mutation analysis has been applied to samples previously determined to be positive by RT-qPCR (Box 1).
  - The aim of mutation analysis is to differentiate FCoV pathotypes (ie, FECV from FIPV) based on differences in the viral genomic sequence, in the hope that this can be used to differentiate cats with FIP from those without [39].

BOX 1
Use of Polymerase Chain Reaction in the Detection of Feline Coronavirus

PCR is the method by which DNA is exponentially amplified using primers to target a specific sequence, enabling sensitive detection down to a very low starting DNA copy number. Post-PCR amplification processing (eg, sequencing) can be applied as well if needed. PCR only amplifies DNA so, because FCoV is an RNA virus, a pre-PCR step using a viral enzyme, RT, is required to generate a strand of cDNA using the original FCoV RNA template, in a process known as reverse transcription. A combination of this process and PCR is known as RT-PCR.

Given that only a very small volume of diagnostic sample is ultimately added to each PCR reaction, this does result in a limit to PCR sensitivity, although it remains a highly sensitivity modality compared with other tests for the presence of a pathogen.

Because of the high frequency of transcriptional errors during replication of RNA viruses and inherently increased variation between viral strains (compared with replication of DNA viruses), primers designed for the detection of FCoV (Fig. 4) predominantly target sections of the genome that are considered to be highly conserved (eg, nonstructural protein 7b; the membrane glycoprotein–nucleocapsid protein border; 3′ untranslated region), as determined by known sequence comparisons. Because of the conserved nature of these sections of the genome, other members of the Alphacoronavirus genus (ie, CCoV, TGEV) may also result in a positive result using assays for FCoV [93]. In contrast, 1 study described a PCR using primers designed on the more variable envelope protein gene on the suspicion that FECV could be differentiated from FIPV based on limited sequence data [94], although this is not supported by more recent data [39]. The shorter the amplified fragment in PCR, the more efficient the assay, which contributes to increased sensitivity; however, this does limit the length of amplified fragment subsequently available for sequencing if required. Regardless of how good primer design is, infrequently genomic variation, even in conserved regions, can result in the failure to detect FCoV (ie, false-negative results) even when likely present at high level [7].

RT-qPCR assays (sometimes known as real-time RT-PCR) that use either DNA-intercalation dyes (eg, SYBR green) or (TaqMan) hydrolysis probes to quantify the DNA within the reaction mixture after every amplification cycle, have been applied to the detection of FCoV [56,95]. If the signal from the reaction exceeds a defined threshold, it is taken to be a positive result and the cycle number at which the sample became positive is usually reported as either a CT (cycle exceeding threshold) or CP (crossing point). Note that the lower the CT/CP value, the higher the starting copy number, such that a CT/CP value of around 20 corresponds to around 10^6 copies per reaction, whereas a CT/CP value of around 40 corresponds to around 10 copies per reaction. Quantitative assays are more easily optimized and may result in them being more sensitive than conventional PCRs (which rely on detection of DNA at the end of the PCR process). Quantitative assays are also subject to less risk of laboratory contamination (a potential cause of false-positive results) than conventional PCRs because the reaction wells containing amplified DNA remain sealed and do not require opening for completion of detection (eg, using a gel) as for conventional PCR. In addition, hydrolysis probes have the potential to increase assay specificity (compared with the use of the PCR amplification primers alone), by providing an additional nucleotide sequence against which the target sequence must match to obtain a positive result. Hydrolysis probes also permit the duplexing of an FCoV assay with another PCR assay, such as one for the detection of host DNA as an internal control.

Because there is a reverse transcription step in the detection of FCoV by PCR, most assays detect both genomic RNA contained within virions and messenger RNA. Produced during active transcription and translation of the virus, messenger RNA may be full length or subgenomic length because of discontinuous transcription [96]. Relative abundance of individual fragments of the genome may therefore vary within a sample depending on the nature of the virus within that sample (eg, cell-free virions vs cell-associated viral replication) [91], which may account for differences in sensitivity between assays targeting different sections of the genome. Differences between the structure of subgenomic mRNA and genomic RNA (see Fig. 4) have been exploited by some assays [91,97], with the premise that detection of active viral transcription would only be present in cats with FIP; however, positive results were obtained from the blood of a small number of cats without FIP [97].

PCR-amplified DNA fragments may be sequenced, either by Sanger sequencing or by pyrosequencing. This technique has been applied to the sequence of the FCoV Spike gene associated with a switch in cell tropism (discussed elsewhere in this article) [7,86,87]. Limitations of Sanger sequencing include lack of data from approximately the first 30 to 50 bases of the fragment, time taken to perform, and need for specialist equipment; however, sequencing of large fragments (eg, 1000+ bases) is possible and the target sequence does not need to be known. Bench-top pyrosequencing is typically used to rapidly sequence short sections (~10–20 bases) on much smaller fragments; this is often facilitated by knowledge of the sequence possibilities of this section of the genome. Sanger sequencing has also been applied to fragments amplified from different regions of the FCoV genome for phylogenetic comparisons of isolates collected from an epizootic outbreak of FIP [98]. An alternative method of FCoV mutation analysis, which has been applied to FCoV RT-qPCR positive samples, is allelic discrimination [89,90,99]. This method is where 2 probes, each containing a different fluorescent dye, corresponding with the alternative FCoV genomic sequence (ie, 1 mutated, 1 not) being targeted are included in an assay, with the ratio of 1 probe to another measured by the relative production of fluorescence during the thermal cycling.

Loop-mediated isothermal amplification (LAMP) is a similar technology to PCR, whereby targeted complementary DNA (cDNA) sequences are amplified; however, because amplification is performed at a constant temperature, there is no longer a requirement for a thermal cycler, and it is therefore potentially considerably cheaper and more robust in the field. DNA amplification is detected by an increase in turbidity, often facilitated by the use of dyes, and postamplification processing is limited (ie, sequencing is not possible). This technology has been applied to the detection of FCoV (ie, RT-LAMP), and although specific (ie, only samples positive for FCoV gave positive results with RT-LAMP), its sensitivity was around half of that of PCR [100,101].

- Presence of mutations M1058L and S1060A within the fragment of Spike gene encoding the putative fusion peptide of the serotype 1 Spike glycoprotein has been most frequently studied for the diagnosis of FIP, albeit using different techniques, different sample types, and with different conclusions (Table 2).
- Inclusion of Spike gene analysis alongside RT-qPCR does not seem to substantially improve specificity; further, a consequence of considering only results with Spike gene mutation as being diagnostic for FIP significantly reduces test sensitivity [7].
- Detection of Spike gene mutations in cats without FIP was expected, because it is estimated that 90% of cats that experience systemic FIPV infection do not go on to develop FIP [36].
- Some investigators remain strongly supportive of the use of Spike gene analysis using allelic discrimination in the diagnosis of FIP where

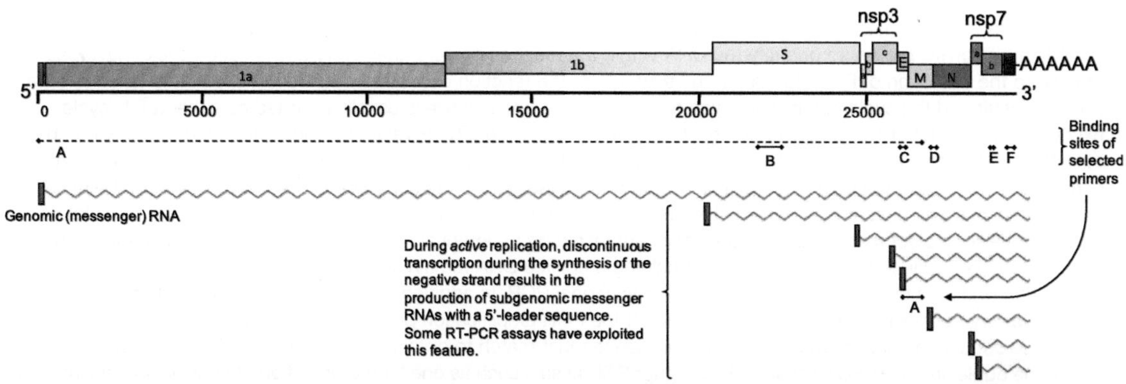

FIG. 4 Primer binding sites of selected RT-PCRs. A: amplifying a 295-bp fragment of subgenomic mRNA of the Membrane gene [97]. B: amplifying a 688-bp fragment of the Spike glycoprotein gene [92]. C: amplifying a 170-bp fragment of the Envelope protein gene [94]. D: amplifying a 171-bp fragment of the Membrane glycoprotein–Nucleocapsid protein gene border [56]. E: amplifying a 102-bp fragment of the nonstructural protein 7b gene [95]. F: amplifying a 223-bp fragment within the 3′ untranslated region [93].

minimizing false-positive results is paramount [47].

TREATMENT

- Until recently, FIP was considered to be a progressive and ultimately fatal disease in almost all cases; however, with the advent of novel antiviral medication (ie, protease inhibitors and nucleoside analogues), there is an argument for considering FIP a potentially curable disease.
- A few cats are thought to have been able to confine the disease locally, at least for some time (months to years) [45,102].
- A paucity of placebo-controlled or current best treatment–controlled clinical trials of cats with definitively diagnosed FIP, along with a lack of licensed drugs with proven efficacy in curing FIP, has limited treatment recommendations.
- Supportive care: appetite stimulants (eg, mirtazapine, up to 2 mg/cat/d), vitamin B_{12} supplementation (0.02 mg/kg by weekly subcutaneous injection, or 0.25 mg/cat orally once daily), antioxidants, fluid therapy.
- Benefit of draining effusions is debated:
  - Thoracocentesis is indicated where dyspnea is present.
  - Therapeutic abdominocentesis is controversial and may be detrimental because of exacerbation of dehydration if large volumes are removed (which often reform rapidly).
  - Some investigators have described fluid drainage followed by intracavitary steroid administration (dexamethasone 1 mg/kg once daily, until resolution of effusion or up to 7 days); in 1 study where this was administered, in addition to other medications, effusions temporarily resolved in 6 of 36 cats, and, although all succumbed to FIP (1 within 7 days of diagnosis, 4 within 21 days to 3 months of diagnosis, and 1 at 200 days post-diagnosis), this compared favorably with the median survival time of 8 to 9 days for all cats treated [103].
- Prednisolone is frequently administered to ameliorate some of the clinical signs associated with the chronic inflammatory process; however, there have been no clinical trials to support its use. A starting dose of 0.5 mg/kg twice daily orally is suggested (some texts suggest up to 1 mg/kg twice daily), then tapered if possible.
  - One study found that survival times of cats with noneffusive FIP were significantly shorter in cats that were treated with corticosteroids (by any route) concurrently with polyprenyl immunostimulant (median survival time, 21.5 days compared with 73.5 days) [59]; however, the investigators could not rule out administration of corticosteroids as an indirect marker of disease severity.
- Feline interferon-omega: often used but lacking convincing evidence of effect in a placebo-controlled trial [103].
- Many other drugs have been suggested but currently lack a robust evidence base for use, including pentoxifylline, propentofylline [104], polyprenyl immunostimulant (20% of cats with dry FIP in recent

TABLE 2
Sensitivity and Specificity of Different Modalities Applied to Spike Gene Mutation Analysis

Methodology	Sample Type (Corresponding Sensitivity ± Specificity Compared with FCoV RT-PCR Alone)					Notes
	Tissue	Effusions	Needle Aspirates (Tissues; Lymph Nodes)	CSF	Aqueous Humor	
Pyrosequencing	Sensitivity = 81% Specificity = 95% (compared with 90% and 93% respectively) 14 out of 19 samples from cats without FIP positive for FCoV were also positive for the Spike gene mutation [7]	Sensitivity = 74% Specificity = 96% (compared with 91% and 96% respectively) The 1 sample from a cat without FIP that was positive by FCoV RT-qPCR (of 28 tested) was also positive for the Spike gene mutation [7]	NA	NA	NA	Spike gene mutations were detected in FCoV-positive tissue from cats without FIP at the same frequency as in cats with FIP Able to obtain results at very low viral loads (down to 1.8×10^3 viral RNA equivalents/mL effusion)
Sanger sequencing	Sensitivity = 70% Specificity = 88% (compared with 91% and 50% respectively) One cat, of the 4 without FIP positive for FCoV (of 8 tested), was positive for the Spike gene mutation [86]	Sensitivity = 40–64% Specificity = 83% (compared with 72%–100% and 83% respectively) [86,87] The 1 sample from a cat without FIP that was positive by FCoV RT-qPCR (of 6 tested) was also positive for the Spike gene mutation [86]	NA	NA	NA	—

(continued on next page)

TABLE 2
(continued)

Methodology	Sample Type (Corresponding Sensitivity ± Specificity Compared with FCoV RT-PCR Alone)					Notes
	Tissue	**Effusions**	**Needle Aspirates (Tissues; Lymph Nodes)**	**CSF**	**Aqueous Humor**	
Allelic discrimination	Sensitivity = 30–71% Specificity = 100% (compared with 65%–95% and 90% respectively) [89,90]	Sensitivity = 64–69% Specificity = 96% (compared with 86%–97% and 88% respectively) [89,99]	Sensitivity = 15–45% (compared with 65%–85%) [89]	Sensitivity = 44% (compared with 63%) [89]	Sensitivity = 10% (compared with 25%) [89]	The copy number below which allelic discrimination is not possible is reported to be 1.5×10^6 viral RNA equivalents/mL effusion [99]; samples that are below the limit of detection are considered negative

Where specificity is not reported, either no cats without FIP were included in those studies or the relevant samples from cats without FIP were negative by FCoV RT-qPCR and therefore Spike gene mutation analysis could not be performed.

Abbreviation: NA, not available.

study had greater survival than expected, gaining more clinical interest) [59], ozagrel hydrochloride [105], cyclophosphamide, ciclosporin A, anti–tumor necrosis factor alpha antibodies [106], itraconazole [107], mefloquine [108], turmeric-based compounds [109], and herbal medication.

- Protease inhibitor GC376:
  - The function of the FCoV protease is to cleave the viral polymerase from polyprotein 1, and is essential for viral replication; GC376 is a reversible, competitive inhibitor of the FCoV protease [110].
  - Administered by subcutaneous injection twice daily, GC376 produced remarkable responses in both experimental and naturally occurring FIP: 6 of 8 cats with experimentally induced FIP were alive at 8 months posttreatment [29], and 19 of the 20 cats with naturally occurring FIP had a positive response (including, where present, rapid resolution of pyrexia, resolution of effusions and associated clinical signs, resolution of icterus, resolution of uveitis, resolution of mass lesions, weight gain) that was sustained in 7 [58].
  - Based on evidence of relapse of clinical signs following withdrawal of short courses of treatment, followed by a sustained response to reinstitution of treatment, in cats with naturally occurring FIP, the minimum duration of treatment was increased and is now recommended as 12 weeks.
  - Reported side effects of GC376 administration included injection reactions (transient pain on administration, occasional foci of subcutaneous fibrosis, hair loss) and interruption of normal dental development in cats aged less than 4 months (delayed development, abnormal eruption of permanent teeth) [58].
  - Eight of the 13 cats that succumbed to naturally occurring FIP did so because of severe neurologic signs, and, although some of these cats had experienced remission of clinical signs following an increase in dose of GC376 administered, ultimately they relapsed [58]. Cats that had initially presented with neurologic FIP had been excluded from this treatment trial based on unpublished experimental studies; presumably poor response to treatment or high frequency of relapse.
- Adenosine nucleoside analogue GS-441524:
  - GS-441524 acts as an alternative substrate and RNA-chain terminator of the viral RNA polymerase, thereby interfering with viral replication.
  - Administered by daily subcutaneous injection, GS-441524 produced remarkable responses in both experimentally induced and naturally occurring FIP: all 10 cats with experimental-induced FIP were alive at 8 months posttreatment [111], and 26 of 31 cats with naturally occurring FIP had a positive response (including, where present, rapid resolution of pyrexia, resolution of effusions and associated clinical signs, resolution of icterus, resolution of uveitis, resolution of mass lesions, weight gain) that was sustained in 25 [112].
  - Based on evidence of relapse of clinical signs following withdrawal of short courses of treatment in cats with naturally occurring FIP treated with GC376 [58] and in cats with experimentally induced FIP treated with GS-441524 [111] (where treatment courses were 2 weeks, with a repeated course in the 2 cats that experienced relapses), the minimum treatment duration for cats with naturally occurring was set at 12 weeks.
  - Cats with neurologic FIP were associated with a poorer outcome and, where successful, required increased doses of GS-441524 (continued for a minimum of 12 weeks) to achieve clinical remission [112,113].
  - Reported side effects of GS-441524 administration included [112] injection reactions (transient pain on administration, lasting 30–60 seconds; ulcerations, progressing to open sores in some cats; scar formation) and development of transient azotemia in 1 cat.
  - A rapid, transient increase in serum globulin level was also found, associated with resolution of effusions.
- Neither protease inhibitor GC376 nor nucleoside analogue GS-441524 are commercially available; however, there are reports that some owners have sourced black-market medication via the Internet (Emi Barker and Séverine Tasker 2019/2020; personal communications).
- Mutian X, an adenosine nucleoside analogue, reported to be different to GS-441524, has been marketed for the treatment of FIP. Mutian X is available as both oral and injectable formulations. Although no evidence has been published to support the use of Mutian X to date, there is limited research describing its use to stop fecal shedding of virus [114].
- Functional changes to the FCoV genome that resulted in in vitro changes in susceptibility to GC376 have been shown following chronic administration of GC376 to a cat with naturally occurring FIP [115]; however, this was not accompanied by

clinical evidence of drug resistance. This report has raised concerns regarding the potential for emergence of resistance to antiviral agents, particularly following chronic administration of treatment or when used in the treatment of enteric FCoV infection (ie, to stop fecal shedding), which may ultimately result in the transmission of resistant strains to other cats.

Prognosis

In the absence of GC376 or GS-441524, prognosis associated with FIP is grave (median survival time, 9 days; range, 3–200 days [103]; most of the cats in that study had effusive disease).

Prevention

- Vaccination:
  - Early immunization studies documented ADE [27], whereby cats experimentally sensitized to 1 strain of FCoV subsequently developed more acute and severe disease than expected following exposure to an alternative strain.
  - An intranasal vaccine (FELOCELL FIP, Zoetis) containing a temperature-sensitive, live-attenuated strain of FCoV is available in the United States and continental Europe.
    - According to manufacturer's guidelines, cats should be seronegative before vaccination, and greater than or equal to 16 weeks at the first dose, with a second dose 3 weeks later.
    - In situations in which FIP is a concern (eg, catteries where FCoV is endemic), and therefore vaccination considered, exposure to FCoV is likely to have occurred before the earliest recommended age of administration (ie, 16 weeks) [116].
    - Variable efficacy has been reported; in 1 study, although vaccination reduced the risk of developing FIP in those cats that had low or negative FCoV antibody titers at time of administration (from 10.7% to 3.3%), it did not eliminate the risk [116].
    - ADE has not been reported for the intranasal vaccine when administered under field conditions [116,117], but was reported under experimental conditions [118].
    - Its use is controversial and routine use is not recommended even where available (ie, it is noncore) [119].
    - It is not possible to differentiate vaccination-induced antibodies from those acquired following natural exposure, potentially limiting interpretation of serologic antibody testing in the future.
- In households or establishments where FIP has been confirmed, efforts should be made to:
  - Reduce transmission of FCoV: good litter tray hygiene, provision of adequate numbers of litter trays, food and water bowls placed away from litter trays (outdoor access for toileting is preferred).
  - Isolation of breeding queens 2 weeks before parturition and separating kittens from the queens (at 5–6 weeks) before MDA level declines to prevent kitten exposure to FCoV has been described, but is controversial:
    - It is often practically difficult for the breeder to maintain strict biosecurity conditions.
    - There are concerns regarding kitten welfare, socialization, and development.
  - Reduce stress: consider stocking density (ie, keep as low as possible) such as rehoming nonbreeding queens/neuters in breeding environment; maintain stable groups of cats; consider environmental provisions for each cat and environmental enrichment.
  - In domestic households (eg, <4 cats), it has been suggested not to introduce any new cats for at least 2 to 3 months after a cat has died of FIP (to allow time for any residual virus to become inactive, and to possibly reduce shedding from remaining cats) [120].
  - In breeding catteries, it is suggested to avoid breeding from cats repeatedly producing kittens that go on to develop FIP (especially stud males, because these have greater capacity to pass on their genetic material to future generations); often breeders are unaware of (or reluctant to admit to) having endemic FCoV within their catteries, because FIP typically only manifests after kittens have been rehomed.
  - Use of serial fecal PCR to identify chronic FCoV shedders may enable segregation of cats, but intermittent shedding and reinfection with FCoV can occur.

PRESENT RELEVANCE AND FUTURE AVENUES TO CONSIDER OR TO INVESTIGATE

Questions remain regarding the pathogenesis, diagnosis, treatment, and prevention of FIP. Many of the articles assessing the utility of specific tests to support the diagnosis of FIP (eg, immunostaining; RT-PCR) have several significant limitations such that interpretation of results might not reflect the reality of clinical practice:

- Many investigators interpret results in isolation from other supportive results such as clinical history, physical examination findings, routine clinic-pathology results, and sample cytology or histology.
- Samples for testing are frequently obtained at post-mortem examination.
- Control populations (ie, cats without FIP) might not necessarily represent cats in which FIP was a significant differential diagnosis (eg, a middle-aged cat with heart failure and thoracic effusion).
- Numbers of cats enrolled in both FIP and non-FIP populations in many studies that use cytologic samples (eg, fine-needle aspirate samples) are small, such that confidence intervals are wide and strong conclusions difficult to make.
- Because different studies perform different assays on subtly different populations, comparison of assay utility on limited numbers of cats remains complicated.

Future studies will ideally compare several different test modalities and assess their utility in the diagnosis of FIP, possibly in combination, as part of a diagnostic algorithm applicable to clinical practice, where less invasive techniques (eg, fine-needle aspirates, needle-core biopsy) are preferred. In recent years, there have also been dramatic leaps forward in the treatment of FIP with novel antiviral agents; more studies are required to determine whether these can be curative. Looking forward, advances in knowledge across all areas, including prevention through vaccination, may occur as a fortuitous consequence of the SARS-2-CoV outbreak in humans.

SUMMARY

Molecular diagnostics (primarily RT-qPCR) are providing increased support for the diagnosis of FIP, although they are not a reference standard for diagnosis. Samples suitable for RT-qPCR analysis are more amenable to minimally invasive diagnostic techniques, compared with biopsy for histology and confirmatory IHC. In the advent of effective antiviral medication for the treatment of FIP, the focus of FIP diagnosis is likely to switch to those modalities that maximize sensitivity, from those that maximize specificity.

FUNDING

E.N. Barker has received financial support for infectious disease research from the British Small Animal Veterinary Association (BSAVA) PetSavers, Langford Trust, Langford Vets Clinical Research Fund, European Society of Veterinary Internal Medicine Clinical Studies Fund grant, Morris Animal Foundation, Winn Feline Foundation, and Zoetis Animal Health. S. Tasker has received financial support for infectious disease research from BSAVA PetSavers, Journal of Comparative Pathology Educational Trust, Langford Trust, Langford Vets Clinical Research Fund, Morris Animal Foundation, NERC/BBSRC/MRC, Petplan Charitable Trust, South West Biosciences DTP, Wellcome Trust, and Zoetis Animal Health.

ACKNOWLEDGMENTS

E.N. Barker and S. Tasker would like to acknowledge the many contributions made by the University of Bristol Feline Coronavirus Research Group and Bristol-Zurich FIP Consortium to the viewpoints and discussions described in this article. Andrew Davidson, Anja Kipar, and Stuart Siddell are also thanked for their valued contributions to past and current FCoV research. Additional thanks go to the veterinary practices, cat owners, cat breeders, and rescue centers that helped in the acquisition of samples used in these research studies and to colleagues, current and past, at the Feline Centre, Langford Vets, and Veterinary Pathology Unit of the Bristol Veterinary School, University of Bristol, who have assisted in obtaining samples. In addition, the authors wish to acknowledge the inspirational work of the late Professor Michael J. Day, because of the large part he played in the diagnosis of cases of FIP and other diseases for samples in the Bristol FIP Biobank.

DISCLOSURE

S. Tasker is a member of the World Forum for Companion Animal Vector Borne diseases, supported by Bayer Animal Health, and of the European Advisory Board on Cat Diseases (supported by Merial/Boehringer Ingelheim, the founding sponsor of the Advisory Board on Cat Diseases, and from November 2018 additionally by Virbac). She is also Chief Medical Officer for the Linnaeus Group. E.N. Barker also works for the Molecular Diagnostic Unit, Langford Vets, University of Bristol.

REFERENCES

[1] Schoeman D, Fielding BC. Coronavirus envelope protein: current knowledge. Virol J 2019;16:69.

[2] Pedersen NC. An overview of feline enteric coronavirus and infectious peritonitis virus-infections. Feline Pract 1995;23:7–20.
[3] Pedersen NC, Black JW, Boyle JF, et al. Pathogenic Differences Between Various Feline Coronavirus Isolates. Adv Exp Med Biol 1984;173:365–80.
[4] Terada Y, Matsui N, Noguchi K, et al. Emergence of pathogenic coronaviruses in cats by homologous recombination between feline and canine coronaviruses. PLoS One 2014;9:e106534.
[5] Le Poder S, Pham-Hung d'Alexandry d'Orangiani AL, Duarte L, et al. Infection of cats with atypical feline coronaviruses harbouring a truncated form of the canine type I non-structural ORF3 gene. Infect Genet Evol 2013;20:488–94.
[6] Herrewegh AA, Smeenk I, Horzinek MC, et al. Feline coronavirus type II strains 79-1683 and 79-1146 originate from a double recombination between feline coronavirus type I and canine coronavirus. J Virol 1998;72: 4508–14.
[7] Barker EN, Stranieri A, Helps CR, et al. Limitations of using feline coronavirus spike protein gene mutations to diagnose feline infectious peritonitis. Vet Res 2017; 48:60.
[8] Reynolds DJ, Garwes DJ, Gaskell CJ. Detection of transmissible gastroenteritis virus neutralising antibody in cats. Arch Virol 1977;55:77–86.
[9] Pedersen NC, Ward J, Mengeling WL. Antigenic relationship of the feline infectious peritonitis virus to coronaviruses of other species. Arch Virol 1978;58:45–53.
[10] Reynolds DJ, Garwes DJ. Virus isolation and serum antibody responses after infection of cats with transmissible gastroenteritis virus. Brief report. Arch Virol 1979; 60:161–6.
[11] Woods RD, Pedersen NC. Cross-protection studies between feline infectious peritonitis and porcine transmissible gastroenteritis viruses. Vet Microbiol 1979;4:11–6.
[12] Barlough JE, Stoddart CA, Sorresso GP, et al. Experimental inoculation of cats with canine coronavirus and subsequent challenge with feline infectious peritonitis virus. Lab Anim Sci 1984;34:592–7.
[13] Barlough JE, Johnson-Lussenburg CM, Stoddart CA, et al. Experimental inoculation of cats with human coronavirus 229E and subsequent challenge with feline infectious peritonitis virus. Can J Comp Med 1985;49: 303–7.
[14] Drechsler Y, Alcaraz A, Bossong FJ, et al. Feline coronavirus in multicat environments. Vet Clin North Am Small Anim Pract 2011;41:1133–69.
[15] Addie DD, Dennis JM, Toth S, et al. Long-term impact on a closed household of pet cats of natural infection with feline coronavirus, feline leukaemia virus and feline immunodeficiency virus. Vet Rec 2000;146: 419–24.
[16] Addie DD, Schaap IA, Nicolson L, et al. Persistence and transmission of natural type I feline coronavirus infection. J Gen Virol 2003;84:2735–44.
[17] Pedersen NC, Allen CE, Lyons LA. Pathogenesis of feline enteric coronavirus infection. J Feline Med Surg 2008;10:529–41.
[18] Addie DD, Jarrett O. A study of naturally occurring feline coronavirus infections in kittens. Vet Rec 1992; 130:133–7.
[19] Addie DD, Toth S, Murray GD, et al. The risk of typical and antibody enhanced feline infectious peritonitis among cats from feline coronavirus endemic households. Feline Pract 1995;23:24–6.
[20] Riemer F, Kuehner KA, Ritz S, et al. Clinical and laboratory features of cats with feline infectious peritonitis - a retrospective study of 231 confirmed cases (2000-2010). J Feline Med Surg 2016;18:348–56.
[21] Norris JM, Bosward KL, White JD, et al. Clinicopathological findings associated with feline infectious peritonitis in Sydney, Australia: 42 cases (1990-2002). Aust Vet J 2005;83:666–73.
[22] Pesteanu-Somogyi LD, Radzai C, Pressler BM. Prevalence of feline infectious peritonitis in specific cat breeds. J Feline Med Surg 2006;8:1–5.
[23] Pedersen NC, Liu H, Gandolfi B, et al. The influence of age and genetics on natural resistance to experimentally induced feline infectious peritonitis. Vet Immunol Immunopathol 2014;162:33–40.
[24] Stoddart ME, Gaskell RM, Harbour DA, et al. The sites of early viral replication in feline infectious peritonitis. Vet Microbiol 1988;18:259–71.
[25] Whittaker GR, Andre NM, Miler A, et al. Detection of feline coronavirus from the respiratory tract and conjunctiva of cats. 2019. Phoenix (AZ): ACVIM Forum; 2019.
[26] Takano T, Yamada S, Doki T, et al. Pathogenesis of oral type I feline infectious peritonitis virus (FIPV) infection: Antibody-dependent enhancement infection of cats with type I FIPV via the oral route. J Vet Med Sci 2019;81:911–5.
[27] Pedersen NC. Virologic and immunologic aspects of feline infectious peritonitis virus infection. Adv Exp Med Biol 1987;218:529–50.
[28] McKeirnan AJ, Evermann JF, Hargis A, et al. Isolation of feline coronaviruses from two cats with diverse disease manifestations. Feline Pract 1981;11:16–20.
[29] Kim Y, Liu H, Galasiti Kankanamalage AC, et al. Reversal of the progression of fatal coronavirus infection in cats by a broad-spectrum coronavirus protease inhibitor. PLoS Pathog 2016;12:e1005531.
[30] Scott FW. Update on FIP. In: 12th Annual Kal Kan Symposium for the Treatment of Small Animal Diseases Columbus, OH, October 1988, p. 43–7.
[31] Addie D, Houe L, Maitland K, et al. Effect of cat litters on feline coronavirus infection of cell culture and cats. J Feline Med Surg 2019. https://doi.org/10.1177/1098612X19848167 1098612X19848167.
[32] Belouzard S, Millet JK, Licitra BN, et al. Mechanisms of coronavirus cell entry mediated by the viral spike protein. Viruses 2012;4:1011–33.

[33] Kipar A, Meli ML, Baptiste KE, et al. Sites of feline coronavirus persistence in healthy cats. J Gen Virol 2010;91: 1698–705.
[34] Desmarets LM, Vermeulen BL, Theuns S, et al. Experimental feline enteric coronavirus infection reveals an aberrant infection pattern and shedding of mutants with impaired infectivity in enterocyte cultures. Sci Rep 2016;6:20022.
[35] Kipar A, Baptiste K, Barth A, et al. Natural FCoV infection: cats with FIP exhibit significantly higher viral loads than healthy infected cats. J Feline Med Surg 2006;8:69–72.
[36] Pedersen NC. Overview of FIP and Current State of FIP. Winn Feline Foundation FIP Symposium: PURRsuing FIP and WINNing. UC Davis, Davis, California. November 16 and 17, 2019.
[37] Acar DD, Olyslaegers DA, Dedeurwaerder A, et al. Upregulation of endothelial cell adhesion molecules characterizes veins close to granulomatous infiltrates in the renal cortex of cats with feline infectious peritonitis and is indirectly triggered by feline infectious peritonitis virus-infected monocytes *in vitro*. J Gen Virol 2016;97: 2633–42.
[38] de Groot-Mijnes JD, van Dun JM, van der Most RG, et al. Natural history of a recurrent feline coronavirus infection and the role of cellular immunity in survival and disease. J Virol 2005;79:1036–44.
[39] Chang HW, Egberink HF, Halpin R, et al. Spike protein fusion peptide and feline coronavirus virulence. Emerg Infect Dis 2012;18:1089–95.
[40] Licitra BN, Millet JK, Regan AD, et al. Mutation in spike protein cleavage site and pathogenesis of feline coronavirus. Emerg Infect Dis 2013;19:1066–73.
[41] Pedersen NC, Liu H, Dodd KA, et al. Significance of coronavirus mutants in feces and diseased tissues of cats suffering from feline infectious peritonitis. Viruses 2009;1:166–84.
[42] Chang HW, de Groot RJ, Egberink HF, et al. Feline infectious peritonitis: insights into feline coronavirus pathobiogenesis and epidemiology based on genetic analysis of the viral 3c gene. J Gen Virol 2010;91: 415–20.
[43] Hsieh LE, Huang WP, Tang DJ, et al. 3C protein of feline coronavirus inhibits viral replication independently of the autophagy pathway. Res Vet Sci 2013; 95:1241–7.
[44] Andre NM, Cossic B, Davies E, et al. Distinct mutation in the feline coronavirus spike protein cleavage activation site in a cat with feline infectious peritonitis-associated meningoencephalomyelitis. J Feline Med Surg Open Rep 2019;5:2055116919856103.
[45] Pedersen NC. A review of feline infectious peritonitis virus infection: 1963-2008. J Feline Med Surg 2009;11: 225–58.
[46] Kipar A, Meli ML. Feline infectious peritonitis: still an enigma? Vet Pathol 2014;51:505–26.
[47] Felten S, Hartmann K. Diagnosis of feline infectious peritonitis: a review of the current literature. Viruses 2019;11. https://doi.org/10.3390/v11111068.
[48] Pedersen NC. The history and interpretation of feline coronavirus serology. Feline Pract 1995;23:46–51.
[49] Addie DD. Utility of feline coronavirus antibody tests. J Feline Med Surg 2014;17:152–62.
[50] Osterhaus AD, Horzinek MC, Reynolds DJ. Seroepidemiology of feline infectious peritonitis virus infections using transmissible gastroenteritis virus as antigen. Zentralbl Veterinarmed B 1977;24:835–41.
[51] Meli M, Kipar A, Muller C, et al. High viral loads despite absence of clinical and pathological findings in cats experimentally infected with feline coronavirus (FCoV) type I and in naturally FCoV-infected cats. J Feline Med Surg 2004;6:69–81.
[52] Bell ET, Toribio JA, White JD, et al. Seroprevalence study of feline coronavirus in owned and feral cats in Sydney, Australia. Aust Vet J 2006;84:74–81.
[53] Meli ML, Burr P, Decaro N, et al. Samples with high virus load cause a trend toward lower signal in feline coronavirus antibody tests. J Feline Med Surg 2013;15: 295–9.
[54] Foley JE, Poland A, Carlson J, et al. Patterns of feline coronavirus infection and fecal shedding from cats in multiple-cat environments. J Am Vet Med Assoc 1997; 210:1307–12.
[55] Foley JE, Poland A, Carlson J, et al. Risk factors for feline infectious peritonitis among cats in multiple-cat environments with endemic feline enteric coronavirus. J Am Vet Med Assoc 1997;210:1313–8.
[56] Dye C, Helps CR, Siddell SG. Evaluation of real-time RT-PCR for the quantification of FCoV shedding in the faeces of domestic cats. J Feline Med Surg 2008; 10:167–74.
[57] Felten S, Matiasek K, Gruendl S, et al. Investigation into the utility of an immunocytochemical assay in body cavity effusions for diagnosis of feline infectious peritonitis. J Feline Med Surg 2017;19:410–8.
[58] Pedersen NC, Kim Y, Liu H, et al. Efficacy of a 3C-like protease inhibitor in treating various forms of acquired feline infectious peritonitis. J Feline Med Surg 2018;20: 378–92.
[59] Legendre AM, Kuritz T, Galyon G, et al. Polyprenyl immunostimulant treatment of cats with presumptive non-effusive feline infectious peritonitis in a field study. Front Vet Sci 2017;4:7.
[60] Dunbar D, Kwok W, Graham E, et al. Diagnosis of non-effusive feline infectious peritonitis by reverse transcriptase quantitative PCR from mesenteric lymph node fine-needle aspirates. J Feline Med Surg 2018;21: 910–21.
[61] Dunbar D, Babayan SA, Addie DD, et al. A machine learning approach for enhancing feline infectious peritonitis diagnosis. ISFM Congress. Cavtat, Croatia: J Feline Med Surg, 26–30th June 2019, p. 848.

[62] Taylor SS, Tappin SW, Dodkin SJ, et al. Serum protein electrophoresis in 155 cats. J Feline Med Surg 2010; 12:643–53.
[63] Stranieri A, Giordano A, Bo S, et al. Frequency of electrophoretic changes consistent with feline infectious peritonitis in two different time periods (2004-2009 vs 2013-2014). J Feline Med Surg 2017;19:880–7.
[64] Jeffery U, Deitz K, Hostetter S. Positive predictive value of albumin: globulin ratio for feline infectious peritonitis in a mid-western referral hospital population. J Feline Med Surg 2012;14:903–5.
[65] Duthie S, Eckersall PD, Addie DD, et al. Value of alpha 1-acid glycoprotein in the diagnosis of feline infectious peritonitis. Vet Rec 1997;141:299–303.
[66] Hazuchova K, Held S, Neiger R. Usefulness of acute phase proteins in differentiating between feline infectious peritonitis and other diseases in cats with body cavity effusions. J Feline Med Surg 2017;19:809–16.
[67] Giordano A, Spagnolo V, Colombo A, et al. Changes in some acute phase protein and immunoglobulin concentrations in cats affected by feline infectious peritonitis or exposed to feline coronavirus infection. Vet J 2004;167:38–44.
[68] Paltrinieri S, Giordano A, Tranquillo V, et al. Critical assessment of the diagnostic value of feline a1-acid glycoprotein for feline infectious peritonitis using the likelihood ratios approach. J Vet Diagn Invest 2007; 19:266–72.
[69] Giori L, Giordano A, Giudice C, et al. Performances of different diagnostic tests for feline infectious peritonitis in challenging clinical cases. J Small Anim Pract 2011; 52:152–7.
[70] Bence LM, Addie DD, Eckersall PD. An immunoturbidimetric assay for rapid quantitative measurement of feline alpha-1-acid glycoprotein in serum and peritoneal fluid. Vet Clin Pathol 2005;34:335–41.
[71] Hartmann K, Binder C, Hirschberger J, et al. Comparison of different tests to diagnose feline infectious peritonitis. J Vet Intern Med 2003;17:781–90.
[72] Fischer Y, Sauter-Louis C, Hartmann K. Diagnostic accuracy of the Rivalta test for feline infectious peritonitis. Vet Clin Pathol 2012;41:558–67.
[73] Gruendl S, Matiasek K, Matiasek L, et al. Diagnostic utility of cerebrospinal fluid immunocytochemistry for diagnosis of feline infectious peritonitis manifesting in the central nervous system. J Feline Med Surg 2017;19:576–85.
[74] Felten S, Matiasek K, Gruendl S, et al. Utility of an immunocytochemical assay using aqueous humor in the diagnosis of feline infectious peritonitis. Vet Ophthalmol 2018;21:27–34.
[75] Giordano A, Paltrinieri S, Bertazzolo W, et al. Sensitivity of Tru-cut and fine needle aspiration biopsies of liver and kidney for diagnosis of feline infectious peritonitis. Vet Clin Pathol 2005;34:368–74.
[76] Kipar A, Koehler K, Bellmann S, et al. Feline infectious peritonitis presenting as a tumour in the abdominal cavity. Vet Rec 1999;144:118–22.
[77] Giuliano A, Watson P, Owen L, et al. Idiopathic sterile pyogranuloma in three domestic cats. J Small Anim Pract 2018. https://doi.org/10.1111/jsap.12853.
[78] Pedersen NC, Eckstrand C, Liu H, et al. Levels of feline infectious peritonitis virus in blood, effusions, and various tissues and the role of lymphopenia in disease outcome following experimental infection. Vet Microbiol 2015;175:157–66.
[79] Cammarata Parodi M, Cammarata G, Paltrinieri S, et al. Using direct immunofluorescence to detect coronaviruses in peritoneal in peritoneal and pleural effusions. J Small Anim Pract 1993;34:609–13.
[80] Paltrinieri S, Parodi MC, Cammarata G. In vivo diagnosis of feline infectious peritonitis by comparison of protein content, cytology, and direct immunofluorescence test on peritoneal and pleural effusions. J Vet Diagn Invest 1999;11:358–61.
[81] Litster AL, Pogranichniy R, Lin TL. Diagnostic utility of a direct immunofluorescence test to detect feline coronavirus antigen in macrophages in effusive feline infectious peritonitis. Vet J 2013;198:362–6.
[82] Felten S, Hartmann K, Gruendl S, et al. Immunocytochemistry of mesenteric lymph node fine-needle aspiration in the diagnosis of feline infectious peritonitis. J Vet Diagn Invest 2019;31:210–6.
[83] Kipar A, Bellmann S, Kremendahl J, et al. Cellular composition, coronavirus antigen expression and production of specific antibodies in lesions in feline infectious peritonitis. Vet Immunol Immunopathol 1998; 65:243–57.
[84] Paltrinieri S, Grieco V, Comazzi S, et al. Laboratory profiles in cats with different pathological and immunohistochemical findings due to feline infectious peritonitis (FIP). J Feline Med Surg 2001;3:149–59.
[85] Fish EJ, Diniz PPV, Juan YC, et al. Cross-sectional quantitative RT-PCR study of feline coronavirus viremia and replication in peripheral blood of healthy shelter cats in Southern California. J Feline Med Surg 2018;20: 295–301.
[86] Stranieri A, Giordano A, Paltrinieri S, et al. Comparison of the performance of laboratory tests in the diagnosis of feline infectious peritonitis. J Vet Diagn Invest 2018;30:459–63.
[87] Felten S, Weider K, Doenges S, et al. Detection of feline coronavirus spike gene mutations as a tool to diagnose feline infectious peritonitis. J Feline Med Surg 2017;19: 321–35.
[88] Doenges SJ, Weber K, Dorsch R, et al. Detection of feline coronavirus in cerebrospinal fluid for diagnosis of feline infectious peritonitis in cats with and

without neurological signs. J Feline Med Surg 2016; 18:104–9.
[89] Emmler L, Felten S, Matiasek K, et al. Feline coronavirus with and without spike gene mutations detected by real-time RT-PCRs in cats with feline infectious peritonitis. J Feline Med Surg 2019. https://doi.org/10.1177/1098612X19886671 1098612X19886671.
[90] Sangl L, Matiasek K, Felten S, et al. Detection of feline coronavirus mutations in paraffin-embedded tissues in cats with feline infectious peritonitis and controls. J Feline Med Surg 2018. https://doi.org/10.1177/1098612X18762883.
[91] Hornyak A, Balint A, Farsang A, et al. Detection of subgenomic mRNA of feline coronavirus by real-time polymerase chain reaction based on primer-probe energy transfer (P-sg-QPCR). J Virol Methods 2012;181:155–63.
[92] Li X, Scott FW. Detection of feline coronaviruses in cell cultures and in fresh and fixed feline tissues using polymerase chain reaction. Vet Microbiol 1994;42:65–77.
[93] Herrewegh AA, de Groot RJ, Cepica A, et al. Detection of feline coronavirus RNA in feces, tissues, and body fluids of naturally infected cats by reverse transcriptase PCR. J Clin Microbiol 1995;33:684–9.
[94] Gamble DA, Lobbiani A, Gramegna M, et al. Development of a nested PCR assay for detection of feline infectious peritonitis virus in clinical specimens. J Clin Microbiol 1997;35:673–5.
[95] Gut M, Leutenegger CM, Huder JB, et al. One-tube fluorogenic reverse transcription-polymerase chain reaction for the quantitation of feline coronaviruses. J Virol Methods 1999;77:37–46.
[96] Sawicki SG, Sawicki DL, Siddell SG. A contemporary view of coronavirus transcription. J Virol 2007;81:20–9.
[97] Simons FA, Vennema H, Rofina JE, et al. A mRNA PCR for the diagnosis of feline infectious peritonitis. J Virol Methods 2005;124:111–6.
[98] Barker EN, Tasker S, Gruffydd-Jones TJ, et al. Phylogenetic analysis of feline coronavirus strains in an epizootic outbreak of feline infectious peritonitis. J Vet Intern Med 2013;27:445–550.
[99] Felten S, Leutenegger CM, Balzer H-J, et al. Sensitivity and specificity of a real-time reverse transcriptase polymerase chain reaction detecting feline coronavirus mutations in effusion and serum/plasma of cats to diagnose feline infectious peritonitis. BMC Vet Res 2017;13:228.
[100] Stranieri A, Lauzi S, Giordano A, et al. Reverse transcriptase loop-mediated isothermal amplification for the detection of feline coronavirus. J Virol Methods 2017; 243:105–8.
[101] Gunther S, Felten S, Wess G, et al. Detection of feline Coronavirus in effusions of cats with and without feline infectious peritonitis using loop-mediated isothermal amplification. J Virol Methods 2018;256:32–6.
[102] Hugo TB, Heading KL. Prolonged survival of a cat diagnosed with feline infectious peritonitis by immunohistochemistry. Can Vet J 2015;56:53–8.
[103] Ritz S, Egberink H, Hartmann K. Effect of feline interferon-omega on the survival time and quality of life of cats with feline infectious peritonitis. J Vet Intern Med 2007;21:1193–7.
[104] Fischer Y, Ritz S, Weber K, et al. Randomized, placebo controlled study of the effect of propentofylline on survival time and quality of life of cats with feline infectious peritonitis. J Vet Intern Med 2011;25:1270–6.
[105] Watari T, Kaneshima T, Tsujimoto H, et al. Effect of thromboxane synthetase inhibitor on feline infectious peritonitis in cats. J Vet Med Sci 1998;60:657–9.
[106] Doki T, Takano T, Kawagoe K, et al. Therapeutic effect of anti-feline TNF-alpha monoclonal antibody for feline infectious peritonitis. Res Vet Sci 2016;104:17–23.
[107] Takano T, Akiyama M, Doki T, et al. Antiviral activity of itraconazole against type I feline coronavirus infection. Vet Res 2019;50:5.
[108] McDonagh P, Sheehy PA, Norris JM. Identification and characterisation of small molecule inhibitors of feline coronavirus replication. Vet Microbiol 2014;174: 438–47.
[109] Ng SW, Selvarajah GT, Hussein MZ, et al. In vitro evaluation of curcumin-encapsulated chitosan nanoparticles against feline infectious peritonitis virus and pharmacokinetics study in cats. Biomed Res Int 2020; 2020:1–18.
[110] Kim Y, Mandadapu SR, Groutas WC, et al. Potent inhibition of feline coronaviruses with peptidyl compounds targeting coronavirus 3C-like protease. Antiviral Res 2013;97:161–8.
[111] Murphy BG, Perron M, Murakami E, et al. The nucleoside analog GS-441524 strongly inhibits feline infectious peritonitis (FIP) virus in tissue culture and experimental cat infection studies. Vet Microbiol 2018;219:226–33.
[112] Pedersen NC, Perron M, Bannasch M, et al. Efficacy and safety of the nucleoside analog GS-441524 for treatment of cats with naturally occurring feline infectious peritonitis. J Feline Med Surg 2019;21:271–81.
[113] Dickinson PJ, Bannasch M, Thomasy SM, et al. Treatment of neurological feline infectious peritonitis using the adensine nucleoside analogue GS-441524. J Vet Intern Med 2020. https://doi.org/10.1111/jvim.15780 JVIM-19-453.
[114] Addie DD, Curran S, Bellini F, et al. Oral Mutian®X stopped faecal feline coronavirus shedding by naturally infected cats. Res Vet Sci 2020;130:222–9.

[115] Perera KD, Rathnayake AD, Liu H, et al. Characterization of amino acid substitutions in feline coronavirus 3C-like protease from a cat with feline infectious peritonitis treated with a protease inhibitor. Vet Microbiol 2019;237:108398.

[116] Fehr D, Holznagel E, Bolla S, et al. Placebo-controlled evaluation of a modified life virus vaccine against feline infectious peritonitis: Safety and efficacy under field conditions. Vaccine 1997;15:1101–9.

[117] Postorino Reeves NC, Pollock RV, Thurber ET. Long-term follow-up study of cats vaccinated with a temperature-sensitive feline infectious peritonitis vaccine. Cornell Vet 1992;82:117–23.

[118] Scott FW, Corapi WV, Olsen CW. Independent evaluation of a modified live FIPV vaccine under experimental conditions (Cornell experience). Feline Pract 1995;23:74–6.

[119] Scherk MA, Ford RB, Gaskell RM, et al. 2013 AAFP feline vaccination advisory panel report. J Feline Med Surg 2013;15:785–808.

[120] Addie D, Belak S, Boucraut-Baralon C, et al. Feline infectious peritonitis. ABCD guidelines on prevention and management. J Feline Med Surg 2009;11:594–604.

Advances in Small Animal Care 1 (2020) 189–206

ADVANCES IN SMALL ANIMAL CARE

Infectious Agents in Feline Chronic Kidney Disease

What Is the Evidence?

Katrin Hartmann, Prof Dr med vet, Dr habil, Dipl ECVIM-CA[a,*],
Maria Grazia Pennisi, Prof Dr med vet, Dr habil, Spec Applied Microbiology[b],
Roswitha Dorsch, Priv-Doz, Dr med vet, Dr habil, Dipl ECVIM-CA[a]

[a]Clinic of Small Animal Medicine, LMU Munich, Veterinaerstrasse 13, Munich 80539, Germany; [b]Department of Veterinary Sciences, University of Messina, via G. Palatucci 13, Messina 98168, Italy

KEYWORDS

• CKD • Cat • Renal • Urine • Glomerulonephritis • Tubulointerstitial nephritis • Chronic persistent infection

KEY POINTS

- Prevalence of chronic kidney disease (CKD) is very high in the feline population.
- Numerous factors have been considered as playing a role in the etiology of CKD.
- An infectious etiology or cofactor should to be considered in cats with a possible exposure.
- Infections that can play a role in CKD recently have emerged or re-emerged.

INTRODUCTION

Chronic kidney disease (CKD) is among the most common diseases of cats and affects in particular the elderly cat population. The overall estimated prevalence in a large study from the United Kingdom, including 142,576 cats in 91 first-opinion practices, was 4% [1]. Prevalence increases with age, and prevalence rates of 28% [2] and 31% [3] in cats older than 12 years and 15 years, respectively, have been reported, but rates also were high in younger cats when nonazotemic cats with CKD (CKD International Renal Interest Society (IRIS) stage 1) were included [4].

CKD is a prolonged process characterized by irreversible loss of kidney function and unpredictable intermittent disease progression. The underlying etiology often remains unknown [5]. Even on histology, a specific cause of disease usually is not identified. In more than half of affected cats, the histologic picture is characterized by chronic tubulointerstitial nephritis (TIN) and renal fibrosis [6,7]. These lesions are nonspecific and represent a final common pathway of a variety of etiologies [8]; thus, CKD currently is considered the result of multiple acute kidney injuries (AKIs) rather than a separate disease entity [9]. Possible underlying etiologies include a variety of factors. These include congenital conditions (eg, polycystic kidney disease and amyloidosis) [10,11], metabolic disorders (eg, hypercalcemia), obstructive nephropathy [12], chronic pyelonephritis, ischemic events [13,14], neoplasia, CKD as a sequela of AKI [9], and also various infectious diseases (Table 1). Apart from age, other known risk factors are frequent vaccinations [15], moderate and severe dental disease [15], and high dietary phosphorus [16].

Chronic interstitial nephritis is regularly associated with secondary glomerular involvement [8,17,18], whereas primary glomerulopathies, an important cause

*Corresponding author, *E-mail address:* hartmann@lmu.de

https://doi.org/10.1016/j.yasa.2020.07.013
2666-4518/20/

TABLE 1
Possible Infectious Causes of Chronic Kidney Disease and Glomerulopathy

Infectious Disease	Proved or Suspected Type of Renal Disease	References
Viral		
FeLV infection	L (H), ICGN (H)	[31–33]
FIV infection	ICGN (H, CP), TIN (H, CP), amyloidosis (H)	[19,34–38,44,54]
FFV infection	small foci of tubular atrophy, mild ultrastructural glomerular changes (H)	[24,30]
FIP	ICGN (H), GI (H)	[74,80,81]
FeMV infection	TIN (H, CP)	[94,95,111]
Bacterial		
Leptospirosis	TIN (H, CP), AKI	[129,132,136]
Lyme borreliosis		
Parasitic		
Leishmaniosis	GI (H), ICGN (CP), TIN (H)	[178,179,183,185]
Heartworm disease	ICGN (CP)	[192]

Abbreviations: AKI, acute kidney injury; CP, clinicopathologic evidence; FeLV, feline leukemiavirus; FIV, feline immunodeficiency virus; FFV, feline foamy virus; FeMV, feline morbillivirus; G, glomerulopathy; GI, granulomatous inflammation; H, histologic evidence; ICGN, immune complex glomerulonephritis; L, lymphoma; TIN, tubulointerstitial nephritis.

of CKD in dogs, are much less common in cats. Generally, glomerulopathies can be categorized as immune complex glomerulonephritis (ICGN) and non-immune complex glomerulopathies, such as glomerulosclerosis, glomerular atrophy, amyloidosis, or glomerular disease as a consequence of severe chronic interstitial nephritis or renal dysplasia [19,20]. For ICGN in general, chronic inflammatory conditions, often associated with chronic persistent infections, primary immune-mediated diseases, and neoplasia, are relevant causes.

SIGNIFICANCE

In this article, the significance of infectious diseases in feline CKD is discussed, including feline retrovirus infections, feline infectious peritonitis (FIP), feline morbillivirus (FeMV) infection, leptospirosis, Lyme borreliosis, leishmaniosis, and heartworm disease.

Feline Retrovirus Infection

Retrovirus infections are common in cats worldwide. In domestic cats, 3 retroviruses have been identified: feline foamy virus (FFV), feline immunodeficiency virus (FIV), and feline leukemia virus (FeLV). All 3 are widespread and cause lifelong infections but differ in their potential to cause disease. FFV (previously known as feline syncytium-forming virus), a spumavirus, is not considered to cause significant illness. FIV, a lentivirus that shares many properties with human immunodeficiency virus (HIV), can lead to increased risk for secondary infections, neurologic diseases, and neoplasia. In most naturally infected cats, however, FIV infection does not cause a severe clinical syndrome. Survival time of FIV-infected cats is not shorter than in uninfected cats [21,22], and quality of life usually is high is over many years or even lifelong. FeLV, an oncornavirus, is the most pathogenic of the 3 viruses, although the prevalence and importance of FeLV as a pathogen in cats have been decreasing since the introduction of vaccines. FeLV can cause neoplasia, bone marrow suppression, neurologic diseases, and reproductive disorders, and life expectancy is shortened in progressively infected cats, although many FeLV-infected cats also can live for years with good quality of life [23]. Although all 3 infections have been discussed as a potential cause of CKD, only FIV plays an important role in the etiology of inflammatory kidney changes.

FFV usually is considered apathogenic but has been isolated from cats with renal and other urinary tract diseases [24–29]. After experimental infection, histopathologic changes in kidneys (and the lung) have been described [24]. In a recent study, ultrastructural kidney changes were demonstrated in all of 5 cats experimentally infected with FFV, and blood urea nitrogen significantly increased after infection compared with preinfection values, although this rise was not above the reference range [30]. In 125 Australian cats with and without CKD, FFV infection was highly prevalent in older cats, particularly in male cats with CKD, although this difference was not significantly different compared with controls [30]. Thus, it is not likely, that FFV plays an important role in the development of CKD.

Cats with progressiv **FeLV** infection can succumb to kidney disease, but this generally is through a parainfectious mechanism. In FeLV-infected cats, kidney disease usually develops because the virus can induce formation of renal lymphoma, and renal function impairment is caused by the neoplasia rather than by the infection. In a recent study, however, cats with ICGN were significantly more frequently FIV-infected or FeLV-infected than cats with non-ICGN [19]. In that study, FIV was 3 times more common among the retrovirus-infected cats and the significance of FeLV by itself was not investigated [19]. In earlier studies, ICGN was described in FeLV-infected cats [31–33] but in most of these cases, cats had FeLV-associated lymphoma and, thus, likely lymphoma-induced immune complex disease. Therefore, FeLV itself does not seem to play a major role in the development of CKD other than being an important neoplasia-promoting factor in cats.

FIV can cause clinical features of CKD resulting from abnormal function or inflammation of affected organs, and virus-associated or immune complex–associated renal changes can be found in FIV-infected cats. Several studies investigated both tubulointerstitial as well as glomerular function in FIV-infected cats, and most investigators identified that proteinuria is a consistent finding, whereas azotemia and low urine specific gravity (USG) was described more inconsistently [21,22,34–43].

Some investigators report an association between FIV and azotemia and abnormal renal function [35,38–42] but prerenal azotemia could not be ruled out in all of these studies because of the lack of concurrent USG data. In 1 study, including 30 cats with FIV infection and 28 healthy cats, FIV-infected cats had a significantly higher creatinine than healthy cats, whereas serum cystatin C estimating glomerular filtration did not differ significantly [37]. Other investigators refute the idea of an association between FIV infection and azotemia [21,22,43]. One study, including client-owned cats (153 FIV-infected cats and 306 noninfected age-matched and sex-matched control cats) and specified pathogen–free research colony cats (95 cats that had been FIV-infected for a variable time period between 0.3 years and 4.9 years [median 2.2 years] and 98 similarly housed noninfected control cats) did not show an association between FIV infection and renal azotemia, neither among client-owned cats nor after experimental infection, although a significantly lower USG was demonstrated in FIV-infected cats, with USG below 1.035 in 44% of the FIV-infected cats [43]. One additional study showed no significant difference in creatinine, urea, or the prevalence of renal azotemia in FIV-infected versus uninfected control cats, but, again, a USG less than 1.035 was observed significantly more often in the FIV-infected group [36]. In an Australian study, young cats with CKD (as defined by an increased creatinine concentration with concurrent low USG) were significantly more likely to be FIV-infected compared with young cats without CKD, although FIV infection was not associated with CKD in older cats [38].

Studies investigating proteinuria in FIV-infected cats describe an increased prevalence of proteinuria but commonly without identifying a specific cause [34,35,37,42,43]. In a study, including 30 FIV-infected cats and 28 healthy cats, cats with FIV infection had a significantly higher urine protein to creatinine (UPC) ratio than healthy cats [37]. Similarly, in a recent study, proteinuria occurred more frequently in FIV-infected cats, and UPC ratio was significantly higher in FIV-infected cats than in controls [36]. In another study investigating client-owned cats (153 FIV-infected cats and 306 noninfected age-matched and sex-matched control cats), a significantly higher proportion of FIV-infected cats was proteinuric (25%) compared with noninfected cats (10%). FIV-infected intact male cats were at higher risk of proteinuria when compared with FIV-infected neutered male cats. In contrast, after experimental infection of specified pathogen–free research colony cats (95 FIV-infected cats and 98 similarly housed noninfected control cats), no association was detected between proteinuria and FIV infection [43].

The putative underlying causes of FIV-associated proteinuria have been discussed intensively. Hypertension, as a potential confounding factor for proteinuria in FIV-infected cats, was investigated in 91 FIV-infected cats and 113 control cats, but FIV-infected cats showed a significantly lower blood pressure and significantly fewer FIV-infected cats were hypertensive compared with control cats, thus excluding hypertension as a cause for the proteinuria [36]. In contrast, the role of immune complexes in FIV-associated kidney disease recently was confirmed when cats with ICGN were significantly more frequently FIV-infected (or FeLV-infected) than cats with non-ICGN

[19]. Also, in earlier studies, mesangioproliferative glomerulonephritis was described as a unique feature in FIV-infected cats [34]. A possible explanation is that FIV infection plays a role in glomerular damage by promoting deposition of immune complexes derived from viral antigens and host antibodies [31,33], and a marked increase of circulating immune complexes has been demonstrated in FIV-infected cats compared with noninfected cats [44,45]. Thus, glomerular disease in FIV-infected cats likely is the result of an immune-mediated response caused by hypergammaglobulinemia [21,46,47] through an excessive antibody response against the chronic persistent infection. Hypergammaglobulinemia, reflecting polyclonal B-cell stimulation, has been demonstrated in experimentally FIV-infected specified pathogen-free healthy cats [46]. The antibodies produced are not neutralizing and, thus, can lead to antigen-antibody complex formation. Hypergammaglobulinemia also can be caused by excessive production of autoantibodies [48]. When comparing plasma electrophoretograms, hypergammaglobulinemia and hyperproteinemia are significantly more common in FIV-infected versus noninfected cats [21,49]. Proteinuria without azotemia also commonly is seen in renal disease in HIV-infected people, particularly in those with HIV-associated nephropathy. Histologic lesions similar to those that define HIV-associated nephropathy have been described in a small number of FIV-infected cats [35,50]. HIV-associated nephropathy, however, often is rapidly progressive and ultimately fatal, with fulminant proteinuric renal disease [51,52], which appears to be rare in FIV-infected cats. The pathogenesis of HIV-associated nephropathy is suspected to be caused by specific genes of HIV, which are not present in FIV [53].

FIV infection also can be associated with structural changes of the kidneys. Renal ultrasonography showed abnormalities in 60/91 FIV-infected cats, with hyperechogenic cortices in 39/91 and enlarged kidneys in 31/91 [36]. At necropsy, TIN has been described in FIV-infected cats. Identified glomerular changes include glomerulonephritis and glomerulosclerosis [35,44,54] as well as amyloid deposition [55]. Histologic changes in 51 experimentally infected cats included mesangial widening and glomerulonephritis as well as tubular and interstitial alterations [34]. Diffuse interstitial infiltrates and glomerular and interstitial amyloidosis were detected in some naturally infected cats [34]. One study found amyloid deposits in different tissues, including the kidneys, in 12/34 (35%) FIV-infected cats and only in 1/30 noninfected field cats [55]. However, 20 experimentally FIV-infected cats showed no amyloid deposits [55].

Feline Infectious Peritonitis

FIP is a fatal disease that occurs worldwide in domestic and wild felids. The etiologic agent, the feline coronavirus (FCoV), which is an alphacoronavirus, exists in 2 different pathotypes that can be distinguished by their biological behavior but not by their morphology. The less pathogenic to nonpathogenic pathotype, sometimes referred to as feline enteric coronavirus, is highly prevalent in multicat environments and highly contagious; however, infection mostly is asymptomatic or causes only mild, transient diarrhea [56–58]. In contrast, the highly pathogenic pathotype, sometimes referred to as feline infectious peritonitis virus, is not infectious via the fecal-oral route but arises by mutation from the nonpathogenic pathotype within a small percentage of FCoV-infected cats to cause the fatal disease FIP [59–61]. It still is unknown which exact genes harbor the mutation(s) leading to the development of FIP but these mutations seem to be responsible for successful virus replication in macrophages [62], which is regarded as a key event in the pathogenesis of FIP [63,64]. Many different genes, including the S, 7a, 7b, and 3c genes, have been discussed as sites for the mutations that are crucial for the pathotype switch [61,65–69] but recently, mutations in the S gene have been identified to play an important role [70,71].

In cats with FIP, kidney disease is relatively common, and ultrasonographic renal changes can be present [72,73]. Kidney changes in FIP derive from 2 different mechanisms, either from granulomatous changes in the kidneys that typically develop within or on the serosal surface of many different organs, including the kidneys, or from ICGN caused by immune complexes through excessive production of non-neutralizing antibodies, which is a typical feature of FIP.

If FIP develops, granulomatous change can occur in many parenchymatous organs, including the kidneys [74,75], leading to impairment of kidney function in cats with or without effusions, although azotemia had been detected more often in cats without effusion [76]. Production of cytokines via infected macrophages and activation of neutrophils [77] results in histologic lesions typical of FIP, consisting of granulomas with focal and perivascular lymphoplasmacytic infiltrates and pyogranulomatous-necrotizing vasculitis [74]. Granulomatous lesions in the target organs are partially caused by overproduction of cytokines by infected macrophages, including neutrophil survival factors (tumor necrosis factor α, granulocyte-macrophage colony-stimulating factor, and granulocyte colony-stimulating factor) [77], that lead to systemic activation of neutrophils, causing them to extravasate and form pyogranulomas [78]. Granulocyte extravasation elicits the inflammation typically associated with these lesions, and recent data indicate that FCoV activates leukocyte-endothelial cells to increase monocyte adhesion by an indirect route, in which proinflammatory factors released from virus-infected monocytes act as key intermediates [79].

FIP has been associated with various types of ICGN, including membranoproliferative glomerulonephritis, membranous glomerulonephropathy, and mesangioproliferative glomerulonephritis [19,80]. Already approximately 40 years ago, depositions of C3 were demonstrated by immunofluorescence in renal glomeruli of cats with FIP. Their localization coincided with IgG deposits, thereby supporting the concept of an immune complex pathogenesis of FIP [81]. Hyperproteinemia is common in cats with FIP and found in approximately 50% of cats with effusion and 70% of cats without effusion [82]. Hyperglobulinemia (that can be present with or without an increase in total serum protein), often in combination with hypoalbuminemia (more frequent in cats with effusion), is common and has been documented in 89% of cats with FIP [76]. Elevated gamma globulin concentrations can be either polyclonal (more common) or monoclonal, as differentiated by serum protein electrophoresis [83]. In experimental infections, an early increase of α_2-globulins was reported [84], whereas gamma globulins and antibody titers increased just before the appearance of clinical signs of FIP [84–86]. The characteristically high levels of gamma globulins [87,88] and the increased antibody titers [85,89] invite the conclusion that hypergammaglobulinemia is due to a specific anti-FCoV immune response, but the wide variation in anti-FCoV titers at a given concentration of gamma globulins indicates additional (immune-mediated) reactions [90,91], and it has been proposed that stimulation of B cells by interleukin-6 contributes to the increase in gamma globulins [92].

Paramyxovirus Infection

Paramyxoviruses are commonly occuring morbilliviruses (RNA viruses) of humans and animals, including measles virus, canine distemper virus (CDV), rinderpest virus, peste-des-petits-ruminants viruses, and viruses affecting marine mammals [93]. In 2012, a new paramyxovirus, named feline morbillivirus (FeMV), was detected in renal tubular cells and lymph nodes of 2 cats affected by TIN [94]. Since then, worldwide studies have identified FeMV with variable prevalences in both healthy cats and sick cats by polymerase chain reaction (PCR) in urine (0.2%–51%) or kidney tissue samples (7%–80%) [94–104]. In addition, other non-FeMV paramyxoviruses were detected in the urine of 3 healthy cats in the United Kingdom [102]. FeMV is characterized by genetic diversity of isolates, and 2 distinct genotypes are known (FeMV-GT1 and FeMV-GT2) [98,105–108]. Epidemiologic data do not yet clarify whether transmission requires close direct contact between cats, but urine PCR positivity was higher in cats from suburban/rural areas and in cats with outdoor access and in colony cats compared with household cats [100,108,109]. Although shelter cats commonly were infected (53%), as detected by urinary PCR in 1 study [99], 1 other study reported a higher prevalence in pet cats compared with shelter cats [103]. Urinary shedding probably is the main source for transmission of FeMV infection between cats, particularly in households where cats are sharing litter trays. Urine of male cats was more frequently PCR positive compared with that of female cats [103] as was urine from intact tomcats compared with neutered male cats [98]. The higher risk of intact tomcats has been explained by the behavior attitude of male cats for territorial fighting and marking [98,103,110]. Presence of anti-FeMV antibodies demonstrating levels of exposure ranged between 19% and 28% [94,98,102,108,109]. In 1 study, old cats were more frequently antibody-positive than younger cats, and this finding is in line with a persistent chronic infection [102]. Although viremia probably is short term [96,101], infection of the urinary tract seems to be chronic as demonstrated by long-lasting viral urinary shedding [106,108]. Interestingly, 2 cats positive for FeMV continued to shed the virus in urine for 6 months and 2 years, respectively, despite high levels of virus-neutralizing antibodies [106]. Similarly, in another study, all cats that were PCR-positive in urine also had antibodies to the FeMV N-protein [102]. Tissue samples, including samples of the urinary tract (kidney and bladder) and less frequently lymphoid tissue and brain, were PCR-positive at necropsy [101,108].

The association between FeMV infection and CKD was the subject of several studies, but so far, the number of cats enrolled in these studies has been small, and longitudinal studies are not available. In 1 case-control study, including a limited number of cats, a significant association between FeMV and TIN was detected [94], whereas other studies did not find a significant association between a positive urine PCR and miscellaneous urinary diseases [95] or azotemia [102,103]. Moreover, concern was raised about potential cross-reactivity between FeMV and CDV [105] as immunoreactivity of anti-FeMV antibodies to CDV and of anti-CDV dog serum to FeMV was demonstrated [105]. Necropsy findings, however, clearly detected associations of FeMV infection and kidney lesions by demonstrating presence of FeMV intralesionally in renal tubular cells using immunohistochemistry [94]. In 1 study, immunohistochemistry detecting FeMV was significantly associated with tubular and interstitial kidney lesions in 38 cats [111]. Moreover, the tissue injury score of tubular lesions was higher in immunohistochemistry-positive tubular sections, and glomerulosclerosis was associated with FeMV positivity [111]. Viral antigen was demonstrated in the cortical tubules associated with small clumps of inflammatory mononuclear cells and in necrotic tubular cells surrounded by inflammatory infiltrate. Additionally, strong and diffuse immunoreactivity was seen in tubules within the medulla with a mild inflammatory mononuclear infiltration [101]. Recently, histopathology and immunohistochemistry evaluations of 7 PCR-positive cats found immunoreactivity within epithelial cells of renal tubuli and lymphoplasmacytic cells infiltrating the tubular and interstitial kidney areas but no association was found between FeMV positivity in kidney tissue (7/35) and evidence of renal lesions (23/35) or of TIN (14/35) [108].

Thus, a role of FeMV in the development of TIN is strongly suspected but still controversial. Associations between FeMV detection and clinical or histopathologic abnormalities do not prove a causative role of FeMV in these disorders. On the other hand, associations between presence of FeMV and TIN and CKD have been suggested for several reasons [110,112]. TIN and CKD can be diagnosed years after the pathogen triggered the pathologic changes, but the infection could have been cleared in the meantime. Some field studies are of limited value if inappropriate clinical criteria are used to select CKD and control cases or if only few cats are enrolled. False-negative PCR results can occur when the primers used are not well optimized or in cross-sectional studies because of intermittent viral shedding. Finally, other infectious and noninfectious factors known to cause feline CKD (www.IRIS-kideny.com) are not easily recognized in field studies. Further studies with larger sample numbers or full genome sequences of the identified strains would be beneficial to understand the effects of FeMV in feline health [110].

Leptospirosis

Leptospirosis is a bacterial disease reported in more than 150 mammalian species, including a variety of domestic and wild animals and humans. It is considered an emerging infectious disease in humans and dogs and is the most prevalent bacterial zoonosis affecting more than 1 million people worldwide [113]. In cats, *Leptospira* spp infection is common, but infection rarely causes disease, although the number of reports on field cats with clinical signs caused by *Leptospira* spp infection is increasing [114]. Antibodies against *Leptospira* spp commonly are present in the feline population, and *Leptospira* spp shedding in cats with outdoor exposure recently has been demonstrated in different regions [115–119]. Prevalence of urinary shedding identified by PCR ranged from 1% in Thailand [115] to 3% in Germany [119] and in Canada [116] to 12% in the United States [115] and 13% in Chile [117] and up to 68% in Taiwan following a natural disaster [120]. Prevalence of urinary shedding is comparable to that of dogs in the same areas [115,119,121]. Recently it was proved that cats not only shed leptospiral DNA but also viable *Leptospira* spp that can be cultured from their urine [117]. Cats usually acquire the infection from hunting rodents [122]. After infection and circulation in the blood for up to 7 days, *Leptospira* spp invade the kidneys as well as other organs (eg, liver, spleen, central nervous system, eyes, and genital tract). They damage these organs by replicating and causing inflammation [123]. An effective immune response can clear *Leptospira* spp from most organs except the kidneys, where the agent can persist long term [124,125]. After experimental infection, clinical signs in cats are mild [126–128]. Some experimentally infected cats showed polyuria and polydipsia (PUPD), diarrhea, and a mild increase in body temperature [129–131]. In addition, at necropsy, 5/7 cats were found to have nonpurulent interstitial nephritis [129]. If clinical signs occur after natural infection, the most common signs of infection also are likely caused by TIN [132–134], and affected cats are presented with acute PUPD, anorexia, and lethargy [132]. In 1 case series of 3 cats with leptospirosis, all cats had acute or chronic signs of renal disease without liver involvement [132].

The association between *Leptospira* spp infection in cats and CKD has been the subject of a few studies. Some studies suggested a relationship between PUPD and the presence of antibodies against *Leptospira* spp in cats [128,135], or an association between the presence of antibodies against *Leptospira* spp and CKD [136]. In 1 of those studies, 14/16 cats with PUPD (88%) had antibodies against *Leptospira* spp, whereas only 32/80 cats without PUPD (40%) were antibody-positive [135]. In another study, 17/114 cats with

CKD (15%) were antibody-positive for *Leptospira* spp compared with 9/125 healthy cats (7%), which represented a significant difference [136]. A third recent study found no such association, with 4/66 azotemic cats being antibody-positive (6%) compared with 8/75 cats without azotemia (11%) [137]. Whether or not *Leptospira* spp urinary shedding and CKD are correlated was investigated when a study comparing 2/125 (2%) clinically healthy cats and 6/113 (5%) cats with CKD found to be urine PCR positive; however, this difference was not significant [136]. In humans, CKD can develop as a continuum of *Leptospira* spp. infection-associated AKI or asymptomatic renal colonization when *Leptospira* spp persist in the renal tubular lumen and interstitium [138,139]. It has been suggested that in field workers with *Leptospira* spp colonization in the kidneys, exposure to extreme heat and dehydration can serve as a second hit in the development of CKD [113]. Chronic *Leptospira* spp kidney infection can lead to TIN and interstitial fibrosis. *Leptospira* spp outer membrane proteins elicit tubular injury and inflammation through a Toll-like receptor–dependent pathway followed by activation of nuclear transcription factor kappa B and mitogen-activated protein kinases as well as a differential induction of chemokines and cytokines associated with tubular inflammation [140]. *Leptospira* spp outer membrane protein also can induce activation of the transforming growth factor–β/Smad–associated fibrosis pathway, leading to accumulation of extracellular matrix [141]. Although the pathogenesis of CKD of *Leptospira* spp infection–associated CKD in cats is not yet clarified, a possible causal relationship is likely.

Lyme Borreliosis

Lyme borreliosis is one of the most common tick-transmitted diseases in humans worldwide. It is caused by infection with *Borrelia* spp—long, helical bacteria that belong to the family Spirochaetaceae and are transmitted to humans and animals via *Ixodes* ticks [142–144]. The *B burgdorferi* sensu lato complex currently includes more than 20 different genospecies, with at least 6 that are pathogenic for humans. In Europe, the species pathogenic for humans include *B afzelii*, *B garinii*, *B bavariensis*, *B burgdorferi* sensu stricto, and occasionally *B spielmanii* and *B mayonii*; in North America, *B burgdorferi* sensu stricto is mainly found as well as *B mayonii* in some areas [145]. The disease is common in humans and its true incidence likely is underestimated. Although infection is common in dogs, disease is much rarer in dogs than in humans and even less common in cats than in dogs [146,147].

Little is known about the pathogenicity of *B burgdorferi* sensu lato for cats. Experimental infection with 3 different *Borrelia* strains induced sporadic intermittent lameness (approximately 5 months after infection) and changes in behavior (irritability, photophobia, and aggression). In histology, multilocalized inflammation in different organs, including the central nervous system and joints, were observed [148]. There are only few reports, however, of naturally infected cats with clinical Lyme borreliosis [149–151], although ticks sampled from cats in Europe and the United States carried *Borrelia* spp [152–155]. The likely reason is a low susceptibility of cats for this infection. Alternatively, feline grooming behavior might explain that cats remove ticks before they are able to transmit pathogens, such as *Borrelia* spp, leading to a lower risk of tick-borne infections [156]. Cats living in areas endemic for *B burgdorferi* sensu lato and testing antibody-positive for *Borrelia* spp have been reported with signs of limb and joint disorders (with or without fever and anorexia), that improved upon antibiotic treatment [149,150]. Associations between infection and clinical signs, however, have not been proved. One study found antibodies against the C6 peptide of *B burgdorferi* sensu lato in 6 of 271 (2%) feline sera from Germany, Sweden, and Belgium by a rapid test based on an enzyme immunoassay technique. The prevalence of *Borrelia* C6 antibody-positive cat sera was significantly lower than the antibody prevalence determined for dogs in the same area during the same time period, which was 3372 of 45,655 (7%) canine sera; 5/6 C6 antibody-positive cats had clinical signs, but a clear causal relationship could not be determined. Also, 2/6 cats had very mildly elevated urea or creatinine values but there was no further renal work-up [157]. One recent study in an endemic area in the United States found *Borrelia* C6 antibodies in 18% of 159 cats [158]. Cats with clinical signs of disease were 4 times more likely to have antibodies against *B burgdorferi* sensu lato (or *Anaplasma phagocytophilum*) than healthy cats [158].

It has been discussed that some cats with *Borrelia* spp infection also might develop kidney disease [157]. Renal involvement has been described in dogs as so-called Lyme nephritis. In contrary, in humans with Lyme borreliosis, renal changes are uncommon, and only a few cases have been reported [159,160]. The involvement is preferentially glomerular; renal biopsies have shown a membranoproliferative glomerulonephritis pattern of injury [159], and histologic forms varied between ICGN and podocytopathy [160]. The pathophysiologic mechanisms appear to be triple, including immune complex deposits, podocytic hyperexpression of the B7-1 membrane protein, and renal infiltration of inflammatory cells [160]. Because the clinical disease is very rare in cats, however, and kidney involvement has not been clarified, *Borrelia* spp infection seems not to play an important role as cause for CKD in cats.

Leishmaniosis

Leishmaniases are a group of sand fly–transmitted diseases caused by protozoal species of *Leishmania* genus, which affect humans and other mammals. Leishmaniosis, caused by *Leishmania infantum*, is a severe, zoonotic, vector-borne disease endemic in many areas worldwide, with the dog serving as the main reservoir host [161]. Most infected dogs do not develop clinical abnormalities but are chronically infected and are infectious to sand fly vectors. A wide spectrum of outcomes is observed in dogs, humans, and other animal hosts, ranging from subclinical infection to mild self-limiting or even severe systemic disease [161,162]. In veterinary medicine, most of research interest has been focused on dogs [163–166]. In contrast to humans, in dogs with leishmaniosis, renal changes are frequent and the kidney usually is the most affected organ [167], and ICGN is more common than tubulointerstitial conditions [168]. The level of circulating immune complexes correlates with the progression of disease [169], with ICGN being (membranous, membranoproliferative, and mesangial) and glomerulosclerosis cause proteinuria and loss of renal function. Glomerular proteinuria can be reduced by antileishmania therapy and it is considered the main prognostic factor for survival in dogs [170–172].

In the past, leishmaniosis was studied infrequently in cats because cats were considered resistant to infection. More recently, however, anti–*Leishmania infantum* antibodies and *L infantum* DNA in blood have been identified in cats in areas endemic for canine leishmaniosis. The prevalence of infection is variable in cats with prevalence of antibodies and/or DNA in blood (measured by PCR), ranging from less than 5% to more than 25% in Brazil, Iran, Israel, Italy, Portugal, and Spain [173]. Prevalence of antibody and parasite DNA positivity in cats, however, usually is lower than that in dogs of the same area [174], and cats also have lower blood parasite loads [175]. Longitudinal observations demonstrated that cats are chronically infected, and the role of cats as reservoir hosts now is recognized [176]. In cats, progression of infection to disease might not occur for years and usually is associated with increasing antibody titers and blood parasite load [176]. Studies about the adaptive feline immune response to *L infantum* infection, however, are scant [177].

Overall, Leishmaniosis is considered an emergent feline vector-borne disease, with clinical cases increasingly reported, particularly in areas endemic for canine leishmaniosis, including Italy, Spain, France, and Portugal, and also sporadically in cats rehomed from these countries to nonendemic areas, sometimes years before [173]. So far, only case reports and a few case series have been published on the clinicopathologic features of feline leishmaniosis [178–180]. The disease is diagnosed mostly in adult to geriatric cats (age range 3–21 years, mean 7 years in 1 study; age range 4–14 years, median 10 years in another study), commonly in the presence of coinfections (in particular, FIV infection), other comorbidities (ie, diabetes mellitus, pemphigus foliaceus, and neoplasia), or immune-suppressive therapies [179,181]. Parasite detection is associated with lesions (usually granulomatous inflammation) in the skin, mucosal membranes (conjunctival, oral, and nasal), lymph nodes (with lymphoid hyperplasia), eye, spleen, bone marrow, liver, lung, and kidney [178,180].

Hyperproteinemia and hypergammaglobulinemia are the biochemical abnormalities reported most frequently [173,180]. Renal proteinuria (mild to severe) and IRIS stage 1 CKD are detected in approximately one-third of feline cases at diagnosis [179,181,182]. Less commonly, azotemia is found [179,181]. Some cats that were followed-up developed CKD over time [179,183,184]. TIN with dominant macrophage infiltration, fibrosis, and tubular proteinuria were identified in post mortem tissues in 1 case [185] and membranous glomerulonephritis in a second [183]. Persistence of *L infantum* infection in cats is likely, although some treated cats become negative on antibody tests and blood PCR [178,184]. Persistency implies a risk for recurrence and for immune complex formation due to chronic antigenic stimulation [184]. Some cats with leishmaniosis lived for several years after diagnosis, and some of these developed CKD [181].

Heartworm disease

Dirofilaria immitis (Spirurida, Onchocercidae), the nematod agent that causes heartworm disease, is transmitted by mosquitos and infects mainly dogs but also cats, ferrets, wild carnivores, and humans [186,187]. *D immitis* has a worldwide distribution. It is endemic in some countries in Europe and in North and South America. *Wolbachia pipientis* is a symbiotic bacterium hosted in filarial worms, which plays an important role in the biology and pathogenicity of the nematode. *D immitis* adults reside in pulmonary arteries and right heart chambers, whereas L1 larvae (microfilariae) live in the blood stream. Mosquitos are the intermediate hosts and become infected by taking a blood meal from a reservoir host carrying an adequate number of circulating microfilariae [186,187]. Dogs and some wild canids are the main reservoir, while cats and humans are scarcely microfilaremic. In susceptible mosquitoes, larvae molt up to the L3 stage, which is infective for the definitive mammal host when inoculated during blood sucking [187]. Compared with dogs, only a low number of L3 larvae develop to the adult stage in cats after inoculation. This occurs in a small percentage of infected cats after approximately 7 to 9 months. The production of microfilariae is rare in cats and, when microfilariae production does occur, it lasts only a few months and at a low load in feline blood [186,187].

Feline heartworm disease is detected in the same areas as canine heartworm disease at approximately 9% to 18% of the rate of those of unprotected dogs [188] but, according to the antibody prevalence in the same area, the rate of exposure to infection is much higher than the disease detected [188,189]. Despite the low parasite load (1–6 adult worms per cat), severe pathologic changes are found early in cats that can be life-threatening. The so-called heartworm-associated respiratory disease of cats is characterized by acute-onset dyspnea and an interstitial pattern on lung radiography. It is secondary to the release of large quantities of *D immitis* antigens from dead parasites. Most cats have, however, an asymptomatic course of the infection or otherwise have transient, recurrent, or chronic heartworm disease with mild to moderate respiratory signs due to chronic bronchoalveolar inflammation persisting even after the parasite death. In experimentally infected cats, presence of circulating *W pipientis* antigens and anti–*W pipientis* antibodies have been associated with inflammation and bronchoconstriction [190].

ICGN is considered a frequent complication of canine heartworm disease, and the localization of *W pipientis* surface protein in glomeruli is suggestive of a role for *W pipientis* in renal pathology [186]. Proteinuria and glomerulonephritis are more severe in dogs with circulating microfilariae [191]. Microfilaremia also was associated with immunohistochemical positivity to *W pipientis* within glomerular capillaries and anti–*W pipientis* antibodies in urine [191]. Proteinuria related to heartworm disease was the objective of a single study evaluating cats with both experimental and natural *D immitis* infections [192]. In this study, proteinuria was significantly associated with the development of adult heartworms in cats but was not associated with microfilaremia. The long-term clinical relevance of the heartworm-associated proteinuria, however, was not investigated [192]. When considering the frequent asymptomatic course of infection, chronic *D immitis* infection likely is underdiagnosed in cats. Infection in cats usually is self-limited within 18 months to 48 months, but this can be long enough for developing ICGN caused by deposition of circulating immune complexes.

CURRENT RELEVANCE AND FUTURE AVENUES TO CONSIDER

CKD is a common disease, particularly in older cats. The International Cat Care/International Society of Feline Medicine recommends health checks, including serum biochemistry and urinalysis, at least annually for all cats older than 7 years [193]. IRIS guidelines should be applied in all cats for diagnosis, staging, and management of CKD (www.iris-kidney.com). In clinical practice, CKD typically is diagnosed based on a persistent elevation of creatinine in combination with an inappropriately concentrated urine (USG <1.035) and quantitative proteinuria, measured by UPC ratio. In addition to creatinine, serum symmetric dimethylarginine as an earlier indicator of decreased kidney function, has been included in IRIS CKD staging guidelines (www.iris-kidney.com). Cats with early CKD are often asymptomatic. Once clinical disease is apparent, PUPD, weight loss, dehydration, small kidney size, or asymmetric kidneys are typical historical and physical examination findings in cats with CKD [5]. A diagnosis of CKD warrants a more extensive diagnostic evaluation of the patient. This includes a complete urinalysis (urine dipstick, urine sediment, UPC ratio, and urine culture if the sediment indicates infection); a serum chemistry, including electrolytes, total protein and albumin, measurement of systolic blood pressure; and diagnostic imaging, with ultrasonography as the most rewarding method. Additional investigations can be necessary to identify potential underlying etiologies, that would require specific therapy and complications that arise from CKD. This is important particularly in animals with a signalment (eg, young cats) that does not fit into the classic CKD picture and cats with findings suggestive for glomerular disease (eg, cats with high-grade proteinuria). Treatment of these diseases might have an effect on the progression of CKD and the prognosis of affected cats. Diagnosis of infectious diseases also influences monitoring and recommendations for the cat owner regarding the cat's lifestyle, health care, disease monitoring and zoonotic aspects.

Therefore, identifying underlying or contributing infectious diseases is highly recommended.

It is well documented that cats with antibodies to *Leptospira* spp can show clinical signs of renal disease or have histopathologic evidence of TIN [129,132–135], and CKD or azotemia have been found significantly more often in cats with antibodies to *Leptospira* spp [135,136]. Therefore, it is recommended to test cats with CKD, especially those with outdoor access for *Leptospira* spp infection, because this has therapeutic consequence. A role of FeMV in feline CKD is also strongly suspected. An infection with FeMV could represent one of a series of insults resulting in CKD or even have a direct causative role in a subset of cats. Due to a lack of reliable noninvasive diagnostic tests, unknown prognostic relevance of a positive urinary PCR, and lack of confirmed effective treatment, however, routine testing of cats for FeMV infection currently is not recommended.

Proteinuria is an important prognostic parameter in cats with CKD [194,195]. A UPC ratio less than 0.2 is considered normal in cats (www.iris-kidney.com). After exclusion of prerenal and postrenal causes, renal proteinuria with a UPC ratio between 0.2 and 0.4 is graded as borderline, and values above UPC ratio of 0.4 indicate pathologic protein loss via the kidney. Proteinuria increases with the severity of CKD and the degree of TIN [19,194]. TIN causes secondary involvement of the glomerulus, and glomerular hypertrophy has been associated with the degree of proteinuria [8]. Tubular proteinuria typically is of low grade, whereas glomerular proteinuria can be of any magnitude, ranging from mild to severe. There is no clear cutoff for the UPC ratio, however, that is diagnostic for any specific renal disease because the overlap in ranges is too broad to be clinically reliable [196]. However, there is a consensus that with increasing magnitude of proteinuria as assessed by UPC ratio, there also is increased likelihood for primary glomerular disease, with a UPC ratio greater than 2 strongly indicative of glomerular disease [196,197]. A search for associated infectious diseases is an important part of the diagnostic work-up for dogs with primary glomerular disease. Analogous guidelines for cats are not yet available, but a similar approach seems reasonable. Although in cats the number of identified infectious diseases associated with glomerulopathies is still small [198], an association between the type of glomerular disease and magnitude of proteinuria was shown in a recent study that included 37 cats with ICGN and 31 cats with glomerulopathies not associated with immune complex deposition, such as end-stage CKD, focal or multifocal glomerulosclerosis, glomerular atrophy, amyloidosis, and renal dysplasia [19]. ICGN was associated with more severe degrees of proteinuria. A UPC ratio of 3.8 had a specificity of 94% and a sensitivity of 92% for diagnosing ICGN. In that study, all retrovirus-infected cats with proteinuria had ICGN. The predominance of glomerular disease in retrovirus-infected cats compared with tubulointerstitial injury was in accordance with previous histopathologic studies [34,35] and with several studies that showed a higher prevalence of proteinuria in FIV-infected cats compared with control cats [34,36,37]. In contrast, a significant difference in creatinine was not a consistent finding [36,199]. Lymphoma is the most common cause of kidney disease in cats with FeLV infection, either primarily via direct neoplastic involvement or secondarily via neoplasia-associated ICGN. FIP can cause renal changes due to formation of granulomas in the kidney and on the serosal surface [74]. Additionally, FIP-associated ICGN was demonstrated in cats with naturally acquired disease [80] and after experimentally induced FIP [81]. FIP-associated renal disease has not been investigated further, probably because of its uniformly fatal course with a poor prognosis and median survival times of 8 days to 9 days [200,201]. New therapies for FIP, however, have recently been shown to improve the prognosis dramatically [202,203], and the type and development of renal disease might become more relevant for cats with FIP in the future. Many cats with *L infantum* infection do not develop clinical disease, but hyperproteinemia and hypergammaglobulinemia are the most common clinicopathologic abnormalities [178,180]. Renal proteinuria and azotemia are present in up to 25% of clinical cases [179,181], and possible immune complex deposition in the kidneys is caused by the to chronic course of infection and common occurrence of hypergammaglobulinemia. Cats with heartworm disease can be asymptomatic or have only very vague clinical signs, and proteinuria can be observed in cats infected with *D immitis*. After experimental infection, 8/10 cats were proteinuric, whereas 9/10 had well concentrated urine [192] indicating that the renal disease in cats with *D immitis* infection is more likely of glomerular origin than TIN. ICGN is a common complication of canine heartworm disease [186] and this likely is the case in cats as well.

Consensus recommendations for standard therapy for glomerular disease in dogs advise that "standard intervention should be considered whenever renal proteinuria is causing the UPC ratio to persistently exceed 0.5 in a dog with glomerular disease, whether the glomerular injury is primary or secondary" [204], and a diagnostic work-up for a potentially underlying infectious disease is strongly recommended. Apart from treatment of the underlying disease (if diagnosed) and antiproteinuric treatment, recommendations for dogs with glomerular disease include dietary therapy with sodium restriction, protein restriction and supplementation with polyunsaturated fatty acids, treatment of hypertension, and treatment of prevention of thromboembolic disease in selected cases. Although guidelines for treatment in case of histologically proved or suspected ICGN in dogs are available, such guidelines for cats in general and also for cats with underlying infectious diseases do not exist. Treatment of the underlying disease is the general recommendation for secondary glomerulopathies. In cats with biopsy-proved or suspected ICGN, risks and benefits of immunosuppressive treatment need to be carefully weighed against each other. Thus, testing for infectious diseases might be indicated, especially in cats with outdoor access before applying immunosuppressive treatment.

SUMMARY

- Prevalence of CKD is very high in the feline population. Depending on the geographic region and climate, local prevalence of infectious agents, signalment, history, clinical signs, and lifestyle (outdoor vs indoor, single-cat household vs multiple-cat household) of a cat with CKD or glomerulopathy, a diagnostic work-up for infectious diseases is indicated.
- In CKD, characterized by TIN, there is considerable evidence that infection with FeMV and *Leptospira* spp. can play a role, even though these might be only some of multiple contributing factors during a cat's life.
- FIV infection, FIP, leishmaniosis, and heartworm disease are important causes of glomerulopathy/renal proteinuria. All cats with renal proteinuria and suspected glomerular disease should be tested for FIV infection, FIP and *Leishmania infantum* and *D immitis* infection in endemic areas.
- Identification of infectious causes of CKD or glomerulopathies is important because it can influence treatment, handling, monitoring, and prognosis of affected cats.
- FeLV infection–associated renal disease typically is due development of lymphoma (neoplastic infiltration of the kidney or ICGN secondary to lymphoma).
- Cats with FIV or FeLV infection need to be prevented from spreading the disease to other cats and need special individualized health care.
- Cats with leptospirosis and leishmaniosis require specific treatment of these infectious diseases. The zoonotic nature of these infections needs to be communicated to the cat owner.
- Cats with heartworm disease should be monitored for clinical signs and presence of proteinuria.
- Currently there is no evidence that *B burgdorferi* sensu lato or FFV infection are associated with kidney disease in cats.

DISCLOSURE

The authors have nothing to disclose.

REFERENCES

[1] O'Neill DG, Church DB, McGreevy PD, et al. Prevalence of disorders recorded in cats attending primary-care veterinary practices in England. Vet J 2014;202:286–91.
[2] Bartlett PC, Van Buren JW, Neterer M, et al. Disease surveillance and referral bias in the veterinary medical database. Prev Vet Med 2010;94:264–71.
[3] Lulich JP, Osborne CA, O`Brien TD, et al. Feline renal-failure - questions, answers, questions. Compend Contin Educ Pract Vet 1992;14:127–53.
[4] Marino CL, Lascelles BD, Vaden SL, et al. Prevalence and classification of chronic kidney disease in cats randomly selected from four age groups and in cats recruited for degenerative joint disease studies. J Feline Med Surg 2014;16:465–72.
[5] Sparkes AH, Caney S, Chalhoub S, et al. ISFM consensus guidelines on the diagnosis and management of feline chronic kidney disease. J Feline Med Surg 2016;18:219–39.
[6] DiBartola SP, Rutgers HC, Zack PM, et al. Clinicopathologic findings associated with chronic renal disease in cats: 74 cases (1973-1984). J Am Vet Med Assoc 1987; 190:1196–202.
[7] Minkus G, Reusch C, Hörauf A, et al. Evaluation of renal biosies in cats and dogs - histopathology in comparison with clinical data. J Small Anim Pract 1994;35:465–72.
[8] Chakrabarti S, Syme HM, Brown CA, et al. Histomorphometry of feline chronic kidney disease and correlation with markers of renal dysfunction. Vet Pathol 2013;50:147–55.
[9] Cowgill LD, Polzin DJ, Elliott J, et al. Is progressive chronic kidney disease a slow acute kidney injury? Vet Clin North Am Small Anim Pract 2016;46:995–1013.
[10] Helps CR, Tasker S, Barr FJ, et al. Detection of the single nucleotide polymorphism causing feline autosomal-dominant polycystic kidney disease in Persians from the UK using a novel real-time PCR assay. Mol Cell Probes 2007;21:31–4.
[11] Nivy R, Lyons LA, Aroch I, et al. Polycystic kidney disease in four British shorthair cats with successful

treatment of bacterial cyst infection. J Small Anim Pract 2015;56:585–9.
[12] Hall JA, Yerramilli M, Obare E, et al. Serum concentrations of symmetric dimethylarginine and creatinine in cats with kidney stones. PLoS One 2017;12:e0174854.
[13] Schmiedt CW, Brainard BM, Hinson W, et al. Unilateral renal ischemia as a model of acute kidney injury and renal fibrosis in cats. Vet Pathol 2016;53:87–101.
[14] Brown CA, Rissi DR, Dickerson VM, et al. Chronic renal changes after a single ischemic event in an experimental model of feline chronic kidney disease. Vet Pathol 2019;56:536–43.
[15] Finch NC, Syme HM, Elliott J. Risk factors for development of chronic kidney disease in cats. J Vet Intern Med 2016;30:602–10.
[16] Dobenecker B, Webel A, Reese S, et al. Effect of a high phosphorus diet on indicators of renal health in cats. J Feline Med Surg 2018;20:339–43.
[17] McLeland SM, Cianciolo RE, Duncan CG, et al. A comparison of biochemical and histopathologic staging in cats with chronic kidney disease. Vet Pathol 2015;52:524–34.
[18] Lawson J, Elliott J, Wheeler-Jones C, et al. Renal fibrosis in feline chronic kidney disease: known mediators and mechanisms of injury. Vet J 2015;203:18–26.
[19] Rossi F, Aresu L, Martini V, et al. Immune-complex glomerulonephritis in cats: a retrospective study based on clinico-pathological data, histopathology and ultrastructural features. BMC Vet Res 2019;15:303.
[20] Cianciolo RE, Brown CA, Mohr FC, et al. Pathologic evaluation of canine renal biopsies: methods for identifying features that differentiate immune-mediated glomerulonephritides from other categories of glomerular diseases. J Vet Intern Med 2013; 27(Suppl 1):10–8.
[21] Gleich SE, Krieger S, Hartmann K. Prevalence of feline immunodeficiency virus and feline leukaemia virus among client-owned cats and risk factors for infection in Germany. J Feline Med Surg 2009;11:985–92.
[22] Liem BP, Dhand NK, Pepper AE, et al. Clinical findings and survival in cats naturally infected with feline immunodeficiency virus. J Vet Intern Med 2013;27:798–805.
[23] Hartmann K. Management of feline retrovirus-infected cats. In: Bonagura JD, Twedt DC, editors. Kirk's current veterinary therapy XV. St Louis (MO): Elsevier Saunders; 2013. p. 1275–83.
[24] German AC, Harbour DA, Helps CR, et al. Is feline foamy virus really apathogenic? Vet Immunol Immunopathol 2008;123:114–8.
[25] Shroyer EL, Shalaby MR. Isolation of feline syncytia-forming virus from oropharyngeal swab samples and buffy coat cells. Am J Vet Res 1978;39:555–60.
[26] Martens JG, McConnell S, Swanson CL. The role of infectious agents in naturally occurring feline urologic syndrome. Vet Clin North Am Small Anim Pract 1984;14:503–11.
[27] Gaskell RM, Gaskell CJ, Page W, et al. Studies on a possible viral aetiology for the feline urological syndrome. Vet Rec 1979;105:243–7.
[28] Fabricant CG, King JM, Gaskin JM, et al. Isolation of a virus from a female cat with urolithiasis. J Am Vet Med Assoc 1971;158:200–1.
[29] Mochizuki M, Konishi S. Feline syncytial virus spontaneously detected in feline cell cultures. Nihon Juigaku Zasshi 1979;41:351–62.
[30] Ledesma-Feliciano C, Troyer RM, Zheng X, et al. Feline foamy virus infection: Characterization of experimental infection and prevalence of natural infection in domestic cats with and without chronic kidney disease. Viruses 2019;11:662.
[31] Glick AD, Horn RG, Holscher M. Characterization of feline glomerulonephritis associated with viral-induced hematopoietic neoplasms. Am J Pathol 1978;92:321–32.
[32] Jeraj KP, Hardy R, O'Leary TP, et al. Immune complex glomerulonephritis in a cat with renal lymphosarcoma. Vet Pathol 1985;22:287–90.
[33] Slauson DO, Lewis RM. Comparative pathology of glomerulonephritis in animals. Vet Pathol 1979;16: 135–64.
[34] Poli A, Tozon N, Guidi G, et al. Renal alterations in feline immunodeficiency virus (FIV)-infected cats: a natural model of lentivirus-induced renal disease changes. Viruses 2012;4:1372–89.
[35] Poli A, Abramo F, Taccini E, et al. Renal involvement in feline immunodeficiency virus infection: a clinicopathological study. Nephron 1993;64:282–8.
[36] Taffin ER, Paepe D, Ghys LF, et al. Systolic blood pressure, routine kidney variables and renal ultrasonographic findings in cats naturally infected with feline immunodeficiency virus. J Feline Med Surg 2017;19:672–9.
[37] Ghys LFE, Paepe D, Taffin ERL, et al. Serum and urinary cystatin C in cats with feline immunodeficiency virus infection and cats with hyperthyroidism. J Feline Med Surg 2016;18:658–65.
[38] White JD, Malik R, Norris JM, et al. Association between naturally occurring chronic kidney disease and feline immunodeficiency virus infection status in cats. J Am Vet Med Assoc 2010;236:424–9.
[39] Hofmann-Lehmann R, Holznagel E, Ossent P, et al. Parameters of disease progression in long-term experimental feline retrovirus (feline immunodeficiency virus and feline leukemia virus) infections: hematology, clinical chemistry, and lymphocyte subsets. Clin Diagn Lab Immunol 1997;4:33–42.
[40] Sparkes AH, Hopper CD, Millard WG, et al. Feline immunodeficiency virus infection. Clinicopathologic findings in 90 naturally occurring cases. J Vet Intern Med 1993;7:85–90.
[41] Thomas E, Overbaugh J. Delayed cytopathicity of a feline leukemia virus variant is due to four mutations in the transmembrane protein gene. J Virol 1993;67: 5724–32.

[42] Ávila A, Reche A, Kogika MM, et al. Occurrence of chronic kidney disease in cats naturally infected with immunodeficiency virus (abstract). J Vet Intern Med 2010;24(3):760–1.
[43] Baxter KJ, Levy JK, Edinboro CH, et al. Renal disease in cats infected with feline immunodeficiency virus. J Vet Intern Med 2012;26:238–43.
[44] Poli A, Falcone ML, Bigalli L, et al. Circulating immune complexes and analysis of renal immune deposits in feline immunodeficiency virus-infected cats. Clin Exp Immunol 1995;101:254–8.
[45] Matsumoto H, Takemura N, Sako T, et al. Serum concentration of circulating immune complexes in cats infected with feline immunodeficiency virus detected by immune adherence hemagglutination method. J Vet Med Sci 1997;59:395–6.
[46] Flynn JN, Cannon CA, Lawrence CE, et al. Polyclonal B-cell activation in cats infected with feline immunodeficiency virus. Immunology 1994;81:626–30.
[47] Ackley CD, Yamamoto JK, Levy N, et al. Immunologic abnormalities in pathogen-free cats experimentally infected with feline immunodeficiency virus. J Virol 1990;64:5652–5.
[48] Pennisi MG, Masucci M, De Majo M. Presenza di anticorpi anti-nucleo in gatti FIV positivi. Messina (Italy): Atti XLVII Congresso Società Italiana di Scienze Veterinarie (SISVet); 1994. p. 973–6.
[49] Miro G, Domenech A, Escolar E, et al. Plasma electrophoretogram in feline immunodeficiency virus (FIV) and/or feline leukaemia virus (FeLV) infections. J Vet Med A Physiol Pathol Clin Med 2007; 54:203–9.
[50] Levy JK, Rottman JB, Ritchey JW, et al. Feline immunodeficiency virus causes nephropathy in cats. FASEB J 1995;A974.
[51] Weiner NJ, Goodman JW, Kimmel PL. The HIV-associated renal diseases: current insight into pathogenesis and treatment. Kidney Int 2003;63:1618–31.
[52] Berliner AR, Fine DM, Lucas GM, et al. Observations on a cohort of HIV-infected patients undergoing native renal biopsy. Am J Nephrol 2008;28:478–86.
[53] Rosenstiel P, Gharavi A, D'Agati V, et al. Transgenic and infectious animal models of HIV-associated nephropathy. J Am Soc Nephrol 2009;20:2296–304.
[54] Poli A, Abramo F, Matteucci D, et al. Renal involvement in feline immunodeficiency virus infection: p24 antigen detection, virus isolation and PCR analysis. Vet Immunol Immunopathol 1995;46:13–20.
[55] Asproni P, Abramo F, Millanta F, et al. Amyloidosis in association with spontaneous feline immunodeficiency virus infection. J Feline Med Surg 2013;15: 300–6.
[56] Pedersen NC, Allen CE, Lyons LA. Pathogenesis of feline enteric coronavirus infection. J Feline Med Surg 2008;10:529–41.
[57] Pedersen NC, Sato R, Foley JE, et al. Common virus infections in cats, before and after being placed in shelters, with emphasis on feline enteric coronavirus. J Feline Med Surg 2004;6:83–8.
[58] Vogel L, Van der Lubben M, te Lintelo EG, et al. Pathogenic characteristics of persistent feline enteric coronavirus infection in cats. Vet Res 2010;41:71.
[59] Pedersen NC, Boyle JF, Floyd K. Infection studies in kittens, using feline infectious peritonitis virus propagated in cell culture. Am J Vet Res 1981;42:363–7.
[60] Pedersen NC, Boyle JF, Floyd K, et al. An enteric coronavirus infection of cats and its relationship to feline infectious peritonitis. Am J Vet Res 1981;42:368–77.
[61] Vennema H, Poland A, Foley J, et al. Feline infectious peritonitis viruses arise by mutation from endemic feline enteric coronaviruses. Virology 1998;243:150–7.
[62] Dewerchin HL, Cornelissen E, Nauwynck HJ. Replication of feline coronaviruses in peripheral blood monocytes. Arch Virol 2005;150:2483–500.
[63] Rottier PJ, Nakamura K, Schellen P, et al. Acquisition of macrophage tropism during the pathogenesis of feline infectious peritonitis is determined by mutations in the feline coronavirus spike protein. J Virol 2005;79: 14122–30.
[64] Stoddart CA, Scott FW. Intrinsic resistance of feline peritoneal macrophages to coronavirus infection correlates with in vivo virulence. J Virol 1989;63:436–40.
[65] Balint A, Farsang A, Zadori Z, et al. Molecular characterization of feline infectious peritonitis virus strain DF-2 and studies of the role of ORF3abc in viral cell tropism. J Virol 2012;86:6258–67.
[66] Balint A, Farsang A, Zadori Z, et al. Comparative in vivo analysis of recombinant type II feline coronaviruses with truncated and completed ORF3 region. PLoS One 2014;9:e88758.
[67] Terada Y, Shiozaki Y, Shimoda H, et al. Feline infectious peritonitis virus with a large deletion in the 5′-terminal region of the spike gene retains its virulence for cats. J Gen Virol 2012;93:1930–4.
[68] Lin CN, Su BL, Huang HP, et al. Field strain feline coronaviruses with small deletions in ORF7b associated with both enteric infection and feline infectious peritonitis. J Feline Med Surg 2009;11:413–9.
[69] Dedeurwaerder A, Olyslaegers DAJ, Desmarets LMB, et al. ORF7-encoded accessory protein 7a of feline infectious peritonitis virus as a counteragent against IFN-alpha-induced antiviral response. J Gen Virol 2014;95: 393–402.
[70] Chang HW, Egberink HF, Halpin R, et al. Spike protein fusion peptide and feline coronavirus virulence. Emerg Infect Dis 2012;18:1089–95.
[71] Bosch BJ, van der Zee R, de Haan CA, et al. The coronavirus spike protein is a class I virus fusion protein: structural and functional characterization of the fusion core complex. J Virol 2003;77:8801–11.
[72] Ferreira A, Marwood R, Batchelor D, et al. Prevalence and clinical significance of the medullary rim sign identified on ultrasound of feline kidneys. Vet Rec 2020; 186:533.

[73] Griffin S. Feline abdominal ultrasonography: what's normal? what's abnormal? The kidneys and perinephric space. J Feline Med Surg 2020;22:409–27.
[74] Kipar A, Bellmann S, Kremendahl J, et al. Cellular composition, coronavirus antigen expression and production of specific antibodies in lesions in feline infectious peritonitis. Vet Immunol Immunopathol 1998; 65:243–57.
[75] Harvey CJ, Lopez JW, Hendrick MJ. An uncommon intestinal manifestation of feline infectious peritonitis: 26 cases (1986-1993). J Am Vet Med Assoc 1996;209: 1117–20.
[76] Riemer F, Kuehner KA, Ritz S, et al. Clinical and laboratory features of cats with feline infectious peritonitis–a retrospective study of 231 confirmed cases (2000-2010). J Feline Med Surg 2016;18:348–56.
[77] Takano T, Azuma N, Satoh M, et al. Neutrophil survival factors (TNF-alpha, GM-CSF, and G-CSF) produced by macrophages in cats infected with feline infectious peritonitis virus contribute to the pathogenesis of granulomatous lesions. Arch Virol 2009; 154:775–81.
[78] Olyslaegers DA, Dedeurwaerder A, Desmarets LM, et al. Altered expression of adhesion molecules on peripheral blood leukocytes in feline infectious peritonitis. Vet Microbiol 2013;166:438–49.
[79] Acar DD, Olyslaegers DAJ, Dedeurwaerder A, et al. Upregulation of endothelial cell adhesion molecules characterizes veins close to granulomatous infiltrates in the renal cortex of cats with feline infectious peritonitis and is indirectly triggered by feline infectious peritonitis virus-infected monocytes in vitro. J Gen Virol 2016; 97:2633–42.
[80] Hayashi T, Ishida T, Fujiwara K. Glomerulonephritis associated with feline infectious peritonitis. Nihon Juigaku Zasshi 1982;44:909–16.
[81] Jacobse-Geels HE, Daha MR, Horzinek MC. Isolation and characterization of feline C3 and evidence for the immune complex pathogenesis of feline infectious peritonitis. J Immunol 1980;125:1606–10.
[82] Hartmann K, Binder C, Hirschberger J, et al. Comparison of different tests to diagnose feline infectious peritonitis. J Vet Intern Med 2003;17:781–90.
[83] Taylor SS, Tappin SW, Dodkin SJ, et al. Serum protein electrophoresis in 155 cats. J Feline Med Surg 2010; 12:643–53.
[84] Stoddart ME, Gaskell RM, Harbour DA, et al. Virus shedding and immune responses in cats inoculated with cell culture-adapted feline infectious peritonitis virus. Vet Microbiol 1988;16:145–58.
[85] Pedersen NC. Serologic studies of naturally occurring feline infectious peritonitis. Am J Vet Res 1976;37: 1449–53.
[86] Gunn-Moore DA, Caney SM, Gruffydd-Jones TJ, et al. Antibody and cytokine responses in kittens during the development of feline infectious peritonitis (FIP). Vet Immunol Immunopathol 1998;65:221–42.
[87] Potkay S, Bacher JD, Pitts TW. Feline infectious peritonitis in a closed breeding colony. Lab Anim Sci 1974; 24:279–89.
[88] Gouffaux M, Pastoret PP, Henroteaux M, et al. Feline infectious peritonitis. Proteins of plasma and ascitic fluid. Vet Pathol 1975;12:335–48.
[89] Horzinek MC, Osterhaus AD, Ellens DJ. Feline infectious peritonitis virus. Zentralbl Veterinarmed B 1977; 24:398–405.
[90] Horzinek MC, Ederveen J, Egberink H, et al. Virion polypeptide specificity of immune complexes and antibodies in cats inoculated with feline infectious peritonitis virus. Am J Vet Res 1986;47:754–61.
[91] Paltrinieri S, Parodi MC, Cammarata G. In vivo diagnosis of feline infectious peritonitis by comparison of protein content, cytology, and direct immunofluorescence test on peritoneal and pleural effusions. J Vet Diagn Invest 1999;11:358–61.
[92] Goitsuka R, Ohashi T, Ono K, et al. IL-6 activity in feline infectious peritonitis. J Immunol 1990;144:2599–603.
[93] Nambulli S, Sharp CR, Acciardo AS, et al. Mapping the evolutionary trajectories of morbilliviruses: what, where and whither. Curr Opin Virol 2016;16:95–105.
[94] Woo PC, Lau SK, Wong BH, et al. Feline morbillivirus, a previously undescribed paramyxovirus associated with tubulointerstitial nephritis in domestic cats. Proc Natl Acad Sci U S A 2012;109:5435–40.
[95] Sieg M, Heenemann K, Ruckner A, et al. Discovery of new feline paramyxoviruses in domestic cats with chronic kidney disease. Virus Genes 2015;51:294–7.
[96] Furuya T, Sassa Y, Omatsu T, et al. Existence of feline morbillivirus infection in Japanese cat populations. Arch Virol 2014;159:371–3.
[97] Sharp CR, Nambulli S, Acciardo AS, et al. Chronic infection of domestic cats with feline morbillivirus, United States. Emerg Infect Dis 2016;22:760–2.
[98] Park ES, Suzuki M, Kimura M, et al. Epidemiological and pathological study of feline morbillivirus infection in domestic cats in Japan. BMC Vet Res 2016;12:228.
[99] Darold GM, Alfieri AA, Muraro LS, et al. First report of feline morbillivirus in South America. Arch Virol 2017; 162:469–75.
[100] Yilmaz H, Tekelioglu BK, Gurel A, et al. Frequency, clinicopathological features and phylogenetic analysis of feline morbillivirus in cats in Istanbul, Turkey. J Feline Med Surg 2017;19:1206–14.
[101] De Luca E, Crisi PE, Di Domenico M, et al. A real-time RT-PCR assay for molecular identification and quantitation of feline morbillivirus RNA from biological specimens. J Virol Methods 2018;258:24–8.
[102] McCallum KE, Stubbs S, Hope N, et al. Detection and seroprevalence of morbillivirus and other paramyxoviruses in geriatric cats with and without evidence of azotemic chronic kidney disease. J Vet Intern Med 2018;32:1100–8.
[103] Mohd Isa NH, Selvarajah GT, Khor KH, et al. Molecular detection and characterisation of feline morbillivirus in

domestic cats in Malaysia. Vet Microbiol 2019;236: 108382.
[104] Stranieri A, Lauzi S, Dallari A, et al. Feline morbillivirus in Northern Italy: prevalence in urine and kidneys with and without renal disease. Vet Microbiol 2019;233:133–9.
[105] Sakaguchi S, Nakagawa S, Yoshikawa R, et al. Genetic diversity of feline morbilliviruses isolated in Japan. J Gen Virol 2014;95:1464–8.
[106] Sieg M, Busch J, Eschke M, et al. A new genotype of feline morbillivirus infects primary cells of the lung, kidney, brain and peripheral blood. Viruses 2019; 11:146.
[107] Donato G, De Luca E, Crisi PE, et al. Isolation and genome sequences of two Feline Morbillivirus genotype 1 strains from Italy. Vet Ital 2019;55:179–82.
[108] De Luca E, Crisi PE, Marcacci M, et al. Epidemiology, pathological aspects and genome heterogeneity of feline morbillivirus in Italy. Vet Microbiol 2020;240: 108484.
[109] Donato G, De Luca E, Pizzurro F, et al. Morbillivirus RNA and antibody prevalence in cats with renal disease investigated by measuring serum SDMA. ISFM European Feline Congress; 2018; Sorrento, Italy.
[110] Choi JC, Ortega V, Aguilar HC. Feline morbillivirus, a new paramyxovirus possibly associated with feline kidney disease. Viruses 2020;12:501.
[111] Sutummaporn K, Suzuki K, Machida N, et al. Association of feline morbillivirus infection with defined pathological changes in cat kidney tissues. Vet Microbiol 2019;228:12–9.
[112] ABCD guidelines. Feline morbillivirus infection. Available at: http://www.abcdcatsvets.org/feline-morbillivirus-infection/. Accessed June 25, 2020.
[113] Yang HY, Chang CH, Yang CW. Leptospirosis and chronic kidney disease. In: Yang CW, Pan MJ, Yang HY, editors. Hrsg. Leptospirosis and the kidney. Basel (Karger): Transl Res Biomed; 2019. p. 27–36.
[114] Murphy K. Leptospirosis: A review to aid diagnosis and treatment. In: MAG Online Library Companion Animal. 2015. Available at: https://www.magonlinelibrary.com/doi/abs/10.12968/coan.2015.20.9.510?af=R&. Accessed April 21, 2020.
[115] Fenimore A, Carter K, Lunn K. Detection of leptospiruria in shelter cats in Colorado. The 30th Annual Congress of the American College of Veterinary Internal Medicine (ACVIM); May 30–June 02, 2012; New Orleans, USA
[116] Rodriguez J, Blais M, Lapointe C, et al. Feline leptospirosis: a serologic and urinary PCR survey in healthy cats and in cats with kidney disease. The 30th Annual Congress of the American College of Veterinary Internal Medicine (ACVIM); May 30–June 02, 2012; New Orleans, USA
[117] Dorsch R, Salgado M, Monti G, et al. Urine shedding of Leptopira species in cats in Southern Chile. The 10th International Leptospirosis Society Meeting; November 27–December 01, 2017; Palmerstone North, New Zealand.
[118] Sprißler F, Jongwattanapisan P, Luengyosluechakul S, Pusoonthornthum R, Prapasarakul N, Kurilung A, Goris M, Ahmed A, Reese S, Bergmann M, Dorsch R, Henricus L, Klaasen M, Hartmann K. Leptospira infection and shedding in cats in Thailand. Transboundary and Emerging Diseases. 2019; 66: 948-956.
[119] Weis S, Rettinger A, Bergmann M, et al. Detection of *Leptospira* DNA in urine and presence of specific antibodies in outdoor cats in Germany. J Feline Med Surg 2017;19:470–6.
[120] Chan KW, Hsu YH, Hu WL, et al. Serological and PCR detection of feline *Leptospira* in Southern Taiwan. Vector Borne Zoonotic Dis 2014;14:118–23.
[121] Llewellyn JR, Krupka-Dyachenko I, Rettinger AL, et al. Urinary shedding of leptospires and presence of *Leptospira* antibodies in healthy dogs from Upper Bavaria. Berl Munch Tierarztl Wochenschr 2016;129: 251–7.
[122] Shophet R, Marshall RB. An experimentally induced predator chain transmission of *Leptospira ballum* from mice to cats. Br Vet J 1980;136:265–70.
[123] Adler B, de la Pena Moctezuma A. *Leptospira* and leptospirosis. Vet Microbiol 2010;140:287–96.
[124] Levett PN. Leptospirosis. Clin Microbiol Rev 2001;14: 296–326.
[125] Schuller S, Francey T, Hartmann K, et al. European consensus statement on leptospirosis in dogs and cats. J Small Anim Pract 2015;56:159–79.
[126] Agunloye CA, Nash AS. Investigation of possible leptospiral infection in cats in Scotland. J Small Anim Pract 1996;37:126–9.
[127] Dickeson D, Love DN. A serological survey of dogs, cats and horses in South-Eastern Australia for leptospiral antibodies. Aust Vet J 1993;70:389–90.
[128] Andre-Fontaine G. Canine leptospirosis-do we have a problem? Vet Microbiol 2006;117:19–24.
[129] Fessler JF, Morter RL. Experimental feline leptospirosis. Cornell Vet 1964;54:176–90.
[130] Semmel M. Über das Vorkommen von Leptospirose bei Katzen in München und Umgebung. Tierärztliche Fakultät der Ludwigs-Maximilians-Universität München; 1954 [Dissertation].
[131] Larsson CE, Santa Rosa CA, Larsson MH, et al. Laboratory and clinical features of experimental feline leptospirosis. Int J Zoonoses 1985;12:111–9.
[132] Arbour J, Blais MC, Carioto L, et al. Clinical leptospirosis in three cats (2001-2009). J Am Anim Hosp Assoc 2012;48:256–60.
[133] Hemsley LA. *Leptospira canicola* and chronic nephritis in cats. Vet Rec 1956;300–1.
[134] Rees HG. Leptospirosis in a cat. N Z Vet J 1964;12:64.
[135] Luciani O. Réceptivité et sensibilité du chat aux leptospires [thesis in French]. France: Thesis École Nationale Vétérinaire de Nantes; 2004.

[136] Rodriguez J, Blais MC, Lapointe C, et al. Serologic and urinary PCR survey of leptospirosis in healthy cats and in cats with kidney disease. J Vet Intern Med 2014;28:284–93.
[137] Shropshire SB, Veir JK, Morris AK, et al. Evaluation of the *Leptospira* species microscopic agglutination test in experimentally vaccinated cats and *Leptospira* species seropositivity in aged azotemic client-owned cats. J Feline Med Surg 2016;18:768–72.
[138] Yang HY, Hung CC, Liu SH, et al. Overlooked risk for chronic kidney disease after leptospiral infection: A population-based survey and epidemiological cohort evidence. PLoS Negl Trop Dis 2015;9:e0004105.
[139] Riefkohl A, Ramirez-Rubio O, Laws RL, et al. *Leptospira* seropositivity as a risk factor for mesoamerican nephropathy. Int J Occup Environ Health 2017;23:1–10.
[140] Tian YC, Hung CC, Li YJ, et al. *Leptospira santorosai* Serovar Shermani detergent extract induces an increase in fibronectin production through a Toll-like receptor 2-mediated pathway. Infect Immun 2011;79:1134–42.
[141] Tian YC, Chen YC, Hung CC, et al. Leptospiral outer membrane protein induces extracellular matrix accumulation through a TGF-beta1/Smad-dependent pathway. J Am Soc Nephrol 2006;17:2792–8.
[142] Paster BJ, Dewhirst FE, Weisburg WG, et al. Phylogenetic analysis of the spirochetes. J Bacteriol 1991;173: 6101–9.
[143] Tijsse-Klasen E, Pandak N, Hengeveld P, et al. Ability to cause erythema migrans differs between *Borrelia burgdorferi* sensu lato isolates. Parasit Vectors 2013;6:23.
[144] Krupka I, Straubinger RK. Lyme borreliosis in dogs and cats: background, diagnosis, treatment and prevention of infections with *Borrelia burgdorferi* sensu stricto. Vet Clin North Am Small Anim Pract 2010;40:1103–19.
[145] Gerold Stanek MD. Lyme borreliosis, ticks and *Borrelia* species. Wien Med Wochenschr 2018;130:459–62.
[146] Bergmann M, Hartmann K. Vector-borne diseases in cats in Germany. Tierarztl Prax Ausg K Kleintiere Heimtiere 2017;45:329–35.
[147] Littman MP, Gerber B, Goldstein RE, et al. ACVIM consensus update on Lyme borreliosis in dogs and cats. J Vet Intern Med 2018;32:887–903.
[148] Gibson MD, Omran MT, Young CR. Experimental feline Lyme borreliosis as a model for testing *Borrelia burgdorferi* vaccines. Adv Exp Med Biol 1995;383:73–82.
[149] Magnarelli LA, Anderson JF, Levine HR, et al. Tick parasitism and antibodies to *Borrelia burgdorferi* in cats. J Am Vet Med Assoc 1990;197:63–6.
[150] Levy SA, O'Connor TP, Hanscom JL, et al. Evaluation of a canine C6 ELISA Lyme disease test for the determination of the infection status of cats naturally exposed to *Borrelia burgdorferi*. Vet Ther 2003;4:172–7.
[151] Peterhans E, Peterhans E. "Lyme disease" as a possible cause for lameness in the cat. Schweiz Arch Tierheilkd 2010;152:295–7.
[152] Geurden T, Becskei C, Six RH, et al. Detection of tick-borne pathogens in ticks from dogs and cats in different European countries. Ticks Tick Borne Dis 2018;9: 1431–6.
[153] Little SE, Barrett AW, Nagamori Y, et al. Ticks from cats in the United States: Patterns of infestation and infection with pathogens. Vet Parasitol 2018;257: 15–20.
[154] Davies S, Abdullah S, Helps C, et al. Prevalence of ticks and tick-borne pathogens: *Babesia* and *Borrelia* species in ticks infesting cats of Great Britain. Vet Parasitol 2017;244:129–35.
[155] Mietze A, Strube C, Beyerbach M, et al. Occurrence of *Bartonella henselae* and *Borrelia burgdorferi* sensu lato co-infections in ticks collected from humans in Germany. Clin Microbiol Infect 2011;17:918–20.
[156] Hamel D, Bondarenko A, Silaghi C, et al. Seroprevalence and bacteremia [corrected] of *Anaplasma phagocytophilum* in cats from Bavaria and Lower Saxony (Germany). Berl Munch Tierarztl Wochenschr 2012; 125:163–7.
[157] Pantchev N, Vrhovec MG, Pluta S, et al. Seropositivity of *Borrelia burgdorferi* in a cohort of symptomatic cats from Europe based on a C6-peptide assay with discussion of implications in disease aetiology. Berl Munch Tierarztl Wochenschr 2016;129:333–9.
[158] Hoyt K, Chandrashekar R, Beall M, et al. Evidence for clinical anaplasmosis and borreliosis in cats in Maine. Top Companion Anim Med 2018;33:40–4.
[159] Mc Causland FR, Niedermaier S, Bijol V, et al. Lyme disease-associated glomerulonephritis. Nephrol Dial Transplant 2011;26:3054–6.
[160] Gueÿe S, Seck SM, Kane Y, et al. Lyme nephritis in humans: Physio-pathological bases and spectrum of kidney lesions. Nephrol Ther 2019;15:127–35.
[161] Solano-Gallego L, Koutinas A, Miro G, et al. Directions for the diagnosis, clinical staging, treatment and prevention of canine leishmaniosis. Vet Parasitol 2009;165: 1–18.
[162] Michel G, Pomares C, Ferrua B, et al. Importance of worldwide asymptomatic carriers of *Leishmania infantum (L. chagasi)* in human. Acta Trop 2011;119:69–75.
[163] Miró G, Petersen C, Cardoso L, et al. Novel areas for prevention and control of canine leishmaniosis. Trends Parasitol 2017;33:718–30.
[164] Solano-Gallego L, Montserrrat-Sangra S, Ordeix L, et al. *Leishmania infantum*-specific production of IFN-gamma and IL-10 in stimulated blood from dogs with clinical leishmaniosis. Parasit Vectors 2016;9:317.
[165] Solano-Gallego L, Cardoso L, Pennisi MG, et al. Diagnostic Challenges in the era of canine *Leishmania infantum* vaccines. Trends Parasitol 2017;33:706–17.
[166] Solano-Gallego L, Miro G, Koutinas A, et al. LeishVet guidelines for the practical management of canine leishmaniosis. Parasit Vectors 2011;4:86.
[167] Miró G, Lopez-Velez R. Clinical management of canine leishmaniosis versus human leishmaniasis due to *Leishmania infantum*: Putting "One Health" principles into practice. Vet Parasitol 2018;254:151–9.

[168] Zatelli A, Borgarelli M, Santilli R, et al. Glomerular lesions in dogs infected with *Leishmania* organisms. Am J Vet Res 2003;64:558–61.
[169] Parody N, Cacheiro-Llaguno C, Osuna C, et al. Circulating immune complexes levels correlate with the progression of canine leishmaniosis in naturally infected dogs. Vet Parasitol 2019;274:108921.
[170] Geisweid K, Mueller R, Sauter-Louis C, et al. Prognostic analytes in dogs with *Leishmania infantum* infection living in a non-endemic area. Vet Rec 2012;171:399.
[171] Proverbio D, Spada E, de Giorgi GB, et al. Proteinuria reduction after treatment with miltefosine and allopurinol in dogs naturally infected with leishmaniasis. Vet World 2016;9:904–8.
[172] Pardo-Marin L, Martinez-Subiela S, Pastor J, et al. Evaluation of various biomarkers for kidney monitoring during canine leishmaniosis treatment. BMC Vet Res 2017;13:31.
[173] Pennisi MG, Cardoso L, Baneth G, et al. LeishVet update and recommendations on feline leishmaniosis. Parasit Vectors 2015;8:302.
[174] Otranto D, Napoli E, Latrofa MS, et al. Feline and canine leishmaniosis and other vector-borne diseases in the Aeolian Islands: Pathogen and vector circulation in a confined environment. Vet Parasitol 2017;236:144–51.
[175] Baneth G, Nachum-Biala Y, Zuberi A, et al. *Leishmania* infection in cats and dogs housed together in an animal shelter reveals a higher parasite load in infected dogs despite a greater seroprevalence among cats. Parasit Vectors 2020;13:115.
[176] Maroli M, Pennisi MG, Di Muccio T, et al. Infection of sandflies by a cat naturally infected with *Leishmania infantum*. Vet Parasitol 2007;145:357–60.
[177] Priolo V, Martinez-Orellana P, Pennisi MG, et al. Leishmania infantum-specific IFN-gamma production in stimulated blood from cats living in areas where canine leishmaniosis is endemic. Parasit Vectors 2019;12:133.
[178] Pennisi MG, Persichetti MF. Feline leishmaniosis: Is the cat a small dog? Vet Parasitol 2018;251:131–7.
[179] Fernandez-Gallego A, Feo Bernabe L, Dalmau A, et al. Feline leishmaniosis: diagnosis, treatment and outcome in 16 cats. J Feline Med Surg 2020;13.
[180] Urbani L, Tirolo A, Salvatore D, et al. Serological, molecular and clinicopathological findings associated with *Leishmania infantum* infection in cats in Northern Italy. J Feline Med Surg 2020. https://doi.org/10.1177/1098612X19895067.
[181] Pennisi MG, Persichetti MF, Migliazzo A, et al. Feline leishmaniosis: clinical signs and course in 14 followed up cases. In: Atti LXX Convegno SISVET. Palermo (Italy): 2016. p. 166–7. Available at: https://www.sisvet.it/joomla30/index.php/archivio-congressi.
[182] Leal RO, Pereira H, Cartaxeiro C, et al. Granulomatous rhinitis secondary to feline leishmaniosis: report of an unusual presentation and therapeutic complications. JFMS Open Rep 2018;4.
[183] Pimenta P, Alves-Pimenta S, Barros J, et al. Feline leishmaniosis in Portugal: 3 cases (year 2014). Vet Parasitol Reg Stud Reports 2015;1-2:65–9.
[184] Pennisi MG, Venza M, Reale S, et al. Case report of leishmaniasis in four cats. Vet Res Commun 2004;28(Suppl 1):363–6.
[185] Navarro JA, Sanchez J, Penafiel-Verdu C, et al. Histopathological lesions in 15 cats with leishmaniosis. J Comp Pathol 2010;143:297–302.
[186] McCall JW, Genchi C, Kramer LH, et al. Heartworm disease in animals and humans. Adv Parasitol 2008;66:193–285.
[187] Simon F, Siles-Lucas M, Morchon R, et al. Human and animal dirofilariasis: the emergence of a zoonotic mosaic. Clin Microbiol Rev 2012;25:507–44.
[188] Venco L, Genchi M, Genchi C, et al. Can heartworm prevalence in dogs be used as provisional data for assessing the prevalence of the infection in cats? Vet Parasitol 2011;176:300–3.
[189] Diakou A, Soubasis N, Chochlios T, et al. Canine and feline dirofilariosis in a highly enzootic area: first report of feline dirofilariosis in Greece. Parasitol Res 2019;118:677–82.
[190] Garcia-Guasch L, Caro-Vadillo A, Manubens-Grau J, et al. Is *Wolbachia* participating in the bronchial reactivity of cats with heartworm associated respiratory disease? Vet Parasitol 2013;196:130–5.
[191] Morchon R, Carreton E, Grandi G, et al. Anti-Wolbachia Surface Protein antibodies are present in the urine of dogs naturally infected with *Dirofilaria immitis* with circulating microfilariae but not in dogs with occult infections. Vector Borne Zoonotic Dis 2012;12:17–20.
[192] Atkins CE, Vaden SL, Arther RG, et al. Renal effects of *Dirofilaria immitis* in experimentally and naturally infected cats. Vet Parasitol 2011;176:317–23.
[193] Hoyumpa Vogt A, Rodan I, Brown M, et al. AAFP-AAHA: feline life stage guidelines. J Feline Med Surg 2010;12:43–54.
[194] Syme HM, Markwell PJ, Pfeiffer D, et al. Survival of cats with naturally occurring chronic renal failure is related to severity of proteinuria. J Vet Intern Med 2006;20:528–35.
[195] Jepson RE, Elliott J, Brodbelt D, et al. Effect of control of systolic blood pressure on survival in cats with systemic hypertension. J Vet Intern Med 2007;21:402–9.
[196] Lees GE, Brown SA, Elliott J, et al. Assessment and management of proteinuria in dogs and cats: 2004 ACVIM Forum Consensus Statement (small animal). J Vet Intern Med 2005;19:377–85.
[197] Lees GE. Early diagnosis of renal disease and renal failure. Vet Clin North Am Small Anim Pract 2004;34:867–85.
[198] Vaden S. Glomerular diseases. In: Ettinger SJ, Feldmann EC, editors. Textbook of veterinar internal medicine. St Louis (MO): Saunders Elsevier; 2010. p. 2021–36.

[199] Gleich S, Hartmann K. Hematology and serum biochemistry of feline immunodeficiency virus-infected and feline leukemia virus-infected cats. J Vet Intern Med 2009;23:552–8.
[200] Fischer Y, Ritz S, Weber K, et al. Randomized, placebo controlled study of the effect of propentofylline on survival time and quality of life of cats with feline infectious peritonitis. J Vet Intern Med 2011;25: 1270–6.
[201] Ritz S, Egberink H, Hartmann K. Effect of feline interferon-omega on the survival time and quality of life of cats with feline infectious peritonitis. J Vet Intern Med 2007;21:1193–7.
[202] Pedersen NC, Perron M, Bannasch M, et al. Efficacy and safety of the nucleoside analog GS-441524 for treatment of cats with naturally occurring feline infectious peritonitis. J Feline Med Surg 2019;21: 271–81.
[203] Pedersen NC, Kim Y, Liu H, et al. Efficacy of a 3C-like protease inhibitor in treating various forms of acquired feline infectious peritonitis. J Feline Med Surg 2018;20: 378–92.
[204] IRIS Canine GN Study Group Standard Therapy Subgroup, Brown S, Elliott J, Francey T, et al. Consensus recommendations for standard therapy of glomerular disease in dogs. J Vet Intern Med 2013;27(Suppl 1):27–43.

Nutrition

Advances in Small Animal Care 1 (2020) 207–225
ADVANCES IN SMALL ANIMAL CARE

Nutrition for the Hospitalized Patient and the Importance of Nutritional Assessment in Critical Care

Yuki Okada, BA, DVM, PhD[a,*], Sean J. Delaney, BS, DVM, MS, DACVN[b]
[a]Veterinary Nutrition Specialty Service, 901 Francisco Boulevard East, San Rafael, CA 94901, USA; [b]Davis Veterinary Medical Consulting, Inc., 350 Pioneer Avenue, Woodland, CA 95776, USA

KEYWORDS

- Critical care nutrition • Enteral nutrition • Feeding tubes • Nutritional assessment • Parenteral nutrition
- Refeeding syndrome • Sarcopenia • Undernutrition

KEY POINTS

- Undernutrition is commonly observed in critical care patients regardless of underlying condition(s), and is associated with longer hospital stay and decreased survival rate. Early identification and management of undernutrition should be practiced.
- A nutritional assessment contributes to identifying patients at risk of developing undernutrition, determining the timing of assisted feeding, the methods of assisted feeding and food type, monitoring patient response, and preventing complications. A detailed nutritional assessment should be performed not only at admission, but often and throughout the hospitalization.
- Feeding methods, rates, and the types of food should be decided based on patient factors, disease factors, availability (technical or logistical), and cost.

INTRODUCTION

Regardless of the underlying etiology, hyporexia (decreased food intake) or anorexia are commonly exhibited by veterinary patients admitted to critical care facilities. As a result, undernutrition is prevalent in hospitalized patients. Multiple published retrospective and prospective studies have indicated that 25% to 65% of hospitalized patients are underfed [1–3]. Notably, one recent extensive prospective study, looking at 498 hospitalized dogs admitted to multiple university veterinary hospitals in Spain over a period of 9 months, showed that 85% of canine patients consumed less than one-quarter of their resting energy requirement (RER), with only 3.4% consuming adequate calories during hospitalization. The same study also showed a positive correlation between anorexia and mortality, and a negative correlation between energy intake and hospitalization length irrespective of the disease type or severity [3], consistent with the principle that inadequate energy intake in hospitalized patients is associated with prolonged hospital stay, increased risk of comorbidity development, and death. In a critical care setting, a greater awareness and earlier identification of undernutrition should exist and be practiced as much as the identification and targeted treatment of the underlying disease(s).

*Corresponding author, *E-mail address:* dryukiokada@vnss.vet

https://doi.org/10.1016/j.yasa.2020.07.014

STARVATION

Starvation is often categorized into 2 processes characterized by their unique metabolic pathways: simple starvation and stress starvation. One is not entirely exclusive of the other, but rather can exist in a continuum of the other process.

Simple Starvation

Regardless of the etiology, when a healthy individual has an eating disturbance, wasting or catabolism follows the metabolic pathway in a reverse order of the natural anabolism pathway that follows food ingestion. First, glycogenolysis is activated in the liver to release glucose into the bloodstream as an energy source [4]. Once glycogen reserves are depleted, the body's glucose metabolism shifts to gluconeogenesis. In obligate carnivores (eg, cats) with minimal liver glycogen, blood glucose concentration is largely maintained by gluconeogenesis. The main substrate for gluconeogenesis is glycerol from lipolysis, and amino acids, lactic acid, and pyruvic acid from proteolysis. During the early stages of starvation, metabolism is temporarily increased to catabolize fat and muscle tissues to maintain blood glucose concentration in support especially of brain cells [4]. If starvation continues, the metabolism is decreased, and the energy source for brain cells shifts from glucose to ketone bodies produced via fatty acid oxidation. This protective shift to ketone bodies minimizes glucose utilization and protein catabolism and thus prevents muscle atrophy [5].

Stress Starvation

In patients with chronic disease, significant inflammation, sepsis, severe wounds, or burns, the normal adaptive responses to minimize glucose utilization and to conserve endogenous substrates (fat and protein) are severely challenged. The body under severe physiologic stress requires immediate energy release, thus excessive glycogenolysis, gluconeogenesis, lipolysis, and proteolysis are promoted. Sympathetic activation stimulates the release of proinflammatory cytokines (eg, tumor necrosis factor-alpha, interleukin [IL]-6, IL-1) or neuroendocrine substances (eg, catecholamine, cortisol, glucagon, growth hormone, antidiuretic hormone), which in turn, causes anorexia and increased metabolic rate and catabolism, and decreased hepatic ketogenesis, leading to loss of body mass or cachexia [6–8]. Metabolism rate is accelerated as a consequence. The body's liver glycogen and adipose tissues are consumed, as is muscle, albumin, and immune cells as sources of protein, all in an effort to meet the demands for both gluconeogenesis and tissue repair [5]. In critical care settings, admitted patients often are already in this hypercatabolic and cachexic state on presentation [7]. Identification of the underlying disease to contain and hopefully reduce the sympathetic activation as well as early provision of nutrition are imperative to conserve endogenous protein [5,8,9].

WHY FEED: PROTEIN CATABOLISM AND SURVIVAL

Sarcopenia (loss of lean body mass) follows prolonged hyporexia or anorexia if not managed properly. It is exacerbated by increased activation of catabolic pathways (resulting in accelerated lipolysis and proteolysis as noted previously) and severe weight loss, as seen in cachexia, which is associated with severe inflammation, malignancy, and/or aging [10]. In recent years, there has been increased interest in the effect of sarcopenia on the overall survival of sick and/or aged humans [10] and veterinary patients. Most published studies examine the prognostic value of sarcopenia and cachexia in cancer, trauma, and cardiac patients, assessing its effect on drug toxicity, surgical wound healing, hospital stay length, and mortality [11,12]. The body needs protein not only as a source of energy and structural support (ie, muscles, tissues, parenchyma), but also for the body's immune system tissue repair and healing (plasma protein) [7]. During wound healing, plasma protein not only supports the immune system by mediating the inflammatory response, but also facilitates wound repair processes by transporting energy sources (ie, carbohydrates, lipids, and amino acids), structural blocks, and trace metal cofactors, and by providing amino acids involved in wound repair stimulation and regulation [13]. As such, sarcopenia is associated with increased morbidity and mortality unrelated to the underlying disease process or patient age.

WHO'S AT RISK OF STARVING OR WHO TO FEED?

In 2011, the World Small Animal Veterinary Association (WSAVA) advocated for adding a nutrition assessment as the fifth vital assessment, following temperature, pulse, respiration, and pain, routinely assessed during physical examinations of veterinary patients [14]. A nutrition assessment is carried out through a multidimensional approach, evaluating animal, diet, and feeding environmental factors to determine the soundness of a patient's nutritional status. Every practitioner should familiarize themselves with the *Nutritional Assessment Checklist* items created by WSAVA [15] and should assess each patient accordingly at admission and reassess often throughout hospitalization (Fig. 1). A thorough understanding and accurate assessment of the patient's weight and weight trends, body condition score (BCS), muscle condition score (MCS), health status (based on diagnosis, diagnostic test results), diet history, and disease process, should assist in early identification and prevention of malnutrition.

The diagnostic criteria for at-risk patients are as follows:

1. Underweight/Recent weight loss

   Unintended weight loss or being underweight can indicate that the body is in or has been in a catabolic state. It is important to note that body weight changes may not be as evident if there is a fluid shift and/or recent fluid replacement.

2. BCS less than 4 of 9 (dog) or less than 5 of 9 (cat)

   BCS is an indirect assessment of the body's fat mass. A patient with decreased BCS is suspected to have low fat reserve and is in or has been in negative energy balance. In-depth descriptions of and instructions on BCS assessment are found in many textbooks and via online resources, such as the WSAVA Web site [16,17].

3. Low MCS

   MCS is an indirect assessment of lean body mass, which reflects protein intake and reserve

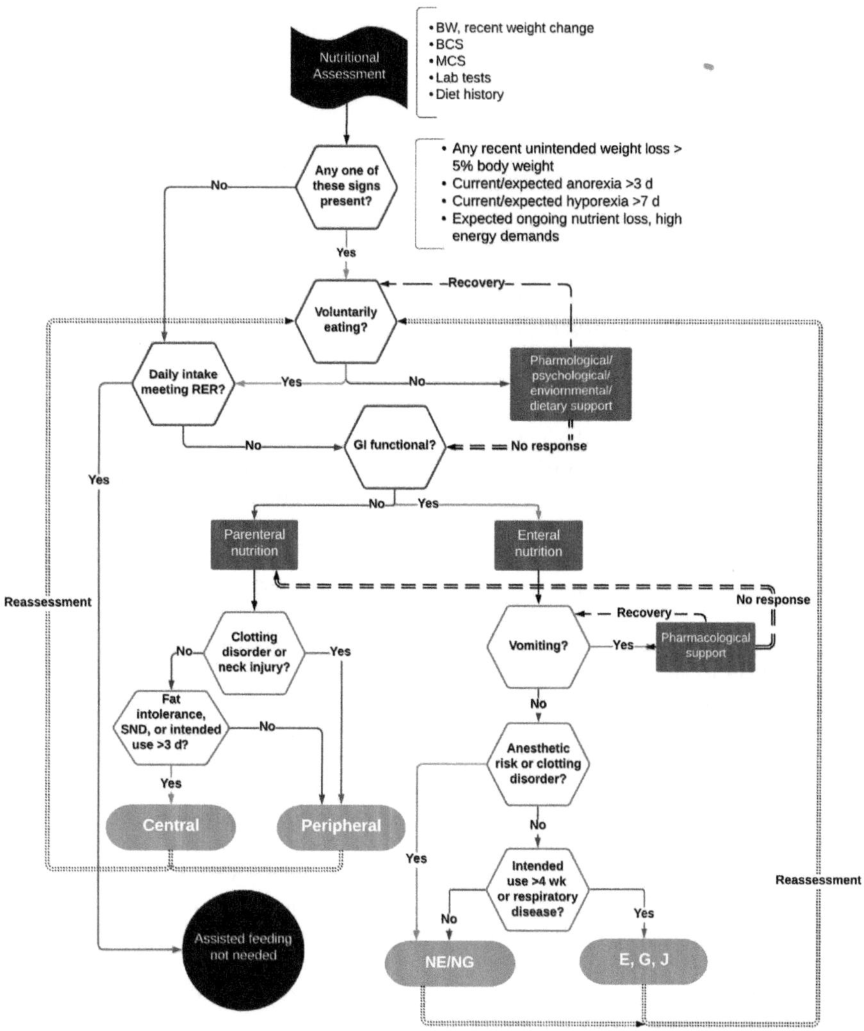

FIG. 1 Nutritional management decision-making flowchart.

[18,19]. When used in conjunction with other parameters, low MCS can be an indicator of ongoing starvation and protein catabolism.

In-depth descriptions of and instructions on MCS assessment are available in multiple textbooks and via online resources, such as the WSAVA Web site [20,21].

4. Abnormal laboratory tests (such as hypokalemia or hypoalbuminemia)

   These blood parameters may reflect recent changes in a patient's nutritional status [22], but careful interpretation is needed, as they also can be affected by certain disease processes that cause excessive losses or failure of synthesis [2].

5. Decreased or Diminished Food Intake

   Patients in prolonged negative energy balance are likely to become malnourished if left untreated. Accurate accounting (via diet history) and comparison of calories ingested before and during hospitalization are the most reliable tools to identify at-risk patients and to trigger early intervention, and to monitor patient response. Theoretically, there is a better chance of collecting an accurate accounting of a patient's caloric intake during hospitalization. Caged patients are under a relatively controlled feeding regimen without the confounding effects of accidental exposure to table scraps, other pets stealing the patient's food, and unaccounted loss of nutrients by unnoticed vomiting.

   - Diet history should include the following:
     - All product(s) a patient consumes, including treats and table scraps
     - Amount(s)
     - Frequency(ies)
     - Recent changes to all the above
   - During hospitalization
     - Patient care team members should be instructed to weigh and record (in grams) how much food was ingested by subtracting the grams left over from the grams of all food items (including treats) offered (eg, food offered − food leftover = food intake).
     - Fresh food that is not eaten readily should not be left exposed for more than 30 minutes, as drying and cooling of the food are not compatible with successful feeding, and food desiccation will affect the net ingestion measurement [23].

6. "At-risk" disease(s)

   A deep understanding of the patient's disease, severity, and its likely course is helpful in predicting the anticipated period of anorexia and accelerated nutrient losses.

   - Diseases that can cause nutrient losses, such as gastrointestinal (GI) disease, diabetes mellitus, protein-losing nephropathy, and/or severe burn
   - Diseases that cause nausea or those managed with medications that can cause nausea or GI dysmotility (eg, phosphate binders, antibiotics, chemotherapy drugs, opioids)
   - Injuries and treatments (including surgeries) that can prevent prehension, mastication, swallowing, and/or digestion/absorption
   - Diseases of a chronic nature or that are irreversible and progressive

Early placement of enteral feeding devices or introduction of the idea of future assisted enteral feeding may be helpful even if the patient is presently eating well.

HOW TO FEED: ORAL AND ENTERAL NUTRITION

Available routes for delivering nutrition therapy include oral (voluntary or force feeding), enteral, and parenteral nutrition. The basic principle of nutrition provision is "when the gut works, use it"; as long as the GI tract can be safely used, it is advised to implement oral and/or enteral/assisted nutrition early.

Early GI tract usage is beneficial in several ways. It prevents disuse atrophy of the GI mucosa and villi. As a result, the digestive function of the GI mucosa is preserved [24,25] for an earlier return of voluntary feeding. Intact GI mucosa further prevents bacterial translocation by acting as a physical barrier to intraluminal toxins and bacteria passing through the lamina propria, and entering mesenteric lymph nodes [26]. The GI tract not only serves as a digestive organ, but also serves as one of the most important immune organs containing 50% to 80% of the body's immune cells, such as lymphocytes that congregate in the periphery [26]. By stimulating the GI tract, the provision of oral and enteral nutrition promotes the body's immune function and limits the risk of secondary infection [24–27].

- Voluntary Feeding

If physically possible, voluntary feeding of a hospitalized patient should always be encouraged.

- Physical and mental hindrance

  Any underlying hindrance to voluntary feeding should be identified and treated whenever possible. Examples of physical and mental hindrance include, but are not limited to E-collars, recumbency, fever, pain, nausea, delayed gastric emptying, and/or vomiting [23]. Temporary removal of physical barriers during feeding should be attempted. Appropriate pharmacologic support, such as analgesics, kinetics, and antiemetics, should be selected to mitigate some of these hindrances.

  In a hospital setting, mental hindrances should not be overlooked. Hospitalized patients are not only physiologically and/or physically compromised, but also are mentally compromised as they are taken out of the comfort of their usual environment and are placed in an environment full of unfamiliar people and animals, noises, smells, sights, and lighting patterns [23]. It is advised to provide physical isolation (ie, a separate feeding area, partition, towel over the cage) from environmental disturbances while feeding and/or have a staff or family member provide hand-feeding. A detailed diet history will help a clinician identify the feeding patterns (ie, solitary feeder vs social feeder, time and frequency of feeding) and diet types, in an effort to mimic the regular feeding pattern and preference(s) of a patient.

- Palatability enhancing techniques

  If not contraindicated, offering high-reward treats or food items (eg, chicken) or increasing the food's palatability through additives may be considered. The strategies that are considered to optimize the food's palatability are as follows: (1) higher protein, (2) higher fat, (3) higher sodium (dogs only), (4) higher sweetness (dogs only), (5) lower or higher moisture, and (6) higher temperature (warm food) [23]. Depending on the patient's condition, some or all of these strategies may be incorporated. Strategies that may be used readily are higher moisture and higher temperature where any food (ie, wet/retorted, dry/extruded, or fresh food) is served warm with the addition of warm water or broth.

- Force Feeding

  Syringe feeding or force feeding with a tongue depressor has been routinely practiced for many years in veterinary medicine. Force feeding, however, is physically and mentally stressful to the patient, as well as to human caretakers, and poses an increased risk of aspiration. Furthermore, it has never been proven effective in delivering enough calories to meet caloric requirement [28]. Therefore, this feeding method is never recommended.

- Enteral-Assisted Feeding
  - Regardless of age and/or body condition, assisted enteral feeding is considered (or implemented or indicated for) in patients meeting any of the following criteria:
    i. Physical inability to prehend, masticate, and/or swallow food
    ii. Long-term hyporexia (>7 days)
    iii. Acute anorexia (>3 days)
    iv. Unintended severe weight loss (>10% in a few days)
    v. Persistent metabolic disturbances (ie, hypoproteinemia or hypermetabolic state)
  - Intervention options include nasoenteral (nasoesophageal [NE] or nasogastric [NG]) tubes, esophagostomy tubes (E tubes), gastrostomy tubes (G tubes), and jejunostomy tubes (J tubes) (Fig. 2) [29,30].

    These interventions involve the use of most or a part of the GI tract for digestion and absorption. Choosing the method that uses the largest area of the GI tract is preferred as long as it is appropriate for the patient's physical and medical status (see Fig. 1). The intervention methods are covered in the order of most extensive use of the GI tract to the least extensive use of the GI tract, and in the order of increasing difficulty and cost in placement.

    - NE or NG Tube

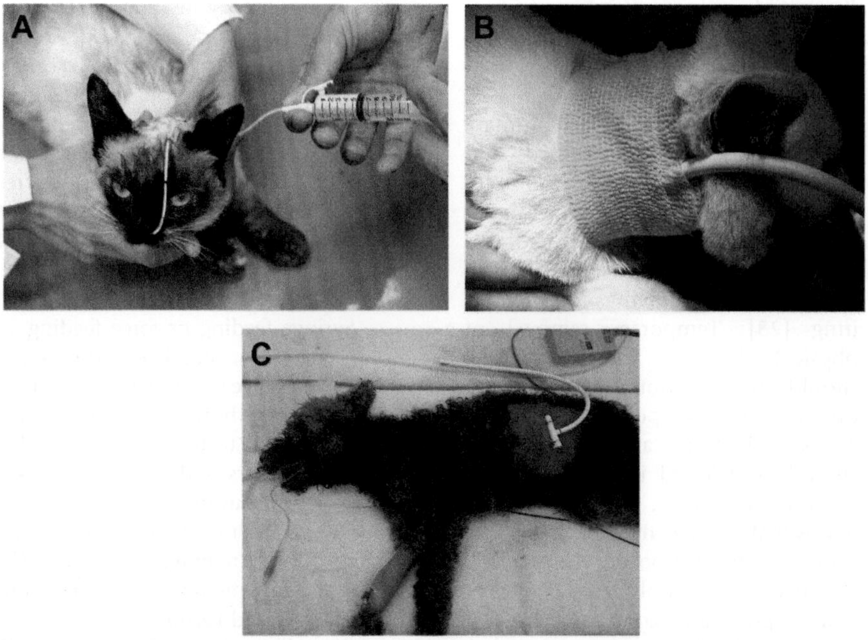

FIG. 2 (**A**) An NE tube feeding of a feline patient. (**B**) An E tube in a feline patient protected with a light bandage around the neck. (**C**) A G tube in an anesthetized canine patient. (*Courtesy of* [*A*] K. Fuji; and [*B*, *C*] H. Mizukami.)

A small tube can be inserted through the nare (see Fig. 2A), passing the nasal cavity, ending in the esophagus or stomach. For an NE tube, the distance from the tip of the nose to the seventh or eighth intercostal space, and for an NG tube, the distance from the tip of the nose to the last rib, should be measured.

The placement is confirmed via radiography, capnography, with the presence of negative pressure with syringe aspiration, and/or with the absence of a cough reflex after injecting air or sterile saline into the tube.

- Indications:
  - Severely ill patients with increased anesthetic risks
  - Short-term use
- Pros:
  - Placement is cheap and easy requiring no incision or anesthesia
  - Can be removed at any time
- Cons:
  - Small bore (5–8 French [FR]) allows only liquid diet feeding
    - Frequent feeding is required to meet RER
  - Not well-tolerated for long-term use
    - Elizabethan collar is required to prevent displacement
  - Contraindicated in trauma, mass, or infection in nose and pharynx

■ E Tube

An E tube is placed through an incision over the ventral-lateral cervical skin (see Fig. 2B) under anesthesia.

- Indications:
  - When long-term use is expected (ie, chronic or progressive diseases)
- Pros:
  - Larger bore (12–14 FR) allows slurry feeding and medication administration

- Well-tolerated in most cases with a light bandage over the tube
- Placement is relatively cheap and safe compared with the latter intervention options
- Can be removed at any time

- Cons:
  - Risk of anesthesia
  - Risk of incision infection or hemorrhage (especially in patients with coagulopathies)
  - Contraindicated in esophageal diseases such as megaesophagus and esophagitis

- G Tube

  A G tube can be inserted through a surgically created fistula (via an endoscopy-guided, laparoscopy-guided, surgical, or fluoroscopy-guided approach) that connects the gastric lumen (through gastric wall and abdominal wall) to a skin opening (see Fig. 2C).

  - Indications:
    - Patients with oral, nasopharyngeal, and/or esophageal disease(s)
    - When long-term use is expected (ie, chronic or progressive diseases)
  - Pros:
    - Very large bore (18–24 FR) allows large volumes of most food types
      - Less frequent feeding required to meet RER
    - Great for long-term use, as it is well-tolerated and feeding is less involved
    - Allows gastric residual volume measurement
  - Cons:
    - Risk of anesthesia
    - Risk of incision site infection or hemorrhage
    - Costly; requires anesthesia, special equipment, and/or experienced practitioner for placement
    - Cannot be removed early; risk of peritonitis development if removed before adhesion of the fistula to the body wall, which can take 7 to 14 days

- J Tube

  A J tube can be inserted through a surgically created fistula (via endoscopy-guided, laparoscopy-guided, or surgical approach) that connects the jejunal lumen (through intestinal wall and abdominal wall) to a skin opening.

  - Indications:
    - Patients with oral, esophageal, gastric, duodenal diseases
    - Used in the case of severe pancreatitis or post-cholecystectomy
  - Pros:
    - It bypasses pancreas and duodenum and prevents stimulation of pancreatic enzyme secretion by dietary fat or protein
    - Well-tolerated, but requires continuous rate infusion (CRI) or very frequent (authors suggest every 1–2 hours), small bolus feedings, as the small intestine does not tolerate bolus introduction of food limiting home use
  - Cons:
    - Small bore allows only liquid feeding
    - Limited to in-hospital use
    - Risk of anesthesia
    - Risk of incision site infection or hemorrhage
    - Costly; requires anesthesia, special equipment, and/or experienced practitioner for placement
    - Cannot be removed early

WHAT TO FEED

An accurate assessment and understanding of the patient's nutritional status and underlying disease are imperative when choosing an appropriate diet for a critically ill patient. Food choice is largely determined by the underlying disease, feeding tube lumen (if applicable), food's energy density, price, and availability.

Critical care diet options available include commercially prepared liquid, canned diets, and human food ingredients (Table 1). For tube feeding, veterinary liquid formulas are available for both dog and cat

TABLE 1
Nutritional Information for Critical Care Diets and Food Items

Nutrient	Unit	RC[a] Recovery Canine, Feline	RC[a] Gastrointestinal Low-Fat Liquid, Canine		RC[a] Renal Support Liquid, Canine	RC[a] Renal Support Liquid, Feline
Protein	% ME	32	35		13	26
Fat	% ME	48	19		51	50
Carbohydrate	% ME	20	46		36	24
Energy density	Cal/mL	0.9	0.9		1.3	0.9
Sodium	g/Mcal	1	1.1		1	0.9
Nutrient	**Unit**	**RC[a] Recovery Ultra Soft Mousse**	**Hill's[b] a/d**	**Purina[c] CN Critical Nutrition**	**Kirkland[d] Signiture Chicken Breast**	**Gerber[e] Chicken and Gravy Baby Food**
Protein	% ME	38	33	28	85	31
Fat	% ME	58	55	63	15	60
Carbohydrate	% ME	4	12	9	0	9
Energy density	Cal/g	1.63	1.15	1.35	1.1	1.26
Sodium	g/Mcal	3	1.65	0.9	3.5	0.4

Shown are the commonly used prescription diets and food items in the United States and their caloric distributions (% on a metabolizable energy [ME] basis), energy densities (Cal/mL [aka kcal/mL], Cal/g [aka kcal/g]), and sodium concentrations (g/1000 kcal [Mcal]). Numbers in red are inappropriately high values if dietary restriction is indicated, whereas numbers in blue are lower and considered safer. *The nutritional information for each product was obtained from the manufacturer's 2019 product guide (for prescription diets) or was calculated based on the nutrition facts provided (as of May 2020) on the labels (for human foods).*

[a] Royal Canin USA, Inc., St. Charles, MO.
[b] Hill's Pet Nutrition, Inc., Topeka, KS.
[c] Nestle Purina PetCare, St. Louis, MO.
[d] Costco Wholesale Corporation, Issaquah, WA.
[e] Gerber Products Company, Arlington, VA.

species, and for some disease conditions, but cost may be prohibitive in chronic cases or for large-breed dogs. Human liquid formulas such as Vivonex and Ensure are less costly alternatives and may be used short-term for dogs (<5 days) to meet their nutritional needs. In cats, the use of human liquid formulas is generally contraindicated, as arginine, which is essential for cats and dogs, may not be supplemented in most human products. In cats, a single protein-containing meal fed without arginine (not likely with natural foodstuffs) can cause death from hyperammonemia [31]. For long-term feeding, a liquid or slurry diet formulated by blending a complete and balanced commercial wet, dry, or homemade diet is recommended as a safe and sustainable option. In certain disease processes, the diet's macronutrient and micronutrient distributions (see Table 1), as well as the ingredients used, should be carefully evaluated to determine appropriateness.

- Anorexic animal without underlying disease(s):
  Most postsurgical patients or hyporexic/anorexic patients without any metabolic diseases requiring dietary restriction(s) (see later in this article for those that commonly do) can be fed as soon as they are sternal and not vomiting. If selective eating is noted, offer the patient's regular diet (if available) or offer high-reward food items such as chicken or tuna, with or without added palatants (see previously). A cottage cheese and rice diet (Table 2) with varied caloric distributions can be easily prepared in the hospital and may serve as a palatable alternative to commercially prepared dog diets, as long as there is no known intolerance to dairy and rice.
- Anorexic patient with protein intolerance:
  - Azotemia/Uremia

TABLE 2
Cottage Cheese and Rice Recipes

2% Fat CC and Rice Prep Table		Normal Protein/Lower Fat for Dogs and Cats				Lower Protein/Higher Fat for Dogs Only			
Weight (kg)	RER (Cal/d)	CC (cup)	Cooked Rice (cup)	Sesame Oil (tsp)	P/F/C (% ME)	Cottage Cheese (cup)	Cooked Rice (cup)	Sesame Oil (tsp)	P/F/C (% ME)
5	234	1/2	3/4	1/4	30/12/58	3 Tbsp	1/2	2 1/4	14/43/43
10	394	3/4	1	3/4	30/16/54	1/4	1	3 1/2	12/39/49
15	534	1	1 1/8	1/2	30/13/58	3/8	1 1/4	5	13/41/46
20	662	1 1/3	1 3/4	1	30/14/56	1/2	1 1/2	6 1/2	14/42/44
25	783	1 1/2	2	1 1/2	30/16/54	1/2	2	7	12/39/49
30	897	1 1/2	2 1/2	2	27/16/57	1/2	2	8 1/2	15/42/44
35	1007	1 3/4	2 3/4	2 1/4	27/17/56	2/3	2 1/2	9	13/39/48
40	1113	2	3	2	29/15/56	2/3	3	9	12/36/52
45	1216	2 1/4	3 1/4	2.5	29/16/55	1	3	10	15/37/48
50	1316	2 2/3	3 1/2	2 1/4	30/15/55	1	3 1/4	11	14/37/49
55	1414	2 3/4	3 3/4	2 1/4	30/15/55	1	3 1/2	12 1/2	13/39/48
60	1509	3	4	2 1/2	30/14/55	1 1/4	3 1/2	13 1/2	15/40/45

Shown are the amounts of 2% low-fat cottage cheese (CC), cooked white rice, and sesame oil needed for normal protein/lower fat and lower protein/normal fat (measured per %ME) diets to meet the resting energy requirement (RER) of patients with varying body weight (5–60 kg). Note this is indicated for short-term use, as they are not complete and balanced diets, and the feeding is contraindicated for patients with dairy or rice intolerance or with sodium restriction.

Abbreviations: ME, metabolizable energy; P/F/C, protein/fat/carbohydrates.

Courtesy of Yuki Okada, DVM, PhD, Veterinary Nutrition Specialty Service, San Rafael, CA.

In the absence of protein loss (ie, GI bleeding) or protein catabolism, dietary protein intake is directly proportional to blood urea nitrogen concentration [32]. As such, protein should be restricted in patients with decreased glomerular filtration rate and resultant azotemia or uremic syndrome, in advanced cases. Moderate and severe uremia directly affects the patient's clinical condition causing polyuria, polydipsia, nausea/inappetence, gastric ulceration, and sometimes altered mentation. As such, restricted protein is indicated for renal patients with azotemia/uremia [33,34].

- Hepatic Encephalopathy

  In hepatic patients exhibiting neurologic signs (ie, hepatic encephalopathy), neurotoxic substances from the GI tract, such as ammonia, bile salts, aromatic amino acids, short-chain fatty acids, manganese, and endogenous benzodiazepines, circulate in increased concentrations, because they are not effectively filtered or eliminated by the failing liver. Generally, the mainstay of nutritional management is moderate restriction of protein (typically at <15% on a metabolizable energy [ME] basis for a dog) to decrease dietary sources of ammonia, amines, and aromatic amino acids, but the dietary protein concentrations should be set as high as the patient can tolerate (ie, without developing neurologic symptoms), as protein deficiency is also a serious concern in liver failure. The diet should be highly digestible, and the protein source should be of high quality (ie, highly bioavailable) and "clean," with lower aromatic amino acid and purine concentrations [35]. Therefore, it is advised to avoid diets composed of organ meats and red meats, whereas diets composed of dairy protein, fish or white meat, and vegetable protein (eg, tofu/soy) are preferred [36]. It is important to note that the use of commercial renal diets should be avoided due to the frequent use of organ meats, although their restricted protein concentrations may be appropriate.

- Anorexic patient with fat intolerance:

  Diseases in which fat restriction is commonly indicated include pancreatitis [37], lymphangiectasia [38], enteritis, colitis, diarrhea, regurgitation, and vomiting. Fat restriction generally varies from less than 15% ME to less than 25% ME depending on the disease type or severity and the patient species (dog vs cat). In fat-intolerant patients, the presence of dietary fat within the GI tract directly causes exacerbation of symptoms via hyperstimulation of pancreatic enzyme secretions (pancreatitis), increasing lymphatic pressure (lymphangiectasia), stimulating colonic water secretion (colitis, diarrhea), and maldigestion (diarrhea) [39,40]. Excessive ingestion of fat also slows gastric emptying time, which may contribute to gastroesophageal reflux and abdominal distension, and cause anorexia, regurgitation, and vomiting [41]. Postoperative patients and critically ill patients are susceptible to having GI dysmotility or ileus [42]. It is the authors' observation that too many critically ill patients with suspected maldigestion, malabsorption, and/or GI dysmotility are inappropriately offered high-fat food items, as these food items are often considered "high-reward" and enticing. In addition, liquid diets and high energy density diets commonly used for liquid/slurry diet formulations are also high in fat (see Table 1) without full awareness of the potential adverse effects. Lower-fat food is indicated, as are less viscous foods (more liquid) to prevent gastroesophageal reflux and abdominal distension.

- Anorexic patient with sodium intolerance, including congestive heart failure, hypertension, ascites, and/or edema:

  Sodium retention can cause or exacerbate increased pressure in the venous circulation and capillaries, increasing cardiac preload and favoring a fluid shift into the interstitium in sodium-intolerant diseases.

  A fluid shift can cause blood albumin loss into the interstitium in some cases and may exacerbate malnutrition and cachexia. The mainstay of hypertension and/or fluid shift management is medication, and although no clear consensus on the timing or degree of dietary sodium reduction is available, a lower-sodium diet is considered effective in reducing medication dosages (ie, diuretics). Reducing medication side effects of nausea or anorexia or water-soluble vitamin losses or electrolyte and mineral imbalances is considered a benefit of lower-sodium diets [43,44].

In cardiac patients, strict sodium restriction is reserved for severe cases exhibiting pulmonary edema or ascites because long-term activation of the renin-angiotension-aldosterone system can increase the load on the compromised heart [43] and accelerate disease progression. In advanced cases of congestive heart failure (CHF), a lower-sodium diet (0.4 g/Mcal or 1000 calories [Cal] or kcal) has been shown to reduce cardiac size in dogs with CHF compared with those fed a diet containing 0.7 g/Mcal of sodium [44]. An even lower-sodium diet of 0.2 g/Mcal is used rarely in cases of severe CHF compared with the noted 0.4 g/Mcal (more commonly used in hypertensive cases with or without minimal third spacing). Lowering sodium often precludes the use of human foods commonly available in veterinary hospitals, like cottage cheese and canned meats, given their inherently higher sodium concentration (see Table 1).

- Anorexic patient with carbohydrate intolerance:

  One of the most common diseases causing carbohydrate intolerance is diabetes mellitus. In the critical care setting, insulin therapy is the mainstay of glycemic control for dogs with type I or insulin-dependent diabetes mellitus and for cats with type II or non–insulin-dependent diabetes mellitus, as hyperglycemia is a negative prognostic indicator in critical care patients [45,46]. Nutritional management may be implemented as an adjunctive therapy to fine tune glycemic control [47], but it is not absolutely necessary especially if other conditions require nutritional management that would be in conflict. High dietary fiber and/or lower carbohydrate foods may improve glycemic control by blunting postprandial glucose spikes [47–49] but are not very palatable and can decrease food intake and energy density. As such, a greater focus is placed on ensuring regular food intake to correspond with insulin therapy rather than on the type of foods offered and to prevent hypoglycemic episodes due to food aversion and insulin overdose.

- Anorexic patient with adverse food reactions:

  Canine and feline inflammatory bowel disease (IBD) is one of the most commonly presented causes of chronic or recurrent GI symptoms [50]. The pathogenesis of canine and feline IBD is not well-defined, but alterations in mucosal immunity to microbiota and/or food antigens have been suggested. GI signs commonly seen are vomiting and diarrhea, but subtle signs such as food aversion, or hyporexia, and/or abdominal discomfort may be seen, which can all exacerbate malnutrition and should immediately be addressed. Because adverse food reaction is considered to be mediated by an immune response to previously presented dietary constituents, the mainstay of diagnosis and treatment is food elimination [50,51]. Novel (new to the patient) or uncommon antigen protein and carbohydrate diets are available commercially or can be formulated after a careful review of the patient's diet history. Hydrolyzed protein therapeutic diets are also available and are considered hypoallergenic, as their protein sources have been broken down (hydrolyzed at the molecular level) to smaller peptides of typically less than 10 KDa in size, decreasing but not eliminating their allergenic potential [52]. Hydrolyzed proteins are also highly digestible and may help alleviate GI signs in some patients.

HOW MUCH AND HOW OFTEN SHOULD I FEED?

In a compromised hospitalized patient that is kept in a cage, its maintenance energy requirement (MER) is initially estimated to be equal to its RER [53]. After prolonged starvation, slow introduction of nutrients over a few days is recommended to prevent complications associated with refeeding (see later in this article).

- Stepwise instructions on how to determine the feeding amount and rate are as follows:
  1. Calculate the patient's MER, which is equal to its RER [53,54].
     - RER = $70\ (BW_{kg})^{3/4}$ (from Kleiber's law) [55].
       A 10-kg canine patient
       1.0*RER = $70\ (10_{kg})^{3/4} = 394\ Cal$
  2. Start at $^1/_4$ to $^1/_3$ of RER, and increase the rate slowly each day if no sign of complications is exhibited:

- Day 1: 25% to 33% of RER; day 2: 50% to 67% RER; day 3: 75% to 100% RER; day 4:100% RER

  A 10-kg canine patient at day 3:

  0.75*394 Cal to 1*394 Cal = 296 *Cal to 394 Cal*

3. The daily feeding amount (in weight or volume) to reach the desired calories can be calculated from the energy density (eg, Cal/g, Cal/mL, or Cal/cup) of the selected commercial or formulated diet. The desired number of calories to feed are divided by the energy density.

   Providing Food A of a known energy density to a 10-kg canine patient at day 3:

   Step 1: The caloric (energy) density of Food A (indicated on its label or Web site) is 3615 Cal/1000 g (or 396 Cal/cup).

   It is always more accurate and recommended to use mass for measurements (ie, *grams or ounces) rather than volume measurements* (eg, *cups, tablespoons, mL).*

   Step 2: The goal caloric provision at day 3 is 296 Cal/d.

   Step 3: 296 Cal/d ÷ 3615 Cal/1000 g (or 396 Cal/cup) = *0.082 kg (or 82 g) per day or 0.75 cup per day.*

4. The feeding amount per meal then can be calculated by dividing the value from step 3 by the desired number of feedings/d (typically 3–6 times daily).

   Providing Food A to a 10-kg canine patient over 4 feedings at day 3:

   82 g/d (from step 3) ÷ 4 feedings/d = *20.5 g per feeding.*

- Formulation of a liquid/slurry diet involves a hands-on trial-and-error mixing of the chosen diet and liquid (eg, water/broth/oil/commercial liquid diet). Liquid is added to the food item(s)/diet of known calories in a blender in small increments. The consistency may need to be tested during the blending process until the slurry/liquid passes through the desired tube without causing any clogging, but without becoming too watery, as that may compromise its energy density. Ideally, the food fed via tube feeding should provide more than 1 Cal/mL. If the energy density is lower, volume intolerance causing complications (ie, regurgitation, vomiting, abdominal distension/pain) or challenging feeding frequency will be encountered when trying to meet the patient's energy requirement.

  Note refrigeration/storage can cause the viscosity of a slurry to change depending on the diet's fat content or starch/soluble fiber content. Thus, the slurry should always be tested at the temperature at which it will be fed and/or prepared fresh at each serving.

- To calculate the energy density of the enteral diet, one must know *the total calories of the slurry/liquid formulated* and *its total volume.*

  1. The total calories may be set based on the specific patient's needs (such as daily target calories) or on a common measuring unit (such as per cup or per can).
  2. Liquid or water is then added to the selected food item or combination of food items of known total calories until the desired consistency (that would pass through the desired feeding tube) is reached.
  3. The total volume of the resultant slurry/liquid (food items and water/liquid blended) is measured using a measuring device such as a measuring cup, beaker, or a graduated cylinder.
  4. Total calories of slurry/liquid ÷ Total volume of the resultant slurry/liquid = energy density (Cal/mL).

     The final volume of the resultant liquid + Food A providing 396 Cal is 425 mL after 188 mL of water is blended to reach the desired consistency:

     396 Cal ÷ *425 mL* = *0.93 Cal/mL*

  5. Divide the target calories by the food's energy density to determine volume of food per day.

     To provide 296 Cal/d to a 10-kg patient using the following:

     I. Liquid + Food A slurry provides 0.93 Cal/mL: 296 Cal ÷ *0.93 Cal/mL* = *318 mL per day*

     II. If instead a slurry provides 1.2 Cal/mL, the volume would be reduced:296 Cal ÷ *1.2 Cal/mL* = *247 mL per day*

  6. For a bolus tube feeding, the liquid/slurry diet should be administered at ~*5 to 10 mL/kg of body weight* over 10 to 15 minutes [30], and given 3 to 6 times/d to meet the targeted feeding amount per day to prevent volume intolerance. For a CRI feeding, a targeted daily amount of feeding is divided by the infusion duration (hours) to calculate per mL/h rate.

     For a 10-kg dog receiving 318 mL of liquid + Food A slurry to reach full RER (at day 3):

I. 318 mL/d divided by *3 boluses/d = 108 mL/bolus* which is greater than 10 mL/kg of body weight per bolus (10 mL/kg/bolus * 10 kg = 100 mL/bolus), so bolus frequency should be more than 3 times/d

II. 318 mL/d divided by *6 boluses/d = 53 mL/bolus*, which is much less than 10 mL/kg per bolus

For a 10-kg dog receiving 247 mL of higher density slurry (1.2 Cal/mL) to reach full RER (on Day 3):

I. 247 mL/d divided by *3 boluses/d = 82 mL/bolus* less than 10 mL/kg body weight per bolus

These examples demonstrate the importance of adjusting the energy density or frequency of feeding to help prevent volume intolerance.

7. Each tube feeding (if bolus feeding) should be preceded by an attempt to encourage voluntary feeding. Once the voluntary intake exceeds 60% of RER, enteral feeding can be gradually decreased, proportional to the caloric intake attained by voluntary feeding/consumption.

   For example, *if on day 5, a 10-kg dog eats 100 Cal voluntarily, only 294 Cal should be given via a feeding tube.*

WHAT TO WATCH FOR: MONITORING FOR COMPLICATIONS

Once assisted feeding is implemented, the patient should be closely monitored for signs of refeeding syndrome, intolerance of enteral feeding, and tube placement complications.

- Refeeding syndrome

  With a sudden introduction of energy (glucose) after a prolonged starvation period, insulin secretion is overstimulated. As a result, sudden intracellular movements and cellular utilizations of phosphorus, potassium, magnesium, and thiamin, which may not have been sufficient during starvation, can cause or exacerbate hypophosphatemia, hypokalemia, hypomagnesemia, and hypothiaminemia [56]. The signs of refeeding syndrome include hemolytic anemia (due to hypophosphatemia), muscle weakness, gait or stance abnormalities, respiratory paralysis (due to hypokalemia and hypomagnesemia), cardiac conduction abnormalities (due to hypokalemia and hypomagnesemia) [56,57], and neurologic signs including seizures and ataxia (due to hypothiaminemia) [56–59]. Serum chemistry and electrolytes as well as complete blood count should be monitored frequently, if not daily, and deficiency should be corrected via supplementation. As thiamine cannot be easily measured, adequate preemptive supplementation/fortification/administration should be ensured to meet requirements.

- Volume intolerance

  GI dysmotility is commonly seen in critically ill or postsurgical patients [42]. Therefore, one of the most common complications of assisted feeding is volume intolerance. If the feeding rate or volume exceeds the patient's ability to empty the stomach, it can result in gastroesophageal reflux, vomiting, and aspiration. Signs of volume intolerance can be assessed by monitoring for clinical signs (eg, regurgitation, burping, vomiting, abdominal discomfort/distention). Vomiting in a critically ill patient that is recumbent or has a feeding tube can increase the risk of aspiration pneumonia, which should be prevented at all cost. Some practitioners may use increased gastric residual volume (GRV) as an indicator of volume intolerance, which can be assessed via ultrasound visualization or by aspirating gastric content via a feeding tube (NG and G tubes). If clinical signs of volume intolerance, increasing GRVs between feedings, or GRV exceeding 10 mL/kg body weight are noted, decrease the rate of CRI or frequency and/or volume of bolus feeding [30]. This may require that the energy density of the food needs to be increased without increasing dietary fat concentration (commonly achieved by use/addition of liquids that provide calories like liquid diets or sugar syrups instead of water when creating a slurry). The use of prokinetics is also recommended.

- Tube placement complications

  Clogging of the tube is a common complication and can be prevented with proper handling of the tube and good feeding practices. Slurry or liquids administered through tubes should have an appropriate consistency for the lumen diameter and the tube should be flushed with an adequate volume of warm water after each feeding. If a clot develops, 1/4 teaspoon of pancreatic enzymes and 325 mg sodium bicarbonate in 5 mL of water has been shown to be an effective clearing solution in one study [60]. Tube dislodgement/accidental removal is also common especially with nasoenteric (NE) and esophageal tubes [61,62]. Feeding tubes should be protected with a protective covering (E-collar for an NE tube and bandage for an E tube) and their use should be avoided in patients that are sneezing (NE) or vomiting (NE, E) [29]. Premature removal (within 7–14 days of placement) of G or J tubes before stroma formation can cause peritonitis and requires immediate medical attention [63]. Incision site infection of E, G, and J tubes is also a risk factor for delayed recovery and should be monitored closely.

HOW TO FEED: PARENTERAL NUTRITION

Parenteral nutrition (PN) provides macronutrients and B vitamins intravenously via a venous catheter. The placement of a catheter needs to be performed aseptically, and handling of the port, line, and the bag, as well as monitoring of the PN solution require extra care by well-trained individuals [64]. Frequent monitoring of laboratory values using in-house laboratory equipment is also recommended to prevent complications. For this reason, PN generally should be provided to hospitalized patients only at secondary or tertiary 24-hour facilities, and for short-term use in veterinary medicine.

- Indications

  With a deeper understanding of the benefits of early enteral feeding, PN has fallen out of favor as the main mode of assisted feeding. However, in specific cases and with special patient needs, PN can be used safely and effectively (see Fig. 1). The common indications include, but are not limited to the following:

  - Hyporexic/anorexic patients with higher risk of anesthesia or tube placement complications:

    When voluntary feeding or tube placement are physically not feasible or contraindicated, PN can be used to provide energy to prevent protein catabolism. E, G, or J tube placement requires anesthesia and surgical incision, and NE tube placement involves a passage of a tube through healthy nasopharyngeal tissue and functional esophagus or stomach, which may not be possible or available in some injured or critically ill patients.

  - For patients with severe maldigestion or malabsorption conditions:

    When severe vomiting, diarrhea, and resultant nutrient losses are exacerbated by voluntary or enteral-assisted feeding, PN can be used short-term to provide energy to prevent protein catabolism.

  - For patients with superficial necrolytic dermatitis (SND; aka hepatocutaneous syndrome):

    SND is an uncommon dog skin disorder with variable forms of skin lesions (eg, erythema, crusting, ulceration) over the footpads, around the eyes or mouth, and pressure points of the limbs or body [65]. Although similar to necrolytic migratory erythema with underlying glucagonoma in humans, hyperglucagonemia and pancreatic tumors are not the common characteristic in affected dogs [65], and the etiopathology is still unclear. The skin lesions are believed to be caused by low circulating amino acids. Hypoaminoacidemia is exhibited in all patients due to excessive catabolism of amino acids by the liver [66]. Parenteral supplementation of amino acids is a preferred method of amino acid repletion as it bypasses the enterohepatic circulation with resultant clearance of amino acids. A combination of periodic amino acid intravenous infusions via a central line and possibly a high-quality protein diet with or without amino acid supplementation has been shown to be effective in some dogs [66,67], but the response to treatment is generally variable and the overall prognosis is poor.

- Methods

  PN can be provided via a central or peripheral venous route. Central venous access is attained via insertion of a catheter through a jugular (more common) or a saphenous vein (less common). Its placement is more challenging than peripheral catheter placement through a cephalic vein, but allows more options for the choice of PN solutions because the central vein tolerates higher osmolarity of PN solutions than the peripheral vein given the risk of thrombophlebitis development. The choice of route access therefore should be determined based on patient factors, disease factors (which in turn, determines the PN solution formulation), as well as availability (of skills and equipment) (see Fig. 1).

  - Patient factors: Peripheral catheter should be selected for patients with coagulopathies and/or neck injuries.
  - Disease factors: A central catheter is preferred for fat-intolerance diseases, as the amino acid and dextrose solutions have lower energy density and higher osmolarity than lipid solutions, thus the need to have a vessel that can tolerate PN solution with a higher osmolarity.
  - Duration: If the expected duration of PN is >3 days, a central catheter is preferred, as it allows for provision of 100% of RER (hence the term, total PN (TPN) is often interchangeably used in veterinary medicine to describe central PN).

- PN components
  - Protein and amino acids (eg, Travasol 10% [Baxter Healthcare Corporation, Deerfield, IL], Aminosyn II 10% [Hospira Inc., Lake Forest, IL])

    An amino acid solution is added to PN to meet the protein and amino acid requirements of a patient. Traditionally, 8.5% or 10% solutions have been used, although currently (as of May 2020), only 10% solutions are commercially available. The energy densities of amino acid solutions range from 0.34 Cal/mL to 0.4 Cal/mL (10% solution), whereas the osmolarities range from 700 to 1000 mOsmol/L. In general, the recommended protein concentration in PN is 16% to 20% protein on an ME basis (% ME) for dogs, and 24% ME for cats; however, the concentrations should be adjusted based on individual needs and underlying disease process(es).
  - Lipids (eg, Intralipid 20% [Baxter Healthcare Corporation])

    Lipid solution is an essential part of PN, not only because it provides essential fatty acids, but also because it supplies energy while negating the effect of the relatively higher osmolarities provided by dextrose and amino acid solutions. A commonly used 20% lipid solution provides 2 Cal/mL with an osmolarity of 260 mOsmol/L. Recommended fat % ME for PN ranges from 30% to 80% [30], but it should be adjusted based on the underlying disease process(es) and patient response.
  - Sugar (5% or 50% Dextrose)

    Dextrose solutions supply carbohydrate energy in PN. The most commonly used solutions are 5% and 50% dextrose solutions, which provide 0.17 Cal/mL and 253 mOsmol/L and 1.7 Cal/mL and 2525 mOsmol/L, respectively. Generally, recommended carbohydrate concentrations in PN range from 20% to 50% ME. As hyperglycemia is one of the most common complications of PN administration [68,69], a provision of a higher carbohydrate PN formulation is reserved for patients in need of protein and/or fat restriction; 50% dextrose solutions are exclusively used in centrally administered PN solutions given their effect on osmolarity.
  - Water-soluble vitamins

    B vitamins are water-soluble and any excess is excreted in the urine, thus daily replenishment is necessary. Most B vitamins act as co-enzymes for energy metabolism and can cause metabolic disturbances when deficient. Most commercially available B complexes contain thiamin, niacin, pyridoxine, pantothenic acid, and riboflavin. Cyanocobalamin is often separately added to PN solutions.
  - Minerals and fat-soluble vitamins

    Because PN is indicated for short-term use in veterinary medicine, PN solutions do not need to be complete and balanced in all essential nutrients. Fat-soluble vitamins and certain minerals that are likely stored in the body or have slower turnover rates, are not commonly added to PN solutions. Phosphorus may be added in the form of potassium phosphate to treat hypophosphatemia from an existing disease or to prevent refeeding syndrome. The needed phosphorus supplementation dosage should be determined by the degree of hypophosphatemia and should be administered separately via an intravenous crystalloid solution to allow for more frequent titration based on monitoring of patient response.

- Electrolytes

  The most common electrolyte added is potassium in the forms of potassium phosphate (see previously) or potassium chloride to treat hypokalemia due to an underlying disease or to prevent refeeding syndrome. Insulin administration indicated for hyperglycemia can also exacerbate or cause hypokalemia, as insulin drives serum potassium into cells. The needed potassium supplementation dosage should be determined by the degree of hypokalemia, and can be provided and more rapidly/easily adjusted in an intravenous crystalloid solution.

- Calculations

  A detailed description of PN formulation is outside the scope of this article. Preparation of lipid-containing solutions requires strict aseptic techniques and, at least, a laminar flow hood. General practitioners should contact local compounding pharmacies to inquire about the availability of PN formulation services or refer cases requiring PN to university or tertiary referral hospitals that more commonly provide PN compounding and administration. Generalized steps to calculate PN formulations are as follows [30,64]:

  1. Determine the daily target calories as a fraction of (for peripheral and central PN) or full RER (only for central PN after 2–4 days of slow introduction).
  2. Determine the daily macronutrient solution volumes (mL) based on the desired caloric distribution.
  3. Determine the daily potassium and/or phosphorus dosages and volumes to correct/prevent deficiency(ies); this may be added separately in crystalloids.
  4. Determine the daily B vitamin complex volume to meet the daily requirement.
  5. Determine the osmolarity per liter of the final solution from step 2 solutions.
     a. Solutions with less than 650 to 700 mOsmol/L: peripheral or central PN are both possible
     b. Solutions with 650 mOsmol/L to 1400 mOsmol/L: only central PN is possible
  6. Calculate the energy density of the final solution by adding the calories provided by the macronutrient solutions and divide the sum by the total volume of the final solution (adding items from steps 2 through 4).
  7. Determine the administration rate (mL/h) based on the daily target calories and the energy density of the final solution.

- Monitoring for complications
  - Hyperglycemia

    Hyperglycemia is one of the most common metabolic complications associated with PN and has been associated with increased mortality in feline [46,68,69] and human patients [70]. However, it is unclear whether hyperglycemia is exacerbated by PN or is caused by the underlying metabolic disturbances commonly seen in critically ill patients. Regardless, the glycemic state should be tightly controlled via adjusting the rate of PN administration (if blood glucose [BG] is persistently 250–300 mg/dL, decrease rate) or via insulin therapy (if BG >300 mg/dL). The authors strongly recommend the use of a separate, dedicated catheter/line/bag for administration of insulin as well as for other medications and electrolyte/mineral supplementations, as frequent and excessive handling of the catheter/port/line may increase the risks of catheter site/admixture contamination and thromboembolism. This separation also enables changes (specifically reductions) in administration without wasting expensive parenteral solutions.

  - Hyperlipidemia

    Hyperlipidemia in dogs receiving PN can be improved or exacerbated by PN [22,68]. In hyporexic/anorexic patients, hyperlipidemia is seen as a result of increased lipid mobilization for gluconeogenesis [4]. In such cases, PN may improve hyperlipidemia by providing an exogenous energy source. Some patients are susceptible to developing hyperlipidemia due to underlying endocrine disease(s) or genetic predilection. If lipemic serum is noted, serum triglycerides should be measured and if present, administration rate or fat concentration of the solution should be adjusted down.

- Refeeding syndrome: see earlier in this article
- Sepsis and infection

Infection at the site of intravenous route access is less common in the hospital setting, but can lead to serious complications [69,71]. PN solutions rich in nutrients provide favorable environments for microbial growth if they are contaminated during handling and/or preparation. Critical care patients that are malnourished, immunosuppressed, or hyperglycemic are prone to developing sepsis as the result of microbial seeding. Preventive measures include close monitoring of the catheter site, and proper handling of the catheter, line, and PN solution bag. These practices are also effective in preventing mechanical complications of PN administration, such as catheter displacement, line torsion, and obstruction. Patients should be frequently evaluated for hyperglycemia from excessive dextrose administration and for signs of sepsis such as fever and catheter site inflammation. Daily nutritional assessment should also guide the practitioners to discontinue PN administration in a timely manner to reduce the chance of sepsis development and other complications.

SUMMARY AND FUTURE DIRECTIONS

Undernutrition is a common condition seen in hospitalized patients and is directly associated with longer hospital stay and increased mortality and morbidity. Whenever possible, enteral feeding is always the preferred method of nutrient provision as it preserves GI mucosa integrity, prevents bacterial translocation, and supports systemic immune function. A systematic decision-making approach, as presented in Fig. 1, should be used to determine the optimal nutritional intervention timing and methods based on patient and disease factors, accessibility, and cost.

The current approach to nutritional management of critically ill veterinary patients focuses on the provision of *calories* to prevent negative energy balance. As some human studies demonstrate the beneficial effects of hyperproteic, hypocaloric nutrition on patient response [72,73], further work is needed to investigate the effects of nutritional status on macronutrient absorption and utilization with or without underlying diseases and the optimal doses of dietary protein versus calories for critically ill veterinary patients.

DISCLOSURE

The authors have nothing to disclose.

REFERENCES

[1] Brunetto MA, Gomes MOS, Andre MR, et al. Effects of nutritional support on hospital outcome in dogs and cats. J Vet Emerg Crit Care 2010;20:224–31.

[2] Chandler ML, Gunn-moore DA. Nutritional status of canine and feline patients admitted to a veterinary internal medicine service. J Nutr 2004;134:2050S–2S.

[3] Molina J, Hervera M, Manzanilla EG, et al. Evaluation of the prevalence and risk factors for undernutrition in hospitalized dogs. Front Vet Sci 2018;5:205.

[4] Berg JM, Tymoczko JL, Stryer L. Food intake and starvation induce metabolic changes. In: Biochemistry. 5th edition. New York: W H Freeman; 2002. Available at: https://www.ncbi.nlm.nih.gov/books/NBK22414/. Accessed May 9, 2020.

[5] Soeters PB. Macronutrient metabolism in starvation and stress. Nestle Nutr Inst Workshop Ser 2015;82:17-25.

[6] von Haehling S, Lainscak M, Springer J, et al. Cardiac cachexia: a systematic overview. Pharmacol Ther 2009; 121:227–52.

[7] Şimşek T, Şimşek HU, Cantürk NZ. Response to trauma and metabolic changes: posttraumatic metabolism. Ulus Cerrahi Derg 2014;30(3):153–9.

[8] Levine B, Kalman J, Mayer L, et al. Elevated circulating levels of tumor necrosis factor in severe chronic heart failure. N Engl J Med 1990;323:236–41.

[9] Laviano A, Inui A, Marks DL, et al. Neural control of the anorexia-cachexia syndrome. Am J Physiol Endocrinol Metab 2008;295:E1000–8.

[10] Cruz-Jentoft AJ, Baeyens JP, Bauer JM, et al. Sarcopenia: European consensus on definition and diagnosis: Report of the European Working Group on Sarcopenia in Older People. Age Ageing 2010;39(4):412–23.

[11] Parker V, Freeman L. Association between body condition and survival in dogs with acquired chronic kidney disease. J Vet Intern Med 2011;25:1306–11.

[12] Freeman L. Cachexia and sarcopenia: emerging syndromes of importance in dogs and cats. J Vet Intern Med 2012;26:3–17.

[13] Powanda MC, Moyer ED. Plasma proteins and wound healing. Surg Gynecol Obstet 1981;153(5):749-755.

[14] Freeman L, Becvarova I, Cave N, et al. WSAVA nutritional assessment guidelines. J Small Anim Pract 2011;52: 385–96.

[15] WASAVA. Nutritional assessment. 2013. Available at: https://wsava.org/wp-content/uploads/2020/01/Nutritional-Assessment-Checklist.pdf. Accessed March 15, 2020.

[16] WASAVA. Body condition score for cats. 2013. Available at: https://wsava.org/wp-content/uploads/2020/01/Cat-Body-Condition-Scoring-2017.pdf. Accessed March 15, 2020.

[17] WASAVA. Body condition score for dogs. 2013. Available at: https://wsava.org/wp-content/uploads/2020/01/Body-Condition-Score-Dog.pdf. Accessed March 15, 2020.

[18] Freeman LM, Michel KE, Zanghi BM, et al. Evaluation of the use of muscle condition score and ultrasonographic measurements for assessment of muscle mass in dogs. Am J Vet Res 2019;80(6):595–600.

[19] Freeman LM, Michel KE, Zanghi BM, et al. Usefulness of muscle condition score and ultrasonographic measurements for assessment of muscle mass in cats with cachexia and sarcopenia. Am J Vet Res 2020;81(3): 254–9.

[20] WASAVA. Muscle condition score for cats. 2013. Available at: https://wsava.org/wp-content/uploads/2020/01/Muscle-Condition-Score-Chart-for-Cats.pdf. Accessed March 15, 2020.

[21] WASAVA, Muscle. Condition score for dogs. 2013. Available at: https://wsava.org/wp-content/uploads/2020/01/Muscle-Condition-Score-Chart-for-Dogs.pdf. Accessed March 15, 2020.

[22] Reuter JD, Marks SL, Rogers QR. Use of total parenteral nutrition in dogs: 209 cases (1988-1995). J Vet Emerg Crit Care 1998;8:201–13.

[23] Delaney SJ. Management of anorexia in dogs and cats. Vet Clin North Am Small Anim Pract 2006;36(6): 1243–9, vi.

[24] Mohr AJ, Leisewitz AL, Jacobson LS, et al. Effect of early enteral nutrition on intestinal permeability, intestinal protein loss, and outcome in dogs with severe parvoviral enteritis. J Vet Intern Med 2003;17(6):791-798.

[25] Li JY, Yu T, Chen GC, et al. Enteral nutrition within 48 hours of admission improves clinical outcomes of acute pancreatitis by reducing complications: a meta-analysis. PLoS One 2013;8(6):e64926.

[26] Hansen SC, Hlusko KC, Matz BM, et al. Retrospective evaluation of 24 cases of gastrostomy tube usage in dogs with septic peritonitis (2009-2016). J Vet Emerg Crit Care 2019;29(5):514–20.

[27] Duran B. The effects of long-term total parenteral nutrition on gut mucosal immunity in children with short bowel syndrome: a systematic review. BMC Nurs 2005; 4(1):2.

[28] Frye CW, Blong AE, Wakshlag JJ. Peri-surgical nutrition: perspectives and perceptions. Vet Clin North Am Small Anim Pract 2015;45(5):1067–84.

[29] Larsen JA. Enteral nutrition and tube feeding. In: Fascetti AJ, Delaney SJ, editors. Applied veterinary clinical nutrition. West Sussex (United Kingdom): Wiley-Blackwell; 2012. p. 329–52. https://doi.org/10.1002/9781118785669.ch20.

[30] Remillard RL, Armstrong PJ, Davenport DJ. Assisted feeding in hospitalized patients: enteral and parenteral. In: Hand MS, Thatcher CD, Remillard RL, et al, editors. Small animal clinical nutrition. 4th edition. Philadelphia: Mark Morris Institute; 2000. p. 352–99.

[31] Morris JG, Rogers QR. Arginine: an essential amino acid for the cat. J Nutr 1978;108(12):1944–53.

[32] Jolliffe N, Smith HW. The excretion of urine in the dog: I. the urea and creatinine clearances on a mixed diet. Am J Physiol 1931;98:572–7.

[33] Jacob F, Polzin DJ, Osborne CA, et al. Clinical evaluation of dietary modification for treatment of spontaneous chronic renal failure in dogs. J Am Vet Med Assoc 2002;220(8):1163-1170.

[34] Ross SJ, Osborne CA, Kirk CA, et al. Clinical evaluation of dietary modification for treatment of spontaneous chronic kidney disease in cats. J Am Vet Med Assoc 2006;229(6):949-957.

[35] Charlton CP, Buchanan E, Holden CE, et al. Intensive enteral feeding in advanced cirrhosis: reversal of malnutrition without precipitation of hepatic encephalopathy. Arch Dis Child 1992;67(5):603-607.

[36] Schaeffer MC, Rogers QR, Leung PMB, et al. Changes in cerebrospinal fluid and plasma amino acid concentrations with elevated dietary protein concentration in dogs with portacaval shunts. Life Sci 1991;48(23): 2215–23.

[37] Backus RC, Rosenquist GL, Rogers QR, et al. Elevation of plasma cholecystokinin (CCK) immunoreactivity by fat, protein, and amino acids in the cat, a carnivore. Regul Pept 1995;57(2):123–31.

[38] Okanishi H, Yoshioka R, Kagawa Y, et al. The clinical efficacy of dietary fat restriction in treatment of dogs with intestinal lymphangiectasia. J Vet Intern Med 2014; 28(3):809–17.

[39] Guilford WG. Nutritional management of gastrointestinal tract diseases of dogs and cats. J Nutr 1994;124: S2663S–2669.

[40] Laflamme DP, Xu H, Long GM. Effect of diets differing in fat content on chronic diarrhea in cats. J Vet Intern Med 2011;25(2):230–5.

[41] Cecil JE, Francis J, Read NW. Comparison of the effects of a high-fat and high-carbohydrate soup delivered orally and intragastrically on gastric emptying, appetite, and eating behaviour. Physiol Behav 1999;67(2): 299–306.

[42] Whitehead K, Cortes Y, Eirmann L. Gastrointestinal dysmotility disorders in critically ill dogs and cats. J Vet Emerg Crit Care 2016;26:234–53.

[43] Freeman LM, Rush JE. Nutritional management of cardiovascular diseases. In: Fascetti AJ, Delaney SJ, editors. Applied veterinary clinical nutrition. West Sussex (United Kingdom): Wiley-Blackwell; 2012. p. 301–13. https://doi.org/10.1002/9781118785669.ch18.

[44] Rush JE, Freeman LM, Brown DJ, et al. Clinical, echocardiographic, and neurohormonal effects of a sodium-restricted diet in dogs with heart failure. J Vet Intern Med 2000;14(5):513–20.
[45] Torre DM, deLaforcade AM, Chan DL. Incidence and clinical relevance of hyperglycemia in critically ill dogs. J Vet Intern Med 2007;21(5):971–5.
[46] Chan DL, Freeman LM, Rozanski EA, et al. Alterations in carbohydrate metabolism in critically ill cats. J Vet Emerg Crit Care 2006;16:S7–13.
[47] Farrow HA, Rand JS, Morton JM, et al. Effect of dietary carbohydrate, fat, and protein on postprandial glycemia and energy intake in cats. J Vet Intern Med 2013;27(5): 1121–35.
[48] Nelson RW, Scott-Moncrieff JC, Feldman EC, et al. Effect of insoluble fiber on control of glycemia in cats with naturally acquired diabetes mellitus. J Am Vet Med Assoc 2000;216:1082–8.
[49] Kimmel SE, Michel KE, Hess RS, et al. Effects of insoluble and soluble dietary fiber on glycemic control in dogs with naturally occurring insulin-dependent diabetes mellitus. J Am Vet Med Assoc 2000;216:1076–81.
[50] Makielski K, Cullen J, O'Connor A, et al. Narrative review of therapies for chronic enteropathies in dogs and cats. J Vet Intern Med 2019;33(1):11–22.
[51] Guilford WG, Jones BR, Markwell PJ, et al. Food sensitivity in cats with chronic idiopathic gastrointestinal problems. J Vet Intern Med 2001;15(1):7–13.
[52] Mandigers PJ, Biourge V, German AJ. Efficacy of a commercial hydrolysate diet in eight cats suffering from inflammatory bowel disease or adverse reaction to food. Tijdschr Diergeneeskd 2010;135(18): 668–72.
[53] O'Toole E, Miller CW, Wilson BA, et al. Comparison of the standard predictive equation for calculation of resting energy expenditure with indirect calorimetry in hospitalized and healthy dogs. J Am Vet Med Assoc 2004;225(1):58–64.
[54] Chan DL. Estimating energy requirements of small animal patients. In: Chan DL, editor. Nutritional management of hospitalized small animals. Oxford: Wiley-Blackwell; 2015. p. 7–13. https://doi.org/10.1002/9781119052951.ch2.
[55] Kleiber M. Body size and metabolism. Hilgardia 1932; 6(11):315–53.
[56] Mehanna HM, Moledina J, Travis J. Refeeding syndrome: what it is, and how to prevent and treat it. Br Med J 2008; 336(7659):1495–8.
[57] National Research Council. Vitamins. In: Nutrient requirements of dogs and cats. Washington, DC: National Academies Press; 2006. p. 193–245.
[58] National Research Council. Minerals. In: Nutrient requirements of dogs and cats. Washington, DC: National Academies Press; 2006. p. 145–92.
[59] Markovich JE, Heinze CR, Freeman LM. Thiamine deficiency in dogs and cats. J Am Vet Med Assoc 2013; 243(5):649–56.
[60] Parker VJ, Freeman LM. Comparison of various solutions to dissolve critical care diet clots. J Vet Emerg Crit Care 2013;23(3):344–7.
[61] Breheny CR, Boag A, Le Gal A, et al. Esophageal feeding tube placement and the associated complications in 248 cats. J Vet Intern Med 2019;33(3):1306–14.
[62] Nathanson O, McGonigle K, Michel K, et al. Esophagostomy tube complications in dogs and cats: Retrospective review of 225 cases. J Vet Intern Med 2019;33(5): 2014–9.
[63] Campbell SJ, Marks SL, Yoshimoto SK, et al. Complications and outcomes of one-step low-profile gastrostomy devices for long-term enteral feeding in dogs and cats. J Am Anim Hosp Assoc 2006;42(3):197–206.
[64] Perea SC. Parenteral Nutrition. In: Fascetti AJ, Delaney SJ, editors. Applied veterinary clinical nutrition. West Sussex (United Kingdom): Wiley-Blackwell; 2012. p. 353–74. https://doi.org/10.1002/9781118785669.ch21.
[65] Gross TL, Song MD, Havel PJ, et al. Superficial necrolytic dermatitis (necrolytic migratory erythema) in dogs. Vet Pathol 1993;30(1):75–81.
[66] Outerbridge CA, Marks SL, Rogers QR. Plasma amino acid concentrations in 36 dogs with histologically confirmed superficial necrolytic dermatitis. Vet Dermatol 2002;13:177–86.
[67] Jaffey JA, Backus RC, Sprinkle M, et al. Successful long-term management of canine superficial necrolytic dermatitis with amino acid infusions and nutritionally balanced home-made diet modification. Front Vet Sci 2020;7:28.
[68] Pyle SC, Marks SL, Kass PH. Evaluation of complications and prognostic factors associated with administration of total parenteral nutrition in cats: 75 cases (1994-2001). J Am Vet Med Assoc 2004;225(2):242–50.
[69] Queau Y, Larsen JA, Kass PH, et al. Factors associated with adverse outcomes during parenteral nutrition administration in dogs and cats. J Vet Intern Med 2011;25(3):446–52.
[70] van den Berghe G, Wouters P, Weekers F, et al. Intensive insulin therapy in critically ill patients. N Engl J Med 2001;345(19):1359–67.
[71] Marra AR, Opilla M. Epidemiology of bloodstream infection associated with parenteral nutrition. Am J Infect Control 2008;36(10):S173.e5-8.
[72] Weijs PJ, Looijaard WG, Beishuizen A, et al. Early high protein intake is associated with low mortality and energy overfeeding with high mortality in non-septic mechanically ventilated critically ill patients. Crit Care 2014;18:701.
[73] Rugeles SJ, Rueda JD, Diaz CE, et al. Hyperproteic hypocaloric enteral nutrition in the critically ill patient: a randomized controlled clinical trial. Indian J Crit Care Med 2013;17:343–9.

Advances in Small Animal Care 1 (2020) 227–238
ADVANCES IN SMALL ANIMAL CARE

The Role of Taurine in Cardiac Health in Dogs and Cats

Jennifer A. Larsen, DVM, MS, PhD, DACVN*, Andrea J. Fascetti, VMD, PhD, DACVIM (SA), DACVN
Department of Molecular Biosciences, School of Veterinary Medicine, University of California, Davis, 1089 Veterinary Medicine Drive, Davis, CA 95616, USA

KEYWORDS
• Taurine • Dilated cardiomyopathy • Nutritional requirements • Sulfur amino acids • Canine • Feline

KEY POINTS

- Taurine deficiency has been linked to development of dilated cardiomyopathy in both cats and dogs.
- In contrast to cats that have a dietary taurine requirement, dogs have the metabolic capacity to synthesize taurine from cysteine and methionine, so taurine is not a required amino acid for them.
- In species able to do so, endogenous synthesis of taurine is highly variable between individuals. Synthesis is impacted by an individual's nutritional state, protein intake, and cysteine availability.
- The precise physiologic roles of taurine remain largely uncharacterized, although a major function is the conjugation of bile acids, for which both dogs and cats are obligated to use solely taurine.
- Dietary factors that influence availability and utilization of sulfur-containing metabolites, pathway intermediates, methyl donors such as choline, and enzyme cofactors such as vitamins potentially also play a role in the development of dilated cardiomyopathy suspected to be related to diet, and full characterization of these impacts largely remain unexplored.

INTRODUCTION

Dilated cardiomyopathy (DCM) is one of the most common acquired cardiovascular diseases in dogs. It is less common in cats following the discovery of an obligate taurine requirement in this species, which led to establishment of regulatory minimum taurine concentrations for commercial feline diets. The finding of DCM related to taurine deficiency appears to be multifactorial and related to nutritional factors, such as protein quality (amino acid profile and bioavailability), biosynthetic rate (in the dog), intake of sulfur amino acid precursors, and energy and fiber intake. Many other interrelated dietary, environmental, genetic, and animal factors also determine taurine status due to impacts on taurine synthesis, metabolism, and utilization. Although not all cases of canine DCM show taurine deficiency based on blood concentrations, taurine is a downstream indicator of overall sulfur amino acid status, and other metabolic intermediates or related pathway molecules also may play a primary or secondary role in the development of DCM. It is clear that DCM in both dogs and cats is a disease highly influenced by nutrition, despite current controversies and uncertainties regarding the precise role of diet. As many veterinary practitioners diagnose and manage DCM in both species, an understanding of what has been defined with regard to the complex etiopathogenesis may help guide clinical decision making as well as provide some foundation for the application of future discoveries.

*Corresponding author, *E-mail address:* jalarsen@vmth.ucdavis.edu

https://doi.org/10.1016/j.yasa.2020.07.015
2666-4518/20/

PHYSIOLOGY AND METABOLISM OF TAURINE IN DOGS AND CATS

Taurine, also known by its chemical name 2-aminoethanesulfonic acid, is an organic compound that can be acquired from food, but it is not a component of peptides. Rather, it is the most abundant of the free amino acids [1]. In species able to do so, endogenous synthesis of taurine is highly variable among individuals. Synthesis is impacted by an individual's nutritional state, protein intake, and cysteine availability [1,2]. Although other tissues, including kidney and brain, also synthesize taurine, among other sulfur amino acid derivatives, only the liver responds to dietary concentrations by altering synthetic rates via enzymatic modulation. Cysteine dioxygenase activity is the major limiting step in taurine biosynthesis and is dependent on cysteine concentration in the portal blood supply [3]. Through modulation of various enzyme activities, the liver is responsible for

1. Disposing of excess sulfur amino acids from the gastrointestinal (GI) tract (deamination and facilitation of the various possible fates of the alpha-keto acids)
2. Transforming some precursors into other substrates (such as synthesis of taurine, glutathione, and proteins, among others)
3. Regulating the systemic concentrations of various metabolites (including taurine) via altered synthesis rates from sulfur amino acid precursors in the GI tract

The availability of cysteine is in turn dependent on the equilibrium between homocysteine and methionine, along with folic acid, vitamin B_{12}, and the efficiency of the enzyme methylenetetrahydrofolate reductase. When hepatic concentrations of cysteine vary, traffic of this precursor through various enzyme pathways is modulated by relative K_m (Michaelis constant) values. For example, synthesis of the tripeptide glutathione is prioritized over that of taurine, such that when cysteine supply is low, a smaller proportion of available cysteine is utilized for taurine biosynthesis, and glutathione synthesis is conserved via the lower K_m of glutamate cysteine ligase [3]. In this situation, altered excretion at the level of the kidney also occurs, which decreases urinary taurine concentrations and conserves taurine in the face of reduced biosynthetic capacity due to inadequate precursor supply.

The precise physiologic roles of taurine remain largely uncharacterized, although a major function is the conjugation of bile acids. Although many other species use both glycine and taurine for this purpose, both dogs and cats are obligated to use only taurine. Outcomes from deficiency and repletion studies, however, that report various clinical signs in deficient animals suggest significant functional importance of other roles. In 1975, Hayes and colleagues [4] discovered that taurine was an essential nutrient in the cat when it was documented that plasma taurine concentrations in cats with central retinal degeneration were only 1% to 2% that of healthy cats. Plasma taurine, along with whole-blood taurine, has been used as a direct measure of taurine status in the cat ever since.

Taurine is highest in animal tissues, especially muscle, viscera, and brain [5,6]. As a strict carnivore, the natural diets of cats typically are high in these components, and because regulatory minimums for taurine concentrations in commercial feline diets have been established, deficiency currently is uncommon. There are other factors, however, that have been shown to increase the risk of suboptimal taurine status or of overt deficiency in the cat even with apparent dietary sufficiency, which appear to have a mostly negative impact on the efficiency of enterohepatic recycling of taurine-conjugated bile salts, both through microbial action and other mechanisms [7–10]. These factors include certain fiber types, indigestible protein, and processing effects, which underlie the differential dietary taurine recommendations for purified diets, commercial dry extruded kibble, and commercial canned products [11,12].

ETIOLOGY AND CHARACTERIZATION OF TAURINE DEFICIENCY

In cats, 3 manifestations of taurine deficiency have been described:

- Central retinal degeneration [4]
- Reproductive failure and impaired fetal development [13]
- DCM [14]

Taurine-deficient cats, however, can show highly variable clinical traits, ranging from no apparent signs to severe fatal DCM or complete blindness from retinal degeneration. Normal echocardiograms and fundic examinations have been reported in both laboratory and pet cats that are taurine-depleted [14,15]. Taurine deficiency also has been linked to DCM and reproductive inefficiency in dogs [16,17]. Although ocular changes have been reported in dogs with low blood taurine concentrations, central retinal degeneration does not appear to be a common finding [18].

Cats have limited ability to synthesize taurine due to low activities of the enzymes cysteine sulfinic acid decarboxylase and cysteine dioxygenase. Taurine supplementation resulted in correction of plasma taurine concentrations and improvement or even resolution of DCM in cats with low taurine concentrations [15]. Taurine also may have a pharmaceutical effect. In addition to deficiency correction with supplementation, it is considered to have ionotropic properties. The mechanism of heart failure in taurine-deficient cats is not well understood, but in the myocardium, taurine appears to participate in many functions, including cellular osmoregulation, free-radical scavenging, and modulation of contractile strength through regulation of calcium concentrations [15,19,20]. Detrimental changes in intracellular calcium dynamics slowing reuptake of calcium by the sarcoplasmic reticulum may be responsible for the slowed myocardium relaxation and diastolic dysfunction in DCM [19,20]. Systolic dysfunction secondary to taurine depletion may be related to a reduction in the calcium sensitivity of the myocardial contractile proteins [19,20]. Reduced taurine concentrations have been associated with an increase in the phosphorylation of troponin I, having a negative impact on calcium sensitivity in myocardial contraction [19,20]. In addition, diminished adenosine triphosphate for cardiac contraction has been associated with low taurine concentrations [20].

Despite the myriad proposed functions of taurine, the mechanisms driving the clinical signs seen in deficiency remain elusive and interpretation has been complicated by unanticipated and sometimes conflicting research findings. For example, in 1 early study, taurine supplementation increased the taurine concentration of the myocardium in cats with naturally occurring DCM, and in healthy cats fed diets with defined taurine concentrations, myocardial taurine content increased according to intake [21]. Myocardial taurine concentrations, however, did not differ among cats with naturally occurring DCM, hypertrophic cardiomyopathy, or volume overload, and the group with DCM had a mean myocardial taurine concentration higher than that of healthy cats given a taurine-free diet [21]. Similarly, another study demonstrated that myocardial taurine concentration was not different in taurine-deficient cats with and without myocardial failure, and the trend was for those with overt DCM to have higher myocardial taurine content [22].

In contrast to cats, dogs have the metabolic capacity to synthesize taurine from cysteine and methionine, and taurine is not considered a required amino acid for the dog (Fig. 1). There is no regulatory requirement for taurine in commercial dog foods [11]. Endogenous synthesis typically is adequate to meet physiologic needs in the dog; however, as in cats, there are dietary factors (such as protein source, fiber type and concentration, and cooking or processing methods) as well as individual dog characteristics (such as breed and calorie needs) that have an impact on the efficiency of taurine syntheses and utilization. Taurine deficiency has been documented in dogs with and without clinical signs, including DCM. In some cases, this was associated with feeding low-protein diets or the feeding of diets apparently limiting in sulfur amino acids [16,17,23]. Both factors appear to have a negative impact on the ability of some dogs to synthesize adequate amounts of taurine to satisfy metabolic needs. However, other cases of taurine-responsive DCM, with or without a carnitine-responsive component, have been reported that appear to be breed related [24,25].

CLINICAL TAURINE DEFICIENCY IN DOGS

Several studies have recognized possible nutritional features associated with taurine deficiency in dogs and that in some cases have been associated with DCM in breeds not documented to have a genetic predisposition to the disease. One published case series described 12 dogs with DCM and taurine deficiency that were consuming diets containing lamb meal, rice, or both [17]. Most affected dogs were consuming their respective diets for long periods of time. Seven dogs surviving beyond a year postdiagnosis only required supplemental taurine with no other cardiac medications. This remarkable improvement in cardiac function is not seen in dogs with heritable DCM, and the similarity with the disease outcomes seen in taurine-deficient cats supported that diet played a major role.

Another retrospective study of 37 dogs with DCM found that 20 (54%) had taurine deficiency based on measurement of whole blood, plasma, or both, and these dogs were more likely to be in congestive heart failure and had a more severe disease classification compared with dogs with adequate taurine status [26]. Based on manufacturer information, there was no difference in dietary taurine content between the taurine-deficient and taurine-adequate groups; 7/20 dogs with deficiency were eating lamb and rice-based diets compared with 3/17 dogs without taurine deficiency. Of the subset of dogs with follow-up assessments, taurine-deficient dogs showed improvements in some but not all echocardiographic measurements, although median survival was not different compared with those without taurine deficiency [26]. Another case series examined the taurine status of 19 Newfoundland dogs eating commercially available diets [16]; 12

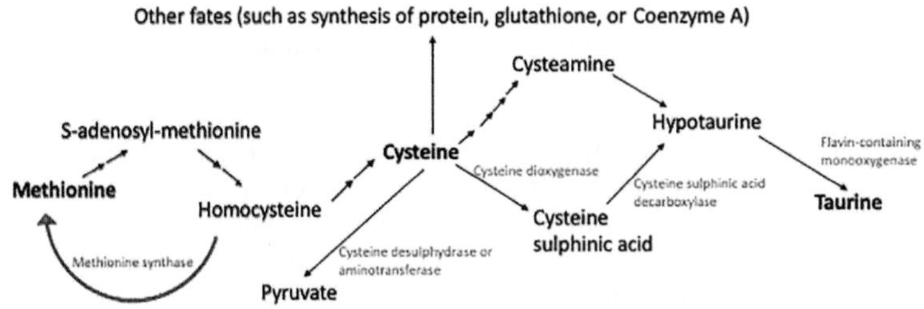

FIG. 1 Simplified schematic of the taurine synthetic pathway. Not all donors, acceptors, or cofactors are shown.

of these dogs were diagnosed with taurine deficiency on the basis of low blood taurine concentrations, and 9/12 were being fed a lamb or lamb meal and rice-based diet. Some of the taurine-deficient dogs either were switched to a different commercial diet or were supplemented with methionine, both of which resulted in increased blood concentrations of taurine. Six of the taurine deficient dogs underwent echocardiographic examination, and none was diagnosed with DCM. In order to further investigate this problem, researchers fed normal dogs either a specific commercially available lamb meal and rice-based diet previously associated with taurine deficiency in clinical cases (diet A) or a commercially available diet not associated with taurine deficiency and that did not contain lamb meal or rice (diet B) [27]. Both diets were analyzed to confirm similar concentrations of methionine, cystine, and taurine. They found that although both groups had similar blood taurine concentrations, the group fed the lamb meal and rice diet appeared to be conserving taurine, because the urinary taurine concentration was much lower compared with the dogs fed diet B. When the dogs were given supplemental methionine, urinary taurine was increased, suggesting that the bioavailability of sulfur amino acid precursors in the lamb meal and rice diet was inadequate to support taurine synthesis [27].

Based on these investigations and the known associations with dietary factors, possible causes for apparent canine taurine deficiency at the time were considered to be related to

1. Insufficient synthesis of taurine due to lack of adequate sulfur amino acid precursors
2. Extraordinary loss of taurine or its precursors in urine
3. Extraordinary GI loss of taurine in bile acid conjugates as found in cats
4. A reduction in global protein digestibility and/or specific amino acid bioavailability

Previous work had documented that relative to other protein sources, lamb meal showed poor ileal nitrogen and cystine digestibility and subsequent poor sulfur amino acid bioavailability in dogs [28].

To further define these relationships, a larger group of Newfoundlands then was investigated by these researchers. Plasma amino acid status was assessed in more than 200 dogs, whereas an additional smaller group of Newfoundlands and beagles were used to measure taurine synthesis [18]. In the large group of dogs, plasma taurine concentrations were correlated with plasma concentrations of its precursors: methionine and cystine. Taurine deficiency was found in 8% (18/209) of the dogs, with this group characterized as "older, less active, and had more medical problems and treatments" compared with the rest of the study population. Nine of those 18 dogs were evaluated further, and 3 were diagnosed with DCM, which resolved with taurine supplementation. Two of the dogs that underwent further evaluation had ocular fundus abnormalities, 1 of which also was diagnosed with DCM.

This study also determined taurine synthesis in a group of 6 Newfoundlands and 6 beagles fed the same diet, adequate in sulfur amino acid concentrations, for 3 weeks prior to assessments [18]. Newfoundlands had significantly lower plasma and whole-blood taurine concentrations and lower urinary taurine to creatinine ratios. Dietary dry matter digestibility did not differ, but Newfoundlands showed higher total fecal bile acid excretion per gram of fecal dry matter. When compared on a metabolic body weight basis, the Newfoundlands required fewer calories to maintain body weight and had a taurine synthetic rate less than half that of the beagles. The effect of body size and, therefore, of food intake relative to weight has since been confirmed to strongly influence taurine synthetic rate [29] and supports that larger breed dogs as well as any dogs with lower than predicted energy requirements may be at risk for taurine deficiency when fed diets limiting in bioavailable sulfur amino acids.

REOCCURRENCE OF CANINE DILATED CARDIOMYOPATHY CASES

After modifications to some commercial diets from the 1990s to 2000s, including those formulated to be lower in protein for management of specific diseases, diagnosis of DCM in dogs of nongenetically predisposed breeds apparently occurred only occasionally. The authors sporadically saw cases of DCM with taurine deficiency in dogs fed a range of diets, including commercial vegetarian diets and home-prepared raw or cooked diets, with or without animal-based protein sources. By late 2016, however, the authors, anecdotally, were noticing higher case numbers of canine DCM seen at their institution, and in early 2017 a cluster of golden retrievers with taurine deficiency and DCM was discussed in the online Veterinary Information Network. The common finding in all cases was that the dogs were fed commercial diets marketed as "grain-free" and containing ingredients, such as potatoes and legumes (chickpeas, lentils, beans, and peas). In response to an increased number of reports, the US Food and Drug Administration (FDA) announced an investigation of the potential connection between diet and canine DCM in July 2018 [30]. Subsequent updates from FDA were provided in February and June 2019 and included more than 500 reports of canine DCM suspected to be related to diet [31,32]. Consequent descriptive and investigative research by multiple groups is ongoing or published, and, although an association with specific diet types is suspected, the role of specific dietary characteristics remains unclear.

Potential Risk Factors

The golden retriever, a breed for which DCM is not a heritable disease, was the breed reported most frequently in the FDA reports as of April 2019 [33]. A multicenter, prospective observational study assessed 24 golden retrievers with DCM and taurine deficiency; 23 of these dogs were consuming diets described as grain-free and/or legume-rich [34]. Almost all dogs improved with diet change and taurine supplementation plus treatment of heart failure when present, which, again, is an outcome not recognized in dogs with heritable DCM and more closely resembles the nutritionally responsive disease seen in cats. A prospective cohort study then was conducted to investigate a larger group of 86 reportedly healthy golden retrievers by these researchers; the group was divided based on diet history [35]. Outcomes of taurine status assessments and echocardiograms showed that dogs consuming grain-free diets containing legumes or potatoes had significantly lower blood taurine concentrations and more frequent cardiac systolic dysfunction compared with those that were consuming grain-inclusive diets lacking legumes or potatoes in the top 5 ingredients. These findings corroborated a previous report of differential echocardiographic findings in 48 dogs of many different breeds with DCM and consuming either grain-free diets (n = 36, 14 of which were fed the same specific brand and formula, which was the most common diet fed in this study, and 22 fed other brands) or grain-inclusive diets (n = 12) [36]. Dogs fed the most common brand of grain-free diet showed more severe cardiac changes suggestive of worsened function and not related to disease stage compared with those consuming grain-inclusive diets; however, there were no echocardiographic variable differences between dogs fed grain-inclusive diets and those fed other brands. Based on plasma and/or whole-blood taurine concentrations of 26/48 dogs in that study, only 2 dogs were classified as taurine deficient, both in the grain-inclusive diet group; 1 of these died in-hospital and 1 improved with diet change and taurine supplementation [36].

The FDA reports, as well as the published case series of both healthy dogs and those with DCM, raise concerns regarding possible adverse effects on cardiac health associated with certain diet categories but do not elucidate the role of any specific nutritional profiles or ingredients. The grain-free diet category is wide and varied, so mechanistic research is needed to define specific characteristics that may play a part in these findings. Grain-free pet foods recently have become popular and now enjoy a large market share. Trends in human nutrition, an increased awareness of pet food manufacturing and ingredients sources, shifts in pet food marketing strategies, and widespread access to online information have contributed to heightened consumer awareness of ingredient-based pet food selections and shifts in pet owner preferences. This effect was enhanced further by unsubstantiated claims that grains cause allergies and other adverse responses in dogs and cats, encouraging more pet owners to select diets lacking grains. There is no evidence, however, of a safety risk of grains for pets or any medical or nutritional indication for grain-free diets per se. One approach to formulating grain-free diets is to utilize ingredients such as legumes, potato, and tapioca. Although a wide range of potential ingredients should be explored for use in pet foods in order to promote sustainability and provide diversity and stability in food production systems, commercial products must be well formulated and adequately researched to ensure safety and nutritional adequacy [37].

Legumes in particular contribute not only dietary carbohydrate but also significant amounts of fiber and protein; however, these ingredients are limiting in sulfur amino acids, and some contain antinutritional factors that have a negative impact on protein digestibility and amino acid bioavailability. Proper manufacturing processes, including adequate cooking times and temperatures, are expected to largely destroy antinutritional factors; however, processing procedures may vary and the result may not be ideally reliable or complete. Because many pet foods marketed as grain-free also include less common animal-based protein sources, the protein concentration overall may be lower, and/or higher proportions of the dietary protein may be contributed by the plant-based ingredients in order to control costs. In addition, under some conditions of pet food production (high heat and pressure), it is well established that amino acids (especially lysine, cysteine, and methionine) undergo nonenzymatic reactions with other dietary constituents to form Maillard reaction products. These compounds impart desirable sensory characteristics to foods but also can result in decreased specific amino acid bioavailability even without negative effects on global protein digestibility [7,38].

Overall, the popularity of grain-free diets in the marketplace has resulted in the increased use of higher amounts of certain pet food ingredients that are limited in sulfur amino acids, that have potentially lower amino acid bioavailability, that may not be as well defined with regard to processing effects, and that may have changed the fiber types and concentrations common in pet foods. These factors all can be expected to have an impact on the overall dietary amino acid balance as well as the microbiome. Among other effects, it is possible the shift of the microbiome may favor the production of microbes containing cholyltaurine hydrolase, which cleaves taurocholic acid to taurine and cholic acid, with subsequent oxidation to taurine and by gut microbes preventing reutilization through the enterohepatic circulation [7,39]. Other dietary factors, however, that influence availability and utilization of sulfur-containing metabolites potentially also play a role in the development of diet-associated DCM. These metabolites include pathway intermediates, methyl donors such as choline, and enzyme cofactors such as vitamins. For example, due to the role of folate in 1-carbon metabolism, this vitamin has an influence on sulfur amino acid status, including in the regeneration of methionine from homocysteine via a cobalamin-requiring process. Folate also is involved in conversion of serine to glycine, formation of pyrimidines, and other biochemical pathways, including homocysteine catabolism, for which rates of substrate flux may differ depending on nutritional status. Due to these interrelationships, inadequate intake of choline, methionine, and cobalamin may increase the metabolic requirement for folate. Characterizations of the deficiency syndromes of both thiamin [40] and pyridoxine [41] in the dog have included descriptions of cardiac chamber dilation with or without congestive failure. Reported assessments are limited, however, to necropsy descriptions rather than premortem evaluation of heart function, and cardiac changes are not reliably seen in all or even most cases. When reported, cardiac changes typically are not consistent with DCM; 1 study described severe congestive failure with both dilation and hypertrophy of the right but not left cardiac chambers [41].

There also is interest in the role of carnitine, a natural, biologically active amino acid derivative, which is both present in food and endogenously synthesized. Deficiency of this micronutrient (based on direct measurements of tissues or response to supplementation) is associated with canine DCM, with or without concurrent taurine deficiency [24,42]. Characterization of carnitine status is complicated by differential plasma and myocardial concentrations, lack of established reference ranges, and scarcity of descriptive clinical data distinct from the effect of taurine. In addition, the regulation of carnitine synthesis in canine health and disease has not been defined. Regardless, carnitine supplementation often is recommended for dogs with DCM even without measurement of blood or myocardial carnitine concentrations [34,43], given that this practice may be beneficial and likely is harmless apart from the cost of the supplement. Full characterization of the impacts of a wide range of nutrients on the development of DCM remains largely unexplored, and much research is needed to accurately define dietary risk factors.

What Is the Role of Taurine?

In the case series published thus far and based on plasma and whole-blood assessments, taurine deficiency is not a universal finding in dogs with cardiac abnormalities or with any particular diet history [34–36]. In addition, of the 560 canine cases reported by the FDA in June 2019, 176 had both an echocardiogram and taurine status evaluation (whole-blood and/or plasma taurine measurements) [32]. A total of 130 of those dogs were diagnosed with DCM, of which 51 (39%)

had a documented low blood taurine concentration. Although a wide range of dog breeds was represented, golden retrievers comprised 37% of the DCM plus taurine-deficient group and made up 48% of dogs with low taurine regardless of echocardiographic diagnosis. It is unknown if blood sampling was performed in all cases prior to or after any changes in diet or supplements and whether sample collection and handling procedures were appropriate for ensuring accurate assessments of taurine concentrations.

As discussed previously, other studies also show discordant taurine assessments in the evaluation of dogs and cats with DCM. Of course, many clinical cases are identified once overt signs of DCM are apparent, which may or may not be accompanied by cardiac failure, and sulfur amino acid metabolism and taurine kinetics under those circumstances have not been characterized. It is possible that tissue damage associated with DCM results in release of taurine, or that other mechanisms that occur with myocardial failure may have an impact on assessments of taurine status. For example, elevated whole-blood taurine concentrations have been reported in people after myocardial infarction with cardiomyocyte injury and death, due to taurine being released and subsequently taken up rapidly by platelets [44,45]. A trend for higher myocardial taurine concentrations was reported for deficient cats with DCM versus those without myocardial failure, which was speculated to be related to a potential compensatory response [22]. Another previous study reported, however, that a group of 28 dogs with acquired valvular disease had higher plasma taurine concentrations compared with those with DCM (n = 76) or healthy controls (n = 47), with no difference when compared on the basis of the presence of congestive heart failure [46]. The mean plasma taurine concentration of the control group was not different than that of the DCM group, although 17% of the dogs with DCM were classified as taurine deficient, and all but 1 of the taurine-deficient dogs in this study had DCM [46].

The presence and progression of DCM in definitive taurine deficiency is not predictable, and not all dogs or cats with known taurine deficiency develop DCM. For example, only 2 of 17 beagles depleted of taurine as the result of consumption of a protein-restricted diet for 2 years had cardiac changes evident of early or overt DCM; this study showed that taurine deficiency preceded the DCM, which then was improved significantly with taurine supplementation [23]. Similarly, cats with experimentally induced taurine deficiency do not inevitably develop DCM (or central retinal degeneration). One research group observed that 11 cats fed experimental purified diets with a marginal taurine content (250 mg/kg or 500 mg/kg dry matter) for 4 years had confirmed deficiency based on very low plasma taurine concentrations (mean 8.4 nmol/mL; normal range >50 nmol/mL) [47]. Regardless, only 3 cats had DCM, whereas 6 had retinal degeneration (1 cat had both and 3 had neither). As such, a more controlled experiment was conducted and involved feeding for 40 weeks of a taurine-free purified diet to 11 cats, an adequate (0.14% taurine dry matter) purified diet to 9 cats, and a commercial canned diet similar to that implicated in the clinical cases (0.15% taurine dry matter [14]) to 9 cats [47]. Cats fed the taurine-free diet and the taurine-depleting commercial diet were taurine-deficient based on very low plasma taurine concentrations and some, but not all, showed evidence of DCM based on echocardiography (significantly decreased fractional shortening and end-systolic diameter was noted in both groups compared with cats fed the adequate purified diet) [47]. Further work done in this laboratory was the basis for current regulatory requirements for higher taurine concentration in commercial canned versus dry cat foods [9–11,39].

The disconnect between the results of taurine status assessments and absence (or presence) of clinical changes in the cardiac muscle may be explained a few other ways. It has been assumed that the kinetics of taurine metabolism in dogs mirrors that characterized in cats. This has not been established, however, and there are many potential differences. In addition, factors such as genetics, breed, sex, and food intake, as well as dietary characteristics, including duration of diet consumption and energy intake, all may play a part in differential clinical phenotypes. A study of plasma amino acids and whole-blood taurine concentrations in healthy dogs suggested the possibility of different ranges for different breeds, because Australian shepherds and Labrador retrievers had distinctly different average values (mean whole-blood taurine; 222 nmol/mL vs 296 nmol/mL, respectively) [48]. More recent work also has postulated that breed-specific reference ranges may be warranted [34,35]. In addition, it should be recognized that taurine has long been used as a readily analyzed marker for sulfur amino acid adequacy and indirectly the adequacy of general methyl donor status. Other markers or more complex assessments, however, may enable a more complete clinical picture of the ability of diets to meet the needs of both dogs and cats long term. The production of other compounds in the sulfur amino acid pathways, including glutathione, has higher priorities than taurine synthesis [3]. Regardless, low plasma or whole-blood taurine concentration values are very good indicators of disease risk and of nutritional inadequacy, even if additional factors also may influence the development of DCM. Nutritional status is dynamic over life stages and among individuals even in health, and the influence of various disease states likely will have a further impact on nutrient requirements. It is critical to avoid conflating the response to supplementation of specific nutrients under the conditions of disease with the role of those nutrients in prevention. Given the complexity of metabolism and physiology, positive responses should not be overinterpreted. Additional research is necessary to investigate the possible role of taurine in canine DCM associated with grain-free diets as well as fully characterize the interrelationships of other potential factors or nutrients that likely influence this disease.

ASSESSMENT OF THE PATIENT WITH DILATED CARDIOMYOPATHY

Individualized patient assessment is a critical aspect of nutritional management of patients with disease, including DCM. Evaluation of the diet history, calorie intake, appetite, medical history, and physical examination findings inform diagnostic and therapeutic plans, including diet options. Detailed questions regarding any treats, supplements, herbs, fish oil, and other products administered are warranted. Current and historical body weights, body condition scores, and muscle condition scores should not be overlooked.

Whole-blood and plasma taurine concentrations should be measured in all cats and dogs with DCM. Both dogs and cats can conserve taurine by reducing renal excretion when whole-body concentrations are low [16,18,27,49]. Therefore, for complete assessment of taurine status, both plasma and whole-blood as well as urine taurine (normalized to creatinine) measurements are necessary. Unfortunately, all 3 samples are uncommonly submitted concurrently for clinical cases. The use of serum taurine concentrations has not been assessed fully but is of questionable clinical value because of the variations in clotting times and methods of serum separation [50]. In the authors' experience, the variability in serum taurine concentrations is greater than the variability in plasma taurine concentrations.

Due to the high taurine content of granulocytes and platelets, clotting and hemolysis can result in substantially, but falsely, increased plasma or serum taurine concentrations; whole-blood taurine concentration is not confounded by these sampling and handling effects [50]. Although blood taurine concentration is only a fraction of the total body concentration, both whole-blood and plasma taurine concentrations do change in proportion with tissue concentrations [51,52]. As such, when plasma taurine concentrations are low, a diagnosis of taurine deficiency can be made; however, with normal or high values, as have been reported in some dogs with DCM, confirmation of taurine status is desirable. Whole-blood taurine concentrations may be used to substantiate a diagnosis of taurine deficiency when plasma concentrations are equivocal. In addition, whole-blood taurine concentrations are only slightly altered after meal consumption, whereas plasma taurine concentration may change substantially depending on species and taurine status [51,53]. When status is adequate, there is not a big influence on time of meals relative to sampling; however, in depleted animals the meal impact may be significant [53] and is expected to be variable depending on the composition of the presampling meal relative to the longer-term diet.

Current reference ranges from the authors' laboratory in cats were established based on blood collection 3 hours to 5 hours after a typical meal [54], because fasting can lower plasma concentrations artificially [53]. In healthy dogs, although fasting does not appear to have an impact on taurine concentrations [55,56], reference ranges from the authors' laboratory also were established based on blood collection 3 hours to 5 hours post meal [27,48]. During taurine depletion in cats, skeletal muscle taurine content is approximated more closely by whole-blood versus taurine concentrations [51]. In both cats and dogs, it appears plasma taurine concentrations decline prior to that of whole blood [27,51]. During taurine repletion in cats, whole-blood concentrations increase faster than plasma [51]. Detailed repletion data currently are not available in dogs, which confounds a reliable answer to the question regarding how quickly taurine assessments will return to normal when supplementing deficient animals. Time to repletion likely is impacted by diet composition, calorie intake, degree of deficiency, and other dietary and animal factors. Reference ranges for plasma amino acids, whole-blood taurine, and urine taurine concentrations vary among laboratories because these are dependent on the specific procedures, equipment, and methodology utilized. Clinicians should contact the specific laboratory directly regarding interpretation of results if necessary.

Plasma concentrations of methionine and cysteine also may be expected to have utility in assessment of sulfur amino acid status. It is well established that accurate measurement of plasma cysteine concentrations requires prompt sample treatment (ideally immediately after plasma separation but definitely within 1 hour of collection) to remove plasma proteins and minimize the typically rapid cysteine loss [57]. One study reported a significant correlation between taurine and both cysteine and methionine plasma concentrations in 131 healthy dogs fed a range of commercial diets [48]. This study also established significant differences between certain plasma amino acids concentrations and specific ingredient combinations (for example, dogs eating diets with lamb meal and rice had lower plasma taurine concentrations); however, interpretation of these associations is challenging without detailed dietary characterizations, including fiber type and content. Another study also found that plasma taurine concentration was weakly but significantly correlated with that of cysteine and methionine in 216 Newfoundlands [18]. In contrast, another study that investigated the effect of intentional taurine depletion over 22 weeks found that plasma methionine, cysteine, and taurine concentrations did not change despite significantly reduced urinary taurine excretion, suggesting that taurine conservation was occurring due to reduced synthetic rate [27]. Presumably with a longer duration of consumption of a taurine depleting diet, poor taurine status would have become evident. All these findings likely reflect the precursor-end metabolite relationship of these sulfur amino acids, but given the tight hepatic metabolic control of synthesis and the resulting weak correlations in plasma concentrations, this underscores that full assessment should not rely on plasma methionine and cysteine concentrations alone.

CORRECTIVE ACTIONS IN PET FOOD FORMULATION

Specific recommendations for product modifications in order to prevent diet-associated DCM in the dog are difficult without a complete understanding of the underlying mechanisms. Faced with recent ongoing concerns of a link to canine DCM, many pet food manufacturers have initiated taurine supplementation in grain-free dog diets. The authors do not support the practice of adding taurine to a commercial diet suspected of being associated with canine DCM. Simply adding taurine may mask the ability to assess for poor sulfur amino acid bioavailability or possibly a sulfur amino acid deficiency [18,58]. Although it is not unreasonable to add taurine to some diets where protein is intentionally restricted (such as in a veterinary therapeutic diet), attention to overall amino acid balance and other nutritional characteristics arguably is more important. It is suggested that correction of poor taurine status in dogs is accomplished most appropriately by increasing the concentration of bioavailable methionine and cysteine [18,58]. Increasing overall protein concentration using sources with low bioavailability of methionine and cysteine also is not effective and may be counterproductive, especially in the case of reduced digestibility and consequently increased fermentable material in the GI tract. Instead, use of high-quality, more digestible protein sources and/or supplementation with purified methionine is recommended, together with consideration for overall amino acid balance and adequate provision of methyl donors necessary for metabolism of sulfur amino acids [37,58].

Formulation of balanced pet foods using a range of ingredients, such as potatoes and legumes, to provide protein and starch in pet foods has been done successfully for years. With judicious use based on published data with regard to amino acid content and availability as well as other physiologic effects established in vivo, these remain appropriate options [59–61]. Any number of available ingredient combinations utilized for pet food formulation do not necessarily pose inherent risks to pet health and longevity; however, much more research is needed to define why some dogs develop DCM while consuming some types of diets as well as the role of specific nutrients, including taurine. Nutritional adequacy of any diet for any population requires a complete understanding of intrinsic nutritional characteristics of all ingredients to ensure appropriate consideration of nutrient digestibility and bioavailability, overall amino acid balance, and micronutrient profile [37].

DISCLOSURE

Dr J.A. Larsen is an investigator in clinical trials sponsored by Royal Canin and Nestlé Purina PetCare. She develops educational materials for Brief Media, Mark Morris Institute, and *HealthyPet* magazine. She participates as a speaker or attendee in continuing education events sponsored or organized by Royal Canin, Nestlé Purina PetCare, and Hill's Pet Nutrition. Dr A.J. Fascetti is the Scientific Director of the Amino Acid Laboratory at the University of California, Davis, which provides amino acid analysis on a fee-for-service basis. She has served as an advisor to Synergy Food Ingredients and received a grant from Nutro. She participated in events and received remuneration for lectures or as an advisor on behalf of the Nestlé Purina PetCare, Mars Petcare, and the Pet Food and Mark Morris Institutes. The Veterinary Medical Teaching Hospital at the University of California, Davis, received funding from Royal Canin to support a residency position, and from Nestlé Purina PetCare to partially support a nutrition technician. A resident trainee of the Nutrition Service received funds through the Hill's Pet Nutrition Resident Clinical Study Grants program, matched by the UCD Center for Companion Animal Health; both authors collaborated on the resulting research project conducted by that trainee.

REFERENCES

[1] Huxtable RJ. Physiological actions of taurine. Physiol Rev 1992;72(1):101–18.

[2] Faggiano A, Melis D, Alfieri R, et al. Sulfur amino acids in Cushing's disease: insight in homocysteine and taurine levels in patients with active and cured disease. J Clin Endocrinol Metab 2005;90:6616–22.

[3] Stipanuk MH. Role of the liver in regulation of body cysteine and taurine levels: A brief review. Neurochem Res 2004;29(1):105–10.

[4] Hayes KC, Carey RE, Schmidt SY. Retinal degeneration associated with taurine deficiency in the cat. Science 1975;188(4191):949–51.

[5] Laidlaw SA, Grosvenor M, Kopple JD. The taurine content of common foodstuffs. JPEN J Parenter Enteral Nutr 1990;14(4):183–8.

[6] Spitze AR, Wong DL, Rogers QR, et al. Taurine concentrations in animal feed ingredients; cooking influences taurine content. J Anim Physiol Anim Nutr (Berl) 2003;87:251–62.

[7] Kim SW, Rogers QR, Morris JG. Maillard reaction products in purified diets induce taurine depletion in cats which is reversed by antibiotics. J Nutr 1996;126(1):195–201.

[8] Stratton-Phelps M, Backus RC, Rogers QR, et al. Dietary rice bran decreases plasma and whole-blood taurine in cats. J Nutr 2002;132(6 Suppl):1745S–7S.

[9] Morris JG, Rogers QR, Kim SW, et al. Dietary taurine requirement of cats is determined by microbial degradation of taurine in the gut. Adv Exp Med Biol 1994;359:59–70.

[10] Hickman MA, Rogers QR, Morris JG. Taurine balance is different in cats fed purified and commercial diets. J Nutr 1992;122(3):553–9.

[11] Association of American Feed Control Officials. Model bill and regulations. Oxford (England): Association of American Feed Control Officials; 2019. p. 107–232.

[12] National Research Council. Nutrient requirements of dogs and cats. Washington, DC: The National Academy Press; 2006.

[13] Sturman JA, Gargano AD, Messing JM, et al. Feline maternal taurine deficiency: Effect on mother and offspring. J Nutr 1986;116:655–67.

[14] Pion PD, Kittleson MD, Rogers QR, et al. Myocardial failure in cats is associated with low plasma taurine: a reversible cardiomyopathy. Science 1987;237:764–8.

[15] Pion P, Kittleson MD, Thomas WP, et al. Dilated cardiomyopathy in the cat: Response to taurine supplementation. J Am Vet Med Assoc 1992;201:275–84.

[16] Backus RC, Cohen G, Pion PD, et al. Taurine deficiency in Newfoundlands fed commercially available complete and balanced diets. J Am Vet Med Assoc 2003;223: 1130–6.

[17] Fascetti AJ, Reed JR, Rogers QR, et al. Taurine deficiency in dogs with dilated cardiomyopathy: 12 cases (1997-2001). J Am Vet Med Assoc 2003;223:1137–41.

[18] Backus RC, Ko KS, Fascetti AJ, et al. Low plasma taurine concentration in Newfoundland dogs is associated with low plasma methionine and cyst(e)ine concentrations and low taurine synthesis. J Nutr 2006;136:2525–33.

[19] Huxtable RJ. From heart to hypothesis: A mechanism for the calcium modulatory actions of taurine. Adv Exp Med Biol 1987;217:371–87.

[20] Schaffer SW, Seyed-Mozaffari M, Kramer J, et al. Effect of taurine depletion and treatment on cardiac contractility and metabolism. Prog Clin Biol Res 1985;179: 167–75.

[21] Fox PR, Sturman JA. Myocardial taurine concentrations in cats with cardiac disease and in healthy cats fed taurine-modified diets. Am J Vet Res 1992;53:237–41.

[22] Pion PD, Kittleson MD, Skiles ML, et al. Dilated cardiomyopathy associated with taurine deficiency in the domestic cat: Relationship to diet and myocardial taurine content. Adv Exp Med Biol 1992;315:63–73.

[23] Sanderson SL, Gross KL, Ogburn PN, et al. Effects of dietary fat and L-carnitine on plasma and whole blood taurine concentrations and cardiac function in healthy dogs fed protein-restricted diets. J Am Vet Med Assoc 2001;62:1616–23.

[24] Kittleson MD, Keene B, Pion PD, et al. Results of the multicenter spaniel trial (MUST): Taurine- and carnitine-responsive dilated cardiomyopathy in American Cocker Spaniels with decreased plasma taurine concentration. J Vet Intern Med 1997;11:204–11.

[25] Alroy J, Rush JE, Sarkar S. Infantile dilated cardiomyopathy in Portuguse water dogs: Correlation of the autosomal recessive trait with low plasma taurine at infancy. Amino Acids 2005;28:51–6.

[26] Freeman LM, Rush JE, Brown DJ, et al. Relationship between circulating and dietary taurine concentrations in dogs with dilated cardiomyopathy. Vet Ther 2001;2(4):370–8.

[27] Torres CL, Backus RC, Fascetti AJ, et al. Taurine status in normal dogs fed a commercial diet associated with taurine deficiency and dilated cardiomyopathy. J Anim Physiol Anim Nutr (Berl) 2003;87(9–10):359–72.

[28] Johnson ML, Parsons CM, Fahey GC, et al. Effects of species raw material source, ash content, and processing temperature on amino acid digestibility of animal by-product meals by cecectomized roosters and ileally cannulated dogs. J Anim Sci 1998;76:1112–22.

[29] Ko KS, Backus RC, Berg JR, et al. Differences in taurine synthesis rate among dogs relate to differences in their maintenance energy requirements. J Nutr 2007;137:1171–5.

[30] FDA Investigating Potential Connection Between Diet and Cases of Canine Heart Disease. Available at: https://www.fda.gov/animal-veterinary/cvm-updates/fda-investigating-potential-connection-between-diet-and-cases-canine-heart-disease. Accessed Aug 19, 2020.

[31] FDA Provides Update on Investigation into Potential Connection Between Certain Diets and Cases of Canine Heart Disease. Available at: https://www.fda.gov/animal-veterinary/cvm-updates/fda-provides-update-investigation-potential-connection-between-certain-diets-and-cases-canine-heart. Accessed Aug 19, 2020.

[32] FDA Provides Third Status Report on Investigation into Potential Connection Between Certain Diets and Cases of Canine Heart Disease. Available at: https://www.fda.gov/animal-veterinary/cvm-updates/fda-provides-third-status-report-investigation-potential-connection-between-certain-diets-and-cases. Accessed Aug 19, 2020.

[33] FDA Investigation into Potential Link between Certain Diets and Canine Dilated Cardiomyopathy. Available at: https://www.fda.gov/animal-veterinary/outbreaks-and-advisories/fda-investigation-potential-link-between-certain-diets-and-canine-dilated-cardiomyopathy.Accessed Aug 29, 2020.

[34] Kaplan JL, Stern JA, Fascetti AJ, et al. Taurine deficiency and dilated cardiomyopathy in Golden Retrievers fed commercial diets. PLoS One 2018;13(12):e0209112.

[35] Ontiveros ES, Whelchel BD, Yu J, et al. Development of plasma and whole blood taurine reference ranges and identification of dietary features associated with taurine deficiency and dilated cardiomyopathy in golden retrievers: A prospective, observational study. PLoS One 2020;15(5):e0233206.

[36] Adin D, DeFrancesco TC, Keene B, et al. Echocardiographic phenotype of canine dilated cardiomyopathy differs based on diet type. J Vet Cardiol 2019;21:1–9.

[37] Mansilla WD, Marinangeli CPF, Ekenstedt KJ, et al. Special topic: The association between pulse ingredients and canine dilated cardiomyopathy: Addressing the knowledge gaps before establishing causation. J Anim Sci 2019;97(3):983–97.

[38] Hendriks WH, Bakker EJ, Bosch G. Protein and amino acid bioavailability estimates for canine foods. J Anim Sci 2015;93:4788–95.

[39] Kim SW, Rogers QR, Morris JG. Dietary antibiotics decrease taurine loss in cats fed a canned heat-processed diet. J Nutr 1996;126:509–15.

[40] Read DH, Jolly RD, Alley MR. Polioencephalomalacia of dogs with thiamin deficiency. Vet Pathol 1977;14(2):103–12.

[41] Street HR, Cowgill GR, Zimmerman HM. Some observations of vitamin B_6 deficiency in the dog. J Nutr 1941; 21(3):275–90.

[42] Keene BW, Panciera DP, Atkins CE, et al. Myocardial L-carnitine deficiency in a family of dogs with dilated cardiomyopathy. J Am Vet Med Assoc 1991;198:647–50.

[43] Sanderson SL. Taurine and carnitine in canine cardiomyopathy. Vet Clin Small Anim 2006;36:1325–43.

[44] Bhatnagar SK, Welty JD, Razzak A, et al. Significance of blood taurine levels in patients with first time acute ischemic cardiac pain. Int J Cardiol 1990;27:361e6.

[45] Lombardini J, Cooper M. Elevated blood taurine levels in acute and evolving myocardial infarction. J Lab Clin Med 1981;849:e59.

[46] Kramer GA, Kittleson MD, Fox PR, et al. Plasma taurine concentrations in normal dogs and in dogs with heart disease. J Vet Intern Med 1995;9:253–8.

[47] Pion PD, Kittleson MD, Rogers QR, et al. Taurine deficiency myocardial failure in the domestic cat. Prog Clin Biol Res 1990;351:423–30.

[48] Delaney SJ, Kass PH, Rogers QR, et al. Plasma and whole blood taurine in normal dogs varying size fed commercially prepared food. J Anim Physiol Anim Nutr (Berl) 2003;87:236–44.

[49] Glass EN, Odle J, Baker DH. Urinary taurine excretion as a function of taurine intake in adult cats. J Nutr 1992; 122(4):1135–42.

[50] Zicker SC, Rogers QR. Use of plasma amino acid concentrations in the diagnosis of nutritional and metabolic diseases in veterinary medicine. Proc IV Congress of the International Society for Animal Clinical Biochemistry July 19-24, 1990 at the University of California-Davis, Davis CA:1-15.

[51] Pacioretty L, Hickman MA, Morris JG, et al. Kinetics of taurine depletion and repletion in plasma, serum, whole blood, and skeletal muscle in cats. Amino Acids 2001;21: 417–27.

[52] Torres CL. The effects of dietary ingredients, bacterial degradation in the gut and amount of food consumed on taurine status of dogs of different body sizes [dissertation]. Davis (CA): University of California; 2003.

[53] Pion PD, Lewis J, Greene K, et al. Effect of meal-feeding and food deprivation on plasma and whole blood taurine concentrations in cats. J Nutr 1991;121: S177–8.

[54] Heinze CR, Larsen JA, Kass PH, et al. Plasma amino acid and whole blood taurine concentrations in cats eating commercially prepared diets. Am J Vet Res 2009; 70(11):1374–82.

[55] Gray K, Alexander LG, Staunton R, et al. The effect of 48-hour fasting on taurine status in healthy dogs. J Anim Physiol Anim Nutr (Berl) 2016;100(3):532–6.

[56] Delaney SJ, Hill AS, Backus RC, et al. Dietary crude protein concentration does not affect the leucine requirement of growing dogs. J Anim Physiol Anim Nutr (Berl) 2001;85:88–100.

[57] Torres CL, Miller JW, Rogers QR. Determination of free and total cysteine in plasma of dogs and cats. Vet Clin Pathol 2004;33:228–33.

[58] Backus RC. Could dietary taurine supplementation in dogs be masking a problem? Montreal (Canada): Amer Coll Vet Intern Med Forum (proc); 2009.

[59] Donadelli RA, Aldrich CG, Jones CK, et al. The amino acid composition and protein quality of various egg, poultry meal by-products, and vegetable proteins used in the production of dog and cat diets. Poult Sci 2019;98(3):1371–8.

[60] Pezzali JG, Acuff HL, Henry W, et al. Effects of different carbohydrate sources on taurine status in healthy Beagle dogs. J Anim Sci 2020;98(2). https://doi.org/10.1093/jas/skaa010.

[61] Reilly LM, von Schaumburg PC, Hoke JM, et al. Macronutrient composition, true metabolizable energy and amino acid digestibility, and indispensable amino acid scoring of pulse ingredients for use in canine and feline diets. J Anim Sci 2020. https://doi.org/10.1093/jas/skaa149.

Advances in Small Animal Care 1 (2020) 239–264
ADVANCES IN SMALL ANIMAL CARE

Combining Nutrition and Physical Rehabilitation to Improve Health Outcomes for Dogs and Cats

Sarah K. Abood, DVM, PhD[a,*], Allison M. Wara, DVM, DACVN[b,c]

[a]Ontario Veterinary College, University of Guelph, 50 Stone Road East, Guelph, Ontario N1G 2W1, Canada; [b]Royal Canin Canada, 100 Bieber Road, Morriston, Ontario, N0B 2C0, Canada; [c]College of Veterinary Medicine at the University of Missouri, 1520 East, Rollins St, Columbia, MO 65211, USA

KEYWORDS

• Nutrition • Dietary management • Physical rehabilitation • Osteoarthritis • Weight loss
• Nutritional assessment • Body condition • Omega-3 fatty acids

KEY POINTS

- Nutrition and physical rehabilitation are important modalities for optimal health and recovery from illness.
- Interventions can be applied to a wide range of clinical conditions seen in small animal general practice.
- Three common case examples outline nutrition assessment tools that veterinary health care teams can use to evaluate a patient's nutritional status and physical status, as well as rehabilitation options for treatment.
- In select cases, supplements may be considered but require a thorough evaluation and understanding of their limitations.
- Referral is not always necessary but should be offered for cases that go beyond the scope of a general practitioner's capabilities.

INTRODUCTION

Poor nutrition and physical activity can directly contribute to pathologic conditions and can significantly decrease quality and quantity of life for companion animals. Malnutrition, which includes obesity, is currently one of the most common clinical conditions seen in veterinary medicine and is associated with negative outcomes caused by alterations in immunity and organ function [1,2]. Specifically, there is a correlation between obesity and various orthopedic, neurologic, and endocrine diseases [3] that can, in turn, exacerbate obesity and negatively affect recovery times (Box 1).

Helping companion animal patients achieve an ideal body condition can directly improve health outcomes and recovery from illness, enhance functional mobility, and reduce the risk of injury. Improvements in quality-of-life measures, such as mobility, can be seen with as little as 6% loss of body weight (BW) [4]. Restricting calories alone can have a profound impact on the management and prevention of chronic, obesity-related disorders, including osteoarthritis. Previous data from a 14-year study showed that dogs with an ideal body condition score (BCS) showed later onset of chronic diseases and greater longevity compared with overweight counterparts [5].

Nutrition and physical rehabilitation are two modalities that are sometimes overlooked in general veterinary practice, despite evidence that shows their utility in improving patient care. Fundamental components of nutritional assessments and rehabilitation treatments, which can be accomplished in day-to-day practice, are presented with guidelines on when to refer to a specialist.

*Corresponding author, *E-mail address:* sabood@uoguelph.ca

https://doi.org/10.1016/j.yasa.2020.07.016
2666-4518/20/

BOX 1
Frequently Encountered Disorders for Which Obesity Is Considered a Risk Factor

- Lameness/osteoarthritis
- Hip dysplasia (dog)
- Cruciate ligament disease (dog)
- Diabetes mellitus
- Hepatic lipidosis (cat)
- Pancreatitis (dog)
- Urinary tract disease
- Oral cavity disease
- Increased risk of neoplasia

This list is not exhaustive. Obesity is associated with several clinical conditions in dogs and cats.

TOOLS AND PROCEDURES FOR GENERAL PRACTITIONERS

In the small animal private practice setting, there are several tools that serve as a minimum database for the assessment of a patient's nutritional and neuromusculoskeletal status. Findings from the diet history and physical assessment can enable the clinician to identify whether risk factors are present and can facilitate the establishment of an appropriate diagnosis. Collecting this information typically does not require specialized equipment and is generally accomplished in conjunction with a routine physical examination.

BODY CONDITION SCORING

Every patient's BW should be recorded at each veterinary visit using a calibrated scale. Because of the large variation of breed sizes in dogs and cats, the use of height-weight tables, similar to those used for humans, is not practical. In contrast, body condition scoring is a standardized, universally accepted technique that has been validated for use in dogs and cats and should be documented during every physical examination. The technique involves both visual assessment and physical palpation of subcutaneous fat deposits over the rib cage, lumbar area, ventral abdomen, and tail base. A score is then assigned according to specific criteria (Figs. 1 and 2). Although several different systems have been developed, the 9-point system is often preferred for consistency in reporting [6]. A BCS of 4 to 5 out of 9 is considered optimal for dogs and a BCS of 5 out of 9 is optimal for cats. The BCS tool is also of value for pet owners, who may have a misperception of their pet's body condition and a tendency to underestimate when obesity is present [7]. Each pet owner can be easily trained on how to use the BCS tool to monitor their pet at home; videos to show how to assign BCS are available online (Box 2).

MUSCLE CONDITION SCORING

Further to evaluating a patient's BCS via assessment of fat mass, evaluation of a patient's muscle condition should also be performed. Muscle condition score (MCS) charts are available for cats (Fig. 3) and dogs (Fig. 4) and should be used at each physical examination. Animals are scored as having normal muscle condition or mild, moderate, or severe muscle loss based on palpation and visualization of the musculature along the spine, scapulae, temporal bones, and wings of the ilia. Evaluating muscle condition is important because changes can indicate injury (eg, cruciate ligament tear) or disease (eg, hyperadrenocorticism) and are independent of body condition scoring. For example, an animal can be obese and have significant muscular atrophy, which can affect the assessment of BCS if not evaluated independently.

NUTRITION ASSESSMENT

In 2011, the World Small Animal Veterinary Association (WSAVA) Global Nutrition Committee (GNC) launched the Nutritional Assessment Guidelines to help veterinary care teams and pet owners ensure pets are receiving an optimal nutrition plan [8]. The GNC's Nutrition Assessment Checklist (Fig. 5) is a means of objectively evaluating a pet's current plane of nutrition and should be part of every veterinary examination. The assessment incorporates the practice of both body condition scoring and muscle condition scoring as described earlier into 1 cohesive tool. Team members can be actively involved in completing this quick screening checklist, which includes, but is not limited to, collection of a diet history, BCS, MCS, physical activity, and historical findings in the home environment. The extended evaluation (see Fig. 5) can then be conducted if, and when, risk factors are identified. The Nutrition Assessment Checklist provides a consistent framework for evaluating a patient's nutritional status and allows the health care team to compare changes from one visit to the next, and also to make specific recommendations for every patient at each visit.

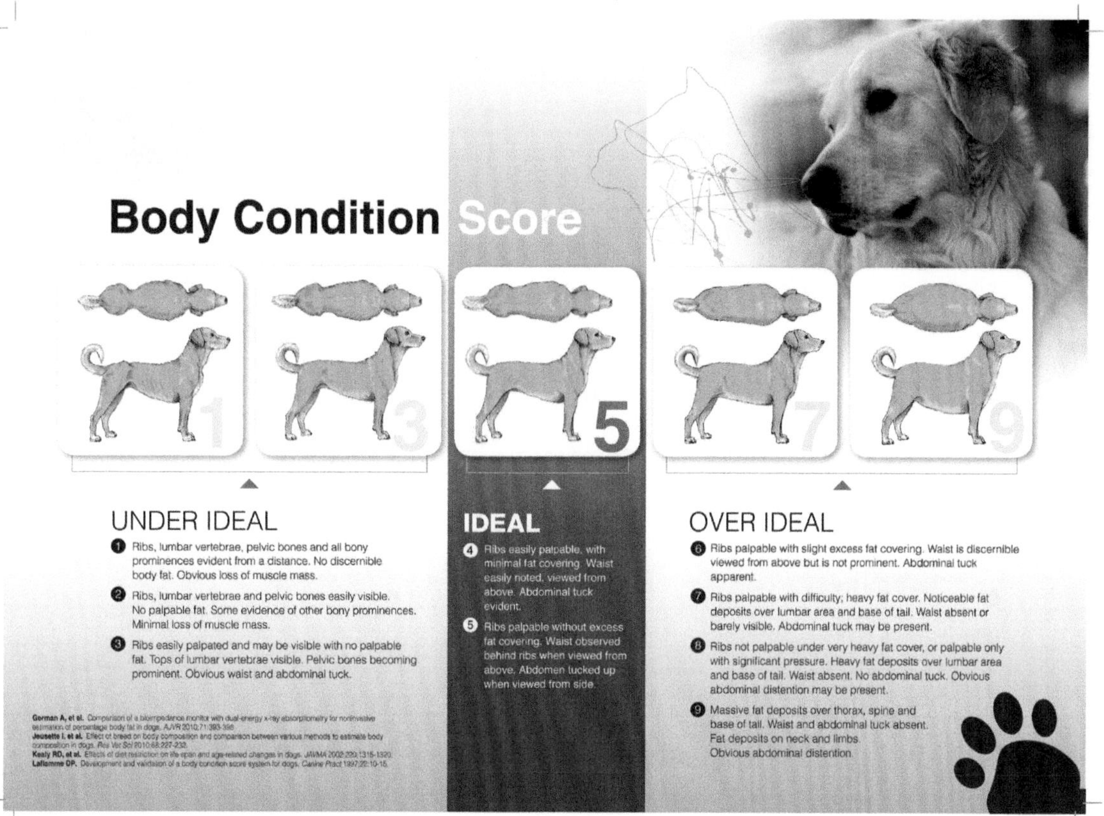

FIG. 1 Canine BCS chart. (Global Nutrition Committee Toolkit material provided courtesy of the World Small Animal Veterinary Association.)

ORTHOPEDIC AND NEUROLOGIC EXAMINATIONS

Based on results of a general physical examination, further assessment of a patient's orthopedic and neurologic status may be warranted. Because lesions associated with either system can manifest with similar clinical signs, a systematic approach is necessary for localization. For example, if a patient is showing evidence of a bilateral hindlimb lameness, the lesion could be neurologic, musculoskeletal, or both.

To evaluate a patient's neurologic function, the clinician must assess the following: mental status, posture, postural reactions, gait, spinal nerve reflexes, and cranial nerve status. The neurologic examination [9,10] is a standard assessment for general practitioners and should be performed on any animal to rule in/out, and localize, those clinical signs suspected to be neurologic. Identification of the anatomic location of the lesion enables the clinician to establish a differential diagnosis.

A methodical approach to the orthopedic examination is also necessary for any patient with abnormal musculoskeletal function. A vital component of this procedure is the ability to detect abnormalities on palpation of the appendicular and axial skeleton, as well as observation of the patient sitting, standing, walking, and running.

Consistency is imperative when evaluating joints; the examiner must assess for pain, range of motion, crepitus, effusion, and instability. The procedure of the orthopedic examination has been widely described and can be referred to for specifics [11,12].

Although other diagnostics may be necessary based on the clinical considerations of the individual, these basic tools can be practically applied to any patient for further evaluation of nutritional and physical status.

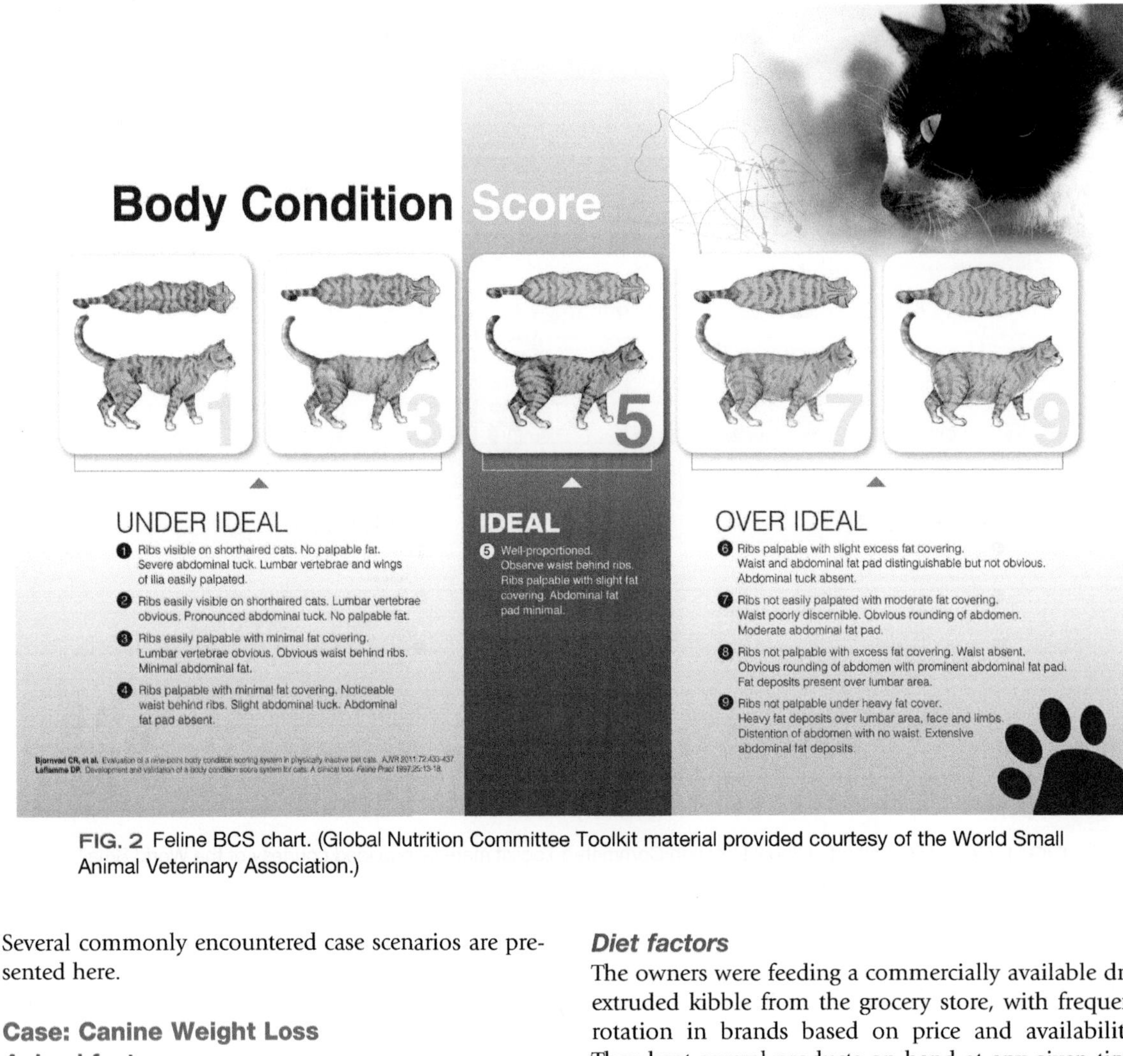

Body Condition Score
1
3
5
7
9
UNDER IDEAL
1 Ribs visible on shorthaired cats. No palpable fat. Severe abdominal tuck. Lumbar vertebrae and wings of ilia easily palpated.
2 Ribs easily visible on shorthaired cats. Lumbar vertebrae obvious. Pronounced abdominal tuck. No palpable fat.
3 Ribs easily palpable with minimal fat covering. Lumbar vertebrae obvious. Obvious waist behind ribs. Minimal abdominal fat.
4 Ribs palpable with minimal fat covering. Noticeable waist behind ribs. Slight abdominal tuck. Abdominal fat pad absent.
IDEAL
5 Well-proportioned. Observe waist behind ribs. Ribs palpable with slight fat covering. Abdominal fat pad minimal.
OVER IDEAL
6 Ribs palpable with slight excess fat covering. Waist and abdominal fat pad distinguishable but not obvious. Abdominal tuck absent.
7 Ribs not easily palpated with moderate fat covering. Waist poorly discernible. Obvious rounding of abdomen. Moderate abdominal fat pad.
8 Ribs not palpable with excess fat covering. Waist absent. Obvious rounding of abdomen with prominent abdominal fat pad. Fat deposits present over lumbar area.
9 Ribs not palpable under heavy fat cover. Heavy fat deposits over lumbar area, face and limbs. Distention of abdomen with no waist. Extensive abdominal fat deposits.
Bjornvad CR, et al. Evaluation of a nine-point body condition scoring system in physically inactive pet cats. AJVR 2011;72:433-437
Laflamme DP. Development and validation of a body condition score system for cats: A clinical tool. Feline Pract 1997;25:13-18.

FIG. 2 Feline BCS chart. (Global Nutrition Committee Toolkit material provided courtesy of the World Small Animal Veterinary Association.)

Several commonly encountered case scenarios are presented here.

Case: Canine Weight Loss

Animal factors

A 3.5-year-old, male neutered Bernese mountain dog presented to the general practitioner for an annual health examination. At 1.5 years of age, the dog was noted to be in ideal body condition with a BCS of 5 out of 9. Since then, his BW had gradually increased each year. On physical examination, the patient was found to be 56.2 kg with a BCS of 8 out of 9 and a normal MCS. No obvious mobility or lameness issues were noted while walking, jogging, or on palpation. The owners reported no concerns in status at home and seemed to be oblivious to changes in BW. As part of a routine health examination, a complete blood cell count, biochemistry panel including T4, and urinalysis were run; results were within normal limits and considered unremarkable.

Diet factors

The owners were feeding a commercially available dry, extruded kibble from the grocery store, with frequent rotation in brands based on price and availability. They kept several products on hand at any given time and were feeding a variety of different formulations and flavors. They offered 2 cups of kibble twice daily regardless of the product or calorie content of the diet. The dog also received many treats and human foods as leftovers from dinner each night.

Feeding management and environmental factors

The dog was the only pet in the household and spent considerable time alone. Both owners had full-time jobs and were away for more than 9 hours at a time. The dog received 2 walks of 10 to 15 minutes each per day but was capable of more. Opportunities for extended exercise were limited to weekends as a result of the owners' demanding work schedules.

BOX 2
Web-Based Resources for Veterinary Health Care Teams to Access Nutrition-Related Tools and Information About Nutraceuticals and Supplements

Organization	Purpose	Web Site URL
Consumerlab.com	Subscription service to evaluate dietary supplements tested for purity, potency, bioavailability	www.consumerlab.com
Canadian Veterinary Medical Association:	BCS video	https://www.youtube.com/watch?v=3qllsZY5hRs
National Animal Supplement Council	Trade organization for pet food and supplement manufacturers demonstrating quality control	https://nasc.cc/
NIH National Center for Complementary and Alternative Medicine	Supports research of alternative therapies, including supplements and nutraceuticals	http://nccam.nih.gov
NIH Office of Dietary Supplements	Evaluates scientific information, disseminates research results, and educates the public	http://dietary-supplements.info.nih.gov
Pet Nutrition Alliance Calculator	Provides nutrition tools and resources for veterinary health care teams to optimize pet health care	https://www.petnutritionalliance.org/
The SkeptVet	Blog established to analyze published research for medical options for dogs and cats using evidence-based medicine	http://skeptvet.com/Blog/
United States Pharmacopeia	Nonprofit that works to ensure quality and safety of medicines and foods	https://www.usp.org/

Nutrition assessment

Key question: how best to evaluate this patient's inconsistent feeding plan?

The first step in managing a patient with obesity is to perform a nutrition assessment. As discussed earlier, the Nutrition Assessment Checklist (see Fig. 5) is a readily available tool that facilitates the process of identifying and documenting risk factors. Important components of the nutrition assessment include measurement of the patient's BW, BCS, and MCS. Another integral component of the nutrition assessment is a complete diet history (Fig. 6). Collecting a diet history is essential for all patients but is especially necessary when obesity and other risk factors are present. This tool ensures that details are not overlooked regarding brands, formulations, treats, snacks, supplements, and amounts. Clients can be sent an electronic history form ahead of a scheduled appointment to complete at home; this approach improves the accuracy of recall for foods and treats being fed. Alternatively, the form can be sent home with pet owners if the information provided at the time of the appointment is insufficient. Recent research suggests that the types of questions posed to pet owners about diet can affect the quality of information collected. Coe and colleagues [13] showed that questions phrased as, "Tell me about..." elicited more information than questions framed as, "What kind of food are you feeding?" As a result, open-ended questions should be emphasized during the examination room visit, to complement the written questionnaire. This technique also allows clinicians to gain more information on the types and quantities of treats fed, because the information provided by the owners was vague and difficult to assess. Ideally, information collected during this stage will enable the health care team to quantify daily caloric intake from all food sources, determine the appropriateness of the feeding plan, and assist in determining initial feeding amounts for weight loss. In cases such

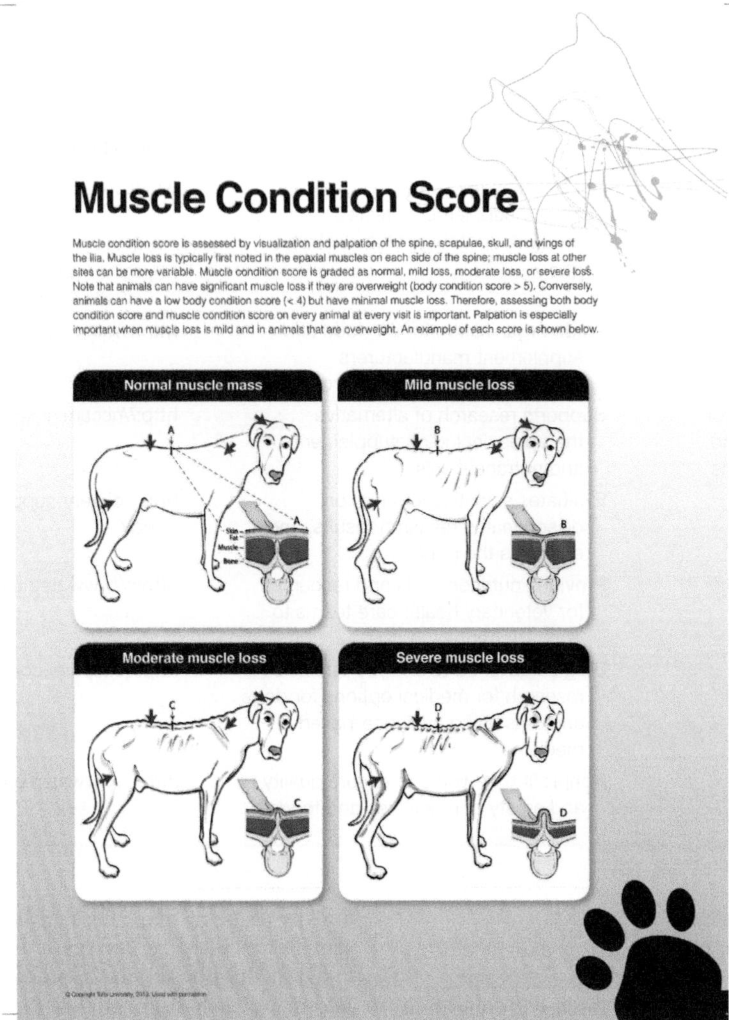

Muscle Condition Score
Muscle condition score is assessed by visualization and palpation of the spine, scapulae, skull, and wings of the ilia. Muscle loss is typically first noted in the epaxial muscles on each side of the spine; muscle loss at other sites can be more variable. Muscle condition score is graded as normal, mild loss, moderate loss, or severe loss. Note that animals can have significant muscle loss if they are overweight (body condition score > 5). Conversely, animals can have a low body condition score (< 4) but have minimal muscle loss. Therefore, assessing both body condition score and muscle condition score on every animal at every visit is important. Palpation is especially important when muscle loss is mild and in animals that are overweight. An example of each score is shown below.
Normal muscle mass
Mild muscle loss
Moderate muscle loss
Severe muscle loss

FIG. 3 Canine MCS chart. (Provided courtesy of the World Small Animal Veterinary Association (WSAVA). Available at the WSAVA Global Nutrition Committee Nutritional Toolkit website: https://wsava.org/global-guidelines/global-nutrition-guidelines/. Accessed February 27, 2020. Copyright Tufts University, 2014.)

as this, inconsistency in feeding can affect the clinician's assessment and can compromise the ability to calculate daily intake. Although this scenario is less ideal, it is frequently encountered in private practice, and therefore clinicians must have the ability to navigate it. Calculating energy requirements for weight loss is discussed later.

Ideal body weight

The next step is to identify the dog's ideal BW (IBW). IBW can be determined in various ways. The preferred method is to use historical medical records to identify the patient's BW that corresponds to a normal BCS of 4 to 5 out of 9. In this case, the dog's BCS was documented as normal at 1.5 years of age when he reached skeletal maturity. Thus, the recorded BW at that hospital visit represents his IBW. This technique is individualized to the patient and is therefore considered the most accurate. When historical records are not available, IBW can be estimated by calculation. Although various calculations exist, a simple method is to use the patient's percentage of excess BW according to

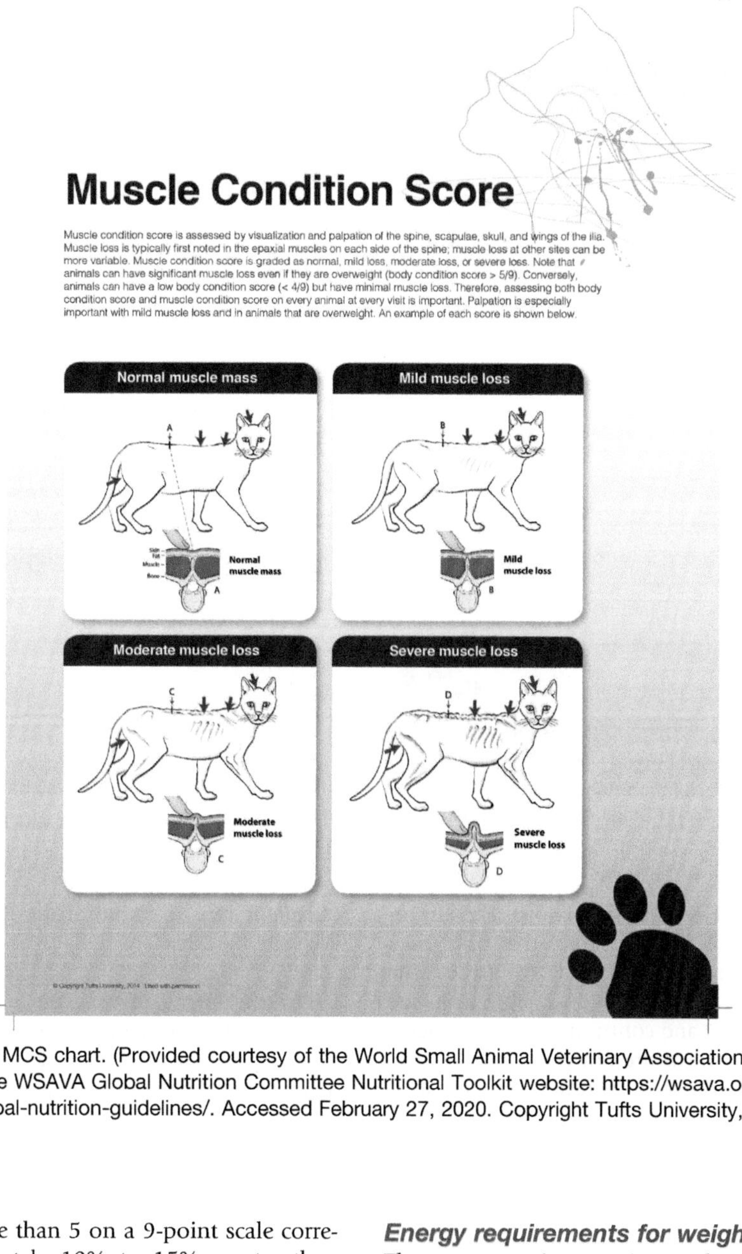
Muscle Condition Score
Muscle condition score is assessed by visualization and palpation of the spine, scapulae, skull, and wings of the ilia. Muscle loss is typically first noted in the epaxial muscles on each side of the spine; muscle loss at other sites can be more variable. Muscle condition score is graded as normal, mild loss, moderate loss, or severe loss. Note that animals can have significant muscle loss even if they are overweight (body condition score > 5/9). Conversely, animals can have a low body condition score (< 4/9) but have minimal muscle loss. Therefore, assessing both body condition score and muscle condition score on every animal at every visit is important. Palpation is especially important with mild muscle loss and in animals that are overweight. An example of each score is shown below.
Normal muscle mass
Normal muscle mass
Mild muscle loss
Mild muscle loss
Moderate muscle loss
Moderate muscle loss
Severe muscle loss
Severe muscle loss

FIG. 4 Feline MCS chart. (Provided courtesy of the World Small Animal Veterinary Association (WSAVA). Available at the WSAVA Global Nutrition Committee Nutritional Toolkit website: https://wsava.org/global-guidelines/global-nutrition-guidelines/. Accessed February 27, 2020. Copyright Tufts University, 2014.)

BCS. Each score more than 5 on a 9-point scale corresponds to approximately 10% to 15% greater than ideal (Box 3). For this canine patient, a BCS of 8 out of 9 is approximately 30% to 45% more than IBW. Regardless of the methodology used, it is important to remember that IBW is not a precise value but a general target that is subject to modification throughout the course of a structured weight loss program.

Energy requirements for weight loss

The next step is to estimate the dog's daily energy requirement for weight loss. When a complete and accurate diet history can be obtained, a simple and useful starting point is to decrease the patient's caloric intake to 80% of the previous intake. For example, if the diet history revealed the patient was consuming ~2000 kcal/d, the starting point for caloric restriction would be 1600 kcal/d, including all treats, snacks, and

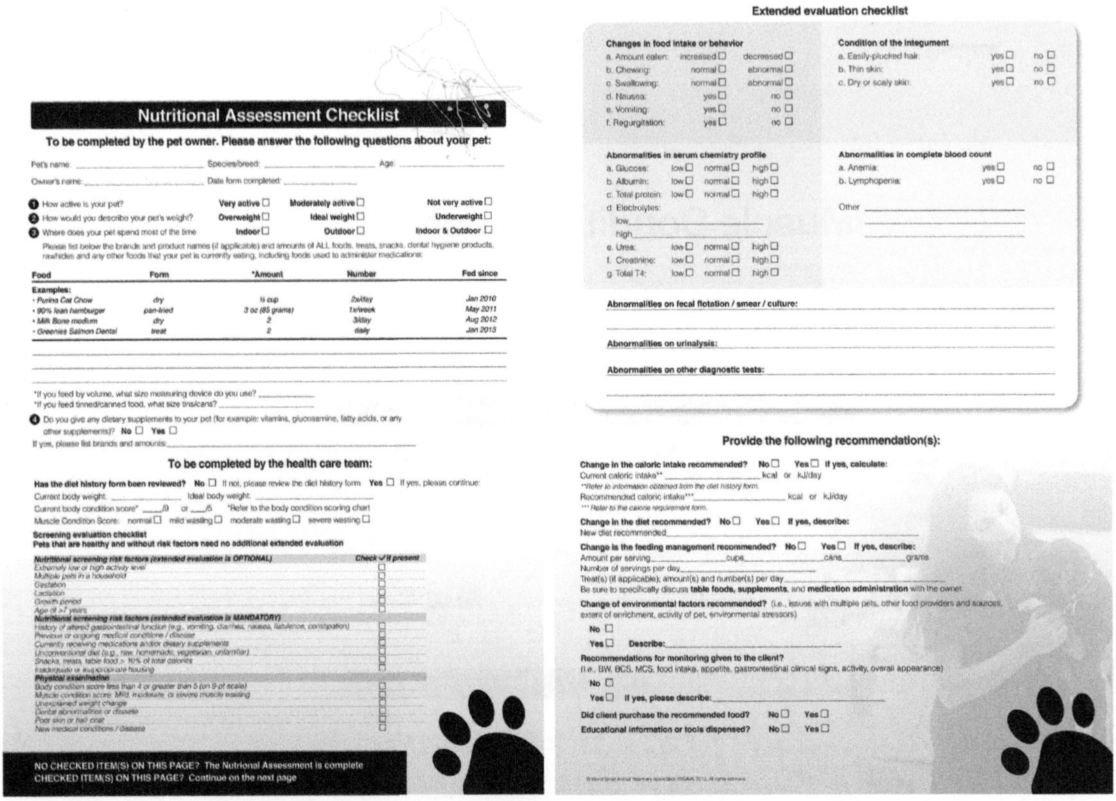

Nutritional Assessment Checklist

To be completed by the pet owner. Please answer the following questions about your pet:

Pet's name: ______ Species/breed: ______ Age: ______

Owner's name: ______ Date form completed: ______

1. How active is your pet? **Very active** ☐ **Moderately active** ☐ **Not very active** ☐
2. How would you describe your pet's weight? **Overweight** ☐ **Ideal weight** ☐ **Underweight** ☐
3. Where does your pet spend most of the time **Indoor** ☐ **Outdoor** ☐ **Indoor & Outdoor** ☐

Please list below the brands and product names (if applicable) and amounts of ALL foods, treats, snacks, dental hygiene products, rawhides and any other foods that your pet is currently eating, including foods used to administer medications:

Food	Form	*Amount	Number	Fed since
Examples:				
· *Purina Cat Chow*	*dry*	*½ cup*	*2x/day*	*Jan 2010*
· *90% lean hamburger*	*pan-fried*	*3 oz (85 grams)*	*1x/week*	*May 2011*
· *Milk Bone medium*	*dry*	*2*	*3/day*	*Aug 2012*
· *Greenies Salmon Dental*	*treat*	*2*	*daily*	*Jan 2013*

*If you feed by volume, what size measuring device do you use? ______

*If you feed tinned/canned food, what size tins/cans? ______

4. Do you give any dietary supplements to your pet (for example: vitamins, glucosamine, fatty acids, or any other supplements)? **No** ☐ **Yes** ☐

If yes, please list brands and amounts: ______

To be completed by the health care team:

Has the diet history form been reviewed? **No** ☐ If not, please review the diet history form **Yes** ☐ If yes, please continue:

Current body weight: ______ Ideal body weight: ______

Current body condition score* ___/9 or ___/5 *Refer to the body condition scoring chart

Muscle Condition Score: normal ☐ mild wasting ☐ moderate wasting ☐ severe wasting ☐

Screening evaluation checklist
Pets that are healthy and without risk factors need no additional extended evaluation

Nutritional screening risk factors (extended evaluation is OPTIONAL)	***Check ✓ if present***
Extremely low or high activity level	☐
Multiple pets in a household	☐
Gestation	☐
Lactation	☐
Growth period	☐
Age of >7 years	☐
Nutritional screening risk factors (extended evaluation is MANDATORY)	
History of altered gastrointestinal function (e.g., vomiting, diarrhea, nausea, flatulence, constipation)	☐
Previous or ongoing medical conditions / disease	☐
Currently receiving medications and/or dietary supplements	☐
Unconventional diet (e.g., raw, homemade, vegetarian, unfamiliar)	☐
Snacks, treats, table food > 10% of total calories	☐
Inadequate or inappropriate housing	☐
Physical examination	
Body condition score less than 4 or greater than 5 (on 9-pt scale)	☐
Muscle condition score: Mild, moderate, or severe muscle wasting	☐
Unexplained weight change	☐
Dental abnormalities or disease	☐
Poor skin or hair coat	☐
New medical conditions / disease	☐

NO CHECKED ITEM(S) ON THIS PAGE? The Nutrional Assessment is complete
CHECKED ITEM(S) ON THIS PAGE? Continue on the next page

Extended evaluation checklist

Changes in food intake or behavior
a. Amount eaten: increased ☐ decreased ☐
b. Chewing: normal ☐ abnormal ☐
c. Swallowing: normal ☐ abnormal ☐
d. Nausea: yes ☐ no ☐
e. Vomiting: yes ☐ no ☐
f. Regurgitation: yes ☐ no ☐

Condition of the integument
a. Easily-plucked hair: yes ☐ no ☐
b. Thin skin: yes ☐ no ☐
c. Dry or scaly skin: yes ☐ no ☐

Abnormalities in serum chemistry profile
a. Glucose: low ☐ normal ☐ high ☐
b. Albumin: low ☐ normal ☐ high ☐
c. Total protein: low ☐ normal ☐ high ☐
d. Electrolytes:
low ______
high ______
e. Urea: low ☐ normal ☐ high ☐
f. Creatinine: low ☐ normal ☐ high ☐
g. Total T4: low ☐ normal ☐ high ☐

Abnormalities in complete blood count
a. Anemia: yes ☐ no ☐
b. Lymphopenia: yes ☐ no ☐

Other ______

Abnormalities on fecal flotation / smear / culture: ______

Abnormalities on urinalysis: ______

Abnormalities on other diagnostic tests: ______

Provide the following recommendation(s):

Change in the caloric intake recommended? **No** ☐ **Yes** ☐ **If yes, calculate:**
Current caloric intake** ______ kcal or kJ/day
***Refer to information obtained from the diet history form.*
Recommended caloric intake*** ______ kcal or kJ/day
**** Refer to the calorie requirement form.*

Change in the diet recommended? **No** ☐ **Yes** ☐ **If yes, describe:**
New diet recommended ______

Change is the feeding management recommended? **No** ☐ **Yes** ☐ **If yes, describe:**
Amount per serving ______ cups ______ cans ______ grams
Number of servings per day ______
Treat(s) (if applicable); amount(s) and number(s) per day ______
Be sure to specifically discuss **table foods, supplements**, and **medication administration** with the owner.

Change of environmental factors recommended? (i.e., issues with multiple pets, other food providers and sources, extent of enrichment, activity of pet, environmental stressors)
No ☐
Yes ☐ **Describe:** ______

Recommendations for monitoring given to the client?
(i.e., BW, BCS, MCS, food intake, appetite, gastrointestinal clinical signs, activity, overall appearance)
No ☐
Yes ☐ **If yes, please describe:** ______

Did client purchase the recommended food? **No** ☐ **Yes** ☐

Educational information or tools dispensed? **No** ☐ **Yes** ☐

FIG. 5 WSAVA Nutrition Assessment Checklist. (Global Nutrition Committee Toolkit material provided courtesy of the World Small Animal Veterinary Association.)

supplements. Most (at least 90% or 1440 kcal) of the total intake should be derived from the base diet, reserving less than 10% (<160 kcal) for treats. The reason for this is 2-fold: (1) many palatable treats are high in calories and fat and contribute to excess energy intake, and (2) most treats are not considered a complete and balanced source of nutrition, so an excess could unbalance the patient's nutrient intake and may risk deficiencies.

When an accurate diet history cannot be determined and the energy intake cannot be calculated as shown in this case example, calorie requirements for weight loss can be estimated by calculation. Various calculations have been reported and used successfully for weight loss. It is noteworthy that any degree of caloric restriction should be considered an initial starting point that is subject to individual variation and response. Many online calculators for weight loss are available and are especially convenient in the constraints of a busy private practice. One example of an easy-to-use online calculator can be found at the Pet Nutrition Alliance Web site (see Box 2).

Diet selection and dosage

An appropriate weight loss diet and a corresponding food dosage must then be selected. Over-the-counter maintenance diets are not recommended for weight loss, because, when they are cut back to the degree required to achieve caloric restriction, essential nutrients are also restricted; this puts an animal at risk of multinutrient deficiencies [14]. In contrast, veterinary therapeutic weight loss diets are enhanced in essential nutrients, including protein and amino acids, vitamins, and minerals, which enables caloric restriction without risking deficits. In combination with a reduction in calories, some therapeutic weight loss diets are also enhanced in fiber, which has been shown to promote satiety and decrease begging (or food-seeking) behaviors [15–17]. When portioning meals, use of an electronic gram scale should be considered standard of

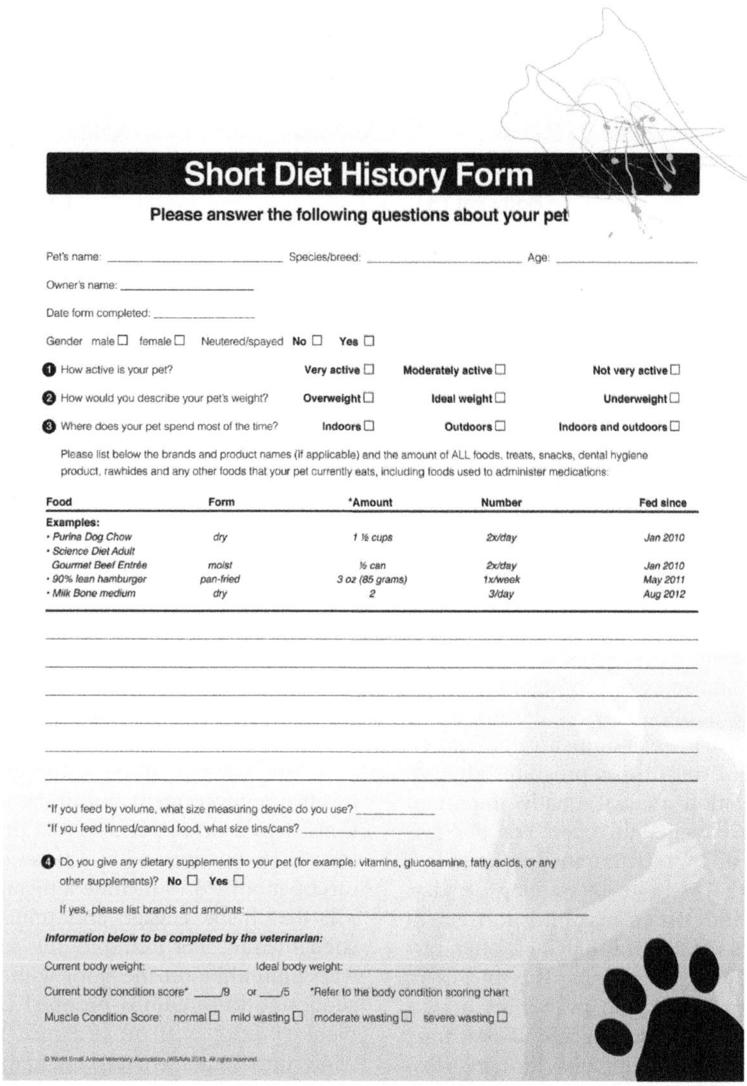

Short Diet History Form

Please answer the following questions about your pet

Pet's name: ____________ Species/breed: ____________ Age: ____________

Owner's name: ____________

Date form completed: ____________

Gender male ☐ female ☐ Neutered/spayed **No** ☐ **Yes** ☐

1. How active is your pet? **Very active** ☐ **Moderately active** ☐ **Not very active** ☐
2. How would you describe your pet's weight? **Overweight** ☐ **Ideal weight** ☐ **Underweight** ☐
3. Where does your pet spend most of the time? **Indoors** ☐ **Outdoors** ☐ **Indoors and outdoors** ☐

Please list below the brands and product names (if applicable) and the amount of ALL foods, treats, snacks, dental hygiene product, rawhides and any other foods that your pet currently eats, including foods used to administer medications:

Food	Form	*Amount	Number	Fed since
Examples:				
• *Purina Dog Chow*	*dry*	*1 ½ cups*	*2x/day*	*Jan 2010*
• *Science Diet Adult Gourmet Beef Entrée*	*moist*	*½ can*	*2x/day*	*Jan 2010*
• *90% lean hamburger*	*pan-fried*	*3 oz (85 grams)*	*1x/week*	*May 2011*
• *Milk Bone medium*	*dry*	*2*	*3/day*	*Aug 2012*

*If you feed by volume, what size measuring device do you use? ____________

*If you feed tinned/canned food, what size tins/cans? ____________

4. Do you give any dietary supplements to your pet (for example: vitamins, glucosamine, fatty acids, or any other supplements)? **No** ☐ **Yes** ☐

If yes, please list brands and amounts: ____________

Information below to be completed by the veterinarian:

Current body weight: ____________ Ideal body weight: ____________

Current body condition score* ____/9 or ____/5 *Refer to the body condition scoring chart

Muscle Condition Score: normal ☐ mild wasting ☐ moderate wasting ☐ severe wasting ☐

FIG. 6 WSAVA Short Diet History Form. (Global Nutrition Committee Toolkit material provided courtesy of the World Small Animal Veterinary Association.)

care. Measuring pet food with a gram scale is significantly more accurate compared with a volumetric measuring cup [18]. Research shows that using a standard measuring cup can result in overestimation of portion sizes by up to 80% [19].

Monitoring and follow-up

Once the diet has been selected and feeding amounts prescribed according to the degree of caloric restriction necessary, monitoring and follow-up are required to ensure a successful outcome. Every 2 weeks, the veterinary care team should schedule a recheck to verify BW, BCS, and client adherence to the feeding regimen. Rechecks also serve as an opportunity to troubleshoot questions or concerns from pet owners. The goal is to achieve a rate of loss of 1% to 2% of BW per week in dogs, and 0.5% to 1% of BW per week in cats [20]. If the degree of weight loss is higher or lower than the desired range, a member of the health care team can review with the client the steps they are taking for measuring food, managing treats, and increasing activity each day. In addition, the clinician can increase or

BOX 3
A Simple Method to Estimate Ideal Body Weight Using the Patient's Percentage of Excess Weight Based on Body Condition Score, with Each Score more than 5 on a 9-Point Scale Corresponding to 10% to 15% more than Ideal Body Weight

BCS	Body Fat (%)	Excess Weight (%>IBW)
5/9	20	Normal BW
6/9	25	10–15
7/9	30	20–30
8/9	35	30–45
9/9	40	40–60

decrease the pet's caloric intake by 5% to 10%, respectively. Because each patient is an individual with unique metabolic differences, it is expected that daily energy requirements will change and require periodic modification throughout the course of the program.

Physical rehabilitation

Key question: what might an exercise program look like for a dog with significant obesity?

Although nutritional interventions are the cornerstone of any successful weight loss program, physical activity and rehabilitation are an equally important means of enhancing patient outcomes. For the case described earlier, the dog was determined to be sedentary with only 20 to 30 minutes of walking per day; therefore, opportunities exist to maximize movement to burn calories. Increased physical activity is often prescribed for overweight dogs and cats as a means of increasing energy expenditure and promoting a state of negative energy balance. Other beneficial outcomes include preservation of lean body mass during fat loss [21] and cognitive benefits from increased social and environmental stimulation. In a study that evaluated obese dogs receiving underwater treadmill therapy, the overall rate of weight loss (1.5% of BW/wk) was faster than previously reported rates in dogs (0.8% of BW/wk) without this intervention [22].

Low-intensity, longer-duration activity is the preferred approach for obese patients on a weight loss program. Compared with strength training exercises performed at aerobic capacity, this strategy helps to minimize the risk of musculoskeletal injury and contributes to the preservation of lean body mass during caloric restriction. Initially, strenuous activities may not be tolerated. The goal with any rehabilitation program is to increase tolerance as the patient progresses. Examples of activities that meet these criteria include sit-to-stand exercises, balance work, targeted core strengthening exercises, controlled walking exercises, and hydrotherapy.

Sit-to-stand exercises and balance work

In sit-to-stand exercises (Fig. 7), the gluteal, hamstring, quadriceps, and gastrocnemius muscle groups are strengthened, without eliciting significant hip extension, which can sometimes be difficult for obese dogs [23]. This exercise can be accomplished at home using positive reinforcement beginning with 5 to 10 repetitions, 1 to 2 times per day, and progressively working toward 15 repetitions 3 to 4 times per day. Movements can be modified to include a therapy ball or a physio-roll that helps engage abdominal muscles for core strengthening. For example, the patient stands or sits with hindlimbs on the floor with or without manual support, and forelimbs propped up by the ball. This plank position can be sustained for several seconds while the animal actively maintains balance (Fig. 8). If an additional challenge is needed, the ball can be slightly rolled or shifted while the position is engaged. Balance work can be further achieved using a balance board or, simply, a board placed over a pipe or broom handle. With all 4 paws on the board, the surface can be rocked back and forth while the patient maintains balance (Fig. 9).

Controlled leash walking

Leash walking is another activity that can be safely executed in the confines of the home environment. It is important that the activity is controlled to avoid injury that may otherwise occur in an off-leash setting with the potential for explosive movements. Depending on the patient's cardiorespiratory capacity, short

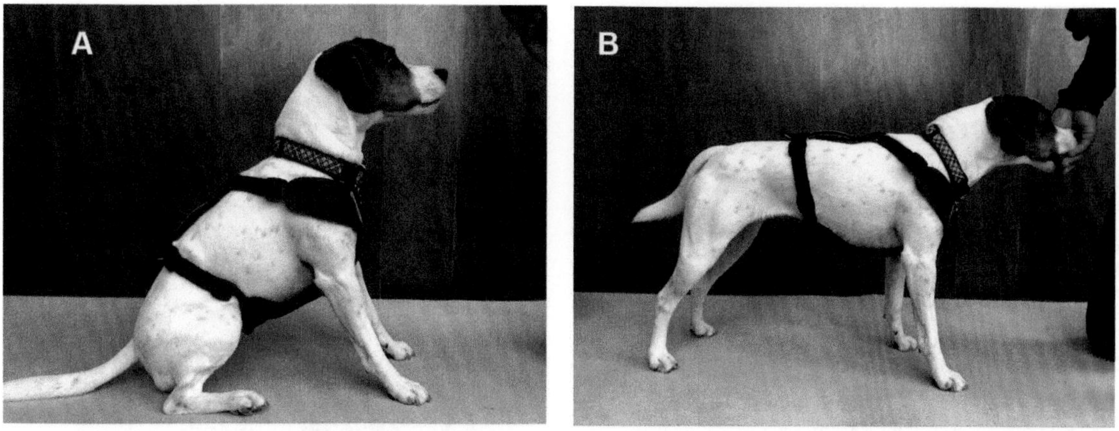

FIG. 7 (**A, B**) Sit-to-stand exercises. The technique of sitting (**A**) then standing (**B**) requires engagement and strengthening of the quadriceps and hamstrings when repetitions are performed. (*Courtesy of* Dr. Stéphanie Keroack.)

walks in greater frequency can be gradually increased in duration as the pet progresses. The program may begin with 2 or 3 10-minute sessions per day, gradually increasing in length as the individual tolerates. To increase the challenge, inclines and declines can be introduced to help strengthen the hindlimb and forelimb musculature, respectively (Fig. 10). The handler can also modify the substrate by walking through grass, snow, or sand to increase resistance and range of motion. A general rule of thumb is to increase the activity time by 10% to 15% each week, if tolerable [24].

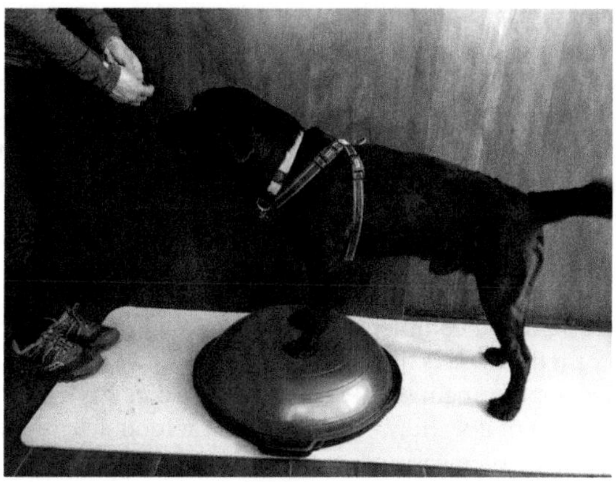

FIG. 8 A balance ball may be used to create a plank position with either forelimbs or hindlimbs propped up by the ball while the patient maintains balance. (*Courtesy of* Dr. Stéphanie Keroack.)

Underwater treadmill therapy

Aquatic therapy using an underwater treadmill is an excellent modality for obese canine patients and should be offered as an adjunctive therapy (Fig. 11). The natural buoyancy of water reduces weight bearing and therefore concussive forces on joints, allowing exercise with a reduced risk of injury. When the water in the tank is filled to the level of the patient's greater trochanter, the patient bears 38% of BW (62% lighter). When the water is filled to the level of the patient's stifle, the patient bears 85% of BW (15% lighter [25]). The increased resistance required to move through water helps strengthen muscles and results in increased caloric expenditure. Typically, 2 to 3 times per week is recommended at intervals of 5 to 20 minutes per session.

When to seek referral

Designing and implementing a weight loss program should be considered a core competency for general practice veterinarians. However, there are times when referral to a specialty service is indicated; examples include (1) when obesity is present alongside other comorbidities (eg, chronic kidney disease), (2) when the patient has unusually low calorie requirements, (3) when the owner has unique demands (eg, homemade diet), and (4) when specialty equipment and expertise are required (eg, an underwater treadmill) (Table 1).

Case: Feline Osteoarthritis

Animal factors

A 12.5-year-old spayed female domestic shorthair cat presented to the family veterinarian for defecating

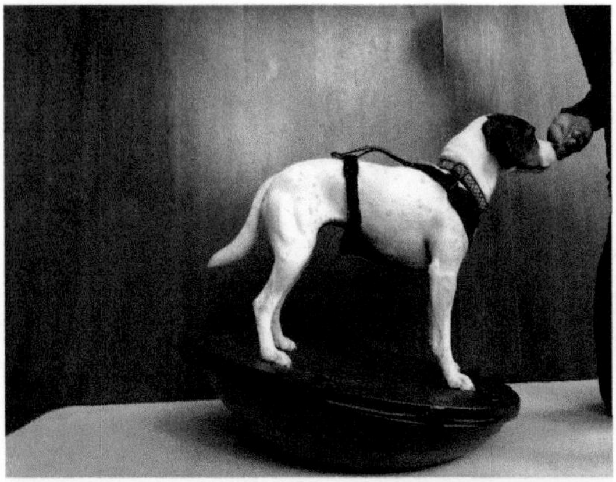

FIG. 9 Using a balance board with all 4 paws on the surface, the board can be rocked back and forth for balance and proprioception. (*Courtesy of* Dr. Stéphanie Keroack.)

outside of the litter box. The owners reported a decrease in her daily activity during the past month but no changes in appetite, water consumption, grooming behavior, or urination in the litter box. The nutritional assessment (Box 4) began with the physical examination, where the cat was noted to have slight muscle wasting in both hindlimbs and a modest amount of pain was elicited in the lumbosacral spine [26]. All other parameters on physical examination were noted to be within normal limits. The cat's BW was 4.54 kg (10 lb) and a BCS of 6 out of 9 was assigned. The clients' concerns focused primarily on the cat's use of her litter box; they did not want to continue picking up feces on

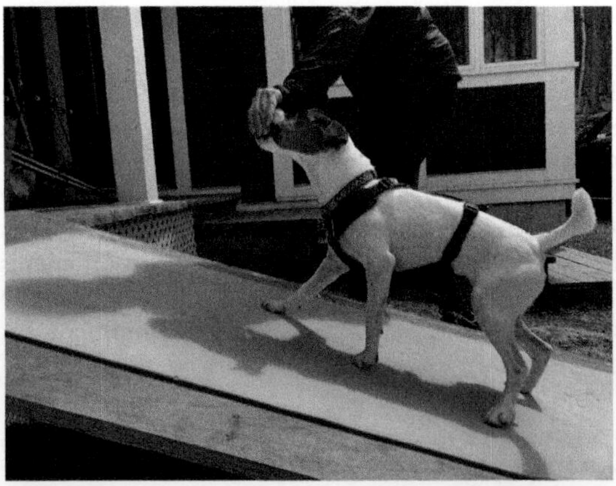

FIG. 10 To increase the challenge of controlled leash walks, an incline is created, which enhances hindlimb strength. (*Courtesy of* Dr. Stéphanie Keroack.)

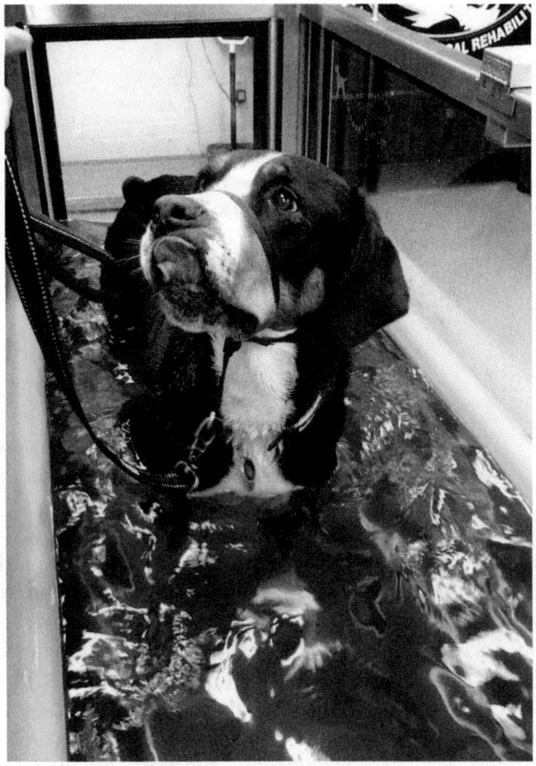

FIG. 11 An underwater treadmill can be a valuable treatment modality to support recovery from disease or to increase athletic performance. (*Courtesy of* Dr. Allison Wara.)

the floor or rug near the litter box. Based on these observations, diagnostics were recommended and the owners agreed. Digital imaging in the form of routine radiographs was performed; osteoarthritic changes to the lumbosacral spine, hips, and right elbow were documented. Using the cat's history, physical examination findings, and radiographs, a diagnosis of uncomplicated osteoarthritis was made. The clients asked about supplementation for the cat's joints; would she benefit from a nutraceutical or a different diet?

Dietary factors

A current and complete diet history was obtained using a form the owners filled out at home before their scheduled appointment (see Fig. 6). The cat's diet was a combination of dry and wet commercial cat food, where dry food was premeasured once in the morning and wet food was offered as 1 level tablespoon each morning and evening. No commercial cat treats or human foods were fed. From the pet food label or Web site, calorie content of each product was identified (Table 2). Using

TABLE 1
Required Qualifications for Nutrition and/or Rehabilitation Services

Specialty or Expertise	Credentials
Nutrition	• PhD in animal nutrition • Board certification by the American College of Veterinary Nutrition • Board certification by the European College of Veterinary Comparative Nutrition
Physical rehabilitation	• Board certification by the American College of Veterinary Sports Medicine and Rehabilitation • Certified canine rehabilitation therapist • Certified canine rehabilitation practitioner

When referring a small animal patient for specialty nutrition and/or physical rehabilitation services, verification of qualifications is essential because of the large number of self-proclaimed experts in these fields. Examples of appropriate credentials for veterinarians that specialize in small animal nutrition and physical rehabilitation are listed. Note: specialty programs also exist for veterinary technicians (not included in the table).

additional information from the label or Web site, an estimate of protein and fat content on an energy basis (eg, grams per 100 kcal) was performed using a previously described technique [27] and a table was created to compare and understand macronutrient intakes (see Table 2).

Environmental factors

The cat was the only pet in the home, with free rein of 2 levels and multiple rooms. There were 2 litter boxes (1 on each floor) and 1 water and food bowl in the kitchen. For enrichment, the cat had a 1.37 m (4.5-foot) climbing tree or cat condo with 3 resting pads or perches; the climbing tree was positioned near a window so the cat could look out into the yard. The cat also had a padded resting bed on each floor in the home and an assortment of toys. During the history taking, it was reported that the owners noticed the cat was not going upstairs or even jumping on the couch as often as before; with further inquiry it was noted that these changes had been observed over the previous 4 weeks.

Assessment

Based on the cat's diagnosis of osteoarthritis, evaluating the use of omega-3 long-chain polyunsaturated fatty acids (eicosapentaenoic acid [EPA] and docosahexaenoic acid [DHA]) was warranted. Sourced primarily from fish oils (eg, salmon, herring, menhaden, or cod liver), EPA and DHA have been used in the nutritional management of various conditions in dogs and cats: cardiovascular, renal, idiopathic hyperlipidemia, inflammatory bowel disease, and osteoarthritis [28]. Table 3 shows several commercial veterinary therapeutic diets positioned to provide joint support for cats with supplemental omega-3 fatty acids; the table is divided into dry kibble and canned products arranged in order from highest to lowest protein content.

Although EPA and DHA supplementation has not been extensively researched in cats with osteoarthritis, 2 randomized controlled, prospective studies have been reported [29,30]. In 1 study, investigators evaluated the impacts of a test diet that contained 1.88 g of EPA and DHA/1000 kcal (supplemented with green-lipped mussel extract and glucosamine-chondroitin sulfate) compared with a control diet containing 0.03 g of EPA and DHA/1000 kcal in cats with radiographic evidence of osteoarthritis [29]. In the second study, investigators assessed the effects of omega-3 fatty

BOX 4
Elements of the Nutritional Assessment Include Diet History and Physical Examination

The nutritional assessment begins during the intake history and physical examination. In order to determine which organ systems are involved, neurologic and musculoskeletal examinations are indicated; reviews on how to perform examinations in older cats are well documented [12]. Collecting information about the type and amount of food fed, treats offered, supplements, and medications is vital to getting a complete diet history. Asking pet owners to complete a diet history form before their appointment saves time and allows the health care team to focus on more specific questions (see Fig. 6). Discussing the patient's pain level with the owner is also valuable; validated pain scales are available [26] and an in-depth review of assessing and managing chronic pain in cats was recently published [29].

TABLE 2
Comparison and Analysis of Feline Feeding Plan

Complete and Balanced Commercial Cat Foods	Energy (kcal/cup or can)	Protein (g/100 kcal)[a]	Fat (g/100 kcal)[a]	Amount to Feed to Meet DER[b]
Dry kibble	333/cup	11.1	5.0	200/333 = 0.6 cup
Wet canned	111/90-mL can	8.8	6.1	20/111 = 0.18 can
—	—	—	—	(220 kcal total)

Abbreviation: DER, daily energy requirement.

Resting energy requirement (RER) = $70(BW_{kg}^{0.75})$ = x kcal/d = $70(4.5^{0.75})$ = 218 kcal/d.

National Research Council (NRC) recommended allowance for protein intake for adult cats: 200 g protein/kg diet at 4.0 kcal metabolizable energy (ME/g).

Rule of thumb for minimum protein intake: 4.4 g/kg BW/d = 19.8 g protein per day for a cat weighing 4.5 kg (9.9 lb).

Assessment: at the current intake of dry and wet food, the cat was getting an appropriate amount of protein each day.

[a] Calculated values based on steps previously outlined [27].

[b] DER = RER × 1.0 to 1.2 = y kcal/d = 218 × 1.0 to 1.2 = 218 to 262 kcal/d.

acid supplementation (1.84 g/1000 kcal of EPA and DHA) compared with corn oil supplementation (0.00 g of EPA and DHA/1000 kcal) in cats with documented osteoarthritis [30]. In both instances, researchers reported improved outcomes and increased mobility in the intervention group compared with the control. Based on these reports, a concentration of 1.8 g of total dietary EPA and DHA/1000 kcal was set as a target for this feline patient.

Key question: using a veterinary therapeutic diet containing supplemental omega-3 fatty acids, what would the cat's intake of EPA and DHA be if consuming sufficient amounts to meet energy needs? What would the intake of glucosamine-chondroitin be?

Diet 2 (see Table 3): this product contains 360 kcal (96 g) per 237-mL (8-oz) cup, as well as 0.18 g of EPA and DHA per 100 kcal (1.8 g EPA and DHA per 1000 kcal), which meets the target as mentioned earlier. If the cat ate 0.6 cups (58 g) to reach 220 kcal/d, this would yield approximately 396 mg of EPA and DHA in the daily food allotment. This diet also contains 25.4 g/100 kcal glucosamine and chondroitin, which yields approximately 56 mg in 220 kcal of food. Although there is no single best diet for all cats with osteoarthritis, factors such as BCS and MCS allow clinicians to individualize a recommendation that is ideal for each pet. In addition to the concentration of EPA and DHA, clinicians should also evaluate energy density and protein content to optimize nutrient intake.

Alternatively, the owner could consider omega-3 fatty acid supplementation in the form of liquid drops or capsules to add to a maintenance diet. Regulations for safety and consistent concentrations of ingredients are lacking in many pet and human supplements, and for this reason pet owners should be guided with a specific recommendation by the veterinary health care team. For example, many products contain additional vitamin A and/or vitamin D, which could inadvertently result in a pet receiving an excessive intake of fat-soluble vitamins. Moreover, each gram of dietary fat contains approximately 9 kcal, which could result in unwanted weight gain if not carefully administered. This possibility is particularly a concern for patients with osteoarthritis, because obesity can exacerbate clinical signs of the disease, and therefore this option may not be ideal for this individual patient. Understanding which nutraceuticals are available and how those products compare with veterinary therapeutic diets containing EPA and DHA is necessary to make informed, evidence-based, and economical recommendations that clients will adhere to for their pets.

Select commercial EPA and DHA supplements are listed in Table 4; several glucosamine-chondroitin supplements are listed in Table 5. Glucosamine-containing products are widely available, can be purchased over-the-counter, and dose ranges have been published [31]; however, studies have failed to show a beneficial effect for the treatment of osteoarthritis in cats or dogs. Ultimately, general practitioners need to stay informed of therapeutic dietary and supplement options and consider available evidence, as well as patient and client needs, when making recommendations; periodic evaluation of patients on long-term supplementation is a key component of any management plan.

Recommendations

Treatment recommendations for this patient focused on (1) monitoring and minimizing pain, (2) improving

TABLE 3
Comparison of Macronutrient, Omega-3 Fatty Acid, and Glucosamine Content of Some Commercial Products Positioned as Senior or Veterinary Therapeutic Diets for Cats

Manufacturer and Formulation	Energy (kcal/237-mL Cup, 163 or 89-mL can)	Protein (g/100 kcal)	Fat (g/100 kcal)	Total Omega-3 Fatty Acids (g/100 kcal)[b]	EPA + DHA (g/100 kcal)[c]	Glucosamine and Chondroitin (mg/100 kcal)[c]
Dry products[a]						
Diet1[e]: Royal Canin Feline Senior Consult	299/cup	7.3	3.7	0.35	0.20	26.3
Diet 2[f]: Royal Canin Feline Mobility Support	360/cup	7.2	3.9	0.33	0.18	25.4
Diet 3[g]: Hill's Prescription Diet k/d + Mobility Feline[d]	484/cup	6.9	5.2	0.35	Not reported	41.1
Canned products[a]						
Diet 4[h]: Royal Canin Feline Mature Consult	134/163-mL can	12	3.0	0.14	0.10	12.5
Diet 5[i]: Royal Canin Feline Senior Consult	150/163-mL can	8.9	4.2	0.23	0.18	24.1
Diet 6[j]: Hill's Prescription Diet k/d + Mobility Feline[d]	68/89-mL can	6.9	5.7	0.38	Not reported	27

[a] Nutrient values obtained from company Web sites; accurate at the time of reporting.
[b] Products reported to have total omega-3 fatty acids could include any combination of alpha-linoleic acid (ALA), EPA and DHA.
[c] If data is not reported, the company can be contacted for further information.
[d] This product is formulated for cats diagnosed with renal disease. To determine if adequate protein intake will be sufficient, protein content per 100 or 1000 Calories should be determined and compared with an individual patient's daily protein requirement.
[e] Royal Canin Feline Senior Consult Dry Cat Food, Royal Canin, Canada, Puslinch, Ontario, Canada.
[f] Royal Canin Veterinary Diet feline mobility support, Royal Canin, Canada, Puslinch, Ontario, Canada.
[g] Hill's Prescription Diet k/d + Mobility Feline, Hill's Pet Nutrition, Inc, Topeka, Kansas.
[h] Royal Canin Feline Mature Consult, Royal Canin, Canada, Puslinch, Ontario, Canada.
[i] Royal Canin Feline Senior Consult, Royal Canin, Canada, Puslinch, Ontario, Canada.
[j] Hill's Prescription Diet k/d + Mobility Feline, Hill's Pet Nutrition, Inc, Topeka, Kansas.

joint mobility and muscle strengthening through physical rehabilitation (discussed later), (3) maintaining a stable BW and appropriate calorie and nutrient intake, and (4) providing an enriched environment to support access to food, water, litter boxes, and bedding. Therapeutic diet and supplement options were discussed; evidence for the use of omega-3 fatty acids (EPA and DHA) was reviewed as well as absence of evidence regarding glucosamine-chondroitin. A recommendation for a 10-package rehabilitation program (including several activities to be done at home) was also made. Improvements to the home environment to support the cat's mobility and access to litter boxes, food/water bowls, and furniture were also discussed during the visit, and a handout with resources was sent home as part of the discharge summary report.

TABLE 4
Examples of 2 Omega-3 Fatty Acid Products for Cats and Estimated Cost per Day

Omega-3 Fatty Acid Products[a]	Amount of EPA and DHA per mL of Product	mL/d to Meet 396 mg/220 kcal[b]	Cost per Container	Days Container Will Last (n)	Cost per Day to Deliver 396 mg/d
—	—	For a 4.5-kg cat = 396 mg/d)[b]	—	—	—
[c]Aventi Omega-3 Complete for Dogs and Cats	825 mg EPA+ 550 mg DHA = 1375 mg/5 mL Or 275 mg/mL	396 mg/275 mg = 1.4 mL	$16.10 per 250 mL	250 mL/1.4 mL = 178 d	$16.10/178 d = $0.09/d
[d]Nordic Naturals Omega-3 Pet	782 mg EPA+ 460 mg DHA = 1242 mg/5 mL or 248.4 mg/mL	396 mg/248 mg = 1.6 mL	$18.86 per 60 mL	60 mL/1.6 mL = 37.5 d	$18.86/37.5 d = 0.50/d

Products selected were those that contained only EPA and DHA, without additional nutrients.

[a] Nutrient values obtained from company Web sites; accurate at the time of reporting.

[b] A cat weighing 4.5 kg was estimated to need 220 kcal/d, and a daily amount of 1.8 g EPA + DHA per 1000 kcal was adapted from published studies [29,30]. Converting 1.8 g EPA + DHA per 1,000 kcal to mg per 220 kcal yields 396 mg per 220 kcal/d.

[c] Aventi Omega-3 Complete for Dogs and Cats, Aventix/Victor Medical Company of Lake Forest, CA.

[d] Nordic Naturals Omega-3 Pet, Nordic Naturals, Watsonville, CA.

Environmental changes in the home setting should be based on making food, water, shelter, and bedding and litter boxes more accessible. Discussing ideas with clients can be educational for the pet owners and insightful for the veterinary health care teams. A variety of suggestions could be offered in the discharge instructions or on the clinic Web site in the form of handouts to be downloaded or short videos. For example, cutting out (removing) a section of the litterbox, if necessary, to allow easy access by the cat is an easy and efficient procedure [32]. Adjusting furniture might include positioning 1 or more pieces in specific places so the animal can use them to reach a higher level or a quiet, secure spot with bedding. Nonslip material, such as yoga mats, on the floor can reduce the risk of slipping or putting stress on joints. Rotating a scratching post so it is in the horizontal position (instead of vertical), as well as elevating food and water bowls, can significantly enhance the environment for cats with stiff elbows, shoulders, and spines.

Physical rehabilitation

Aging changes associated with joints (eg, osteoarthritis), postorthopedic surgeries, neurologic conditions, or injuries related to trauma are all conditions for which middle-aged and older pets could benefit from physical rehabilitation. Two general types of rehabilitation modalities to consider for small animal patients with osteoarthritis are noninvasive or invasive. Cold laser therapy, massage, floor exercises, and hydrotherapy are in the noninvasive category, whereas acupuncture and joint injections of a disease-modifying osteoarthritis drug are considered invasive. Details of each of these modalities have been well described for cats in several publications during the past decade [23,33–35].

A thorough understanding of feline behavior as well as training in physical rehabilitation are necessary to achieve a successful outcome. Customized programs should be designed with individual patient needs in mind, and treatment modalities should not be avoided just because it is assumed that cats will not comply with treatment. Cultivating patience and an open-minded attitude is necessary for engagement or participation of feline patients in rehabilitation therapy. Members of the rehabilitation team need to be competent in their manual skills, free of anxiety and distractions, and be able to create a calm environment that is separated from hospital traffic and loud noises [35]. Minimal patient handling is ideal (use a hands-off approach when possible) and close monitoring of pain is important so the patient does not develop resistance to treatment. Although some pets may be food motivated, it cannot be assumed that every cat (or dog) will work for food. Clients may consider delaying feeding on the day of a

TABLE 5
Examples of 3 Glucosamine and Chondroitin Products for Cats and Estimated Cost per Day

Glucosamine and Chondroitin Products[a]	Amount of Glucosamine and Chondroitin per Tablet, Chew or Capsule[b]	Tablets, Chews, or Capsules per Daily Dose (n)	Cost per Container	Days 1 Container Will Last (n)	Cost per Day to Meet Daily Dose
Capsules					
[c]Piping Rock.com Hip & Joint Chewables for Pets	350 mg/tablet glucosamine 100 mg/tablet chondroitin sulfate	4.5 × 80 mg/kg = 360 mg = 1 tablet/d	$18.88/120 tablets	120 tablets/1 per day = 120 d	$18.88/120 d = $0.16/d
[d]Pet Naturals of Vermont, Hip + Joint Chews for Cats	200 mg/2 chew glucosamine 75 mg/2 chews chondroitin sulfate	4.5 × 80 mg/kg = 360 mg/200 mg per 2 chews per day = 1.8 or 4 chews total	$9.83/30 chews	30 chews/4 per day = 7.5 d	$9.83/7.5 d = $1.31/d
Powder					
[e]Glucosamine, Chondroitin and Vitamin C for Cats by VitaPaws (sprinkle capsules)	700 mg/cap glucosamine 445 mg/capsule chondroitin sulfate	4.5 × 80 mg/kg = 360 mg/700 mg per capsule = 0.5 capsule/d	$15.95/120 sprinkle capsules	120/0.5 = 240 d	$15.95/240 d = $0.07/d

Calculations are based on a daily dose for a 4.5-kg cat (80 mg/kg/d).

[a] Nutrient values obtained from company Web sites; accurate at the time of reporting.

[b] Veterinarians should be practicing evidence-based medicine. Although there are numerous over-the-counter glucosamine/chondroitin products currently available in the marketplace, there is no evidence to support their efficacy in the treatment of osteoarthritis for dogs or cats.

[c] Piping Rock.com Hip & Joint Chewables for Pets, Piping Rock Health Products, Ronkonkoma, NY.

[d] Pet Naturals of Vermont, Hip + Joint Chews for Cats, Pet Naturals, Williston, VT.

[e] Glucosamine, Chondroitin and Vitamin C for Cats by VitaPaws (sprinkle capsules), Simply Supplements, Peterborough, United Kingdom.

rehabilitation appointment so the pet is hungry and more likely to work for some kibble during the procedure. This approach also avoids a surplus of calories, which could contribute to unwanted weight gain. Rehabilitation teams should determine whether pet owners want to be involved in structured activities done in the home setting; their participation can help allow continuation of therapy between scheduled clinic sessions.

Analgesic use in cats with osteoarthritis

Pharmacologic interventions, including antiinflammatories (eg, meloxicam), analgesics (tramadol), and injectable chondroprotective agents (eg, Adequan) are a component of multimodal management of osteoarthritis in cats and have been reviewed [32,36]. A patient's age, medical history, current medications, individual drug tolerance, and potential for side effects should all be considered before formulating a treatment plan. Although pharmacologic therapies may be required, further discussion of their merits and use is beyond the scope of this article.

Supplements and nutraceuticals for cats and dogs

Across North America, there are various commonly recommended nutritional supplements or nutraceuticals for dogs and cats (Box 5). At present the gold standard of scientific evidence is considered to be the prospective, randomized, blinded, placebo-controlled clinical trial. Although not impossible, it can be challenging and expensive to perform this type of research to study the effects of individual nutrients (or nutritional supplements), or when trying to examine the effect of one diet versus another in a group of client-owned animals.

However, there are few studies (in terms of objective evidence) to support the use of most nutritional supplements (or nutraceuticals) in veterinary practice. One exception is omega-3 fatty acids in the form of capsules or liquid drops, or provided directly in dry or canned pet food products. Certain omega-3 fatty acid supplements provide EPA and DHA, but they may also contain omega fatty acids that are not easily converted or used by cats and dogs (eg, alpha-linoleic acid [ALA]). Specific recommendations should be made by examining product concentrations of EPA and DHA and by calculating an appropriate dose for individual patients.

Key question: what criteria should be used to make decisions on prescribing a supplement or nutraceutical?

First, perform a literature search (via PubMed, Google Scholar, or some other search engine) for a prospective, randomized, blinded, controlled feeding trial in the patient population of interest. If that level of scientific evidence is not available, ask 1 or more manufacturers of products you are researching for the evidence they have published (other than testimonials). If objective, peer-reviewed evidence is not available, you should question whether the supplement is safe and effective for your patient.

Unlike pharmaceuticals sold across North America, nutritional supplements and nutraceuticals are not tightly regulated, which means it is much more likely that the contents of a nutritional supplement will not match the concentration written on the label or Web site. It is also possible that contaminants may be included in these products. For these reasons, using a third-party evaluator, such as Consumerlab.com (see Box 2), can be worth the annual subscription fee. ConsumerLab.com is an independent certifying organization that tests nutritional supplements and nutraceuticals for both people and pets. However, this service does not extend to evaluating every product in the marketplace.

For human supplements, consumers can look on brand labels for the seal of the United States Pharmacopeia (USP) Verification Program (see Box 2). The USP-verified mark on a label means the product contains ingredients listed in the amount and potency claimed by the manufacturer. It also means the product was made under controlled manufacturing processes and that it has no harmful levels of contaminants. In addition, the USP-verified mark means the product will break down and release into the body within a designated amount of time. For animal supplements, consumers can look on brand labels for the National Animal Supplement Council (NASC) seal (see Box 2). The NASC is a nonprofit industry group that has a quality seal program for member manufacturers willing to submit to an independent audit to ensure compliance with quality standards. Participating companies must have a quality control manual with standard operating procedures in place; they must also have an adverse event reporting system and must follow proper labeling guidelines. With so few regulations of pet supplements or nutraceuticals, this is 1 way that manufacturers can attempt to show quality control efforts.

BOX 5
Common Supplements or Nutraceuticals Used in Small Animal Veterinary Practice in North America

- Coenzyme Q
- Digestive enzymes
- Fish oil (omega-3 fatty acids: EPA + DHA)
- Glucosamine and chondroitin sulfate
- Lysine
- Milk thistle (silymarin)
- Multivitamins
- Probiotics
- S-adenosyl methionine
- Taurine
- Yunnan baiyao

The next level of criteria includes both the patient's health and medical condition, as well as owner preferences. For owners determined to try a nutritional supplement for their pet, it is important for the family veterinarian to discuss how to conduct a dietary trial with an N of 1, as well as about the power of the placebo response.

Conducting a dietary trial for a single pet (N of 1)

Establish with your client what the perceived value of the nutritional supplement or nutraceutical might be for the pet. It is critical for clients to understand that, during any trial period, there should no other new diets, treats, supplements, or alternative treatments initiated.

Establish a baseline period before the introduction of the nutritional supplement or nutraceutical being tested. During this baseline period of 5 or 7 days, the owner should closely monitor and document the pet's appetite, daily activity, fecal score, urine output, pain level, or whatever clinical signs the veterinarian (or owner) is attempting to manage with the inclusion of the nutritional supplement. Discussing and implementing a numerical scoring system between 0 and 4 is an easy method for most owners to manage in the home environment.

Prescribe the nutritional supplement or nutraceutical as per any drug: instruct the owner on a specific dose (with or without food), specific time of day for dosing, specific length of time for total treatment, what to look for in terms of a positive therapeutic response, what to look for in terms of a negative response, when to call the clinic if there are concerns, and when to bring the animal to the clinic for a recheck.

Instruct the owner to document the pet's behaviors and responses each day throughout the test period (often this is 2 months or longer); the length of the test period should be discussed with owners to make sure they understand and are able to adhere to the recommendations. The health care team should encourage owners to bring their documentation from home at each recheck or office visit.

Stop the treatment after a predetermined time period that you and the owner have agreed on. During the posttreatment period, it will be just as critical for the owner to continue monitoring and recording the animal's behaviors and responses in order to compare and contrast between baseline, treatment period, and the posttreatment period. Only by completing all 3 phases of the dietary trial can the veterinarian and owner attempt to objectively determine whether the supplementation had an impact.

Case: Canine Athlete

Animal factors

Signalment: a 5-year-old, spayed female German shepherd dog presented to the family veterinarian for specific guidance on muscle conditioning and strength training. The owner planned to enter the dog in several agility competitions later in the year (in 9 months' time). On physical examination, the dog was noted to be healthy and fit; other than mild tartar in the oral cavity, all other parameters were within normal limits. The dog's BW was 32 kg; she was well muscled and had a BCS of 5 out of 9. In addition to daily walks of 30 to 60 minutes, the dog was exercised or trained between 3 and 5 days each week; training periods lasted between 15 and 45 minutes each. The owner also had questions about potential supplements, such as omega-3 fatty acids and glucosamine–chondroitin sulfate to support the dog's joints.

Dietary factors

A current and complete diet history was obtained using a diet history form that the owners filled out at home before their scheduled appointment (see Fig. 6). The dog's primary diet consisted of an over-the-counter commercial kibble marketed for performance. The food was premeasured by the owners at 2 cups in the morning and another 2 cups about 11 hours later (calories/cup = 475 × 4 cups = 1900 kcal/d). Two different commercial training treats were used for rewards, which were calculated to deliver ~14% of the dog's total daily calorie needs (300 kcal).

From the pet food label or Web site, the respective calorie contents of the food and treats were identified. The dry kibble product contained 475 kcal (417 g) per 237-mL (8-oz) cup and the 2 training treats provided 69 kcal and 5 kcal per treat, respectively. Using additional information from the label or Web site, an estimate of protein and fat content on an energy basis (eg, grams per 100 kcal) was calculated and a table was created to more clearly understand macronutrient intakes (Table 6) [27].

According to the Association of American Feed Control Officials [37], the minimum dietary protein requirement for adult dogs is 4.5 g of protein per 100 kcal of metabolizable energy. So, if the dog's daily energy intake was 2200 kcal, and the food contained 7.4 g of protein per 100 kcal, the dog would be consuming more than enough protein from the base diet. The dry kibble contained 0.12% omega fatty acids (EPA + DHA) on an as-fed basis, and a minimum of 500 ppm glucosamine. With the wide diversity in energy expenditures and lifestyles of athletic and working dogs, an objective or formalized standard for nutrient levels for canine athletes has not been established. However, a review of macronutrients used by sled dogs and racing greyhounds highlights how different work types (sprinting vs endurance running) use different macronutrients [38]. Additional research is needed to better understand the unique nutritional requirements of other types of athletic or performance dogs (eg, search and rescue, herding, military, detection, competitive agility).

Environmental factors

The dog in this case is the only animal in the home and is fed in the kitchen; she has her own dog bed on the main floor and upstairs in the bedroom. The backyard is fenced with enough space to toss a ball and play fetch. One owner works outside the home, whereas the other owner works from home and has a flexible schedule, so adequate time can be devoted to exercising the dog.

Assessment and questions

The dog is in ideal body condition, has maintained a stable BW, and eats a complete and balanced commercial diet. However, collection of a thorough diet history (and calculation of calories consumed) revealed that an excessive number of calories were provided from treats (~14%). Recall that when more than 10% of the pet's daily calories are derived from treats, it risks unbalancing the feeding plan. Excessive treating is a common finding among dog owners that rely on food rewards for training and should be addressed through client education. In this case, the total number of calories consumed per day can be maintained (2200 kcal/d) but treats should only comprise less than 220 kcal of the total. The owner can also be coached to use portions of the dog's own kibble as training treats to avoid exceeding the recommended target.

One approach to consider is whether the owners should switch to a veterinary therapeutic diet that provides long-chain omega-3 fatty acids (EPA and DHA) for joint health, or whether they should add a supplement to the current diet. An additional approach is whether there would be any benefit to using a veterinary therapeutic diet that contains glucosamine and chondroitin sulfate, or whether that should be provided as a separate supplement. As was mentioned earlier, there is evidence to support the use of EPA and DHA, but no consistently repeatable evidence to support the use of glucosamine. Some veterinary therapeutic diets marketed for mobility and containing EPA and DHA are listed in Table 7. Comparison charts of omega-3 fatty products (Table 8) and glucosamine products (Table 9) can be created in order to better understand concentrations and relative costs before making a specific recommendation to clients.

Key question: using a veterinary therapeutic diet, what would the dog's intake of EPA and DHA be if meeting its energy needs? What would its intake of glucosamine be from the diet?

There is a minimum recommended allowance for EPA and DHA in adult dogs (30 mg/kg$^{0.75}$) and published recommendations for EPA and DHA

TABLE 6
Comparison and Analysis of Macronutrient Content, Total Calorie Intake, and Total Protein Intake of the Canine Patient's Current Feeding Plan

Complete and Balanced Commercial Dog Foods	Energy (kcal/cup or per Treat)	Protein (g/100 kcal)[a]	Fat (g/100 kcal)[a]	Amount to Feed to Meet DER**
Performance Pet Foods kibble	475	7.4	4.9	1900/475 = 4 cups per day
Treat 1	69	19	1.85	210/69 = 3 treats
Treat 2	5	18.1	1.7	90/5 = 18 treats
—	—	—	—	Total: 2200 kcal/d

RER = $70(BW_{kg}^{0.75}) = 70(32^{0.75}) = 942$ kcal/d.

DER** = RER × 2.4 = 942 × 2.4 = 2200 kcal/d.

NRC recommended allowance for protein intake for adult dogs: 100 g protein/kg diet at 4.0 kcal ME/g.

Rule of thumb for minimum protein intake: 2.2 g/kg BW/d = 70 g protein per day for a dog weighing 32 kg (70.4 lb).

Assessment: at the current intake of dry food only, the dog was consuming considerably more than the minimum amount of protein each day; total calories as treats was more than the general rule of no more than 10% of total estimated daily calories.

[a] Calculated values based on steps previously outlined [27].

supplementation for dogs with various clinical conditions, including osteoarthritis (310 mg/kg$^{0.75}$) [28]; the safe upper limit has been established as 370 mg/kg$^{0.75}$ [39]. However, there is no published dose for the prevention of joint disease in healthy dogs. An empiric dose of 25 to 45 mg/kg EPA and DHA has been suggested for otherwise healthy dogs (Dr Joe Wakshlag, personal communication, 2020), which would result in a 32-kg dog needing between 800 and 1440 mg; the midpoint of this dosing range would be 1120 mg of EPA and DHA per day.

Two examples of calculations follow, in which full nutrient data were available to address the question of whether or not the dog would be able to meet the omega-3 fatty acid target by consuming the diet according to energy requirements.

Diet 1 (see Table 7): if the food contains 0.22 g per 100 kcal of EPA and DHA and 401 kcal (423 g) per 237-mL (8-oz) cup, then there will be approximately 0.88 g in 1 cup. If the dog needs to eat 5.5 cups/d (616 g/d) to meet daily energy requirement (DER) of 2200 kcal, that will equal 4.84 g or 4840 mg of EPA and DHA. This amount meets the calculated target dose of 1120 mg/d. If the food contains 28 mg/100 kcal glucosamine, there will be approximately 616 mg in 5.5 cups, which is within the published dosage range of 480 to 960 mg/d [31].

Diet 3 (see Table 7): if the food contains 0.17 g of EPA and DHA per 100 kcal and 313 kcal (91g) per cup, and the dog eats 7.0 cups (637 g) (enough to meet DER of 2200 kcal/d), then the dog will be receiving 3740 mg/d. This amount also meets the calculated target dose of 1120 mg/d.

Alternatively, the owner could consider omega-3 fatty acid supplementation in the form of capsules, softgels or liquid drops. Pet owners should be guided with a specific recommendation by the veterinary health care team, because the concentration of

TABLE 7
Comparison of Macronutrient, Omega-3 Fatty Acid, and Glucosamine Content of Some Commercial Products Positioned as Veterinary Therapeutic Mobility Diets for Dogs

Manufacturer and Formulation[a]	Energy (kcal/237-mL cup)	Protein (g/100 kcal)	Fat (g/100 kcal)	Total Omega 3 Fatty Acids (g/100 kcal)[c]	EPA + DHA (g/100 kcal)	Glucosamine (mg/100 kcal)[d]
Diet 1[e]: Purina Pro Plan Veterinary Diets JM Joint Mobility Dry Canine Formula	401	8.2	3.5	0.25	0.22	28
Diet 2[f]: Hill's Prescription Diet j/d	353	5.0	4.2	0.82	0.12[b]	Not listed
Diet 3[g]: Royal Canin Advanced Mobility Support	313	7.0	3.3	0.28	0.17	Not listed
Diet 4[h]: Royal Canin Mobility Support	324	6.6	3.2	0.22	0.14	Not listed

[a] Nutrient values obtained from company Web sites; accurate at the time of reporting.
[b] Amount for EPA only as per product guide reporting.
[c] Products reported to have total omega-3 fatty acids could include any combination of ALA, EPA, and DHA.
[d] If data are not reported, the company can be contacted for further information.
[e] Purina Pro Plan Veterinary Diets JM Joint Mobility Dry Canine Formula, Nestle Purina PetCare, St Louis, MO.
[f] Hill's Prescription Diet j/d, Hill's Pet Nutrition, Inc, Topeka, KS.
[g] Royal Canin Advanced Mobility Support, Royal Canin, Canada, Puslinch, Ontario, Canada.
[h] Royal Canin Mobility Support, Royal Canin, Canada, Puslinch, Ontario, Canada.

TABLE 8
Five Omega-3 Fatty Acid Products for Dogs and Estimated Cost per Day

Omega-3 Fatty Acid Products[a]	EPA and DHA (mg) per mL, Softgel or Capsule	Amount (mg), Softgels or Capsules per Day (mL)	Cost per Container	Days Container Will Last	Cost per Day
Liquids					
[b]Nordic Naturals Omega-3 Pet	782 mg EPA+ 460 mg DHA = 1242 mg/5 mL or 248.4 mg/mL	1120 mg/248 mg = 4.5 mL	$18.86/60 mL	60 mL/4.5 mL = 13 d	$18.86/13 d = $1.45/d
[c]Ascenta NutraSea Omega-3 Liquid	750 EPA + 500 mg DHA = 1250 mg/5 mL or 250 mg/mL	1120 mg/250 mg/ mL = 4.5 mL	$41.97/500 mL	500 mL/4.5 mL = 111 d	$41.97/111 d = $0.38/d
[d]Aventi Omega-3 Complete for Dogs and Cats	825 mg EPA+ 550 mg DHA = 1375 mg/5 mL Or 275 mg/mL	1120 mg/275 mg = 4.0 mL	$22.00/500 mL	500 mL/4.0 mL = 125 d	$22/125 d = $0.18/d
Softgels					
[e]Nordic Naturals Omega-3 Pet	165 mg EPA + 105 mg DHA per softgel cap	1120 mg/370 mg = 3 softgels/d	$47.23 for 180 softgel caps	180/3 per day = 60 d	$47.23/60 d = 0.79/d
[f]Nature Made Burp-Less Mini Omega-3	500 mg EPA + DHA/softgel cap	1120 mg/500 mg = 2.25 softgels/d	$16.27/120 softgels	120/2.25 = 53 d	$16.27/53 d = 0.3/d

Calculations are based on a daily dose for an otherwise healthy 32-kg dog (1120 mg/d).
[a] Nutrient values obtained from company Web sites; accurate at the time of reporting.
[b] Nordic Naturals Omega-3 Pet, Nordic Naturals, Watsonville, CA.
[c] Ascenta NutraSea Omega-3 Liquid, Nature's Way of Canada, Richmond Hill, Ontario, Canada.
[d] Aventi Omega-3 Complete for Dogs and Cats, Aventix Animal Health, Burlington, Ontario, Canada.
[e] Nordic Naturals Omega-3 Pet, Nordic Naturals, Watsonville, CA.
[f] Nature Made Burp-Less Mini Omega-3, Pharmavit, Northridge, CA.

EPA and DHA in pet and human products varies widely, and regulations for safety and consistent concentrations is lacking for many (if not most) products. Understanding which nutraceuticals are available and how those products compare with veterinary therapeutic diets containing EPA and DHA is necessary to make informed, economical recommendations that clients will adhere to over time for their pets.

Rehabilitation

In addition to a targeted diet plan, exercise and athletic conditioning are necessary to minimize risks associated with injury and to prepare dogs for optimal performance.

Key question: what activities should the owner focus on in the dog's home environments?

In general, the type and duration of exercise should be based on the components of work the dog participates in. In this case, the dog is a competitive agility athlete, which involves performing a series of obstacles in a timed manner. Therefore, aerobic endeavors such as running, cavaletti rails, tunnels, stair climbing, weave polls, and jumps are examples of activities that could be incorporated into the dog's exercise plan.

Walking/running

The dog is currently walked for 30 to 60 min/d. Walking is a commonly used activity for conditioning that can be easily modified to increase the challenge

TABLE 9
Five Glucosamine and Chondroitin Sulfate Products for Dogs and Estimated Cost per Day

Product[a]	Amount (mg) per Tablet or Chew[b]	Tablets/d (n)	Cost per Container ($)	Days 1 Container Will Last (n)	Cost per Day to Meet Dose ($)
[c]Dasuquin with MSM Chewable Tablets (large dog)	900 mg/tablet, 150 tablets	960/900 = 1.06	74.99	150	0.49
[d]Cosequin Maximum Strength Plus MSM Chewable Tablets	600 mg/tablet, 250 tablets	960/600 = 1.6	54.99	125	0.44
[e]NaturVet Glucosamine DS Plus Tabs	500 mg/chew, 120 chews	960/500 = 1.92	24.99	60	0.42
[f]NaturVet ArthriSoothe-GOLD	500 mg/chew, 70 chews	960/500 = 1.92 chews	19.98	35	0.57
[g]Paw-Preferred Hip and Joint Glucosamine Dog Supplement	250 mg/tablet, 60 tablets	960/250 = 3.84	16.99	15	1.13

Calculations are based on a daily dose for a 32-kg dog (960 mg/d).

[a] Nutrient values obtained from company Web sites; accurate at the time of reporting.

[b] Veterinarians should be practicing evidence-based medicine. Although there are numerous over-the-counter glucosamine/chondroitin products currently available in the marketplace, there is no evidence to support their efficacy in the treatment of osteoarthritis for dogs or cats.

[c] Dasuquin with MSM Chewable Tablets (large dog), Nutramax Laboratories Veterinary Sciences, Inc, Lancaster, SC.

[d] Cosequin Maximum Strength Plus MSM Chewable Tablets, Nutramax Laboratories Veterinary Sciences, Inc, Lancaster, SC.

[e] NaturVet Glucosamine DS Plus Tabs, Garmon Corporation, Temecula, CA.

[f] NaturVet ArthriSoothe-GOLD, Garmon Corporation, Temecula, CA.

[g] Paw-Preferred Hip and Joint Glucosamine Dog Supplement, Downtown Pet Supply, Woodbridge, IL.

over time. If the owner has a land treadmill, the dog can be exercised consistently, regardless of the weather or time of day. Many treadmills also have an incline setting to adapt the slope of the ramp and therefore increase the workload (Fig. 12). Shoulder extension and range of motion are greater when walking or trotting at an incline (eg,10%) compared with on level surfaces [40]. Note that the dog should not be left unattended on the treadmill, regardless of level of comfort. Underwater treadmill therapy could also be considered, using a dedicated veterinary practice with specialized equipment to facilitate sessions (eg, 2–3 treatments per week). In this setting, the resistance imposed by water increases the cardiovascular demand and improves strength; the degree of resistance can be adapted by changing the depth of the water. Much like a land treadmill, the speed of the underwater treadmill belt may also be increased to enhance the conditioning program.

Cavaletti rails

Cavaletti rails are another modality that can be used safely in the confines of the home environment and mimic the movements required on the agility course. Cavaletti rails are essentially poles that are spaced apart at equal distances at a particular height from the ground (Fig. 13). This technique is used to enhance proprioception, balance, and coordination and increase range of

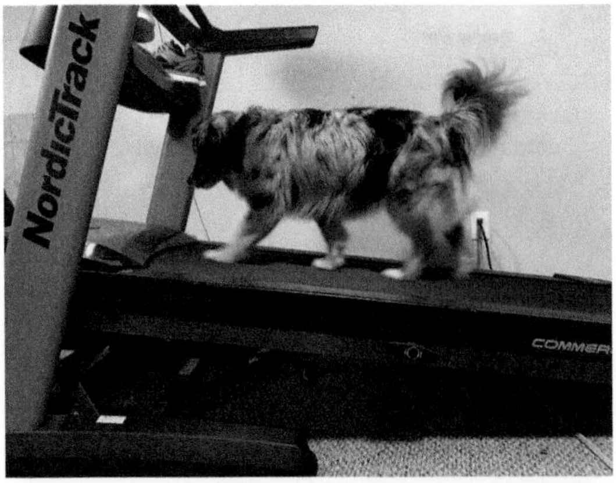

FIG. 12 Dogs can be trained to use a land treadmill, which allows consistent exercise with measurable targets. Here, the incline is set at 15%. (*Courtesy of* Dr. Sara Ritzie.)

motion. Cavaletti rails can be purchased commercially or can be assembled at home using broom sticks or even a ladder. The goal is to space the poles apart to allow for 1 single step in between, according to the natural stride of the animal. Maintaining the rails at approximately the height of the carpus is a typical starting point and can be increased as the animal progresses. The owner can start by walking the dog 3 to 5 times over the rails at each session, working up to 8 to 10 times. From there, further challenges can be imposed by trotting the dog across the rails.

Agility tunnels

Tunnels for agility training can be purchased commercially and incorporated into the activity plan. The goal is to select a tunnel size that results in a slightly crouched posture while the dog navigates through the tunnel. This posture requires increased flexion of the joints in the forelimbs and hindlimbs, while also enhancing muscular strength [23]. To intensify the challenge over time, the owner can work the dog toward faster speeds, starting first with a walk, progressing to a trot, and ultimately to a run. Another modification is to experiment with different heights; the lower the height of the tunnel, the tighter the crouch, and the higher the muscular demand. An initial goal of 15 to 20 repetitions can targeted.

Other activities can be performed at home according to the dog's ability and the demands of the work performed in agility trials. Figure-of-eight walking, weave polls, stair climbing, and jumps can all be integrated into the dog's daily walking routine to enhance strength, balance and proprioception. Environmental obstacles such as trees, logs, hills, and fences can all be leveraged to facilitate these activities.

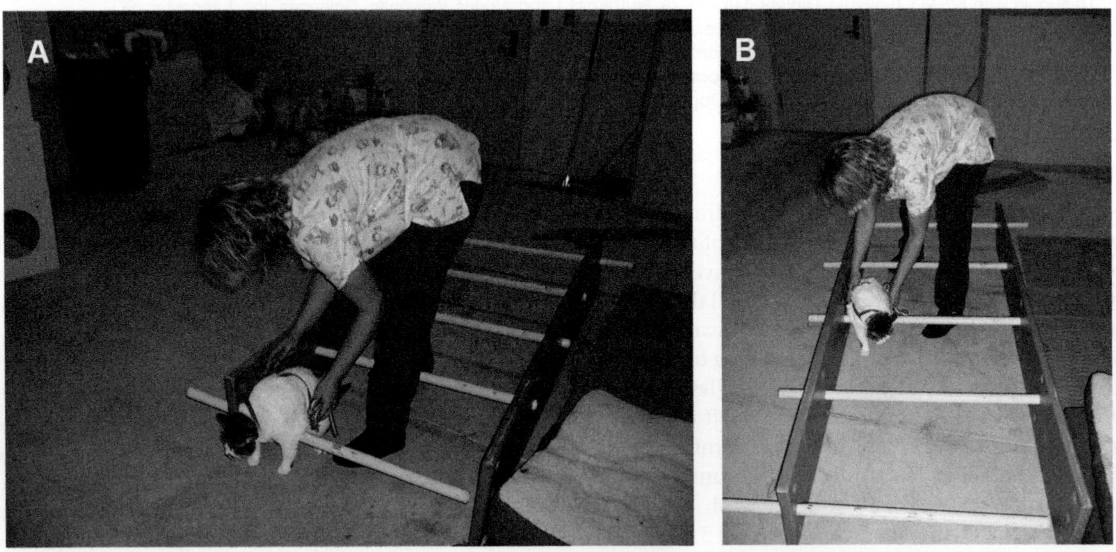

FIG. 13 (**A, B**) This feline patient is guided over cavaletti rails to encourage increased range of motion compared with ground walking. (*Courtesy of* Dr. Sarah Abood.)

SUMMARY

Sound nutrition and regular physical activity are necessary components of everyday health and wellness; they are also critical treatment modalities for patient recovery from disease. When paired together, these interventions act synergistically to enhance the quality and duration of life of companion animals. Assessment of the patient's nutritional and musculoskeletal status can be efficiently conducted on every patient at every visit; tools to facilitate these assessments are readily accessible to general practitioners. Experience, comfort level, and the time required to research and evaluate over-the-counter or therapeutic veterinary diets and supplements, and to formulate homemade diets, may influence the veterinary health care team's desire to seek a qualified professional. When the clinical considerations of a case are beyond the scope of a practitioner's abilities, referral to specialty services can, and should, be pursued.

DISCLOSURE

Dr A.M. Wara is employed by Royal Canin Canada as a veterinary clinical nutritionist. Dr. S.K. Abood does contract work with Veterinary Nutritional Consultations, Inc. and has her own consulting business called Sit, Stay, Speak Nutrition.

REFERENCES

[1] Remillard RL, Darden DE, Michel KE, et al. An investigation of the relationship between caloric intake and outcome in hospitalized dogs. Vet Ther 2001;2:301–10.

[2] Brunetto MA, Gomes MO, Andre MR, et al. Effects of nutritional support on hospital outcome in dogs and cats. J Vet Emerg Crit Care 2010;20:224–31.

[3] German A. Weight control and obesity in companion animals. Vet Focus 2012;22(2):38–46.

[4] Marshall WG, Hazewinkel HA, Mullen D, et al. The effect of weight loss on lameness in obese dogs with osteoarthritis. Vet Res Commun 2010;34:241–53.

[5] Kealy RD, Lawler DF, Ballam JM, et al. Effects of diet restriction on life span and age-related changes in dogs. J Am Vet Med Assoc 2002;220(9):1315–20.

[6] Ward E, German AJ, Churchill JA. The Global Pet Obesity Initiative Position Statement. 2018. Available at: https://static1.squarespace.com/static/597c71d3e58c621d0683 0e3f/t/5da311c5519bf62664dac512/1570968005938/ Global+pet+obesity+initiative+position+statement.pdf.

[7] Eastland-Jones RC, German AJ, Holden SL, et al. Owner misperception of a canine body condition persists despite use of a body condition score chart. J Nutr Sci 2014;3:e45.

[8] Freeman L, Becvarova I, Cave N, et al. WSAVA Nutritional Assessment Guidelines. J Small Anim Pract 2011; 52(7):385–96.

[9] de Lahunta A. Neurological Examination. In: Cohn LA, Cote E, editors. Cote's clinical veterinary advisor dogs and cats. 4th edition. St Louis (MO): Elsevier Inc.; 2020. p. 1136–7.

[10] Nye C, Troxel M. The Neurological Examination. In: Clinicians Brief. 2017. Available at: https://files.brief.vet/migration/article/40256/prop_the-neurologic-examination-40256-article.pdf. Accessed February 20, 2020.

[11] Trout NJ. Orthopedic Examination. In: Cohn LA, Cote E, editors. Cote's clinical veterinary advisor dogs and cats. 4th edition. St Louis (MO): Elsevier Inc.; 2020. p. 1143–4.

[12] Kerwin S. Orthopedic examination in the cat: Clinical tips for ruling in/out common musculoskeletal disease. J Feline Med Surg 2012;14:6–12.

[13] Coe JB, O'Connor RE, MacMartin C, et al. Effects of three diet history questions on the amount of information gained from a sample of pet owners in Ontario. Canada 2020;256(4):469–78.

[14] Gaylord L, Remillard R, Saker K. Risk of nutritional deficiencies for dogs on a weight loss plan. J Small Anim Pract 2018;59(11):695–703.

[15] Bissot T, Servet E, Vidal S, et al. Novel dietary strategies can improve the outcome of weight loss programmes in obese client-owned cats. J Feline Med Surg 2010; 12(2):104–12.

[16] Flanagan J, Bissot T, Hours M, et al. Success of a weight loss plan for overweight dogs: The results of an international weight loss study. PLoS One 2017;12(9): e0184199.

[17] Flanagan J, Bissot T, Hours M, et al. An international multi-centre cohort study of weight loss in overweight cats: Differences in outcome in different geographical locations. PLoS One 2018;13(7): e0200414.

[18] Coe JB, Rankovic A, Edwards TR, et al. Dog owner's accuracy measuring different volumes of dry dog food using three different measuring devices. Vet Rec 2019; 185(19):599.

[19] German AJ, Holden SL, Mason SL, et al. Imprecision when using measuring cups to weigh out extruded dry kibbled food. J Anim Physiol Anim Nutr 2011;95: 368–73.

[20] Toll P, Yamka R, Schoenherr WD, et al. Obesity. In: Hand MS, Thatcher, Remillard, et al, editors. Small animal clinical nutrition. 5th edition. Kansas: Mark Morris Institute; 2005. p. 501–42.

[21] Vitger AD, Stallknecht BM, Nielsen DH, et al. Integration of a physical training program in a weight loss plan for overweight pet dogs. J Am Vet Med Assoc 2016;248(2): 174–82.

[22] Chauvet A, Laclair J, Elliot D, et al. Incorporation of exercise, using an underwater treadmill, and active client

education into a weight management program for obese dogs. Can Vet J 2011;52:491–6.

[23] Millis DL, Drum M, Levin D. Therapeutic Exercises: Joint Motion, Strengthening, Endurance, and Speed Exercises. In: Millis DL, Levine D, editors. Canine rehabilitation and physical therapy. 2nd edition. Philadelphia: Elsevier Inc; 2014. p. 506–25.

[24] Millis DL, Drum M, Levine D. Therapeutic Exercises: Early Limb Use Exercises. In: Millis DL, Levine D, editors. Canine rehabilitation and physical therapy. 2nd edition. Philadelphia: Elsevier Inc; 2014. p. 495–505.

[25] Levine D, Marcellin-Little D, Millis D, et al. Effects of partial immersion in water on vertical ground reaction forces and weight distribution in dogs. Am J Vet Res 2010;71:1413–6.

[26] Benito J, Hansen B, DePuy V, et al. Feline musculoskeletal pain index (FMPI): responsiveness and criterion validity testing. J Vet Intern Med 2013;27(3):474–82.

[27] Shmalberg J. Beyond the Guaranteed Analysis. Todays Vet Pract 2013;3(1):38–9. Available at: https://mydigitalpublication.com/publication/?i=597074&p=&pn=. Accessed May 1, 2020.

[28] Bauer J. Therapeutic use of fish oil in companion animals. J Am Vet Med Assoc 2011;239(11):1441–51.

[29] Lascelles B, DePuy V, Thomson A, et al. Evaluation of a therapeutic diet for feline degenerative joint disease. J Vet Intern Med 2010;24:487–95.

[30] Corbee RJ, Barnier MC, van de Lest CA, et al. The effect of dietary long-chain omega-3 fatty acid supplementation on owner's perception of behaviour and locomotion in cats with naturally occurring osteoarthritis. J Anim Physiol Anim Nutr 2012;97(2013):846–53.

[31] VIN Veterinary Drug Handbook. 2017. Available at: https://www.vin.com/doc/?pid=13468&id=7923492. Accessed May 30, 2020.

[32] Bennett D, Zainal A, Johnston P. Osteoarthritis in the cat: 2. How should it be managed and treated? J Feline Med Surg 2012;14:76–84.

[33] Bockstahler B, Levine D. Physical therapy and rehabilitation. In: Schmeltzer LE, Norsworthy GD, editors. Nursing the feline patient. Ames (IA): John Wiley & Sons; 2012. p. 138–44.

[34] Drum MG, Bockstahler B, Levine D. Feline rehabilitation. Vet Clin North Am Small Anim Pract 2015;45:185–201.

[35] Sharp B. Feline physiotherapy and rehabilitation. 2. Clinical application. J Feline Med Surg 2012;14:633–45.

[36] Goldberg ME. A look at chronic pain in cats. Vet Nurs J 2017;32(3):67–77.

[37] AAFCO. 2019 Official publication. Champaign: Association of American Feed Control Officials; 2019.

[38] Hill RC. Nutritional and energy requirements for performance. In: Fascetti AJ, Delaney SJ, editors. Applied veterinary clinical nutrition. West Sussex (UK): Wiley-Blackwell; 2012. p. 47–56.

[39] National Research Council. Nutrient requirements of dogs and cats. Washington, DC: The National Academies Press; 2006.

[40] Weigel JP, Millis D. Biomechanics of Physical Rehabilitation and Kinematics of Exercise. In: Millis DL, Levine D, editors. Canine rehabilitation and physical therapy. 2nd edition. Philadelphia: Elsevier Inc; 2014. p. 401–30.

Advances in Small Animal Care 1 (2020) 265–277

ADVANCES IN SMALL ANIMAL CARE

Vitamin D in Health and Disease in Dogs and Cats

Ronald Jan Corbee, DVM, PhD, Dipl ECVCN
Department of Clinical Sciences, Faculty of Veterinary Medicine, Utrecht University, Yalelaan 108, Utrecht 3584 CM, the Netherlands

KEYWORDS
• Calcidiol • Cholecalciferol • Calcitriol • Canine • Feline

KEY POINTS

- 25-hydroxyvitamin D is not a sensitive indicator of vitamin D status in dogs and cats.
- Food intake and food ingredient analysis are often absent in studies on vitamin D in dogs and cats.
- 1,25-dihydroxyvitamin D is the most potent vitamin D metabolite with the greatest binding affinity to the vitamin D receptor.
- Determination of other vitamin D metabolites rather than 25-hydroxyvitamin D in vitamin D studies will provide better insight in cause-effect relationships.

INTRODUCTION

Vitamin D plays an important role in several organ systems, especially in bone metabolism. However, the role of vitamin D extends well beyond bone metabolism. A low vitamin D status has been linked to different kinds of diseases, such as chronic kidney disease [1–5], chronic enteropathy [6–8], congestive heart failure [9], infectious diseases [10–15], cancer [16–18], and chronic liver disease [19]. This corresponds with recent findings that vitamin D receptors are expressed in various tissues in dogs [20]. Other reviews [21,22] of vitamin D status (mostly expressed by 25-hydroxyvitamin D [calcidiol, or 25OHD]) and its correlation with diseases in dogs and cats have already been published. However, the underlying pathophysiological mechanisms are not discussed, which is essential to determine the clinical relevance of the correlations that were found. The aim of this review was to investigate the clinical relevance of the vitamin D status for health and disease in dogs and cats, and its practical implications.

SIGNIFICANCE

Vitamin D Metabolism

Most animal species meet their vitamin D content by consuming plants (ergocalciferol), prey (cholecalciferol), or they synthesize vitamin D under the influence of sunlight (ultraviolet B light). Vitamin D is bound to vitamin D binding protein and transported to target organs. Dietary vitamin D is absorbed from the gut by protein-mediated and passive diffusion. As vitamin D is a fat-soluble vitamin, it is transported to the liver in chylomicrons [23]. Vitamin D is first metabolized in the liver by 25-hydroxylase, which is weakly regulated, and therefore, 25OHD is thought to reflect dietary vitamin D intake in dogs and cats, as they are unable to synthesize sufficient of amounts of vitamin D under the influence of sunlight and use pro-vitamin D for cholesterol synthesis instead [24,25]. 25OHD can be further metabolized into the most active metabolite 1,25-dihydroxyvitamin D (calcitriol) under the influence of 1-alpha-hydroxylase, which is predominantly present in the proximal tubules

E-mail address: r.j.corbee@uu.nl

https://doi.org/10.1016/j.yasa.2020.07.017
2666-4518/20/

of the kidney, or 25OHD is metabolized to 24,25-dihydroxyvitamin D (24,25DHCC) by 24-hydroxylase, which is present in several tissues, or 25OHD will be stored in the liver [26]. Calcitriol formation is stimulated by parathyroid hormone (PTH), growth hormone, insulinlike growth factor-1, and inhibited by 24-hydroxylase and fibroblast growth factor 23 (FGF-23) [26]. Calcitriol is the vitamin D metabolite with the greatest binding affinity to the vitamin D receptor (VDR) [27]. 25OHD and 24,25DHCC are also able to bind to the VDR, but are 100-fold less potent compared with calcitriol [28]. Under the influence of PTH, 1-alpha hydroxylase is stimulated, and calcitriol formation is enhanced when plasma calcium level drops. The effects of calcitriol are used to restore plasma calcium level, as PTH enhances urinary phosphate excretion. Calcitriol has a negative feedback on PTH formation to prevent a perpetuating cycle. Calcitriol also stimulates 24-hydroxylase, which metabolizes calcitriol into 1,24,25-trihydroxyvitamin D (1,24,25THCC), which can be excreted by the urine. High plasma phosphorus levels stimulate FGF-23, which stimulates 24-hydroxylase to form 24,25DHCC, which stimulates mineralization of bone [29], FGF-23 also inhibits 1-alpha-hydroxylase and promotes excretion of calcitriol by enhancing 1,24,25THCC formation. On the cellular level, vitamin D actions are mediated by the VDR, a ligand-activated transcription factor that functions to control gene expression. Following ligand activation, the VDR binds directly to specific sequences located near promoters and recruits a variety of coregulatory complexes that perform the additional functions required to modify transcriptional output. Recent advances in transcriptional regulation, which permit the unbiased identification of the regulatory regions of genes, are providing new insight into how genes are regulated. The vitamin D target genes play important roles in calcium and phosphorus homeostasis, and additional targets important to these processes continue to be discovered [30].

Vitamin D Requirements

The Association of American Feed Control Officials [31], Fédération Européenne de l'Industrie des Aliments pour Animaux Familiers [32], and National Research Council [23] have determined nutritional requirements of vitamin D for dogs and cats, which are summarized in Table 1. The minimum requirement for dogs is determined based on a study demonstrating no adverse effects on bones in growing Great Dane puppies when raised on a diet with 110 IU vitamin D per 1000 kcal metabolizable energy (ME) [33]. The maximum amount for dogs is based on the same study, as adverse effects on bone were seen in puppies raised on a diet with 1000 IU vitamin D per 1000 kcal ME. Minimum requirements for cats are based on a study demonstrating no adverse effects on 25OHD plasma levels in growing kittens raised on a diet with 28 IU per 1000 kcal ME [34]. The maximum amount for cats is based on a study demonstrating no adverse effects in cats and kittens that were fed a diet with 7520 IU vitamin D per 1000 kcal ME during 18 months [35].

Vitamin D in Bone Metabolism, and Calcium and Phosphorus Homeostasis

The main function of calcitriol in bone metabolism is bone growth and remodeling. For vitamin D (ie,

TABLE 1
Nutritional Requirements of Vitamin D for Dogs and Cats

	Puppies Minimum	Adult Dogs Minimum	Dogs Maximum
AAFCO	500/125/29.9	500./125/29.9	3000/750/179
FEDIAF	552/138/33	639/159/38	2270[a]/800/191
NRC	552/136/32.5	552/136/32.5	3200/800/191
	Kittens Minimum	**Adult Cats Minimum**	**Cats Maximum**
AAFCO	280/70/16.7	280/70/16.7	30,080/7520/1798
FEDIAF	280/70/16.7	333/83.3/19.9	2270[a]/7500/1793
NRC	224/56/13.4	280/70/16.7	30,000/7500/1793

Data are expressed as amounts of vitamin D3 in IU per kg dry matter/1000 kcal metabolizable energy (ME)/MJ ME, respectively.

Abbreviations: AAFCO, Association of American Feed Control Officials; FEDIAF, Fédération Européenne de l'Industrie des Aliments pour Animaux Familiers; NRC, National Research Council.

[a] FEDIAF has defined a legal maximum for vitamin D, on dry matter basis only.

predominantly calcitriol) to be able to mineralize osteoid and cartilage, it needs calcium and phosphate. Therefore, calcitriol enhances the uptake of calcium and phosphorus from the gastrointestinal tract, the reabsorption of calcium and phosphorus from the pre-urine (filtrate) and release of calcium and phosphorus from metabolically inactive bone (ie, bone that is not frequently remodeled). Vitamin D assists PTH in maintaining plasma calcium levels, and assists FGF-23 in maintaining plasma phosphorus levels, as described previously.

Vitamin D deficiency

Vitamin D deficiency results in classic rickets. On radiographs, changes will be most apparent at epiphyseal growth plates. These changes include enlarged growth plates, hazy metaphyseal borders, ragged and cup-shaped calcification borders, thinned trabecular pattern of diaphysis, and bowed bone shafts. The changes will be most prominent in parts where growth is maximal, such as the distal growth plate of the ulna [36]. Bone pain, stiff gait, metaphyseal swelling, bowed limbs, fractures, and low serum vitamin D and calcium concentrations, are typical clinical symptoms for rickets. Symptoms of rickets are often more severe because of combined deficiencies in calcium and/or phosphorus, and aggravated by an inverse Ca:P ratio, also known as "all-meat syndrome," resulting in decreased mineralization of bone, thin cortices, greenstick fractures, and compression fractures [26].

All-meat syndrome has also been described in an adult dog, where low intake of vitamin D and calcium did not result in fractures, but instead, bone tissue was replaced by fibrous tissue, similar as in cases of renal secondary hyperparathyroidism [37].

Non–nutrition-related are the genetic types of rickets, which are also referred to as vitamin D-dependent rickets type 1 (VDDR-1) and type 2 (VDDR-2). In VDDR-1, the renal enzyme 1-alpha-hydroxylase is lacking, resulting in insufficient calcitriol production. In VDDR-2, the VDR is not responding to calcitriol due to a defective VDR (and therefore also referred to as hereditary vitamin D resistant rickets). In case of VDDR-2, high serum levels of calcitriol will coincide with low serum calcium levels. In both dogs and children with VDDR-2, alopecia is reported, but the underlying mechanism is poorly understood [38].

Vitamin D toxicity. Acute vitamin D toxicity is characterized by hypercalcemia and calcifications in bone and soft tissues. Whether these symptoms can be explained by increased levels of 25OHD, 1,25DHCC, 24,25DHCC, and/or 1,24,25THCC remains speculative. In one report, 2 dogs were diagnosed with acute vitamin D toxicity due to a commercial diet with 92.30 IU/g of vitamin D were described. Clinical findings were lethargy, polydipsia, and polyuria (due to hypercalcemia), and a stiff gait. Hypercalcemia, elevated 25OHD and calcitriol plasma concentrations, and PTH levels below the detection limit were found. The successful treatment in this case included a dietary change. Serum concentrations of calcium were within the reference range after 28 days. Serum 25OHD concentrations remained slightly elevated even after the clinical signs were gone at day 180. Serum calcitriol concentrations were within the reference range at day 150 [39].

Chronic vitamin D toxicity is not extensively studied. Previous studies demonstrated mild disturbances of endochondral ossification and irregular growth plates in puppies that were fed 135 times the recommended levels of vitamin D from 3 until 21 weeks of age. Serum concentrations of calcitonin, PTH, and all vitamin D metabolites were increased, although calcitriol was not. Instead, calcitriol serum concentrations decreased, probably due to low PTH levels or increased metabolic clearance [33].

Non–nutrition-related cases of acute vitamin D intoxication are described and related to ingestion of rodenticides. Clinical signs of vitamin D toxicosis is reported with an intake of greater than 0.5 mg (= 20,000 IU) per kg body weight in dogs and cats, but treatment is recommended from 0.1 mg (= 4000 IU) per kg body weight [40]. With suspicion of excessive intake, the author recommends to start treatment in any case, to prevent possible clinical signs. Usually, after a toxic intake of vitamin D, hyperphosphatemia, hypercalcemia and azotemia (raised blood urea nitrogen and serum creatinine levels) will develop within respectively 12, 24, and 72 hours. Other causes of hypervitaminosis that have been reported are due to treatment with the vitamin D analogues calcipotriol and tacalcitol for conditions such as psoriasis or after treatment of hypoparathyroidism [39]. Calcipotriol is a synthetic structural analogue of calcitriol; 40 to 60 μg calcipotriol per kg of body weight is reported to be the toxic dosage. Clinical signs are similar to those in rodenticide intoxication, but also soft tissue mineralization, which usually occurs within 36 hours of intoxication [41]. Fewer reports can be found on the intoxication of tacalcitol. A case report of a 21 kg dog who consumed approximately 80 μg of tacalcitol 36 to 48 hours was described. Clinical signs were mostly the same as in the calcipotriol cases, although soft tissue mineralization appeared more severe and the lungs were filled with fluid, probably due to congestive heart failure. In this particular case, it was unclear whether the dog had ingested more tacalcitol, so whether tacalcitol intoxication is more severe compared with calcipotriol intoxication remains inconclusive [42].

Treatment of vitamin D toxicity. Treatment of vitamin D toxicity depends on the time that it is ingested, the amount that is ingested, and the severity of the clinical signs. When the toxicity is acute and consumption was within approximately 4 hours, emesis can be induced. This is only useful when clinical signs are not present, otherwise the excessive amounts of vitamin D are already taken up. Activated charcoal can be given additionally to prevent further absorption of vitamin D that was not excreted by emesis. Administration of active charcoal should be repeated every 4 to 8 hours for 1 or 2 days in case of cholecalciferol toxicity, because vitamin D recirculates through the liver and small intestine. Monitoring blood serum concentrations of calcium, phosphorus, blood urea nitrogen, and creatinine is recommended for 4 days. When clinical signs are present, immediate treatment is necessary. When clinical signs are severe or if treatment is delayed, the prognosis is guarded. Treatment of hypervitaminosis D would include the following: aggressive fluid therapy with a 0.9% saline solution, until the serum calcium concentration is back within the reference range. Fluids that contain calcium should be avoided. Decreased dietary calcium intake is prescribed to prevent further accumulation of calcium. Corticosteroids reduce vitamin D–mediated calcium absorption from the intestine, reduce bone resorption, and increase renal calcium excretion, probably due to an effect on PTH regulation. Furthermore, furosemide can be administered to promote calcium excretion by the kidneys. When the fluid therapy is not effective, treatment with bisphosphonates, such as pamidronate disodium, should be considered (1.3–2.0 mg/kg diluted in 0.9% saline, administered slowly, over 2 hours, intravenously). Bisphosphonates inhibit bone resorption through a direct effect on the osteoclast itself and by interfering hydroxyapatite crystal dissolution. Because this treatment is expensive, it is mostly applied in severe cases that do not respond well to other treatments [40].

Serum vitamin D levels

Current consensus among nutritionists is that 25OHD is not a very sensitive indicator of vitamin D status. Despite this fact, many nutrition researchers explore associations of 25OHD levels with diseases [22]. 25OHD levels are easier to measure compared with calcitriol, because calcitriol has a short half-life, and is present at much lower levels compared with 25OHD. In human medicine, especially in the western world at higher latitudes, people are vitamin D deficient in winter times because of deprivation of UVB from sunlight combined with insufficient dietary vitamin D intake. Most dogs and cats eat standardized diets largely meeting their vitamin D requirement on a daily basis in all life stages [43,44], which makes it difficult to extrapolate findings of studies in people from the western world to dogs and cats. Furthermore, there are several explanations for low 25OHD in diseased animals and people, such as low food intake, low dietary vitamin D, deprivation of UVB from sunlight (in people and several other animals than dog and cat), inadequate absorption from the gut, leakage of vitamin D in the gut (eg, when suffering from protein loosing enteropathy), reduced reabsorption from the filtrate, increased use of 25OHD for formation of calcitriol, 24,25DHCC, and or 1,24,25THCC, and increased use of vitamin D metabolites for the immune system. To be able to elucidate cause-effect relations, we need to measure all the vitamin D metabolites, which were not determined in most studies, and their results should therefore be interpreted with caution.

Another issue with interpretation of 25OHD values is variations between methodology (ie, different assays), which makes it difficult to compare results and set a normal range.

Other factors than differences in methodology can also play a role, such as the presence of epimers [45]. Serum 25OHD concentrations between 9.5 and 249.2 ng/mL in healthy dogs were demonstrated [22]. This variation has several possible explanations such as differences between breeds and sexes. An interesting finding was that intact male dogs had significantly higher serum 25OHD concentrations compared with neutered male dogs and neutered female dogs. Sexually intact female dogs had slightly higher 25OHD serum concentrations compared with neutered female dogs, but this was not significant. These findings demonstrated that either sex hormones affect 25OHD serum concentrations (and male sex hormones do so more than female sex hormones), or that gender and neutering had an effect on the amount of food eaten [46].

Although vitamin D is a fat-soluble hormone, which can be distributed and stored within adipose tissue, no significant effects of adiposity on serum 25OHD concentrations have been demonstrated [47]. When evaluating dog and cat studies on serum 25OHD concentrations, the variation in control groups is 9.5 to 249 ng/mL in dogs, and 14.9 to 83.1 ng/mL in cats, whereas in diseased animals, serum 25OHD concentrations vary between 0 to 151 ng/mL, and 1.7 to 97.1 ng/mL, respectively [22]. In human medicine, levels of greater than 20 ng/mL are considered sufficient, but 75 to 90 ng/mL are associated with better outcome in case of disease [22]. In dogs, 100 to 120 ng/mL was suggested to be the minimum concentration to inhibit PTH secretion, which, based on the current studies, implies many dogs being vitamin D deficient according to that definition despite being fed complete and balanced diets. Unfortunately, calcitriol, 24,25DHCC, and 1,24,25THCC levels were not determined in this study, so it is difficult to draw strong conclusions [17]. Similarly, the optimal feline serum 25OHD concentrations have yet to be determined.

Associations Between Vitamin D Status and Diseases

Vitamin D and chronic kidney disease

Lower calcitriol and 25OHD concentrations were observed in dogs with acute renal failure and chronic kidney disease (CKD) [1,3]. Furthermore, significantly lower calcitriol, 25OHD, and 24,25DHCC concentrations were found in dogs with CKD IRIS (International Renal Interest Society) stages 3 and 4 [4].

As 1-alpha hydroxylase is mostly expressed in the kidney, renal disease may result in lower formation of calcitriol. In addition, loss of nephron mass increases serum phosphorus due to decreased renal excretion, which promotes FGF-23 and inhibits 1-alpha-hydroxylase activity.

An increase in PTH concentration leads to upregulation of 1-alpha-hydroxylase, which should normally increase calcitriol production, however due to progressive loss of nephron mass, the 1-alpha-hydroxylase activity remains low despite increased levels of PTH, resulting in renal secondary hyperparathyroidism. Low calcitriol, together with increased renal loss of vitamin D metabolites, can provide an explanation as to why lower vitamin D metabolite concentrations (25OHD, calcitriol and 24,25DHCC) were only observed in CKD IRIS stages 3 and 4 and not in earlier stages [4].

The endocytic receptor megalin binds to 25OHD to enter the proximal tubules in the kidney.

After binding to the megalin receptor, 25OHD can be hydroxylated to form calcitriol, or can re-enter the circulation to maintain the serum 25OHD concentration. In renal disease, decreased megalin expression contributes to lower 25OHD and calcitriol concentrations [48]. When there is a decrease in 25OHD concentration and subsequent decrease in calcitriol formation, more vitamin D metabolites will be lost via the urine due to decreased megalin expression. Additionally, decreased megalin expression is related to proteinuria.

Lower 25OHD concentration in renal disease can also be caused by decreased intake of vitamin D due to a dietary deficiency or reduced intake due to decreased appetite, vomiting, and/or diarrhea [3].

Vitamin D and gastrointestinal diseases

Lower 25OHD concentrations were found in dogs with chronic enteropathy (CE) and hypoalbuminemia, and in cats with CE or intestinal small cell lymphoma [6,7]. Furthermore, low 25OHD concentrations are linked to systemic inflammation in dogs with protein losing enteropathy, and a poor prognosis [49,50].

Decreased dietary intake because of reduced appetite or malabsorption have been suggested as contributing factors to a lower vitamin D status in dogs and cats with CE [6–8]. Inflammation of the intestinal epithelium can impair both the absorption of dietary vitamin D and reabsorption of 25OHD as a part of the enterohepatic circulation [51], however, this was not demonstrated in dogs [52].

Vitamin D signaling is important for maintenance of the intestinal mucosal barrier [53]. This barrier is essential to prevent infiltration of pathogenic microorganisms, which can evoke an immune response which can finally result in chronic inflammation. In human patients with CE, the amount of VDR in the intestinal epithelium was decreased [54], suggesting a possible correlation between gastrointestinal health and VDR expression and function. However, this was not demonstrated in dogs [20]. Vitamin D also helps to maintain a normal intestinal microbiome, as calcitriol can enhance antimicrobial activity by inducing antimicrobial peptides (AMPs) [55]. In mice, Vitamin D deficiency predisposed for colitis due to microbiome alterations [56].

Vitamin D and cardiovascular diseases

A low vitamin D status has been associated with cardiovascular diseases in humans and dogs. Significantly lower 25OHD concentrations were found in dogs with chronic valvular heart disease (CVHD) stages B2 and C/D (ACVIM Consensus Classification System for Canine Chronic Valvular Heart Disease) compared with dogs with CVHD stage B1, and in dogs with chronic heart failure (CHF) compared with healthy dogs [9,57]. Low 25OHD concentrations were also correlated to poor outcome in dogs with CHF. There are no published studies of cardiovascular diseases in relation to vitamin D in cats. In humans, lower vitamin 25OHD concentrations were associated with higher risk of cardiovascular disease [58]. For example, an association between low 25OHD concentrations and reduced left ventricle function was found in geriatric patients [59]. This can be explained by the role of calcitriol in signal transduction.

Calcitriol can activate voltage-gated calcium channels in cardiomyocytes and improve the contractility of the myocardium [60,61]. Other cardio-protective effects of calcitriol includes inhibition of PTH and renin angiotensin aldersterone system (RAAS) activity [62], decrease in atrial natriuretic peptide expression [63] and direct, and indirect (as a consequence of PTH suppression) inhibition of hypertrophy of the myocardium [64]. Furthermore, vitamin D increases endothelial function, as serum 25OHD concentrations and flow mediated dilatation of the brachial artery were positively correlated, and therefore vitamin D could prevent the progression of coronary artery disease [65].

Vitamin D and immune function and infectious diseases

Lower 25OHD and calcitriol concentrations were found in dogs with immune-mediated diseases, such as immune-mediated thrombocytopenia, immune-mediated polyarthritis, and immune-mediated hemolytic anemia [66]. In addition, hospitalized cats with neutrophilia had lower 25OHD levels compared with hospitalized cats with normal neutrophil concentrations [67]. An in vitro study with blood of critically ill dogs showed that calcitriol has anti-inflammatory effects by suppressing the production of tumor necrosis factor alpha (a proinflammatory cytokine) and enhancing the production of interleukin (IL)-10 (an anti-inflammatory cytokine) [68].

Calcitriol enhances the antimicrobial activity by inducing AMPs and activating (the synthesis of) macrophages, supporting the first line of defense against pathogens. Furthermore, calcitriol stimulates the anti-inflammatory response by increasing Th2 response and the development of regulatory T cells, and inhibiting Th1 response, Th17 response, as well as B-cell development and differentiation [66,69–71].

A possible synergistic effect of vitamin D in prednisolone therapy in dogs with atopic dermatitis (AD) was postulated [72], as prednisolone therapy was more effective in dogs with higher serum 25OHD concentrations. A possible underlying mechanism for this finding might be found in the expression of cytokines, as over-expression of Th1 and Th2 cytokines are important in the pathogenesis of AD [73].

Various pathogenic microorganisms and parasites in relation to vitamin D status have been studied. Significantly lower 25OHD concentrations were found in cats with feline immunodeficiency virus (FIV) and mycobacteriosis compared with healthy cats and in dogs with blastomycosis, babesiosis, leishmaniasis and neoplastic spirocercosis compared with healthy dogs [10–15].

A possible explanation for the relation between lower 25OHD concentrations and bacterial infection might be a decrease in expression of cathelicidins (AMPs). Another explanation might be decreased macrophage synthesis and activation. On the contrary, increased use of 25OHD for calcitriol synthesis can be the cause of lower 25OHD levels in infectious or auto-immune diseases.

Vitamin D status in relation to viral infection was studied in humans. In patients with human immune-deficiency virus (HIV) type-1 calcitriol induced autophagocytosis, leading to inhibition of the virus in macrophages [74]. HIV closely resembles FIV and therefore a possible role for calcitriol supplementation in cats with FIV might be postulated [75].

Vitamin D in cancer and other diseases

The vitamin D status is not only linked to tumors related to bone metabolism, like osteosarcoma, but also to other tumors. Lower serum 25OHD concentrations were found in dogs with mast cell tumors (MCT) [18], and in dogs with splenic hemangiosarcoma [17]. In dogs with cancer, serum 25OHD concentrations increased with increasing serum calcium concentrations [16]. Whereas healthy dogs showed the opposite, indicating that the vitamin D metabolism is altered in patients with cancer and that serum calcium concentrations are involved in this change. These increased calcium concentrations can be caused by increased levels of PTH-related peptide, as was demonstrated in dogs with anal sac adenocarcinoma and in dogs with lymphoma. Calcitriol concentrations were increased, normal, or decreased in these dogs, but calcitriol levels decreased in these dogs after successful cancer treatment [76]. Antiproliferative effects of calcitriol in relation to tumor growth were described, including stimulation of G1/G0 cell-cycle arrest and cell death, reduction of epidermal growth factor, and suppression of invasive growth [77].

Alterations in vitamin D status also occurred in patients with liver disease. The liver is an important part of the vitamin D metabolism, as hydroxylation of cholecalciferol to form 25OHD takes place in the liver. Impaired liver function affects the vitamin D metabolism, resulting in lower serum 25OHD concentrations. Lower 25OHD concentrations were found in cats with cholestatic liver disease, and in dogs with chronic liver disease [19,78].

In addition, lower serum 25OHD concentrations were found in dogs with acute pancreatitis [79]. In humans, it was found that CYP24A1 expression, also known as 24-hydroxylase, correlated with VDR expression in patients with chronic pancreatitis [80]. If dogs with pancreatitis have increased levels of 24,25DHCC, which is responsible for the lower 25OHD, remains speculative.

Finally, the vitamin D status has been linked to mortality. A correlation was found between low 25OHD concentrations and a poor prognosis in hospitalized dogs and cats [81–83].

A decreased vitamin D status in hospitalized patients can, however, be caused by many factors altering vitamin D metabolism, such as reduced intake and/or malabsorption, decreased immune function, or decreased liver and/or kidney function, which impairs the formation of 25OHD and calcitriol, all of which can affect prognosis.

The Role of Supplementation

It is important to understand which metabolite is most effective to administer. Recent studies have demonstrated that supplementation with vitamin D is often not effective. In humans and dogs, supplementation with 25OHD is much more effective in rising serum 25OHD concentrations compared with vitamin D. The amount of vitamin D had to be 10 times higher compared with 25OHD to obtain similar effects [84]. Most pet food ingredients contain vitamin D2 or D3, but not the other metabolites. For cats, it is important to determine whether a product contains vitamin D2 or vitamin D3, as they use D3 more effectively [85].

Vitamin D supplementation in renal disease

In renal disease, vitamin D or 25OHD supplementation is less effective compared with calcitriol, as calcitriol formation is impaired, due to reduced 1-alpha-hydroxylase activity. Calcitriol supplementation in dogs and cats with CKD has several beneficial effects. Calcitriol inhibits PTH and the renin-angiotensin-aldosterone-system [86] by suppressing the expression of the renin gene and the activation of VDR [62]. Calcitriol also decreases injury and loss of podocytes [87], possibly by increasing nephrin and Wilms tumor suppressor gene 1 (WT1) protein expression [88]. In addition, calcitriol slows down the progression of fibrosis in patients with CKD by reducing transforming growth factor-β synthesis and increasing antifibrotic factors [89]. Furthermore, calcitriol suppresses tumor necrosis factor alpha-converting enzyme, a factor involved in the mechanism of developing proteinuria, glomerulosclerosis, tubular hyperplasia, mononuclear cell infiltration, and fibrosis [90]. Finally, calcitriol therapy is associated with increased appetite, increased physical activity, and a longer life expectancy due to its inhibitory effects on PTH secretion [91].

Calcitriol therapy can be used to control renal secondary hyperparathyroidism and to slow down the progression of CKD. It is often combined with a phosphorus restricted diet to prevent hyperphosphatemia and to reduce the risk of soft tissue mineralization [89]. Calcitriol treatment should be monitored closely to prevent hypercalcemia, which is one of the consequences of vitamin D toxicosis [1,39]. Calcitriol should be supplemented when the patient is in a fasted state to prevent increased intestinal calcium and phosphorus absorption [92]. In dogs and cats, oral administration of calcitriol starts with a daily initial dose of 2.0 to 3.5 ng/kg with a maximum dose of 5.0 ng/kg [92]. An initial calcitriol dose of 2.5 to 3.5 ng/kg per day (if serum creatinine is 176–265 μmol/L) or 3.5 ng/kg per day (if serum creatinine is higher than 265 μmol/L) is described for cats [93]. No supporting evidence was given for these doses for dogs and cats.

For dogs with CKD IRIS stages 3 and 4, calcitriol therapy is recommended [92], as they have lower vitamin D levels [4], and calcitriol treatment was associated with increased survival in 37 dogs with stage 3 and 4 CKD55. Positive or negative results of calcitriol therapy in cats have yet to be demonstrated, although an experiment involving 10 cats with CKD failed to demonstrate an increase in serum PTH [2].

Vitamin D supplementation in gastrointestinal disease

The effects of 25OHD or calcitriol therapy in dogs and cats with gastrointestinal diseases have not yet been determined. In humans with Crohn's disease, a decrease in severity of symptoms was observed after oral cholecalciferol supplementation for 24 weeks [94]. A possible explanation might be reduced inflammation because of the immunomodulatory effects of calcitriol. Another study, evaluating humans with various gastrointestinal diseases, demonstrated no increase in 25OHD levels after vitamin D supplementation [55]. Calcitriol induces VDR expression in the ileum of humans and rats [95], which suggests that calcitriol could stimulate vitamin D uptake or affect the immune system in the intestinal tract.

Vitamin D supplementation in cardiovascular disease

Studies on the effects of vitamin D supplementation on the cardiovascular system in dogs and cat have not yet been performed. One case report of a cat presented with primary hypoparathyroidism and CHF demonstrated possible effects of calcitriol on the cardiovascular system. This cat received medication and calcitriol for 4 weeks. After 4 weeks, only oral calcitriol administration (twice a week) was continued. A year later, the patient had not shown symptoms of CHF nor did it need medication [96]. In humans, vitamin D supplementation resulted in a better outcome in patients with heart failure (HF), and an increased ejection fraction in geriatric patients with low vitamin D levels and HF [97,98]. In addition, oral cholecalciferol supplementation in children with CHF showed anti-inflammatory effects [99]. Vitamin D supplementation in patients with coronary artery disease has also been studied; however, cholecalciferol supplementation did not always result in significantly positive effects (such as improved endothelial function and vascular inflammation and prevention of myocardial injury) [65]. Patients with coronary artery disease supplemented with calcitriol instead of cholecalciferol demonstrated anti-inflammatory effects, but there was also an increase in severity of coronary artery disease possibly due to reduced RAAS activity [100]. Although calcitriol is negatively correlated to RAAS activity, supplementation with vitamin D, its metabolites, or analogues should not be used as a drug to control hypertension, as experimental studies failed to show beneficial effects [101].

Vitamin D supplementation in immune diseases

Calcitriol inhibits Th1 response [73], which indicates that calcitriol might have beneficial effects in patients with AD in the chronic phase of disease. In humans, possible beneficial effects of vitamin D administration in patients with immune-mediated disease have been suggested, for example, in patients with psoriasis. Topical treatment of the skin with maxacalcitol (a vitamin D3 analogue) in mice resulted in decreased inflammation of the skin, due to an increase of regulatory T cells and a decrease in IL-23 and IL-17 synthesis [102].

Vitamin D supplementation in cancer

An in vitro study observed that oral calcitriol administration improves the effects of chemotherapy in canine MCTs [103]. This might be due to the activation of VDR, as VDR expresses broadly in canine neoplastic mast cells [104]. Another possible explanation might be a decrease in receptor tyrosine kinase activity [103]. In addition, calcitriol and calcipotriol (a calcitriol analogue) showed cytotoxic effects on multidrug resistance protein-1 overexpressing cells in a study using cytotoxicity assays [105]. Impairment of the transport function of ATP-binding cassette transporters, which are related to proteins involved in multidrug resistance (P-glycoprotein, MRP1 and breast cancer resistance protein) was also observed. Another study observed synergistic effects of calcitriol and cisplatin on inhibition of proliferation of canine tumor cells in vitro [106]. This study also conducted a noncontrolled clinical trial that showed antitumor effects of intravenous calcitriol/cisplatin administration in 3 of 8 dogs with tumors that had a measurable size. In humans, a systematic review and meta-analysis concluded no evidence was found to support the use of vitamin D supplementation to decrease mortality in patients with cancer, or to decrease cancer incidence [107].

Vitamin D supplementation in liver disease

Vitamin D supplementation was found to decrease inflammation and fibrosis in cats with chronic vitamin A intoxication [108]. No evidence for effects of vitamin D supplementation on liver disease has been reported in dogs.

PRESENT RELEVANCE AND FUTURE AVENUES TO CONSIDER OR TO INVESTIGATE

Vitamin D requirements are based on a limited number of studies that were characterized by absence of disease, rather than demonstrating pathology. Differences between institutes are based on different safety margins, as all of them are referring to the same studies. More research should be done to determine true requirement intervals. Furthermore, the minimum requirement for cats is based on maintenance of 25OHD levels. As 25OHD levels are not a sensitive marker for vitamin D status, other metabolites should be included in future studies. Nutrient interactions also warrants inclusion of PTH, calcium, and phosphorus.

Food intake, amount of vitamin D, form of vitamin D (ie, D2 or D3, or metabolites) all have an effect on 25OHD levels and should therefore be measured and reported in future studies.

Several relations between low 25OHD levels and diseases have been reported, but underlying mechanisms are mostly hypothetical and need further evaluation.

Most evidence is present for calcitriol supplementation in dogs with IRIS stage 3 and 4 renal disease.

To determine whether or not enteric loss of protein-bound vitamin D is a significant factor in low serum 25OHD concentrations in CE, it is necessary to compare VDBP serum concentrations between dogs and cats with CE and a control group consisting of healthy dogs and cats. Even though the effects of vitamin D on the gastrointestinal system have been studied, it is still unknown if vitamin D has a (significant) role in the pathogenesis of CE or is just a result of CE. This requires an experimental study design, which determines if supplementation of 25OHD or calcitriol significantly improves the described effects of vitamin D in patients with CE.

Clinical trials are required to determine the use of vitamin D supplementation in dogs and cats with cardiovascular disease regarding in which form and dosage it should be administered. It is postulated that calcitriol might be more potent than cholecalciferol because calcitriol acts directly on the cardiovascular system.

It might be useful to determine if calcitriol therapy in patients with immune-mediated diseases is more potent than vitamin D3 supplementation. Calcitriol seems to enhance the immune function. However, additional studies are required to determine the differences of calcitriol effects on the immune system in humans, dogs, and cats. In addition, it has yet to be proven that vitamin D (metabolite) supplementation can have significant beneficial effects in dogs and cats with various infectious diseases.

SUMMARY

Vitamin D is an important nutrient which has a vital role in bone metabolism as well as in other vital functions. Low vitamin D intake often coincides with low calcium intake, and is characterized by bone deformities, especially during the growth period. Bent legs, retarded growth, altered locomotion, enlarged growth plates, and decreased bone mineralization are the most common clinical and radiological findings. Dogs and cats seem to be quite resistant to excessive vitamin D intake, but calcitriol supplementation can cause hypercalcemia and renal disease. Early and thorough detoxification is important to prevent permanent damage and guarded prognosis. 25OHD is often used to evaluate vitamin D status; however, this is only a rough estimation and reflects dietary intake. Other vitamin D metabolites, especially calcitriol, provide more insight in vitamin D metabolism and effects on target tissues, but are often not reported. Associations of low 25OHD levels and several diseases have been reported, but underlying mechanisms are mostly theoretic, and not well studied. Most evidence is available for effectiveness of calcitriol supplementation in dogs with IRIS stage 3 and 4 CKD, for all other disease conditions the level of evidence is preliminary.

ACKNOWLEDGMENTS

The author thanks Graciela van Schaik and Saskia van der Vaart for their valuable contributions to the manuscript, which were part of their bachelor theses.

DISCLOSURE

The author has nothing to disclose.

REFERENCES

[1] Galler A, Tran JL, Krammer-Lukas S, et al. Blood vitamin levels in dogs with chronic kidney disease. Vet J 2012; 192(2):226–31.

[2] Hostutler RA, DiBartola SP, Chew DJ, et al. Comparison of the effects of daily and intermittent-dose calcitriol on serum parathyroid hormone and ionized calcium concentrations in normal cats and cats with chronic renal failure. J Vet Intern Med 2006;20(6):1307–13.

[3] Gerber B, Hässig M, Reusch CE. Serum concentrations of 1,25-dihydroxycholecalciferol and 25-hydroxycholecalciferol in clinically normal dogs and dogs with acute and chronic renal failure. Am J Vet Res 2003;64(9): 1161–6.

[4] Parker VJ, Harjes LM, Dembek K, et al. Association of vitamin D metabolites with parathyroid hormone, fibroblast growth factor-23, calcium, and phosphorus in dogs with various stages of chronic kidney disease. J Vet Intern Med 2017;31(3):791–8.

[5] Rudinsky AJ, Harjes LM, Byron J, et al. Factors associated with survival in dogs with chronic kidney disease. J Vet Intern Med 2018;32(6):1977–82.

[6] Lalor S, Schwartz AM, Titmarsh H, et al. Cats with inflammatory bowel disease and intestinal small cell lymphoma have low serum concentrations of 25-hydroxyvitamin d. J Vet Intern Med 2014;28(2): 351–5.

[7] Gow AG, Else R, Evans H, et al. Hypovitaminosis D in dogs with inflammatory bowel disease and hypoalbuminaemia. J Small Anim Pract 2011;52(8):411–8.

[8] Titmarsh H, Gow AG, Kilpatrick S, et al. Association of vitamin D status and clinical outcome in dogs with a chronic enteropathy. J Vet Intern Med 2015;29(6): 1473–8.

[9] Kraus MS, Rassnick KM, Wakshlag JJ, et al. Relation of Vitamin D status to congestive heart failure and cardiovascular events in dogs. J Vet Intern Med 2014;28(1): 109–15.

[10] Erdogan H, Ural K, Pasa S. Relationship between mean platelet volume, low-grade systemic coagulation and Vitamin D deficiency in canine visceral leishmaniasis. Medycyna Weterinaryjna 2019;75(8):493–6. https://doi.org/10.21521/mw.6252.

[11] O'Brien MA, McMichael MA, Le Boedec K. 25-Hydroxyvitamin D concentrations in dogs with naturally acquired blastomycosis. J Vet Intern Med 2018;32(5):1684–91.

[12] Rosa CT, Schoeman JP, Berry JL, et al. Hypovitaminosis D in dogs with spirocercosis. J Vet Intern Med 2013;27(5):1159–64.

[13] Titmarsh HF, Lalor SM, Tasker S, et al. Vitamin D status in cats with feline immunodeficiency virus. Vet Med Sci 2015;1(2):72–8.

[14] Lalor SM, Mellanby RJ, Friend EJ, et al. Domesticated cats with active mycobacteria infections have low serum vitamin D (25(OH)D) concentrations. Transbound Emerg Dis 2012;59(3):279–81.

[15] Dvir E, Rosa C, Handel I, et al. Vitamin D status in dogs with babesiosis. Onderstepoort J Vet Res 2019;86(1):e1–5.

[16] Weidner N, Woods JP, Conlon P, et al. Influence of various factors on circulating 25(OH) vitamin d concentrations in dogs with cancer and healthy dogs. J Vet Intern Med 2017;31(6):1796–803.

[17] Selting KA, Sharp CR, Ringold R, et al. Serum 25-hydroxyvitamin D concentrations in dogs - correlation with health and cancer risk. Vet Comp Oncol 2016;14(3):295–305.

[18] Wakshlag JJ, Rassnick KM, Malone EK, et al. Cross-sectional study to investigate the association between vitamin D status and cutaneous mast cell tumours in Labrador retrievers. Br J Nutr 2011;106(S1):S60–3.

[19] Galler A, Tran JL, Krammer-Lukas S, et al. Blood vitamin levels in dogs with chronic liver disease. Wien Tierarztl Monatsschr 2013;100(5–6):133–9.

[20] Cartwright JA, Gow AG, Milne E, et al. Vitamin D receptor expression in dogs. J Vet Intern Med 2018;32(2):764–74.

[21] Parker VJ, Rudinsky AJ, Chew DJ. Vitamin D metabolism in canine and feline medicine. J Am Vet Med Assoc 2017;250(11):1259–69.

[22] Zafalon RVA, Risolia LW, Pedrinelli V, et al. Vitamin D metabolism in dogs and cats and its relation to diseases not associated with bone metabolism. J Anim Physiol Anim Nutr 2020;104(1):322–42.

[23] National Research Council. Nutrient requirements of dogs and cats. Washington D.C. National Academy Press; 2006.

[24] How KL, Hazewinkel HA, Mol JA. Dietary vitamin D dependence of cat and dog due to inadequate cutaneous synthesis of vitamin D. Gen Comp Endocrinol 1994;96(1):12–8.

[25] Morris JG. Ineffective vitamin D synthesis in cats is reversed by an inhibitor of 7-dehydrocholestrol-δ7-reductase. J Nutr 1999;129(4):903–8.

[26] Hazewinkel HAW, Tryfonidou MA. Vitamin D3 metabolism in dogs. Mol Cell Endocrinol 2002;197(1):23–33.

[27] Haddad JG Jr. Transport of vitamin D metabolites. Clin Orthop Relat Res 1979;142:249–61.

[28] Brown AJ, Dusso A, Slatopolsky E. Vitamin D. Am J Physiol 1999;277(2):F157–75.

[29] Norman AW, Okamura WH, Bishop JE, et al. Update on biological actions of 1alpha,25(OH)2-vitamin D3 (rapid effects) and 24R,25(OH)2-vitamin D3. Mol Cell Endocrinol 2002;197(1–2):1–13.

[30] Pike JW, Meyer MB. The vitamin D receptor: new paradigms for the regulation of gene expression by 1,25-dihydroxyvitamin D3. Endocrinol Metab Clin North Am 2010;39(2):255–69.

[31] AAFCO. AAFCO dog and cat food nutrient profiles. AAFCO; 2014.

[32] FEDIAF. FEDIAF nutritional guidelines for complete and complementary pet food for cats and dogs. FEDIAF; 2019.

[33] Tryfonidou MA, Holla MS, Stevenhagen JJ, et al. Dietary 135-fold cholecalciferol supplementation severely disturbs the endochondral ossification in growing dogs. Domest Anim Endocrinol 2003;24(4):265–85.

[34] Morris JG, Earle KE, Anderson PA. Plasma 25-hydroxyvitamin D in growing kittens is related to dietary intake of cholecalciferol. J Nutr 1999;129(4):909–12.

[35] Sih TR, Morris JG, Hickman MA. Chronic ingestion of high concentrations of cholecalciferol in cats. Am J Vet Res 2001;62(9):1500–6.

[36] Malik R, Laing C, Davis PE, et al. Rickets in a litter of racing greyhounds. J Small Anim Pract 1997;38(3):109–14.

[37] de Fornel-Thibaud P, Blanchard G, Escoffier-Chateau L, et al. Unusual case of osteopenia associated with nutritional calcium and vitamin D deficiency in an adult dog. J Am Anim Hosp Assoc 2007;43(1):52–60.

[38] LeVine DN, Zhou Y, Ghiloni RJ, et al. Hereditary 1,25-Dihydroxyvitamin D-Resistant rickets in a pomeranian dog caused by a novel mutation in the vitamin D receptor gene. J Vet Intern Med 2009;23(6):1278–83.

[39] Mellanby RJ, Mee AP, Berry JL, et al. Hypercalcaemia in two dogs caused by excessive dietary supplementation of vitamin D. J Small Anim Pract 2005;46(7):334–8.

[40] DeClementi C, Sobczak BR. Common rodenticide toxicoses in small animals. Vet Clin North Am Small Anim Pract 2018;48(6):1027–38.

[41] Fan TM, Simpson KW, Trasti S, et al. Calcipotriol toxicity in a dog. J Small Anim Pract 1998;39(12):581–6.

[42] Hilbe M, Sydler T, Fischer L, et al. Metastatic calcification in a dog attributable to ingestion of a tacalcitol ointment. Vet Pathol 2000;37(5):490–2.

[43] Corbee RJ, Tryfonidou MA, Beckers IP, et al. Composition and use of puppy milk replacers in German Shepherd puppies in the Netherlands. J Anim Physiol Anim Nutr 2012;96(3):395–402.

[44] Kritikos G, Weidner N, Atkinson JL, et al. Quantification of vitamin D3 in commercial dog foods and comparison with Association of American Feed Control Officials recommendations and manufacturer-reported concentrations. J Am Vet Med Assoc 2018;252(12):1521–6.

[45] Hurst EA, Homer NZ, Denham SG, et al. Development and application of a LC–MS/MS assay for simultaneous analysis of 25-hydroxyvitamin-D and 3-epi-25-hydroxyvitamin-D metabolites in canine serum. J Steroid Biochem Mol Biol 2020;199:105598.

[46] Sharp CR, Selting KA, Ringold R. The effect of diet on serum 25-hydroxyvitamin D concentrations in dogs. BMC Res Notes 2005;8:442.

[47] Hookey TJ, Backus RC, Wara AM. Effects of body fat mass and therapeutic weight loss on vitamin D status in privately owned adult dogs. J Nutr Sci 2018;7:e17.

[48] Dusso AS, Brown AJ. Mechanism of vitamin D action and its regulation. Am J Kidney Dis 1998;32(4, Supplement 2):S13–24.

[49] Titmarsh HF, Gow AG, Kilpatrick S, et al. Low vitamin D status is associated with systemic and gastrointestinal inflammation in dogs with a chronic enteropathy. PLoS One 2015;10(9).

[50] Allenspach K, Rizzo J, Jergens AE, et al. Hypovitaminosis D is associated with negative outcome in dogs with protein losing enteropathy: A retrospective study of 43 cases. BMC Vet Res 2017;13(1).

[51] Bikle D. Vitamin D insufficiency/deficiency in gastrointestinal disorders. J Bone Miner Res 2008;22(Suppl 2):50.

[52] Wennogle SA, Priestnall SL, Suárez-Bonnet A, et al. Comparison of clinical, clinicopathologic, and histologic variables in dogs with chronic inflammatory enteropathy and low or normal serum 25-hydroxycholecalciferol concentrations. J Vet Intern Med 2019;33(5):1995–2004.

[53] Yamamoto EA, Jorgensen TN. Relationships between vitamin D, gut microbiome, and systemic autoimmunity. Front Immunol 2020;21(10):3141.

[54] Li YC, Chen Y, Du J. Critical roles of intestinal epithelial vitamin D receptor signaling in controlling gut mucosal inflammation. J Steroid Biochem Mol Biol 2015;148:179–83.

[55] Nielsen OH, Hansen TI, Gubatan JM, et al. Managing vitamin D deficiency in inflammatory bowel disease. Frontline Gastroenterol 2019;10(4):394.

[56] Lagishetty V, Misharin AV, Liu NQ, et al. Vitamin D deficiency in mice impairs colonic antibacterial activity and predisposes to colitis. Endocrinology 2010;151(6):2423–32.

[57] Osuga T, Nakamura K, Morita T, et al. Vitamin D status in different stages of disease severity in dogs with chronic valvular heart disease. J Vet Intern Med 2015;29(6):1518–23.

[58] Wang TJ, Pencina MJ, Booth SL, et al. Vitamin D deficiency and risk of cardiovascular disease. Circulation 2008;117(4):503–11.

[59] Fall T, Shiue I, Bergea af Geijerstam P, et al. Relations of circulating vitamin D concentrations with left ventricular geometry and function. Eur J Heart Fail 2012;14(9):985–91.

[60] Simpson RU, Weishaar RE. Involvement of 1,25-dihydroxyvitamin D3 in regulating myocardial calcium metabolism: physiological and pathological actions. Cell Calcium 1988;9(5):285–92.

[61] De Boland AR, Boland RL. Non-genomic signal transduction pathway of vitamin D in muscle. Cell Signal 1994;6(7):717–24.

[62] Li YC, Qiao G, Uskokovic M, et al. Vitamin D: a negative endocrine regulator of the renin–angiotensin system and blood pressure. J Steroid Biochem Mol Biol 2004;89-90:387–92.

[63] Li Q, Gardner DG. Negative regulation of the human atrial natriuretic peptide gene by 1,25-dihydroxyvitamin D3. J Biol Chem 1994;269(7):4934–9.

[64] Kim HW, Park CW, Shin YS, et al. Calcitriol regresses cardiac hypertrophy and QT dispersion in secondary hyperparathyroidism on hemodialysis. Nephron Clin Pract 2006;102(1):21.

[65] Legarth C, Grimm D, Krüger M, et al. Potential beneficial effects of vitamin D in coronary artery disease. Nutrients 2019;12(1).

[66] Mick PJ, Peng SA, Loftus JP. Serum vitamin D metabolites and CXCL10 concentrations associate with survival in dogs with immune mediated disease. Front Vet Sci 2019;6.

[67] Titmarsh HF, Cartwright JA, Kilpatrick S, et al. Relationship between vitamin D status and leukocytes in hospitalised cats. J Feline Med Surg 2017;19(4):364–9.

[68] Jaffey JA, Amorim J, DeClue AE. Effect of calcitriol on in vitro whole blood cytokine production in critically ill dogs. Vet J 2018;236:31–6.

[69] Lemire JM, Archer DC, Beck L, et al. Immunosuppressive actions of 1,25-dihydroxyvitamin D3: preferential inhibition of Th1 functions. J Nutr 1995;125(6 Suppl):1704S–8S.

[70] Boonstra A, Barrat FJ, Crain C, et al. 1alpha,25-Dihydroxyvitamin d3 has a direct effect on naive CD4(+) T cells to enhance the development of Th2 cells. J Immunol 2001;167(9):4974–80.

[71] Tang J, Zhou R, Luger D, et al. Calcitriol suppresses antiretinal autoimmunity through inhibitory effects on the Th17 effector response. J Immunol 2009;182(8):4624–32.

[72] Kovalik M, Thoday KL, Berry J, et al. Prednisolone therapy for atopic dermatitis is less effective in dogs with lower pretreatment serum 25-hydroxyvitamin D concentrations. Vet Dermatol 2012;23(2):125–e28.

[73] Marsella R, Sousa CA, Gonzales AJ, et al. Current understanding of the pathophysiologic mechanisms of canine atopic dermatitis. J Am Vet Med Assoc 2012;241(2):194–207.

[74] Campbell GR, Spector SA. Vitamin D inhibits human immunodeficiency virus type 1 and Mycobacterium

tuberculosis infection in macrophages through the induction of autophagy. PLoS Pathog 2012;8(5):e1002689.
[75] Miller C, Abdo Z, Ericsson A, et al. Applications of the FIV model to study HIV pathogenesis. Viruses 2018;10(4). https://doi.org/10.3390/v10040206.
[76] Rosol TJ, Nagode LA, Couto CG, et al. Parathyroid hormone (PTH)-related protein, PTH, and 1,25-dihydroxy vitamin D in dogs with cancer-associated hypercalcemia. Endocrinology 1992;131(3):1157–64.
[77] Raditic DM, Bartges JW. Evidence-based integrative medicine in clinical veterinary oncology. Vet Clin North Am Small Anim Pract 2014;44(5):831–53.
[78] Kibler L, Heinze CR, Webster CRL. Serum vitamin D status in sick cats with and without cholestatic liver disease. J Feline Med Surg 2020. https://doi.org/10.1177/1098612X19895081.
[79] Kim D, Kim H, Son P, et al. Serum 25-hydroxyvitamin D concentrations in dogs with suspected acute pancreatitis. J Vet Med Sci 2017;79(8):1366–73.
[80] Hummel D, Aggarwal A, Borka K, et al. The vitamin D system is deregulated in pancreatic diseases. J Steroid Biochem Mol Biol 2014;144:402–9.
[81] Titmarsh H, Kilpatrick S, Sinclair J, et al. Vitamin D status predicts 30 day mortality in hospitalised cats. PLoS One 2015;10(5):e0125997.
[82] Cazzolli DM, Prittie JE, Fox PR, et al. Evaluation of serum 25-hydroxyvitamin D concentrations in a heterogeneous canine ICU population. J Vet Emerg Crit Care (San Antonio) 2019;29(6):605–10.
[83] Jaffey JA, Backus RC, McDaniel KM, et al. Serum vitamin D concentrations in hospitalized critically ill dogs. PLoS One 2018;13(3):e0194062.
[84] Young LR, Backus RC. Oral vitamin D supplementation at five times the recommended allowance marginally affects serum 25-hydroxyvitamin D concentrations in dogs. J Nutr Sci 2016;5:e31.
[85] Morris JG. Cats discriminate between cholecalciferol and ergocalciferol. J Anim Physiol Anim Nutr 2002;86:229–38.
[86] Pörsti IH. Expanding targets of vitamin D receptor activation: Downregulation of several RAS components in the kidney. Kidney Int 2008;74(11):1371–3.
[87] Kuhlmann A, Haas CS, Gross ML, et al. 1,25-Dihydroxyvitamin D3 decreases podocyte loss and podocyte hypertrophy in the subtotally nephrectomized rat. Am J Physiol Renal Physiol 2004;286(3):526.
[88] Shi W, Guo L, Liu G, et al. Protective effect of calcitriol on podocytes in spontaneously hypertensive rat. J Chin Med Assoc 2018;81(8):691–8.
[89] de Brito Galvao JF, Nagode LA, Schenck PA, et al. Calcitriol, calcidiol, parathyroid hormone, and fibroblast growth factor-23 interactions in chronic kidney disease. J Vet Emerg Crit Care (San Antonio) 2013;23(2):134–62.
[90] Dusso A, González EA, Martin KJ. Vitamin D in chronic kidney disease. Best Pract Res Clin Endocrinol Metab 2011;25(4):647–55.
[91] Nagode LA, Chew DJ, Podell M. Benefits of calcitriol therapy and serum phosphorus control in dogs and cats with chronic renal failure. Both are essential to prevent or suppress toxic hyperparathyroidism. Vet Clin North Am Small Anim Pract 1996;26(6):1293–330.
[92] Polzin DJ. Chronic kidney disease in small animals. Vet Clin North Am Small Anim Pract 2011;41(1):15–30.
[93] Korman RM, White JD, Feline CKD. Current therapies - what is achievable? J Feline Med Surg 2013;15(Suppl 1):29–44.
[94] Yang L, Weaver V, Smith JP, et al. Therapeutic effect of vitamin d supplementation in a pilot study of Crohn's patients. Clin Transl Gastroenterol 2013;18(4):e33.
[95] Khan AA, Dragt BS, Porte RJ, et al. Regulation of VDR expression in rat and human intestine and liver–consequences for CYP3A expression. Toxicol In Vitro 2010;24(3):822–9.
[96] Lie AR, MacDonald KA. Reversible myocardial failure in a cat with primary hypoparathyroidism. J Feline Med Surg 2013;15(10):932–40.
[97] Dalbeni A, Scaturro G, Degan M, et al. Effects of six months of vitamin D supplementation in patients with heart failure: A randomized double-blind controlled trial. Nutr Metab Cardiovasc Dis 2014;24(8):861–8.
[98] Gotsman I, Shauer A, Zwas DR, et al. Vitamin D deficiency is a predictor of reduced survival in patients with heart failure; vitamin D supplementation improves outcome. Eur J Heart Fail 2012;14(4):357–66.
[99] Shedeed SA. Vitamin D supplementation in infants with chronic congestive heart failure. Pediatr Cardiol 2012;33(5):713–9.
[100] Wu Z, Wang T, Zhu S, et al. Effects of vitamin D supplementation as an adjuvant therapy in coronary artery disease patients. Scand Cardiovasc J 2016;50(1):9–16.
[101] Beveridge LA, Witham MD. Controversy in the link between vitamin D supplementation and hypertension. Expert Rev Cardiovasc Ther 2015;13(9):971–3.
[102] Hau CS, Shimizu T, Tada Y, et al. The vitamin D3 analog, maxacalcitol, reduces psoriasiform skin inflammation by inducing regulatory T cells and downregulating IL-23 and IL-17 production. J Dermatol Sci 2018;92(2):117–26.
[103] Malone EK, Rassnick KM, Wakshlag JJ, et al. Calcitriol (1,25-dihydroxycholecalciferol) enhances mast cell tumour chemotherapy and receptor tyrosine kinase inhibitor activity in vitro and has single-agent activity against spontaneously occurring canine mast cell tumours. Vet Comp Oncol 2010;8(3):209–20.
[104] Russell DS, Rassnick KM, Erb HN, et al. An immunohistochemical study of vitamin D receptor expression in canine cutaneous mast cell tumours. J Comp Pathol 2010;143(2–3):223–6.
[105] Tan KW, Sampson A, Osa-Andrews B, et al. Calcitriol and calcipotriol modulate transport activity of ABC transporters and exhibit selective cytotoxicity in

MRP1-overexpressing cells. Drug Metab Dispos 2018;46(12):1856–66.

[106] Rassnick KM, Muindi JR, Johnson CS, et al. In vitro and in vivo evaluation of combined calcitriol and cisplatin in dogs with spontaneously occurring tumors. Cancer Chemother Pharmacol 2008;62(5):881–91.

[107] Goulao B, Stewart F, Ford J, et al. Cancer and vitamin D supplementation: a systematic review and meta-analysis. Am J Clin Nutr 2018;107:652–63.

[108] Corbee RJ, Tryfonidou MA, Grinwis GC, et al. Skeletal and hepatic changes induced by chronic vitamin A supplementation in cats. Vet J 2014;202(3):503–9.

Printed and bound by CPI Group (UK) Ltd, Croydon, CR0 4YY
08/05/2025
01864697-0008